Latina Health in the United States

Latina Health in the United States

A Public Health Reader

Marilyn Aguirre-Molina
Carlos W. Molina
Editors

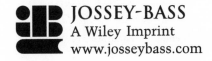

JOSSEY-BASS
A Wiley Imprint
www.josseybass.com

Published by Jossey-Bass
A Wiley Imprint
989 Market Street, San Francisco, CA 94103-1741   www.josseybass.com

Jossey-Bass books and products are available through most bookstores. To contact Jossey-Bass directly call our Customer Care Department within the U.S. at 800-956-7739, outside the U.S. at 317-572-3986 or fax 317-572-4002.

Jossey-Bass also publishes its books in a variety of electronic formats. Some content that appears in print may not be available in electronic books.

Library of Congress Cataloging-in-Publication Data
Latina health in the United States : a public health reader / Marilyn Aguirre-Molina and Carlos W. Molina, editors.
p. ; cm.
Includes bibliographical references and index.
1. Hispanic American women—Health and hygiene. 2. Hispanic American women—Medical care.
[DNLM: 1. Women's Health—United States—Collected Works. 2. Disease—ethnology—United States—Collected Works. 3. Health Services Needs and Demand—United States—Collected Works. 4. Health Status—United States—Collected Works. 5. Hispanic Americans—United States—Collected Works. WA 309 L357 2003] I. Aguirre-Molina, Marilyn.
II. Molina, Carlos W.
RA778.4.H57L38 2003
613'.04244'08968073—dc21
2003006260

Printed in the United States of America
FIRST EDITION
PB Printing   10 9 8 7 6 5 4 3 2 1

CONTENTS

TABLES, FIGURES, AND EXHIBITS

TABLES

FIGURES

EXHIBITS

SOURCES

Chapter Two: Hortensia Amaro and Adela de la Torre, "Public Health Needs and Scientific Opportunities in Research on Latinas," *American Journal of Public Health, 92*(4): 525–529, 2002.

Chapter Three: Lourdes Baezconde-Garbanati, Carmen J. Portillo, and James A. Garbanati, "Disparities in Health Indicators for Latinas in California," *Hispanic Journal of Behavioral Sciences, 21*(3): 302–329, 1999.

Chapter Five: Aida L. Giachello, "The Reproductive Years," in Marilyn Aguirre-Molina, Carlos W. Molina, and Ruth Zambrana (eds.), *Health Issues in the Latino Community.* San Francisco: Jossey-Bass, 2001.

Chapter Six: Iris Lopez, "Agency and Constraint: Sterilization and Reproductive Freedom Among Puerto Rican Women in New York City," in Louise Lamphere, Helena Ragone, and Patricia Zavella (eds.), *Situated Lives: Gender and Culture in Everyday Lives.* New York: Routledge, 1997.

Chapter Seven: Blanca Ortiz-Torres, Irma Serrano-García, and Nélida Torres-Burgos, "Subverting Culture: Promoting HIV/AIDS Prevention Among Puerto Rican and Dominican Women," *American Journal of Community Psychology, 28*(6): 859–881, 2000.

Chapter Eight: Youlian Liao, Richard S. Cooper, Guichan Cao, Jay S. Kaufman, Andrew E. Long, and Daniel L. McGee, "Mortality from Coronary Heart Disease and Cardiovascular Disease Among Adult U.S. Hispanics: Findings from the National Health Interview Survey (1986 to 1994)," *Journal of the American College of Cardiology, 30*(5): 1200–1205.

Chapter Nine: Ruth E. Zambrana, Nancy Breen, Sarah A. Fox, and Mary Lou Gutierrez-Mohamed, "Use of Cancer Screening Practices by Hispanic Women: Analyses by Subgroup," *Preventive Medicine, 29:* 466–477, 1999.

Chapter Ten: Anna Nápoles-Springer, Eliseo J. Pérez-Stable, and Eugene Washington, "Risk Factors for Invasive Cervical Cancer in Latino Women," *Journal of Medical Systems, 20*(5): 277–293, 1996.

Chapter Eleven: Edith C. Kieffer, Sharla K. Willis, Natalia Arellano, and Ricardo Guzman, "Perspectives of Pregnant and Postpartum Latino Women on Diabetes, Physical Activity, and Health," *Health Education and Behavior, 29*(5): 542–556, 2002.

Chapter Twelve: Glorisa Canino, "Alcohol Use and Misuse Among Hispanic Women: Selected Factors, Processes and Studies," *International Journal of the Addictions, 29*(9): 1083–1100, 1994.

Chapter Thirteen: Juana Mora, "The Treatment of Alcohol Dependency Among Latinas: A Feminist, Cultural and Community Perspective," *Alcoholism Treatment Quarterly, 16*(1/2): 163–177, 1998.

Chapter Fourteen: Jon F. Kerner, Nancy Breen, Mariella C. Tefft, and Joscelyn Silsby, "Tobacco Use Among Multi-Ethnic Latino Populations," *Ethnicity and Disease, 8:* 165–183, 1998.

Chapter Fifteen: William A. Vega, Ethel Alderete, Bohdan Kolody, and Sergio Aguilar-Gaxiola, "Illicit Drug Use Among Mexicans and Mexican Americans in California: The Effects of Gender and Acculturation," *Addiction, 93*(12): 1839–1850, 1998.

Chapter Sixteen: Hortensia Amaro, Rita Nieves, Sergut Wolde Johannes, and Nirzka M. Labault Cabeza, "Substance Abuse Treatment: Critical Issues and Challenges in the Treatment of Latina Women," *Hispanic Journal of Behavioral Sciences, 21*(93): 266–282, 1999.

Chapter Seventeen: Melba J. T. Vasquez, "Latinas," in Lillian Comas-Diaz and Beverly Greene (eds.), *Women of Color: Integrating Ethnic and Gender Identities in Psychotherapy.* New York: Guilford Press, 1994.

Chapter Eighteen: Jill Denner, Douglas Kirby, Karin Coyle, and Claire Brindis, "The Protective Role of Social Capital and Cultural Norms in Latino Communities: A Study of Adolescent Births," *Hispanic Journal of Behavioral Sciences, 23*(1): 3–21, 2001.

Chapter Nineteen: Celia P. Kaplan, Anna Nápoles-Springer, Susan L. Stewart, and Eliseo J. Pérez-Stable, "Smoking Acquisition Among Adolescents and Young Latinas: The Role of Socioenvironmental and Personal Factors," *Addictive Behaviors, 26:* 531–550, 2001.

Chapter Twenty: María Félix-Ortiz, Alicia Fernandez, and Michael D. Newcomb, "The Role of Intergenerational Discrepancy of Cultural Orientation in Drug Use Among Latina Adolescents," *Substance Use and Misuse, 33*(4): 967–994, 1998.

Chapter Twenty-One: Robert E. Roberts and Yuan-Who Chen, "Depressive Symptoms and Suicidal Ideation Among Mexican-Origin and Anglo Adolescents," *Journal of the American Academy of Child Adolescent Psychiatry, 34*(1): 81–90, 1995.

Chapter Twenty-Two: Tracy L. Skaer, Linda M. Robison, David A. Sclar, and Gary H. Harding, "Cancer-Screening Determinants Among Hispanic Women Using Migrant Health Clinics," *Journal of Health Care for the Poor and Underserved, 7*(4): 338–354, 1996.

Chapter Twenty-Three: Ethel Alderete, William A. Vega, Bohdan Kolody, and Sergio Aguilar-Gaxiola, "Lifetime Prevalence of and Risk Factors for Psychiatric Disorders Among Mexican Migrant Farmworkers in California," *American Journal of Public Health, 90*(4): 608–614, 2000.

Chapter Twenty-Four: Joe Gorton and Nikki R. Van Hightower, "Intimate Victimization of Latina Farm Workers: A Research Summary," *Hispanic Journal of Behavioral Sciences, 21*(4): 502–507, 1999.

Chapter Twenty-Five: Ellen B. Gold, Barbara Sternfeld, Jennifer L. Kelsey, Charlotte Brown, Charles Mouton, Nancy Reame, Loran Salamone, and Rebecca

Stellato, "Relation of Demographic and Lifestyle Factors to Symptoms in a Multi-Racial/Ethnic Population of Women 40–55 Years of Age," *American Journal of Epidemiology, 152*(5): 463–473, 2000.

Chapter Twenty-Six: Beverly Greene, "Lesbian Women of Color: Triple Jeopardy," in Lillian Comas-Diaz and Beverly Greene (eds.), *Women of Color: Integrating Ethnic and Gender Identities in Psychotherapy.* New York: Guilford Press, 1994.

Chapter Twenty-Seven: E. Anne Lown and William A. Vega, "Prevalence and Predictors of Physical Partner Abuse Among Mexican American Women," *American Journal of Public Health, 91*(3): 441–445, 2001.

Chapter Twenty-Eight: Rebeca Chamorro and Yvette Flores-Ortiz, "Acculturation and Disordered Eating Patterns Among Mexican American Women," *International Journal of Eating Disorders, 28*(1): 125–129, 2000.

THE AUTHORS

Noilyn Abesamis, M.P.H., Heilbrunn Department of Population and Family Health, Mailman School of Public Health, Columbia University, New York

Sergio Aguilar-Gaxiola, M.D., Ph.D., M.S., Department of Psychology, California State University, Fresno

Marilyn Aguirre-Molina, Ed.D., Heilbrunn Department of Population and Family Health, Mailman School of Public Health, Columbia University, New York

Ethel Alderete, Dr.P.H., Center for Mental Health Services Research, Institute of Business and Economic Research, University of California, Berkeley

Hortensia Amaro, Ph.D., School of Health Professions, Bouve College of Health Sciences, Northeastern University, Boston

Natalia Arellano, M.S.W., School of Social Work, University of Michigan, Ann Arbor

Lourdes Baezconde-Garbanati, Ph.D., M.P.H., M.A., Department of Preventive Medicine, University of Southern California, Los Angeles

Nancy Breen, M.D., Applied Research Program, Health Services and Economics Branch, National Institutes of Health, Bethesda, Maryland

Claire Brindis, Dr.P.H., M.P.H., Division of Adolescent Medicine, Center for Reproductive Health Research and Policy, University of California, San Francisco

Charlotte Brown, Ph.D., Department of Psychiatry, School of Medicine, University of Pittsburgh

Guichan Cao, M.S., Department of Biometry and Epidemiology, Medical University of South Carolina, Charleston

Glorisa Canino, Ph.D., Behavioral Sciences Research Institute, University of Puerto Rico, San Juan

Olveen Carrasquillo, M.D., M.P.H., College of Physicians and Surgeons, Columbia University, New York

Michelle Castro, Centers for Disease Control Fellow, Department of Sociomedical Sciences, Mailman School of Public Health, Columbia University, New York

Rebeca Chamorro, Ph.D., Department of Psychiatry, Beth Israel Deaconess Medical Center, Harvard Medical School, Boston

Yuan-Who Chen, Ph.D., Department of Psychiatry and Behavioral Sciences, School of Medicine, University of Texas, Health Sciences Center, Houston

Richard S. Cooper, M.D., Department of Preventive Medicine and Epidemiology, Loyola University Chicago Stritch School of Medicine, Maywood, Illinois

Karin Coyle, Ph.D., Education, Training, and Research Associates, Santa Cruz, California

Adela de la Torre, Ph.D., Chicana/o Studies Program, University of California, Davis

Jill Denner, Ph.D., Education, Training, and Research Associates, Santa Cruz, California

María Felíx-Ortiz de la Garza, Ph.D., Department of Psychology, University of Southern California, Los Angeles

Alicia Fernandez, University of Southern California, Los Angeles

Yvette Flores-Ortiz, Ph.D., Department of Chicana/o Studies, University of California, Davis

Sarah A. Fox, Ed.D., M.Sc., Department of Medicine, University of California, Los Angeles, and Rand Corporation, Santa Monica, California

James A. Garbanati, Ph.D., California School of Professional Psychology, Alhambra

Aida L. Giachello, Ph.D., M.S.W., Jane Addams College of Social Work, Midwest Latino Health Research Training and Policy Center, University of Illinois, Chicago

Ellen B. Gold, Ph.D., Department of Epidemiology and Preventive Medicine, University of California, Davis

Joe Gorton, Ph.D., Department of Sociology, Anthropology and Criminology, University of Northern Iowa, Cedar Falls

Beverly Greene, Ph.D., St. John's University, New York

Mary Lou Gutierrez-Mohamed, Ph.D., Jackson Heart Study, Jackson State University, Jackson, Mississippi

Ricardo Guzman, M.P.H., M.S.W., Community Health and Social Services, Detroit

Gary H. Harding, M.D., M.P.H., Civil Surgeon, Wenatchee Community Health, Wenatchee, Washington

Sergut Wolde Johannes, M.P.J., Ed.M. School of Public Health, Boston University, Boston

Celia P. Kaplan, Dr.P.H., Internal Medicine, University of California, San Francisco

Jay S. Kaufman, Ph.D., Department of Epidemiology, School of Public Health, University of North Carolina, Chapel Hill

Jennifer L. Kelsey, Ph.D., Division of Epidemiology, Stanford University, Palo Alto, California

Jon F. Kerner, Ph.D., Division of Cancer Control and Population Sciences National Cancer Institute, Rockville, Maryland

Edith C. Kieffer, Ph.D., M.P.H., Department of Health Behavior and Health Education, School of Public Health, University of Michigan, Ann Arbor

Douglas Kirby, Ph.D., Education, Training, and Research Associates, Santa Cruz, California

Bohdan Kolody, Ph.D., Department of Sociology, San Diego State University, San Diego, California

Nirzka M. Labault Cabeza, M.S., M.P.H., Ph.D., Department of Human Development, School of Public Health, University of Puerto Rico, San Juan

Youlian Liao, M.D., Department of Biometry and Epidemiology, Medical University of South Carolina, Charleston

Andrew E. Long, Ph.D., Department of Epidemiology, School of Public Health, University of Michigan, Ann Arbor

Iris Lopez, Ph.D., Department of Sociology, Latin American and Hispanic Caribbean Studies Program, City College, City University of New York, New York

E. Anne Lown, M.P.H., Dr.P.H., Alcohol Research Group, Berkeley, California

Daniel L. McGee, Ph.D., Department of Biometry and Epidemiology, Medical University of South Carolina, Charleston

Juana Mora, Ph.D., College of Humanities and Department of Chicana/o Studies, California State University, Northridge

Charles Mouton, M.D., University of Texas, Health Sciences Center, San Antonio

Anna Nápoles-Springer, Ph.D., M.P.H., Division of General Internal Medicine, Department of Medicine, Medical Effectiveness Research Center for Diverse Populations, University of California, San Francisco

Michael D. Newcomb, Ph.D., Department of Counseling Psychology, USC Rossier School of Education, University of Southern California, Los Angeles

Rita Nieves, R.N., M.P.H., Entre Familia, Boston Public Health Commission, Mattapan, Massachusetts

Blanca Ortiz-Torres, Ph.D., J.D., M.A., University Center for Psychological Services and Research, University of Puerto Rico, San Juan

Eliseo J. Pérez-Stable, M.D., Division of General Internal Medicine, Department of Medicine, Medical Effectiveness Research Center for Diverse Populations, University of California, San Francisco

Carmen J. Portillo, R.N., Ph.D., Department of Community Health Systems, School of Nursing, University of California, San Francisco

Nancy Reame, Ph.D., M.S.N, R.N., School of Nursing, University of Michigan, Ann Arbor

Robert E. Roberts, Ph.D., Department of Behavioral Sciences, School of Public Health, Department of Psychiatry and Behavioral Sciences, School of Medicine, Social Psychiatry Research Group, University of Texas, Health Science Center, Houston

Linda M. Robison, M.S.P.H., Pharmacoeconomics and Pharmacoepidemiology Research Unit, Washington State University, Pullman

Estelamari Rodriguez, M.D., M.P.H., Health Science Center, State University of New York, Downstate Medical Center, Brooklyn

Diana Romero, Ph.D., M.A., Finding Common Ground Project, Heilbrunn Department of Population and Family Health, Mailman School of Public Health, Columbia University, New York

Loran Salamone, Ph.D., School of Medicine, University of Pittsburgh, Pittsburgh, Pennsylvania

David A. Sclar, Ph.D., Pharmacoeconomics and Pharmacoepidemiology Research Unit, Washington State University, Pullman

Irma Serrano-García, Ph.D., M.A., Department of Psychology, University of Puerto Rico, Río Piedras

Joscelyn Silsby, M.P.H., Public Health Informatics Research Laboratory, Department of Health Education, University of Maryland, College Park

Tracy L. Skaer, PharmD., Pharmacoeconomics and Pharmacoepidemiology Research Unit, Washington State University, Pullman

Rebecca Stellato, M.A., New England Research Institute, Watertown, Massachusetts

Barbara Sternfeld, Ph.D., Division of Research, Kaiser Permanente, Oakland, California

Susan L. Stewart, Ph.D., Northern California Cancer Center, Union City, California

Mariella C. Tefft, R.N., M.S., Lombardi Cancer Center, Georgetown University Medical Center, Washington, D.C.

Nélida Torres-Burgos, M.A., University Center for Psychological Services and Research, University of Puerto Rico, San Juan

Nikki R. Van Hightower, Ph.D., M.A., Department of Political Sciences, Texas A&M University, College Station

Melba J. T. Vasquez, Ph.D., psychologist in independent practice, Austin, Texas

William A. Vega, Ph.D., University of Medicine and Dentistry of New Jersey, Robert Wood Johnson Medical School, New Brunswick, New Jersey

Eugene Washington, M.D., Department of Obstetrics, Gynecology, and Reproductive Sciences and Department of Epidemiology and Biostatistics, School of Medicine, University of California, San Francisco

Sharla K. Willis, Dr.P.H., Department of Health Behavior and Health Promotion, School of Public Health, Ohio State University, Columbus

Ruth E. Zambrana, Ph.D., University of Maryland College Park and Department of Family Medicine, School of Medicine, University of Maryland, Baltimore

THE EDITORS

Marilyn Aguirre-Molina is a professor of population and family health at the Mailman School of Public Health, Columbia University, in New York City. Prior to joining the Columbia faculty, she served as the executive vice president of the California Endowment and as a senior program officer at the Robert Wood Johnson Foundation. Preceding her work within philanthropy, she was an associate professor in the University of Medicine and Dentistry of New Jersey–Robert Wood Johnson Medical School, Department of Environmental and Community Medicine. In this capacity, she taught within the M.D./M.P.H. program and engaged in applied research.

The focus of Aguirre-Molina's work is on program development and applied research that address public health approaches to the prevention of alcohol, tobacco, and other drug problems among young people. She has published in this area of study. Aguirre-Molina is or has been a member of various national boards and committees, including the National Institutes of Health–National Advisory Council of the National Institute of Alcohol Abuse and Alcoholism (NIAAA), the NIAAA Panel on College Drinking, and the national council of the Center for Substance Abuse Prevention. She is the cofounder of the National Latino Council on Alcohol and Tobacco Prevention. She also served on the National Board of the Alliance to End Childhood Lead Poisoning. She was elected to the executive board of the American Public Health Association, where she served for four years and was the board's vice chair. She currently serves on the Institute of Medicine's Committee on Developing a Strategy to Reduce and Prevent Underage Drinking, on the editorial board of the *Journal of Public Health Policy,* and the Editorial Advisory Board of the *Harvard Journal of Hispanic Policy.* In addition, she is a consultant to the Robert Wood Johnson Foundation and serves on the selection panel of the Johnson & Johnson Community Health Care Program (corporate giving).

As a Kellogg Foundation Fellow, Aguirre-Molina traveled extensively and studied the political economy of selected developing countries, with a primary emphasis on the Caribbean and Latin America.

In addition to her interest in substance abuse, Aguirre-Molina has worked extensively on and written about Latino health policy issues. This is her third edited book on the health of Latino populations in the United States. *Latino Health in the U.S.: A Growing Challenge* was published in 1994, and *Health Issues in the Latino Community* was published in 2001.

Aguirre-Molina received a B.S. in health sciences from Hunter College-City University of New York, an M.S. in community health and an Ed.D. in health education and administration from Columbia University.

Carlos W. Molina is the Dean for Special Programs in the Office of Academic Affairs at Eugenio Maria de Hostos Community College of the City University of New York (CUNY) and professor of public health education at York College, CUNY. The foci of his teaching and scholarship have been on Latino health, administration, and behavioral health. This is his third edited text on Latino health; this one is coedited with Marilyn Aguirre-Molina. The other two are *Latino Health in the U.S.: A Growing Challenge* (1994) and *Health Issues in the Latino Community* (2001).

In the early 1990s, Molina served as the CEO of Lincoln Hospital of the Health and Hospitals Corporations of New York City, the country's largest public hospital system. He is a cofounder and currently a board member of the National Latino Council on Alcohol and Tobacco Prevention. Among the many national boards on which Molina has served are the national Planned Parenthood Federation of America, Alan Guttmacher Institute, SIECUS, as well as numerous other local boards and committees. From 1993 to 1997 he served as an elected member of the executive board of the American Public Health Association. He serves as a member of the editorial board of the *Journal of Public Health Policy.* Molina received a B.S. in health education from the City College of New York, the City University of New York, and an M.A. and Ed.D. in community health education from Columbia University.

In the memory of Helen Rodriguez-Trias and Antonia Pantoja.
Within five months, the Latino community experienced the passing of two of its
most important Latinas in recent history: Helen Rodriguez-Trias, M.D. (December
2001) and Antonia Pantoja, Ph.D. (May 2002). Each of these extraordinary
women made enormous contributions to our Latino communities and provided
magnificent role models for Latinas.

Dr. Rodriguez-Trias was a pediatrician who graduated from the University of Puerto
Rico Medical School in 1960, the same year her fourth child was born. During her
residency training at the university hospital, she created the island's first center for
neonatal care. After moving to New York City, she devoted her life to the health
and well-being of women and children. She became an outspoken leader in the
women's health movement and cofounded the Campaign to End Sterilization
Abuse. These efforts led to the federal guidelines requiring that a woman's consent
for sterilization be obtained in a language she understands and be documented in
writing and that surgeons observe a specific waiting period after obtaining a
woman's consent for sterilization. Chapter Six in this book, written by Iris Lopez,
provides an informative analysis of the situation that existed at the time the
guidelines were developed.

Helen had an unequaled career in medicine and public health and made numerous
contributions as a teacher, director of pediatric services at major urban hospitals,
and a policy advocate. As medical director of the New York State Department of
Health's AIDS Institute, she developed programs directed at families affected by
HIV. She also made history in 1991 when she was elected president of the
American Public Health Association (APHA)—the first Latino/a to serve in this
position. The organization has created an award in her name, building on the
Helen Rodriguez-Trias Latino Caucus of APHA Annual Breakfast that was estab-
lished in her honor. In 1996, when Helen "retired" to California, she
remained active and there helped found the Pacific Institute for Women's Health, a
Los Angeles–based nonprofit organization dedicated to improving women's
health and well-being.

In January 2001, Helen received the Presidential Citizen's Medal from President
Bill Clinton for her work on behalf of women, children, and people with AIDS.
Helen was a guiding light to hundreds of Latino men and women to whom she
selflessly gave of herself. We are honored to have been recipients of her wisdom
and love. It is our wish that others will be equally nourished by the legacy she
leaves behind.

Dr. Pantoja was an educator, activist, and community leader who has left a legacy of institutions that have made enormous contributions to the development of the Puerto Rican/Latino community. After graduating from the University of Puerto Rico, she worked as a school teacher, where her early interests in education and the needs of disadvantaged children were cultivated. In 1944, she went from the classrooms of Puerto Rico to a welding factory in New York City, making lamps for children. This experience awakened her consciousness of the injustice with which people of color were treated. She became an activist in the factory where the women organized to "weld together a fragmented community" much in need of leadership. This laid the foundation for what was to become her life's work

In 1958, Tony joined a group of young professionals to create the Puerto Rican Forum, which paved the way for the establishment of a Latino educational organization, ASPIRA, in 1961. This was her dream and one of the greatest contributions made to the lives of young Latinos. Although Tony founded many other organizations in the Puerto Rican community—Puerto Rican Association for Community Affairs, Universidad Boricua, Puerto Rican Research and Resource Center in Washington, D.C., and Graduate School for Community Development in San Diego—she will always be best known for the establishment of ASPIRA. Through local affiliates and its national office, this organization has assisted students through educational support and mentoring programs, facilitating students' access to college, leadership development, and policy advocacy. Many of today's leaders in the Puerto Rican/Latino community were at one time "Aspriantes"; many of them would not have accessed higher education were it not for Tony's dream.

In 1996, Tony received the Presidential Medal of Freedom from President Bill Clinton, the highest honor bestowed on civilians by the U.S. government. It was given in recognition of her legendary role in education and leadership development.

After nearly sixty years as an educator and activist, Tony continued to pursue her life's work with the same vigor and passion as when she first came to New York from Puerto Rico. This is reflected in a statement she made in 1999: "One cannot live a lukewarm life. You have to live life with passion." Tony touched the lives of thousands, and the fruits of her labor continue today. She is best characterized as a woman who built institutions, leaving behind a legacy that will benefit future generations.

For all of these reasons, we dedicate this anthology on Latina health to the accomplishments and memories of these two extraordinary women. There is no doubt that those who were privileged to have known or worked with either of them will forever be grateful for the many contributions that they made to our individual and collective lives. But it is for those women who follow that we share their memory so that they may remember the roads Helen and Tony have paved for us in education and in health. It is our hope that the example of these women's lives will serve as a beacon that lights the way for others on which to fashion their work.

PREFACE

The process of reviewing and critiquing the numerous articles gathered for this book resulted in an initial list of seventeen areas of focus for inclusion. Through several revisions and discussions, the list was narrowed to the following topic areas:

Part One: Overview and Critical Issues Affecting Latina Health

Part Two: Risk Factors and Disparities Among Latinas

Part Three: Sexual and Reproductive Health Issues

Part Four: Chronic Conditions: Heart Disease, Cancer, and Diabetes

Part Five: Alcohol, Tobacco, and Other Drugs

Part Six: Mental Health

Part Seven: The Next Generation: Latina Adolescents

Part Eight: Rural and Migrant Farmworker Latinas

Part Nine: Special Issues

Demographic and profile data may differ from one chapter to another due to the publication date of the original article and the data available at the time. For example, Chapter One by Aguirre-Molina, Abesamis, and Castro, as well as others, contain data from the 2000 Census, while chapters written prior to the 2000 Census use older data that are at variance with the more recent information presented. Please be aware of these variations.

Each chapter gives readers a perspective on the issues that Latinas face in addressing their health care needs and concerns. As will be observed, the factors affecting their health are both highly complex and multilayered. Given this situation, the goals of the anthology are (1) to identify a number of critical issues of importance and relevance to Latinas; (2) present an overview of the existing literature on Latina health; (3) highlight the leading indicators of morbidity and mortality (where the data exist) affecting various subgroups of Latinas; (4) provide a document for students, practitioners, and decision makers alike who seek to address the challenge of the growing health disparities among communities of color; and (5) identify gaps in research, policy issues, program planning, and practice.

With the growing numbers and diversity occurring within the Latino community in the United States, health and public health communities must move beyond simplistic and inadequately informed views of the health needs of this population. A more resolute and strategic effort is especially crucial when tackling Latinas' health disparities. We hope that *Latina Health in the United States* will serve as a stepping-stone for prospective efforts that ensure Latinas are included in the dialogues of addressing health inequity. In doing so, this would not only secure their future health and well-being but the nation's as well.

Marilyn Aguirre-Molina
Carlos W. Molina

New York
July 2003

ACKNOWLEDGMENTS

We are deeply grateful to Noilyn Abesamis, research assistant in the Heilbrunn Department of Population and Family Health at the Mailman School of Public Health, Columbia University, for her invaluable assistance in the preparation of the final manuscript and to the impeccable attention she gave to the myriad follow-up details required during this period. We extend our thanks and acknowledgment to Michelle Castro, a Centers for Disease Control Fellow and M.P.H. candidate at the Mailman School of Public Health, who worked with Marilyn Aguirre-Molina during the early stages in the development of this project. Special thanks also to our colleague Marita Murman of the Department of Sociomedical Sciences at the Mailman School of Public Health. She was especially helpful to us in the process of identifying experts on Latina health within schools of public health across the country. We extend special thanks to Jesse Orleans, a summer intern, for the many hours he spent in the library in the search for the elusive literature on Latina health, and for his assistance in its review.

PART ONE

INTRODUCTION
Overview and Critical Issues
Affecting Latina Health

CHAPTER ONE

The State of the Art

Latinas in the Health Literature

Marilyn Aguirre-Molina
Noilyn Abesamis
Michelle Castro

One of the editors of this book and two colleagues review the process of identifying and selecting literature on Latina health for inclusion in this book. Although the lack of adequate, commendable, or relevant literature on Latinas posed challenges, it also presented an opportunity to assess what exists (in terms of both strengths and limitations) and to identify needed areas of research and what there is of merit from which to build. The authors transform the inadequate attention to the health of Latinas and a weak existing literature into an opportunity to inform the research and practice communities of a course of action that might fill gaps and improve our understanding of the health of Latinas.

This anthology represents another point on the continuum of efforts to bring the complex issues affecting the health of Latinos in the United States to the attention of the health and public health communities. In earlier books, *Latino Health in the U.S.: A Growing Challenge* (1994) and *Health Issues in the Latino Community* (2001), we faced the challenge of filling a gap in the literature while endeavoring to impart a comprehensive picture of the health needs of Latinos in the United States—the fastest-growing, youngest, and what is becoming the most heterogeneous ethnic/racial group in the country. In many instances, the challenge was finding ways to prepare a survey text that included topic areas and critical health issues in an environment of limited research and inadequate data on Latinos. Nevertheless, since the first volume, some gains have been made in the availability of Latino data, and more studies have been conducted on this population.

Like earlier efforts, the goal of *Latina Health in the United States: A Public Health Reader* is to provide an integrated understanding of Latina health at a time when their numbers are growing in our society and the subgroups are becoming more diverse (for example, by country of origin and levels of acculturation). But the challenge is heightened by several factors. Specifically, Latinas are underrepresented in the research literature, which is a reflection of the paucity of studies that focus on these women. What does exist in general does not address the primary issues affecting their health and health status.

So why attempt to assemble an anthology constructed from the current literature when relevant research and literature are scarce? The reason is that the growing ethnic/racial diversity and demographic changes that are occurring in the United States have significant implications for public health, health care, and health policy. Latinas are prominent within these changes. They are part of the growing sector for which policy and programmatic interventions are needed to the address disparities in health status and health care.

Latinas make up approximately half of the Latino community and 6 percent of the total U.S. population. By the year 2050, they will make up 25 percent of the U.S. total female population: one in four women will be a Latina. Furthermore, they represent the youngest population of women in the United States; 40 percent are under the age of 21 years. (See Exhibit 1.1 and Figures 1.1 and 1.2 for additional information.)

Beyond demographic changes, Latinas represent the social capital of the community as mothers, daughters, family caretakers, partners to their *compañeros* (partners or husbands), and contributors to the economic well-being of their family. Latinas also make major contributions to society as they enter the workforce and, more important, as they nurture future generations.

Despite data limitations, a publication is needed that works from what there is to identify promising studies on which to build and areas of need that are yet to be examined.

Many of the chapters in this book were selected because they highlight and review issues that are relevant but often neglected, and thus begin the process of identifying the multiplicity of issues affecting Latinas that the research and provider sectors do not take into consideration. Among these are the combined stressors affecting Latinas as migrant farmworkers, as adolescents attempting to mediate conflicting cultural worlds, as mothers seeking health insurance for themselves and their children, and as health care consumers in search of culturally and linguistically responsive services. Many of these stressors place them at high risk for health and related problems but are not adequately acknowledged in studies or the literature.

Notwithstanding prevailing health issues that have implications for the well-being of Latinas, this group has not captured the attention of those who contribute to the literature. Furthermore, Latinas have not been immune to the narrow focus on women's health that concentrates primarily on the biological processes of reproductive health. Therefore, there exists a need to look beyond

Exhibit 1.1. Profile of Latinas in the United States

- Forty percent are under 21 years old.

- Latina fertility rates per 1,000 women aged 15–44 years is (105.9 versus 66.5 for Whites, 71.7 for Blacks, and 70.7 for Asian Pacific Islanders) and birthrates (25.1 versus 14.1 for Whites, 17.6 for African Americans, and 17.8 for Asian Pacific Islanders) are the highest in the United States, which contributed to the growth of the Latino population, as did the high rates of immigration in the decade 1990–2000.[a]

- Sixty percent of Latinas were born in the United States compared to 96 percent of White women.

- Twenty-three percent of Latinas are heads of households compared to 14 percent of White women.

- Twenty-five percent of Latinas live below the poverty level compared to 9 percent of White women.

- Forty-three percent of Latinas have a twelfth-grade education or less compared to 12 percent of White women.

- Eleven percent of Latinas have a bachelor's degree or more compared to 26 percent of White women.

- Ninety-two percent of Latinas 16 years and older are employed compared to 97 percent of White women.

- Although the majority of Latinas are in the workforce, they are concentrated in low-paying, part-time, or seasonal jobs and experience twice the rate of unemployment compared to White women (7.7 percent versus 3.3 percent).

Sources: U.S. Bureau of the Census (2001); Anderson (2002).

[a]The birth, fertility, and total fertility rates for Central and South Americans include other and unknown Latino.

what there is in the literature to what is needed to inform policy and program development.

Often Latina sexual and reproductive health studies are guided by incomplete or inaccurate assumptions and cultural conjecture. Or they are studied outside a structural context and without adequate acknowledgment of the influence of subgroup variations, acculturation, gender relations, and other factors. When these variables are not taken into consideration, they often have adverse implications for Latinas, as negative stereotypes are reinforced and perpetuated.

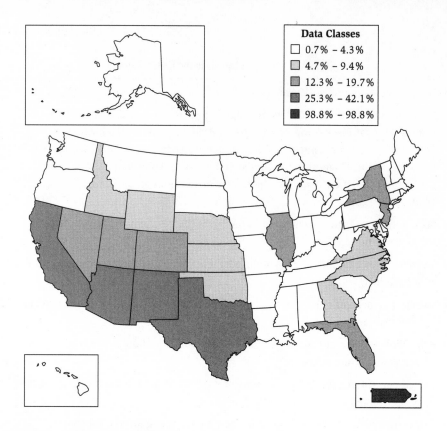

Data Classes

☐ 0.7% – 4.3%
▨ 4.7% – 9.4%
▨ 12.3% – 19.7%
▨ 25.3% – 42.1%
■ 98.8% – 98.8%

Figure 1.1. Geographic Distribution of Latinos

Source: U.S. Bureau of the Census (2000).

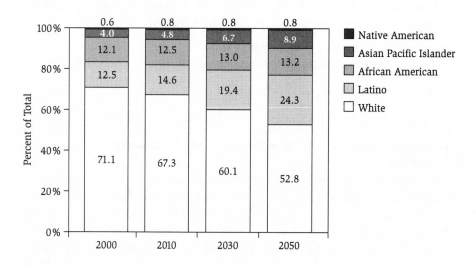

Figure 1.2. Projection of U.S. Resident Population, 2000–2050

Source: Day (1996).

6

MOVING BEYOND A SIMPLISTIC VIEW OF LATINAS' HEALTH

It is important to share how these observations and conclusions were reached, and the process used to identify, select, and assemble the chapters in this anthology. This was a learning process that is worth sharing because it makes known the state of the field and state of the literature on Latina health in the early years of the new millennium. The findings can help to identify a course of action that informs research, program development, health practices, and policies as they affect Latinas.

Interview of Content Experts

An open-ended questionnaire was used to interview eleven experts on Latina health. The experts were identified through their prominence in the literature, the recommendations of others who are knowledgeable in the field, and the assistance of a colleague who contacted schools of public health across the country to assist in the process. The intent of this process was to identify essential topics for inclusion in this anthology and peer-reviewed articles that were both informative and of merit for a publication that would be of value to a professional audience.

The experts identified forty-eight topics, the majority of which focused on reproductive health, sexually transmitted diseases, mental health, and socioeconomic status and its impact on health. The literature recommended by this group primarily addressed substance abuse, HIV/AIDS, sexuality, and gender roles.

Review of Latinas' Health and Health Care Needs

Simultaneous with the interview of experts, morbidity and mortality data and patterns were reviewed to determine the leading causes of death and illness among Latinas, as well as issues related to access to care. (See Tables 1.1 through 1.4, Figures 1.3 and 1.4, Exhibits 1.2 and 1.3, and Chapter Five for more details.) This was conducted for the purpose of assessing the extent to which experts identified areas and topic of need that corresponded to the health and health care needs of Latinas, and determining the extent to which the peer-reviewed literature reflected the situation of Latinas.

Review of the experts' opinion of priority health issues did not correspond with the leading causes of illness and death among Latinas as reflected in national vital statistics (Anderson, 2002) or other reports regarding access to care (Salganicoff, Beckerman, Wyn, and Ojeda, 2002; Wyn, Solis, Ojeda, and Pourat, 2001).

Assessing and Selecting Work for Inclusion

The next step was an assessment of the peer-reviewed literature and other reports to determine the extent to which they reflected the health and health care needs of Latinas, or, stated differently, the attention to which Latina health needs were reflected in studies reported in the research literature.

Table 1.1. Health Insurance Coverage of Latina Subgroups by Poverty Level,
18–64 Years, 1997 and 1998

	Population (in thousands)	Uninsured	Medicaid	Job Based
Central and South American				
All women	1,578	42%	8%	46%
200% or below of poverty	738	57	15	24
200% or more of poverty	840	28	NA	65
Cuban				
All women	441	20%	NA	58%
200 or less of poverty	150	34	NA	NA
200% or more of poverty	290	NA	NA	76
Mexican origin				
All women	5,638	41%	13%	43%
200% or less of poverty	3,160	53	20	24
200% or more of poverty	2,478	25	4	68
Puerto Rican				
All women	960	21%	28%	46%
200% or less of poverty	485	26	48	20
200% or more of poverty	475	17	NA	74

Note: Poverty designations are based on the 1998 U.S. Census Bureau poverty thresholds. The incomes corresponding to 100 percent of the total federal poverty threshold are $10,972 for a family of two and $16,660 for a family of four. Population totals are for 1998 only. NA (not available): The sample size was too small to produce a reliable estimate.

Source: Average of March 1998 and March 1999 Current Population Surveys.

A comprehensive literature review and database search were conducted to assess the quantity and quality of relevant information on Latinas. Peer-reviewed journals, book chapters, and other publications on women's health that were published between 1984 and 2002 were reviewed. Approximately two hundred articles were retrieved. The majority of this work was written between 1994 and 2002, with the year 2000 yielding the largest number of articles, thus reflecting a growing interest in this group of women (see Figure 1.5).

All of the peer-reviewed articles and other publications were assessed and ranked on a scale from 1 to 5, with 5 reflecting the highest score using the following criteria:

- Extent to which the focus of the study reflected Latinas' health needs and priorities (reflective of morbidity and mortality data, access to health care, other determinants of health)

Text continued on page 17.

Table 1.2. **Access and Barriers to Care Issues for Women Ages 18–64 Years, by Race/Ethnicity**

	All Women %	Latinas %	Whites %	Blacks %
Experiences with provider in past two years				
Doctor did not usually take time to answer all questions	10	14[a]	9	8
Left doctor's office and did not understand or remember some of the information given	17	20	17	14
Out-of-pocket costs of doctor visit higher than expected	28	31	28	26
Concerns about quality of care (in past year)	22	34[a]	20	24
Barriers to care in past year				
General access problem:				
Had a problem and needed to see a doctor but did not	27	32[a]	25	32[a]
Provider availability:				
Difficulty getting care due to lack of doctors and clinics	9	12[a]	8	9
Referral issue:				
Was not able to see specialist when thought needed one	15	22	12	15
Cost of care:				
Did not fill prescription medication due to cost	21	20	21	21
Reasons for delaying or not getting needed care in past year				
Could not afford it	24	31[a]	22	25
Hard to take time off	24	25	23	26
Could not get appointment with doctor wanted to see	22	23	21	21
Transportation	7	18[a]	5	10
No child care[b]	10	15[a]	9	11

[a]Significantly different from reference group (White women) at $p < .05$.

[b]Among women with children.

Source: Henry J. Kaiser Family Foundation (2001).

Table 1.3. Top Ten Leading Causes of Mortality for Latinas and Non-Hispanic White Women, All Ages

	Latinas					Non-Hispanic White Women			
Rank[a]	Cause of Death[b]	Number[c]	Percentage of Total Deaths	Rate[c]	Rank[a]	Cause of Death[b]	Number[c]	Percentage of Total Deaths	Rate[c]
...	All causes	47,082	100.0	291.5	...	All causes	1,015,138	100.0	1,011.7
1	Diseases of the heart	12,253	26.0	75.9	1	Diseases of the heart	307,255	30.3	306.2
2	Malignant neoplasms	10,022	21.3	62.0	2	Malignant neoplasms	222,268	21.9	221.5
3	Cerebrovascular diseases	3,322	7.1	20.6	3	Cerebrovascular diseases	86,210	8.5	85.9
4	Diabetes mellitus	2,821	6.0	17.5	4	Chronic lower respiratory diseases	56,670	5.6	56.5
5	Accidents (unintentional injuries)	2,134	4.5	13.2	5	Alzheimer's disease	32,123	3.2	32.0
6	Influenza and pneumonia	1,322	2.8	8.2	6	Influenza and pneumonia	31,526	3.1	31.4
7	Chronic lower respiratory diseases	1,238	2.6	7.7	7	Accidents (unintentional injuries)	27,066	2.7	27.0
8	Certain conditions pertaining to perinatal period	951	2.0	5.9	8	Diabetes mellitus	26,698	2.6	26.6
9	Chronic liver disease and cirrhosis	875	1.9	5.4	9	Nephritis, nephritic syndrome, and nephrosis	14,357	1.4	14.3
10	Nephritis, nephritic syndrome, and nephrosis	841	1.8	5.2	10	Septicemia	13,461	1.3	13.4
...	All other causes	11,303	24.0	70.0	...	All other causes	197,504	19.5	196.8

[a]Rank based on number of deaths.

[b]Causes of death based on the *Tenth Revision, International Classification of Diseases, 1992.*

[c]Figures for age not stated are included in "all ages" but not distributed among age groups.

Source: Anderson (2002).

Table 1.4. Top Ten Leading Causes of Mortality for Latinas, by Age Group

Latinas, 15–19 Years

Rank[a]	Cause of Death[b]	Number[c]	Percentage of Total Deaths	Rate[c]
...	All causes	425	100.0	31.0
1	Accidents (unintentional injuries)	195	45.9	14.2
2	Malignant neoplasms	50	11.8	3.6
3	Assault (homicide)	42	9.9	3.1
4	Intentional self-harm (suicide)	35	8.2	2.6
5	Diseases of the heart	13	3.1	*
6	Congenital malformations, deformations, and chromosomal abnormalities	5	1.2	*
7	Nephritis, nephritic syndrome, and nephrosis	4	0.9	*
8	HIV	3	0.7	*
8	Cerebrovascular disease	3	0.7	*
8	Influenza and pneumonia	3	0.7	*
...	All other causes	72	16.9	5.3

Latinas, 20–24 Years

Rank[a]	Cause of Death[b]	Number[c]	Percentage of Total Deaths	Rate[c]
...	All causes	531	100.0	39.6
1	Accidents (unintentional injuries)	183	34.5	13.6
2	Assault (homicide)	70	13.2	5.2
3	Malignant neoplasms	63	11.9	4.7
4	Diseases of the heart	25	4.7	1.9
5	Intentional self-harm (suicide)	25	4.7	1.9
6	Pregnancy, childbirth and the puerperium	22	4.1	1.6
7	Cerebrovascular diseases	11	2.1	*
8	Congenital malformations, deformations, and chromosomal abnormalities	10	1.9	*
9	Influenza and pneumonia	8	1.5	*
10	Septicemia	5	0.9	*
10	Diabetes mellitus	5	0.9	*
...	All other causes	104	19.6	7.8

(Continued)

Table 1.4. Top Ten Leading Causes of Mortality for Latinas, by Age Group (Continued)

		Latinas, 25–34 Years					Latinas, 35–44 Years		
Rank[a]	Cause of Death[b]	Number[c]	Percentage of Total Deaths	Rate[c]	Rank[a]	Cause of Death[b]	Number[c]	Percentage of Total Deaths	Rate[c]
. . .	All causes	1,309	100.0	50.8	. . .	All causes	2,488	100.0	103.0
1	Accidents (unintentional injuries)	277	21.2	10.8	1	Malignant neoplasms	761	30.6	31.5
2	Malignant neoplasms	235	18.0	9.1	2	Accidents (unintentional injuries)	301	12.1	12.5
3	Assault (homicide)	113	8.6	4.4	3	Diseases of the heart	210	8.4	8.7
4	HIV	91	7.0	3.5	4	HIV	159	6.4	6.6
5	Diseases of the heart	81	6.2	3.1	5	Cerebrovascular diseases	122	4.9	5.0
6	Intentional self-harm (suicide)	50	3.8	1.9	6	Chronic liver disease and cirrhosis	102	4.1	4.2
7	Cerebrovascular diseases	43	3.3	1.7	7	Assault (homicide)	88	3.5	3.6
8	Pregnancy, childbirth, and puerperium	36	2.8	1.4	8	Intentional self-harm (suicide)	65	2.6	2.7
9	Influenza and pneumonia	21	1.6	0.8	9	Diabetes mellitus	59	2.4	2.4
10	Congenital malformations, deformations, and chromosomal abnormalities	20	1.5	0.8	10	Septicemia	33	1.3	1.4
. . .	All other causes	342	26.1	13.3	. . .	All other causes	588	23.6	24.3

Latinas, 45–54 Years

Rank[a]	Cause of Death[b]	Number[c]	Percentage of Total Deaths	Rate[c]
. . .	All causes	3,548	100.0	223.5
1	Malignant neoplasms	1,343	37.9	84.6
2	Diseases of the heart	447	12.6	28.2
3	Accidents (unintentional injuries)	203	5.7	12.8
4	Diabetes mellitus	199	5.6	12.5
5	Cerebrovascular diseases	197	5.6	12.4
6	Chronic liver disease and cirrhosis	147	4.1	9.3
7	HIV	105	3.0	6.6
8	Viral hepatitis	53	1.5	3.3
8	Assault (homicide)	53	1.5	3.3
10	Chronic lower respiratory diseases	52	1.5	3.3
. . .	All other causes	749	21.1	47.2

Latinas, 55–64 Years

Rank[a]	Cause of Death[b]	Number[c]	Percentage of Total Deaths	Rate[c]
. . .	All causes	4,973	100.0	525.0
1	Malignant neoplasms	1,746	35.1	184.3
2	Diseases of the heart	1,008	20.3	106.4
3	Diabetes mellitus	430	8.6	45.4
4	Cerebrovascular diseases	289	5.8	30.5
5	Chronic liver disease and cirrhosis	177	3.6	18.7
6	Accidents (unintentional injuries)	145	2.9	15.3
7	Nephritis, nephritic syndrome and nephrosis	117	2.4	12.4
8	Chronic lower respiratory diseases	98	2.0	10.3
9	Influenza and pneumonia	72	1.4	7.6
10	Septicemia	65	1.3	6.9
. . .	All other causes	826	16.6	87.2

(Continued)

Table 1.4. Top Ten Leading Causes of Mortality for Latinas, by Age Group (Continued)

Latinas, 65 Years and Over

Rank[a]	Cause of Death[b]	Number[c]	Percentage of Total Deaths	Rate[c]
. . .	All causes	30,881	100.0	2,741.5
1	Diseases of the heart	10,406	33.7	923.8
2	Malignant neoplasms	5,709	18.6	506.8
3	Cerebrovascular diseases	2,638	8.5	234.2
4	Diabetes mellitus	2,109	6.8	187.2
5	Influenza and pneumonia	1,101	3.6	97.7
6	Chronic lower respiratory diseases	1,033	3.3	91.7
7	Alzheimer's disease	732	2.4	65.0
8	Nephritis, nephritic syndrome and nephrosis	634	2.1	56.3
8	Accidents (unintentional injuries)	474	1.5	42.1
10	Chronic liver disease and cirrhosis	436	1.4	38.7
. . .	All other causes	5,609	18.2	497.9

[a]Rank based on number of deaths.

[b]Causes of death based on the *Tenth Revision, International Classification of Diseases, 1992.*

[c]Figures for age not stated are included in "all ages" but not distributed among age groups.

Source: Anderson (2002).

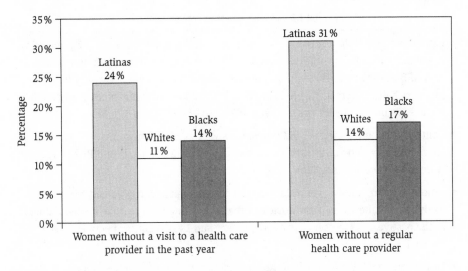

Figure 1.3. Provider Visits for Women by Race/Ethnicity, Ages 18 to 64

[a]Significantly different from the reference group (White women) at $p < 0.05$.

Source: Henry J. Kaiser Family Foundation (2001).

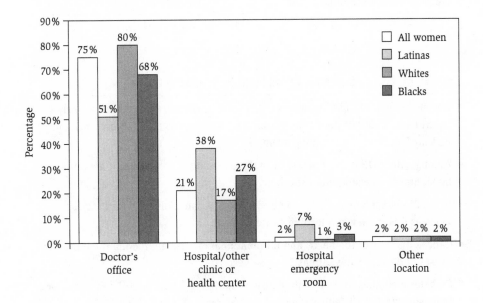

Figure 1.4. Site of Care by Race/Ethnicity, Women Ages 18 to 64 Years

[a]Significantly different from reference group (White women) at $p < .05$.

Source: Henry J. Kaiser Family Foundation (2001).

Exhibit 1.2. Access Barriers to Care for Latinas

- Latinas are at the highest risk for being uninsured; nearly four in ten (37 percent) are without health coverage compared to 16 percent of White women and 20 percent of Black women. Among poor Latinas (below 200 percent of poverty level), just over half (51 percent) were insured in 1999, and they experienced a 5 percent increase in uninsurance rates between 1994 and 1999.

- Central and South American (42 percent) as well as Mexican women (41 percent) are more likely to be uninsured compared to Cuban (20 percent) and Puerto Rican women (21 percent) (see Table 1.1).

- Among Latinas, a little over a third do not have a regular provider and are more likely than White women and African American women not to have visited a doctor in the past year (24 percent versus 11 percent and 14 percent, respectively) (see Figure 1.3).

- Latinas are more likely to rely on hospital clinics and health centers (38 percent) and hospital emergency rooms (7 percent) for medical care than other women see Figure 1.4).

- Compared to other women, Latinas reported higher levels of difficulty when communicating with their providers and faced considerable access problems and barriers to care (see Table 1.2).

Sources: Salganicoff, Beckerman, Wyn, and Ojeda (2002); Wyn, Solis, Ojeda, and Pourat (2001).

Exhibit 1.3. Critical Health Issues Affecting Latinas

- Despite being a younger population, Latinas (29 percent) were the most likely to report being in fair or poor health compared to White women (13 percent) and African American women (20 percent).

- Among Latinas 15 to 34 years, the top three leading causes of death are unintentional injuries, assault, and cancer.

- In the 25–34 age range, HIV is the fourth leading cause of death for Latinas, whereas it is the seventh leading cause of death among White women.

- Cancer, diseases of the heart, and unintentional injuries are the top three leading causes of death among Latinas 35 to 54 years.

- Diabetes continues to be a major cause of morbidity for Latinas 45 years and older. More specifically, it is either the third (55–64 years old) or fourth (45–54 years old) leading cause of death for these women.

Sources: Salganicoff, Beckerman, Wyn, and Ojeda (2002); Anderson (2002).

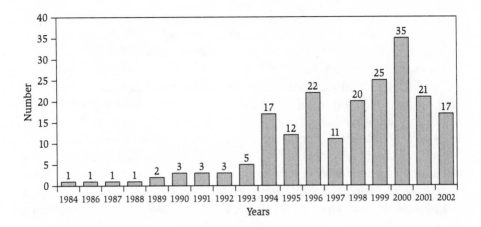

Figure 1.5. Articles Retrieved by Year ($n = 200$).

- Soundness and rigor of methodology employed in the study (valid and reliable study methods, identification of subgroup variations and acculturation where relevant)
- Sample size and selection process (for example, a sufficient number of Latinas in studies)
- Conclusions that are supported by study findings and studies that provided informative insights or have the potential of informing future studies and stimulating research questions and issues to build on

Studies that did not meet at least three of the five criteria were eliminated from further consideration. This resulted in 105 studies that received a second review and ranking by four readers. The outcome is the inclusion of 26 articles in the reader, plus an additional two commissioned papers and this introductory chapter, resulting in a total of 29 chapters for the book.

WHAT WAS LEARNED FROM THE PROCESS

Limited Focus of Studies on Latinas

In spite of the growing numbers of Latinas and what is known about their health status, there continues to be limited research and literature reflective of their health and health care needs. In spite of the data from national registries and surveillance reports documenting the leading causes of morbidity and mortality among Latinas, as well as reports on health indicators, there continues to be a disconnect between researchers' focus and interests, and the health needs of Latinas. There is limited attention in the literature to chronic conditions, even though chronic diseases such as cancer and heart disease are the leading causes of death (age specific) for Latinas. Neither is there adequate attention to issues such as barriers to care and the impact of welfare reform.

For example, although Mexican American women represent the largest subgroup of Latinas in the United States and are the subgroup most represented in the research literature, their specific needs are still underdocumented. Although they suffer from one of the highest rates of diabetes in the country (10.9 percent versus 4.5 percent for White women and 9.1 percent for African American women) (Harris and others, 1998), it was extremely difficult to identify a study for inclusion in this book that adequately addressed this issue. Therefore, we included a small focus group study of Latinas with pregnant or postpartum diabetes that raises a number of preliminary insights for future research.

Research attention is heavily weighted toward reproductive health and some to substance abuse. More specifically, following are the topics most frequently addressed in the literature on Latinas (see Figure 1.6):

- Reproductive health (for example, contraception, pregnancy, abortion, prenatal and perinatal care, and sexuality issues)
- Alcohol, tobacco, and other drug use
- Sexually transmitted diseases (including HIV/AIDS)

Limitations of the Studies

One of the two most obvious limitations across the many studies reviewed is the failure to adequately account for the effects of acculturation. When taken into consideration, the definition and variables used to measure acculturation vary tremendously. This is a significant limitation in the light of what is known about the influence of increased acculturation and the negative effect on health behaviors and health status. Among the studies reviewed, one sought to identify the reasons that Latinas do not seek prenatal care. Only English-speaking Latinas were recruited for the study. The authors posit that the ability to understand and speak English was an indicator of acculturation, implying that speaking English would enable the women to learn about available health services in the health care facilities they frequent. The methodology employed is problematic for many reasons. Acculturation cannot be measured by English comprehension alone. Other variables that go beyond language need to be considered (for example, length of residence and media language preference). Furthermore, limiting the study to Latinas who speak only English can lead to misguided assumptions that should not be generalized.

The second most obvious limitation of most studies is the failure to disaggregate data by Latina subgroups. Most studies report data in aggregate form, with no indication of the ethnic origin of women in the study. Preliminary studies

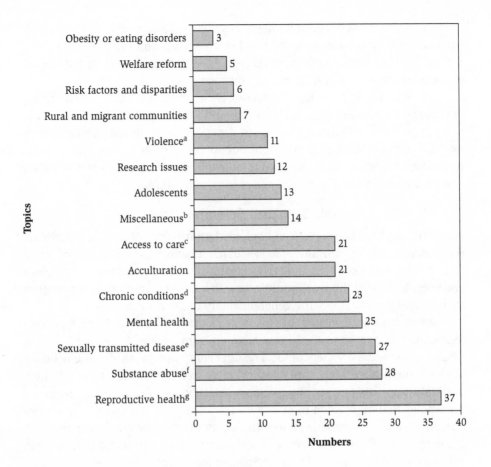

Figure 1.6. List of Topics and Frequency, 1984–2002

Note: Each topic covered in the article was included in the final count and does not equal the total of articles retrieved (*n* = 200).

[a]Violence includes assault, domestic or intimate partner violence, abuse, and rape.

[b]Miscellaneous includes topics on midlife women (45–64 years old), workforce issues, self-perception of health status, general minority health, lesbian women of color, transnational motherhood, health issues among Southwest Latinos, and policies affecting health status.

[c]Access to care includes access issues in general, barriers to care, insurance, quality of care, and patient-provider interaction.

[d]Chronic conditions include cancer, cardiovascular disease, and diabetes.

[e]Sexually transmitted disease also includes HIV/AIDS.

[f]Substance abuse includes substance abuse in general, alcohol, tobacco, other drug use, and recovery and treatment.

[g]Reproductive health includes family planning, perinatal care, prenatal care, sexuality issues, teen pregnancy, forced sterilization, abortion, and other topics.

indicate that there are significant differences across Latina groups that may result from acculturation levels, educational level, socioeconomic status, and other factors. In some cases, the failure to disaggregate data homogenizes the finding to the extent that the meaning and significance are lost.

There are very few studies that focus on Puerto Rican, Cuban, Dominican, or Central or South American women primarily. The last two represent growing numbers for which data and studies are almost nonexistent, but whose growth over the past decade and presence in our society require the attention of the public health and medical care communities. In many cases, these groups are almost invisible when it comes to the research literature.

Sample Size and Selection Process

A number of the studies reviewed contained an insufficient sample of Latinas. For example, a study on health practices of adult Latinas used a sample of seven respondents who were each interviewed four to seven times about their health practices. In spite of the small sample size, the authors reported the findings in such a manner as to imply the generalizability of the results.

In another instance, a study of what was reported to be of Mexican American women in Chicago, the sample was selected from a list of Spanish-surnamed women who visited a variety of local health centers and hospitals. The majority of the women were then contacted by telephone or recruited during their hospital stays. This process of participant selection by surname is problematic. It assumes that all women interviewed were Mexican American; the survey instrument did ask respondents to self-identify their ethnic group. A portion of the women may have not been of Mexican origin or Latino for that matter; Filipinos and Guamanians also have Spanish surnames.

Conclusion Reached by Research

The use of small sample sizes, lack of comparison groups, or use of Spanish surnames as the primary method of sample selection can lead to a number of limitations regarding the generalizability of the findings, adequacy of the sampling process, and validity of the conclusions reached. In general, these limitations can mask certain inter- and intraethnic differences, misdirect research efforts, and result in erroneous assumptions about the health behaviors and needs of Latinas. We observed several cases where conclusions did not correspond to findings.

Inclusion of Latina Health Topics in Leading Journals

During the review process, another interesting finding was the limited number of journals that include Latina health issues among the articles published. The articles retrieved by the research team were most commonly found in the *American Journal of Public Health* and the *Hispanic Journal of Behavioral*

Sciences. Other journals where articles on Latinas were published were the *American Journal of Obstetrics and Gynecology, Harvard Review of Psychiatry, Journal of Adolescent Health, Journal of Pediatrics,* and *Public Health Reports.* Although these journals should be commended for covering materials relevant to Latina health, the focus has been narrow and often concentrated on reproductive issues or substance use.

NEEDED COURSE OF ACTION

Ideally, more studies of Latinas are needed in a broader range of peer-reviewed journals and publications. They are needed for professionals, providers, and policymakers to inform the process of addressing and reducing health disparities. However, the research team realizes that the paucity of literature on Latina health is ultimately a reflection of public and private sector funders' lack of attention to or awareness of Latinas' health needs. Although it is easy to look to the journals and publications that publish these works, a more critical assessment needs to be conducted with respect to the support provided to researchers who choose to do work in this community. The paucity of available funding for minority women's health issues in turn shapes the interests and studies conducted by investigators, and thus may be contributing to the continued underrepresentation of Latinas in the research literature. It is vital that the philanthropic and public funding sectors become more cognizant of the need and act accordingly.

Funders, researchers, and advocates for women's health alike can play an integral role in bringing to the forefront the health needs of Latinas to policymakers and decision makers. Collaboration across these groups can help facilitate the needed advocacy to convey the importance of the health needs of Latinas so that they may understand the benefit it will serve these women, society, and future generations of Latino children and families as well.

References

Aguirre-Molina, M., Molina, C. W., and Zambrana, R. E. *Health Issues in the Latino Community.* San Francisco: Jossey-Bass, 2001.

Anderson, R. N. "Deaths: Leading Causes for 2000." *National Vital Statistics Reports,* 2002, *50,* 16.

Day, J. C. *Population of the United States by Age, Sex, Race, and Hispanic Origin, 1995–2050.* Washington, D.C.: U.S. Government Printing Office, 1996.

Harris, M. I., and others. "Prevalence of Diabetes, Impaired Fasting Glucose, and Impaired Glucose Tolerance in U.S. Adults. The Third National Health and Nutrition Examination Survey, 1988–1994." *Diabetes Care,* 1998, *21*(4), 518–524.

Henry J. Kaiser Family Foundation. *Kaiser Women's Health Survey.* Menlo Park, Calif.: Henry J. Kaiser Family Foundation, 2001.

Molina, C. W., and Aguirre-Molina, M. *Latino Health in the U.S.: A Growing Challenge.* Washington, D.C.: American Public Health Association, 1994.

Salganicoff, A., Beckerman, J. Z., Wyn, R., and Ojeda, V. D. *Women's Health in the United States: Health Coverage and Access to Care.* Washington, D.C.: Henry J. Kaiser Family Foundation, May 2002.

U.S. Bureau of the Census. *Current Population Survey.* Washington, D.C.: U.S. Government Printing Office, 1998.

U.S. Bureau of the Census. *Current Population Survey.* Washington, D.C.: U.S. Government Printing Office, 1999.

U.S. Bureau of the Census. *Percentage of Persons Who Are Hispanic or Latino (of Any Race): 2000:* Washington, D.C.: American Factfinder, 2000.

U.S. Bureau of the Census. *Current Population Survey.* Washington, D.C.: U.S. Government Printing Office, 2001.

Wyn, R., Solis, B., Ojeda, V. D., and Pourat, N. *Falling Through the Cracks: Health Insurance Coverage of Low-Income Women.* Washington, D.C.: Kaiser Family Foundation, 2001.

CHAPTER TWO

Public Health Needs and Scientific Opportunities in Research on Latinas

Hortensia Amaro
Adela de la Torre

Chapter One established that the public health needs of Latinas are significantly underrepresented in the research literature. In response, Amaro and de la Torre map out a cogent research agenda to address the public health needs of Latinas. The paradigm they propose serves to guide the formation of a research agenda that could make significant contributions toward an understanding of this population of women.

The last three decades have brought increasing attention to women's health research, both in the United States and internationally. Through its incorporation of various theoretical perspectives, the emerging body of research has resulted in a growing and rich understanding of factors affecting the health of women (Ruzek, Clarke, and Olesen, 1997). Despite some exceptions, however, much of the research on women's health has not contributed to a deeper understanding of the health issues affecting Latinas (Zambrana and Ellis, 1995; Amaro, 1993). The limitations of existing knowledge regarding the health of Latinas result from lack of attention to this population in studies of women's health; they also stem from broader problems involved in collecting health data on all Latinos, although we will not discuss those problems here (Amaro and Zambrana, 2000).

The integration of research on Latinas into the women's health agenda is important for at least two reasons. First, there are critical public health issues facing Latinas that must be better understood if interventions to eliminate racial and ethnic disparities in health are to be developed and implemented. Second, research on the health of Latinas presents unique opportunities to advance scientific understandings of underlying processes relevant to the health of other populations.

H. Amaro had primary responsibility for the conceptualization and writing of the chapter. A. de la Torre contributed to the writing of various sections of the chapter.

23

PUBLIC HEALTH NEEDS

According to the 2000 census, Latinos are now the largest minority group in the United States, composing 12.5 percent of the population; in comparison, 12 percent of U.S. residents are African Americans (U.S. Bureau of the Census, 2000a, 2000b). Latinos living in the continental United States and its territories total more than 40 million, as compared with 34 million African Americans. By the year 2050, Latinos are expected to constitute 25 percent of the U.S. population (Day, 1996; Falcon, Aguirre-Molina, and Molina, 2001). Thus, the mere size of the Latina population should be sufficient to increase its emphasis in the women's health research agenda. From a public health perspective, however, there are other compelling reasons for deepening our understanding of the health of Latinas.

The public health literature often highlights the "paradox" that Latinos, while sharing many of the demographic risk characteristics of African Americans, exhibit overall life expectancy and mortality rates that compare favorably to those of non-Hispanic Whites (Day, 1996; Falcon, Aguirre-Molina, and Molina, 2001; Vega and Amaro, 1994). However, a closer look reveals important health disparities not reflected in global and aggregate measures of health status. For example, the age-adjusted mortality rate (255.5 per 100,000) among Latinas is lower than that among non-Hispanic White women (359.1) (Murphy, 2000). Yet mortality data specific to Latino subgroups (Day, 1996) show that Mexican American girls younger than 1 year (559.4 per 100,000) and between the ages of 1 and 4 years (29.5 per 100,000) have higher death rates than their non-Hispanic White counterparts (544.6 and 27.0 per 100,000, respectively).

Similarly, death rates among female Puerto Ricans are higher than death rates among their non-Hispanic White counterparts in the 5- to 14-year (17.1 versus 14.9 per 100,000), 25- to 34-year (89.0 versus 58.7 per 100,000), 35- to 44-year (167.7 versus 123.7 per 100,000), and 45- to 54-year (353.0 versus 280.5 per 100,000) age groups. Furthermore, more Latinos (15.3 percent) than non-Hispanic Whites (9.3 percent) perceive themselves as being in fair or poor health (Hajat, Lucas, and Kington, 2000). Self-perceptions of health differ among Latino subgroups, with larger percentages of Puerto Ricans (17.5 percent) and Mexican Americans (16.2 percent) than members of other Latino groups reporting fair or poor health (Hajat, Lucas, and Kington, 2000).

Both the Latino "paradox" and the higher mortality rates among some Latino age cohorts and subgroups present important opportunities for research. First, the factors responsible for the apparent overall lower mortality among Latinas are not well understood, and research in this area might prove uniquely useful in understanding whether and how contextual and cultural factors have a salutary effect on the overall health status of populations that would otherwise be deemed to be at higher risk. Second, we know little about why some Latino age cohorts and subgroups might have higher mortality risks than others, and investigation of this question could prove important in understanding elevated risks for specific health problems among population subgroups. Research in both of these areas can offer unique scientific opportunities for informing the epidemiology of health problems not only among Latinas but also among other populations.

Research on Latinas also is important because there are clear health conditions that disproportionately affect this population, and studies are needed to inform public health efforts to eliminate such health disparities. For example, relative to non-Hispanic White women, Latinas have disproportionately high rates of cervical cancer (Wingo and others, 1998), sexually transmitted diseases (Centers for Disease Control and Prevention, 1998), HIV/AIDS (Centers for Disease Control and Prevention, 1999), teenage pregnancy (Ventura and Tappel, 1985), obesity (Kuczmarski, Flegal, Campbell, and Johnston, 1994), diabetes (Flegal and others, 1991), and violence and unintentional injuries (Rodriguez and Brindis, 1995; U.S. Department of Health and Human Services, 2000a). At the same time, Latinas face significant obstacles to health care. For instance, they are less likely than women in other racial or ethnic groups to have a regular source of health care (U.S. Department of Health and Human Services, 2000b) or to have health insurance coverage (de la Torre, Friis, Hunter, and Garcia, 1996). Furthermore, they may experience problems in communicating with English-speaking providers, which represents a major deterrent to seeking care (Derose and Baker, 2000). Research is needed on the factors that contribute to elevated health risks and disease patterns among Latinas and on effective prevention and intervention strategies for this population.

CULTURAL TRANSFORMATION AND HEALTH

Latinas are in the midst of major transformations that present opportunities for studying immigrant and intergenerational patterns in gender roles, family patterns, social support, socialization, and other factors (Baca-Zinn, 1995; Vega, 1995) and their effects on health. The dynamic roles of Latinas within their families and communities and the changing gender roles within Latino families (Baca-Zinn, 1995; Vega, 1995) provide a powerful opportunity for research on the effects of these changes on the health of Latinas throughout the life cycle.

The impact of intergenerational differences in assimilation and identity formation among Latinas is also an important emerging area that must be considered if there is to be a better understanding of the health status of Latinas. Studies focusing on the impact of differentiated trajectories of assimilation will provide needed data on risk factors affecting the health of Latinas. Models such as segmented assimilation theory (Portes and Zhou, 1993) bring attention to the critical interplay of individual, family, and community forces that shape the life

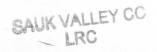

opportunities and experiences of Latinos and their adaptation to life in the United States (Rumbaut, 1994).

Public health research on Latinas and cultural adaptation has focused largely on acculturation, health status, and health behaviors. In most studies, acculturation has been measured via proxy variables such as place of birth, years of residence in the United States, and language use. Consistently, these studies (Zambrana and Ellis, 1995; Giachello, 2001; Guendelman, 1998) have demonstrated that as women become more acculturated, they are more at risk for adverse birth outcomes (Guendelman and Abrams, 1994; Guendelman and English, 1995); younger age at first intercourse (Marcell, 1994; Reynoso, Felice, and Shragg, 1993), first use of birth control (Brindis, Wolfe, and McCarter, 1995), and first pregnancy (Ventura and others, 2000); partner violence (Caetano and others, 2000; Kantor, Jasinski, and Aldarondo, 1993; Sorenson and Telles, 1991); tobacco (Palinkas and others, 1993; Coreil, Ray, and Markides, 1991; Marin and others, 1989; Stephen, Foote, Hendershot, and Schoenborn, 1994), alcohol (Stephen, Foote, Hendershot, and Schoenborn, 1994; Black and Markides, 1993), and illicit drug use (Stephen, Foote, Hendershot, and Schoenborn, 1994; Amaro, Whitaker, Coffman, and Heeren, 1990; Nyamathi and others, 1993; Khoury and others 1996); depression (Vega and Alegria, 2001); sexual activity with multiple partners (Nyamathi and others, 1993; Sabogal, Faigeles, and Catania, 1993); and negative attitudes toward condom use (Marin, Tschann, Gomez, and Kegeles, 1993).

While less acculturated Latinas experience fewer health problems and risk factors, they are also less likely to have access to health care services when they need them. In comparison with more acculturated Latinas, those with lower levels of acculturation are less likely to seek prenatal care (Ventura and others, 2000), to use needed mental health services (Vega, Kolody, Aguilar-Gaxiola, and Catalano, 1999), to have had annual Papanicolaou tests or mammograms (Elder and others 1991; Harlan, Bernstein, and Kessler, 1991), and to have health insurance coverage (Solis, Marks, Garcia, and Shelton, 1990) and a regular source of health care (Estrada, Treviño, and Ray, 1990).

Despite the significance of these findings that link levels of acculturation of Latinas to health status and health care access, there still is a dearth of conceptual and empirical attention focused on the mechanisms underlying the relationships between cultural change, risk factors, and health status. Empirical studies readily incorporate existing acculturation variables but do not fully explore the more complex domain of Latina identity formation.

In the case of many Latinas, linear acculturation models fall short of explaining the complex and fluid nature of identity formation and maintenance of bicultural identities despite external assimilation pressures (Romero, Cuéllar, and Roberts, 2000). Cultural changes do occur for many of these women and their families, but often these changes are measured primarily through variables such as immigrant status and language of origin. Clearly, these variables do not effectively measure degrees of bicultural identity formation or shifting identity roles; rather, they merely provide a glimpse of the possible effects of identity formation among Latinas and their children.

Moreover, there is a real danger that we may be confounding narrower acculturation and assimilation variables with items that actually predict economic trajectories of immigrant groups. It is clear that the class position of Latinas affects their overall health status, yet we still need to capture the extent to which these women and their families maintain cultural practices intergenerationally, creating resilient models of bicultural identity formation. We also need to know how these identities and practices may protect Latinas and their children from the degrading effects of racism within American society, as well as the effects on their overall mental and physical health. Both qualitative and quantitative studies on Latina identity formation and health status are needed to develop this emerging area of scholarship further.

SOCIAL STATUS AND HEALTH

Cultural factors such as familism, gender roles, *respeto* (the value of respect toward others, especially those deemed to have positions of authority based on age and role in the family and community), and *personalismo* (the value of maintaining smooth social relationships and interactions) are thought to be relevant in shaping Latinas' health-related beliefs, attitudes, and practices and deserve further investigation (Marin, Pérez-Stable, Otero-Sabogal, and Sabogal, 1990; Marin and Marin, 1991; Angel and Angel, 1997; Williams, Mourey, and Warren, 1994). While there continues to be a need for research that provides a more in-depth understanding of the role of culture in the health of Latinas, there is an equally pressing need for research on the effects of socially constructed arrangements based on gender, class, and race/ethnicity.

With the exception of those advocating purely biological models of women's health, a number of researchers acknowledge the relevance of gender, race, and class to the health of women (Krieger, 1999; Ruzek, Clarke, and Olesen, 1997). Yet Reid points out that most feminist theory and research have been "directed to the explication of women's essential experience of gender, as if this could be separated from the confounds of class and race" (Reid, 1993). It is critical to build an understanding of health that considers the extent to which Latinas most at risk for health problems are affected by oppression based on gender, race/ethnicity, and class.

The framework of oppression invites us to consider the role of social institutions and their participation in oppression, the dynamics through which social control is exerted at the group and individual levels, and group and individual coping responses to oppression. Amaro and Raj (2000) described and applied such a framework in the understanding of the disproportionate risk of HIV among African American women and Latinas. They noted the influences of gender bias, racism, and class bias in psychological and health research and public health programs, as evidenced in the history of the eugenics movement and sterilization campaign in Puerto Rico and among women of color in the United States.

More recently, policies that have sought to block access to health care among immigrants, including legal immigrants, have had an impact on use of health care services among some groups of Latinas (de la Torre, Friis, Hunter, and Garcia, 1996). Yet with few exceptions (Krieger, 1999), research on women who are members of racial and ethnic "minority groups," including Latinas, has lagged in terms of conceptualization and measurement of the effects of socially defined status and oppression.

A common hallmark of oppression is ascription by the dominant group of the oppressed group's negative and disempowering characteristics (Amaro and Raj, 2000). The characteristics ascribed to socially subordinate groups both reflect and reinforce the lower power status of these groups. Because these dynamics can pervasively define the life experiences of lower-status groups, they are likely to be relevant to our understanding of the context of Latinas' health. The work of Williams and colleagues (Williams, Mourey, and Warren, 1994; Williams, Yu, Jackson, and Anderson, 1997; Williams and Collins, 1995), Krieger (1999), and Leveist (1993) has begun to document the relationship between discrimination and jeopardized health. However, much of this work has focused on African Americans, with few studies documenting the role of discrimination in the health status of Latinas (Amaro, Russo, and Johnson, 1987; Salgado de Snyder, 1987).

Research is needed that investigates the nature of discrimination experienced by Latinas through the process of cultural adaptation and the resulting effects on health and experiences in the health care delivery system. One important line of research involves stereotypes held by service providers and their impact on the health care received by Latinas. Scrimshaw, Zambrana, and Dunkel-Schetter (1997) found that stereotypes held by medical providers negatively affect the obstetrical and gynecological care received by Latinas. Further research is needed to assess the frequency of negative ascriptions of Latinas among health care providers and the effects on quality of care.

Latinas' development of an ethnic identity as a "minority" group within U.S. society has been overlooked as a facet of oppression that may have an impact on their health. A number of researchers who study development of racial and ethnic identity among U.S. "minority" groups have documented that in early stages of ethnic identity development, members of oppressed racial and ethnic groups internalize negative views of their groups that have been prescribed by the larger, dominant group. This negative internalization may result in a desire of individuals to distance themselves from their racial or ethnic group (Helms, 1990; Phinney, 1993; Russell, Wilson, and Hall, 1992; Powell-Hopson and Hopson, 1988).

Alternatively, exploration, knowledge, and acceptance of one's cultural group have been linked to healthier psychological development. Studies on the health of Latinas have generally categorized these women solely in terms of their reported ethnic identification. However, we know relatively little about the ways in which Latinas cope with the meaning of being a member of a socially defined subservient group and how varying coping responses are related to health behaviors and risk factors. The responses of groups ascribed lower social status in a society are complex and depend on many historical and situational contextual factors.

Berry (1984) proposed four strategies adopted by members of nondominant cultural groups in response to domination: integration, assimilation, separation, and marginalization. These strategies have important implications for identity, values, attitudes, and abilities, and they are expressed in behaviors and social relations. Marginalization, which involves disengagement from one's culture of origin as well as lack of integration into one's new culture, has been associated with the most negative outcomes. In a study of illicit drug use, Amaro, Whitaker, Coffman, and Heeren (1990) found that Latinos who were highly acculturated but were not integrated into the U.S. mainstream (as reflected in their poverty status) had by far the highest rates of illicit drug use. The literature suggests that marginalization might be a health risk factor deserving attention in future studies on Latinas.

CONCLUSION

Innovative and practical studies will be required to reduce health disparities in the United States. Beyond its public health practice value, research on factors affecting the health of Latinas will provide opportunities to further our understanding of a number of more universal contextual factors affecting immigrant and socially marginalized populations. Given the status of current research on this population as well as promising new scientific opportunities for research, we offer the following suggestions:

1. Although aggregate and global measures of Latina health may provide useful benchmarks of Latinas in relation to other groups, these measures mask important differences that could explain the Latino "paradox" in health as well as differential mortality rates among some Latina age cohorts and subgroups. Developing research studies that address the impact of contextual and cultural factors on the health status of Latina age cohorts and subpopulations may prove valuable in identifying the health needs of this rapidly growing group.

2. The impact of Latina identity formation and cultural transformation on health behaviors, health risks, and protective coping strategies represents an emerging area of study that requires further conceptual and empirical

development. There is a significant amount of public health research primarily addressing the impact of acculturation on health status and health behaviors; thus, there is a real opportunity to disentangle aggregate acculturation measures that focus on immigrant status or language of origin and to expand them to include variables that measure identity formation, perceived discrimination, and cultural negotiation. The representation of both U.S.-born and immigrant populations among Latinas provides an additional opportunity for this type of research.

3. Methods of measuring the impact of oppression and power dynamics based on how Latinas experience the intersections of gender, race, and class must be developed if there is to be a full understanding of the health status and access issues faced by this group. For example, by developing research on discrimination, coping, and resistance strategies, researchers could shed light on how these affect the health status of Latinas.

4. Finally, given a broader conceptual framework of oppression for assessing Latina health, researchers may develop a better understanding of the negative effects of social institutions, as well as of actors within these institutions, on access to health care services.

References

Amaro, H. "Health Data on Hispanic Women: Methodological Limitations." In *Proceedings of the Public Health Conference on Records and Statistics, Washington, D.C., July 19–21, 1993.* Hyattsville, Md.: National Center for Health Statistics, 1993.

Amaro, H., and Raj, A. "On the Margin: Power and Women's HIV Risk Reduction Strategies." *Psychology of Women Quarterly,* 2000, *24,* 723–749.

Amaro, H., Russo, N. F., and Johnson, J. "Family and Work Predictors of Psychological Well-Being Among Hispanic Women Professionals." *Psychology of Women Quarterly,* 1987, *11,* 505–521.

Amaro, H., Whitaker, R., Coffman, G., and Heeren, T. "Acculturation and Marijuana and Cocaine Use: Findings from the Hispanic HANES." *American Journal of Public Health,* 1990, *80* (suppl.), 54–60.

Amaro, H., and Zambrana, R. E. "Criollo, Mestizo, Mulatto, Latinegro, Indígena, White, or Black? The U.S. Hispanic/Latino Population and Multiple Responses in the 2000 Census." *American Journal of Public Health,* 2000, *90,* 1724–1727.

Angel, R., and Angel, J. *Who Will Care for Us? Aging and Long-Term Care in Multicultural America.* New York: New York University Press, 1997.

Baca-Zinn, M. "Social Science Theorizing for Latino Families." In R. E. Zambrana (ed.), *Understanding Latino Families.* Thousand Oaks, Calif.: Sage, 1995.

Berry, J. W. "Cultural Relations in Plural Societies: Alternatives to Segregation and Their Socio-Psychological Implications." In N. Baker Miller and M. B. Brewer (eds.), *Groups in Contact.* Orlando, Fla.: Academic Press, 1984.

Black, S. A., and Markides, K. S. "Acculturation and Alcohol Consumption in Puerto Rican, Cuban-American, and Mexican-American Women in the United States." *American Journal of Public Health*, 1993, *83*, 890–893.

Brindis, C., Wolfe, A., and McCarter, V. "The Associations Between Immigrant Status and Risk-Behavior Patterns in Latino Adolescents." *Journal of Adolescent Health*, 1995, *17*, 99–105.

Caetano, R., and others. "Intimate Partner Violence, Acculturation, and Alcohol Consumption Among Hispanic Couples in the United States." *Journal of Interpersonal Violence*, 2000, *15*, 30–45.

Centers for Disease Control and Prevention. *Sexually Transmitted Disease Surveillance 1997*. Atlanta, Ga.: Centers for Disease Control and Prevention, 1998.

Centers for Disease Control and Prevention. *HIV/AIDS Surveillance Report: U.S. HIV and AIDS Cases Reported Through June 1999*. Atlanta, Ga.: Centers for Disease Control and Prevention, 1999.

Coreil, J., Ray, L. A., and Markides, K. S. "Predictors of Smoking Among Mexican-Americans: Findings from the Hispanic HANES." *Preventive Medicine*, 1991, *20*, 508–517.

Day, J. C. *Population Projections of the United States by Age, Sex, Race, and Hispanic Origin: 1995–2050*. Washington, D.C.: U.S. Bureau of the Census, 1996.

de la Torre, A., Friis, R., Hunter, H. R., and Garcia, L. "The Health Insurance Status of U.S. Latino Women: A Profile from the 1982–1984 Hispanic HANES." *American Journal of Public Health*, 1996, *86*, 534–537.

Derose, K. P., and Baker, D. W. "Limited English Proficiency and Latinos' Use of Physician Services." *Medical Care Research and Review*, 2000, *57*, 76–91.

Elder, J. P., and others. "Differences in Cancer-Risk-Related Behaviors in Latino and Non-Hispanic Adults." *Preventive Medicine*, 1991, *20*, 751–763.

Estrada, A. L., Treviño, F. M., and Ray, L. A. "Health Care Utilization Barriers Among Mexican-Americans: Evidence from the HHANES 1982–1984." *American Journal of Public Health*, 1990, *80* (suppl.), 27–31.

Falcon, A., Aguirre-Molina, M., and Molina, C. W. "Latino Health Policy: Beyond Demographic Determinism." In M. Aguirre-Molina, C. W. Molina, and R. E. Zambrana (eds.), *Health Issues in the Latino Community*. San Francisco: Jossey-Bass, 2001.

Flegal, K. M., and others. "Prevalence of Diabetes in Mexican Americans, Cubans, and Puerto Ricans from the Hispanic Health and Nutrition Examination Survey, 1982–1984." *Diabetes Care*, 1991, *14*, 628–638.

Giachello, A. "The Reproductive Years: The Health of Latinas." In M. Aguirre-Molina, C. W. Molina, and R. E. Zambrana (eds.), *Health Issues in the Latino Community*. San Francisco: Jossey-Bass, 2001.

Guendelman, S. "Health and Disease Among Hispanics." In S. Loue (ed.), *Handbook of Immigrant Health*. New York: Plenum Press, 1998.

Guendelman, S., and Abrams, B. "Dietary, Alcohol, and Tobacco Intake Among Mexican-American Women of Childbearing Age: Results from the HHANES Data." *American Journal of Health Promotion*, 1994, *8*, 363–372.

Guendelman, S., and English, P. "The Effects of United States Residence on Birth Outcomes Among Mexican Immigrants: An Exploratory Study." *American Journal of Epidemiology,* 1995, *142,* 530–538.

Hajat, A., Lucas, J., and Kington, R. "Health Outcomes Among Hispanic Subgroups: United States, 1992–95." *Advance Data from Vital and Health Statistics,* Feb. 10, 2000, p. 310.

Harlan, L. C., Bernstein, A. B., and Kessler, L. G. "Cervical Cancer Screening: Who Is Not Screened and Why?" *American Journal of Public Health,* 1991, *81,* 885–890.

Helms, J. *Black and White Racial Identity: Theory, Research, and Practice.* Westport, Conn.: Greenwood Press, 1990.

Kantor, J., Jasinski, J., and Aldarondo, E. *Incidence of Hispanic Drinking and Intra-Family Violence.* San Antonio, Tex.: Research Society on Alcoholism, 1993.

Khoury, E. L., and others. "Gender and Ethnic Differences in Prevalence of Alcohol, Cigarette, and Illicit Drug Use Among an Ethnically Diverse Sample of Hispanic, African American, and Non-Hispanic White Adolescents." *Women and Health,* 1996, *24,* 21–40.

Krieger N. "Embodying Inequality: A Review of Concepts, Measures, and Methods for Studying Health Consequences of Discrimination." *International Journal of Health Services,* 1999, *29,* 295–352.

Kuczmarski, R. J., Flegal, K. M., Campbell, S. M., and Johnston, C. L. "Increasing Prevalence of Overweight Among U.S. Adults." *JAMA,* 1994, *272,* 205–211.

Leveist, T. A. "Segregation, Poverty, and Empowerment: Health Consequences for African Americans." *Milbank Quarterly,* 1993, *71,* 42–64.

Marcell, A. "Understanding Ethnicity, Identity Formation, and Risk Behavior Among Adolescents of Mexican Descent." *Journal of School Health,* 1994, *64,* 323–327.

Marin, B. V., Pérez-Stable, E. J., Otero-Sabogal, R., and Sabogal, F. "Cultural Differences in Attitudes Toward Smoking: Developing Messages Using the Theory of Reasoned Action." *Journal of Applied Social Psychology,* 1990, *20,* 478–493.

Marin, B. V., Tschann, J. M., Gomez, C. A., and Kegeles, S. M. "Acculturation and Gender Differences in Sexual Attitudes and Behaviors: Hispanic Versus Non-Hispanic White Unmarried Adults." *American Journal of Public Health,* 1993, *83,* 1259–1261.

Marin, G., and Marin, B. V. *Research with Hispanic Populations.* Newbury Park, Calif.: Sage, 1991.

Marin, G., and others. "The Role of Acculturation in the Attitudes, Norms, and Expectancies of Hispanic Smokers." *Journal of Cross-Cultural Psychology,* 1989, *20,* 399–415.

Murphy, S. L. "Deaths: Final Data for 1998." *National Vital Statistics Report,* 2000, *48,* 11.

Nyamathi, A., and others. "AIDS-Related Knowledge, Perceptions, and Behaviors Among Impoverished Minority Women." *American Journal of Public Health,* 1993, *83,* 65–71.

Palinkas, L., and others. "Cigarette Smoking Behavior and Beliefs of Hispanics in California." *American Journal of Preventive Medicine,* 1993, *9,* 331–337.

Phinney, J. S. "A Three-Stage Model of Ethnic Identity Development in Adolescence." In M. B. Bernal and G. P. Knight (eds.), *Ethnic Identity: Formation and Transmission Among Hispanics and Other Minorities.* Albany: State University of New York Press, 1993.

Portes, A., and Zhou, M. "The New Second Generation: Segmented Assimilation and Its Variants." *Annals of the American Academy of Political Social Science,* 1993, *530,* 74–96.

Powell-Hopson, D., and Hopson, D. S. "Implications of Doll Color Preferences Among Black Preschool Children and White Preschool Children." *Journal of Black Psychology,* 1988, *14,* 57–63.

Reid, P. "Poor Women in Psychological Research: Shut Up and Shut Out." *Psychology of Women Quarterly,* 1993, *17,* 143.

Reynoso, T., Felice, M., and Shragg, G. "Does American Acculturation Affect Outcome of Mexican-American Teenage Pregnancy?" *Journal of Adolescent Health,* 1993, *14,* 257–261.

Rodriguez, M., and Brindis, C. "Violence and Latino Youth: Prevention and Methodological Issues." *Public Health Report,* 1995, *110,* 260–267.

Romero, A. J., Cuéllar, I., and Roberts, R. E. "Ethnocultural Variables and Attitudes Toward Cultural Socialization of Children." *Journal of Community Psychology,* 2000, *28,* 79–89.

Rumbaut, R. G. "The Crucible Within: Ethnic Identity, Self-Esteem, and Segmented Assimilation Among Children of Immigrants." *International Migration Review,* 1994, *28,* 748–794.

Russell, K., Wilson, M., and Hall, R. "Embracing Whiteness." In K. Russell, M. Wilson, and R. Hall (eds.), *The Color Complex: The Politics of Skin Color Among African Americans.* New York: Doubleday, 1992.

Ruzek, S. B., Clarke, A. E., and Olesen, V. L. "Social, Biomedical, and Feminist Models of Women's Health." In S. B. Ruzek, V. L. Olesen, and A. E. Clarke (eds.), *Women's Health: Complexities and Differences.* Columbus: Ohio State University Press, 1997.

Sabogal, F., Faigeles, B., and Catania, J. A. "Data from the National AIDS Behavioral Surveys, II: Multiple Sexual Partners Among Hispanics in High Risk Cities." *Family Planning Perspectives,* 1993, *25,* 257–262.

Salgado de Snyder, N. V. "Factors Associated with Acculturative Stress and Depressive Symptomatology Among Married Mexican Immigrant Women." *Psychology of Women Quarterly,* 1987, *11,* 457–488.

Scrimshaw, S.C.M., Zambrana, R. E., and Dunkel-Schetter, C. "Issues in Latino Women's Health: Myths and Challenges." In S. B. Ruzek, V. L. Olesen, and A. E. Clarke (eds.), *Women's Health: Complexities and Differences.* Columbus: Ohio State University Press, 1997.

Solis, J. M., Marks, G., Garcia, M., and Shelton, D. "Acculturation, Access to Care, and Use of Preventive Services by Hispanics: Findings from HHANES 1982–1984." *American Journal of Public Health,* 1990, *80*(suppl.), 11–19.

Sorenson, S. B., and Telles, C. A. "Selfreports of Spousal Violence in a Mexican-American and Non-Hispanic White Population." *Violence and Victims,* 1991, *6,* 3–15.

Stephen, E., Foote, K., Hendershot, G., and Schoenborn, C. *Health of the Foreign-Born Population: United States, 1989–1990.* Atlanta, Ga.: Centers for Disease Control and Prevention, 1994.

U.S. Bureau of the Census. *Census 2000 Redistricting Data.* Washington, D.C.: U.S. Bureau of the Census, 2000a.

U.S. Bureau of the Census. *Projections of the Resident Population by Race, Hispanic Origin and Nativity.* Washington, D.C.: U.S. Bureau of the Census, 2000b.

U.S. Department of Health and Human Services. *National Health Interview Survey, 1997.* Washington, D.C.: U.S. Department of Health and Human Services, 2000a.

U.S. Department of Health and Human Services. *National Vital Statistics System, 1998.* Washington, D.C.: U.S. Department of Health and Human Services, 2000b.

Vega, W. A. "The Study of Latino families." In R. E. Zambrana (ed.), *Understanding Latino Families.* Thousand Oaks, Calif.: Sage, 1995.

Vega, W. A., and Alegria, M. "Latino Mental Health and Treatment in the United States." In M. Aguirre-Molina, C. W. Molina, and R. E. Zambrana (eds.), *Health Issues in the Latino Community.* San Francisco: Jossey-Bass, 2001.

Vega, W. A., and Amaro, H. "Latino Outlook: Good Health, Uncertain Prognosis." *Annual Review of Public Health,* 1994, *15,* 39–67.

Vega, W. A., Kolody, B., Aguilar-Gaxiola, S., and Catalano, R. "Gaps in Service Utilization by Mexican-Americans with Mental Health Problems." *American Journal of Psychiatry,* 1999, *156,* 928–934.

Ventura, S. J., and Tappel, S. M. "Childbearing Characteristics of U.S. and Foreignborn Hispanic Mothers." *Public Health Report,* 1985, *100,* 647–652.

Ventura, S. J., and others. "Births: Final Data for 1998." *National Vital Statistics Report,* 2000, *48,* 3.

Williams, D. R., and Collins, C. "U.S. Socioeconomic and Racial Differences in Health: Patterns and Explanations." *Annual Review of Sociology,* 1995, *21,* 349–386.

Williams, D. R., Mourey, R., and Warren, R. "The Concept of Race and Health Status in America." *Public Health Report,* 1994, *109,* 26–41.

Williams, D. R., Yu, Y., Jackson, J. S., and Anderson, N. B. "Racial Differences in Physical and Mental Health: Socioeconomic Status, Stress, and Discrimination." *Journal of Health Psychology,* 1997, *2,* 335–351.

Wingo, P. A., and others. "Cancer Incidence and Mortality, 1973–1996." *Cancer,* 1998, *82,* 1197–1207.

Zambrana, R., and Ellis, B. K. "Contemporary Research Issues in Hispanic/Latino Women's Health." In D. L. Adams (ed.), *Health Issues for Women of Color.* Thousand Oaks, Calif.: Sage, 1995.

PART TWO

RISK FACTORS
AND DISPARITIES
AMONG LATINAS

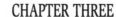

CHAPTER THREE

Disparities in Health Indicators for Latinas in California

Lourdes Baezconde-Garbanati
Carmen J. Portillo
James A. Garbanati

This chapter provides an excellent overview and analysis of the health indicators and disparities that Latinas (primarily Mexican American women) in California face. The authors also provide comparisons with White women in the state and Mexican women in Mexico, while acknowledging the limitations of some of these data. Although the focus is on a single state, California is the home of the largest number of Latinos in the United States; they compose almost half of the state's total population. Therefore, in spite of what may be perceived as a geographic limitation, the chapter represents one of the few efforts to address and examine disparities as well as risk factors among Latinas. This work provides important insights from which to build.

Research on Latina health shows positive outcomes for some indicators, such as life expectancy, low birth weight babies, depression, alcohol abuse, and smoking among Latinas when compared to their non-Latino White or African American counterparts (Baezconde-Garbanati, 1994; Hayes-Bautista,

This chapter is based in part on a report of the Latina Health Policy Project at the Latino Coalition for a Healthy California titled "Ensuring Health Access for Latinas," and is part of an ongoing study. The information is printed with permission from the Latino Coalition for a Healthy California. The study is supported through the generous support of the James Irvine Foundation to the Latino Coalition for a Healthy California. We wish to acknowledge the support of Marty Campbell, program director, and Avon Swofford, program associate, at the James Irvine Foundation. At the Latino Coalition for a Healthy California, we wish to acknowledge Martha Jimenez, Patricia Barrera, Julie Davidson Gomez, and former staff Carmela Castellanos, Sandra Camacho, and Brenda Solorzano, who provided guidance, expertise, and technical support. In addition, we want to thank Latina Health Leadership Council members: Adela de la Torre, Helen Rodriguez-Trias, Kathleen Torres, Martha Torres Montoya, Luz Alvarez Martinez, Liz Torres, Martha Jazo-Bajet, Marielena Lara, Barbara Marquez, and Sylvia Villareal who through multiple council meetings provided leadership and input on various stages of this project. Special thanks are also due to the Policy Committee, staff, volunteers, interns, and consultants who worked on different phases of this project.

Baezconde-Garbanati, Schink, and Hayes-Bautista, 1994; Hayes-Bautista, 1997). In some areas, Latinas in the United States have better outcomes than do women in Mexico. For others, immigrant Latinas have more positive health outcomes than more acculturated Latinas (Hayes-Bautista, 1990a; Vega and others, 1998). This overall scenario of wellness tends to mask critical areas of health for which Latinas are clearly disadvantaged (Latino Coalition for a Healthy California, 1999). The U.S. Department of Health and Human Services, Public Health Service (1997) is currently working on Healthy People 2010 objectives. But as we enter the twenty-first century, many of the Year 2000 objectives for Latinos have not been met. Although some progress has been made, disparities still exist in many factors. According to the U.S. Department of Health and Human Services, at least 10 percent of Year 2000 Latino objectives show no improvements, and for another 21 percent, there are no data to assess progress. This complex picture poses both challenges and opportunities for health care policy, programs, and research in the twenty-first century (Hayes-Bautista, 1997).

The purpose of this research is to investigate disparities among Latinas when compared to other ethnic/racial groups, for which advocacy and policy action may be needed. Recommendations for future policy research are presented, calling for culturally and linguistically appropriate prevention efforts that target improvements in Latina health.

BACKGROUND

This study was conducted as part of ongoing research of the Latina Health Policy Project at the Latino Coalition for a Healthy California (LCHC). The Latina Health Policy Project is a statewide policy and advocacy program funded by the James Irvine Foundation. The goals of the project are to gather information on Latina health, monitor and analyze health-related legislative policies, meet with policymakers, and maintain a clearinghouse on Latina health information.

METHOD

With guidance from the Latina Health Policy Project's Leadership Council, existing data were identified, prioritized, and analyzed on demographics and selected health indicators for which Latino advocacy is needed (LCHC, 1999). Secondary data analyses were conducted using data tapes and printed files from the California Department of Finance, *Interim County Population Projections* (1997), the summary data tape and Current Population Survey (CPS), and the U.S. Bureau of the Census (1996). Education and dropout data were obtained from the California Basic Educational Data System's database (CBEDS) (California Department of

Education, 1995). Labor force and occupational data were obtained through special analytic requests from the California Employment Development Department (EDD) (1995). Health data were compiled from existing and special analyses requested of the California Department of Health Services' (CDHS) vital statistics section (1993, 1994, 1997, 1998), 1997 California Women's Health Survey, the Tobacco Control Section, and the Planning and Data Analysis Section

Various government reports were also reviewed. These included the following: the Cardiovascular Disease Outreach, Resources and Epidemiology (CORE) Program's *Cardiovascular Disease Risk Factors Among California Adults 1984–1996* (Gazzaniga and others, 1998), the 1998 Los Angeles County Women's Health Policy Summit Report of the Los Angeles County Commission for Women (1998), several policy briefs from the Center for Health Policy Research (Brown, Pourat, Wyn, and Solis, 1997; Wyn, Leslie, Glick, and Solis, 1997), and the Center for the Study of Latino Health at the University of California, Los Angeles (Hayes-Bautista, 1990b, 1997).

DATA ANALYSIS

A detailed description of data analyses for this project is presented elsewhere (LCHC, 1999). For these Latino Coalition data, univariate and descriptive analyses were performed. Crude age and race-specific rates were calculated. In addition, various printed sources were systematically reviewed for inclusion. A schema for cultural specificity in Latino research (Castro and Baezconde-Garbanati, 1987) provided the context for examining information that met one or more of the following criteria: (1) inclusion of women of Latino heritage in the sample; (2) comparison with non-Latino White, African American, Asian, Native American, or other women in California; (3) data on national origin (Mexican versus Central and or South American); (4) acculturation and or immigration status; (5) language of preference; (6) rural versus urban differences; (7) county-specific data in areas with high Latina concentration; (8) data on Latinas by age group (younger than 15, 15–17, 18–20, 21–44, 45–64, 65 and older years); (9) factors that place Latinas at risk for disease; and (10) as available, comparable data on women in Mexico.

RESULTS

Latina Demographics in California

The Number of Latinas in California. There are close to 5 million Latinas in California (4,846,257) (California Department of Finance, 1997), representing 29 percent of the female population in the state. Of these, the majority (approximately 60 percent) are of Mexican origin. This population in California is increasing at an accelerated pace when compared to other groups. California Department of Finance data (1997) for 1990 to 1996 show a 31 percent increase among Latinas, compared to 4 percent for non-Latino White women, 9 percent for African American women, and 13 percent for the total female population in California. This growth is fueled by a high birth rate and immigration. For example, in 1993, 45 percent of births in California were to Latinas, compared to 29 percent of births in 1980 (California Department of Finance, 1993). In some counties, such as Los Angeles County, Latinas already account for the majority of births (61 percent) (Los Angeles County Department of Health Services, 1997).

Immigration from Mexico and Central America also contributes to the increasing numbers of Latinas in California. These women are very heterogeneous in nature, coming from various countries, such as Nicaragua, El Salvador, Honduras, and Mexico. Women from Mexico, for example, are very heterogeneous. According to data from the Secretaría de Gobernación (1996), in Mexico there are 46.5 million women, with 28.7 percent living in rural areas with fewer than 2,500 inhabitants. Among them, indigenous women constitute approximately half of the 8 million indigenous people of Mexico.

In California, Latinas tend to concentrate in five counties: Los Angeles (2,032,344), Orange (333,771), San Diego (322,831), San Bernardino (278,117), and Riverside (260,965). In Los Angeles, Latinas surpass the numbers of non-Latina White and African American women (42 percent versus 36 percent and 10 percent, respectively). Although in lesser numbers, Latinas represent a large percentage of the total female population in Fresno (38 percent), Riverside (34 percent), Kern (33 percent), San Bernardino (31 percent), Ventura (29 percent), Orange (25 percent), Santa Clara (22 percent), and San Diego (23 percent) Counties (California Department of Finance, 1997).

Youthfulness of the Latina Population. Latinas are a young population, with a median age of 25, compared to 30 for African Americans, 32 for Asian women, and 41 for non-Latina Whites (U.S. Bureau of the Census, 1996). This is consistent with the median age for women in Mexico, 25 years (Secretaría de Gobernación, 1996). In California, the majority of Latinas (82 percent) are younger than 44 years of age, with a large concentration in the 0- to 19-year-old group (42 percent), versus 40 percent among the 20- to 44-year-old group, and 18 percent of those 45 years of age or older.

Labor Force Participation. Although many Latinas participate in the labor force in large numbers and enter the labor force at an early age (Hayes-Bautista, Baezconde-Garbanati, and Hayes-Bautista, 1994; Hayes-Bautista, Baezconde-Garbanati, Schink, and Hayes-Bautista, 1994), the nature of the jobs they occupy prevents them from having adequate access to health insurance and other benefits that would decrease their risk for disease. Regardless, labor force participation among Latinas does ensure a certain level of contribution to the life and economy of California for which investment in this population is needed (Hayes-Bautista, 1990a, 1990b, 1997).

Labor force participation also provides Latinas with several roles and resources, some outside the traditional family resources and roles expected within the culture (Golding and Baezconde-Garbanati, 1990). This, combined with her ability to contribute to the maintenance of the family, may raise self-esteem and provide additional emotional and instrumental resources and support to obtain needed goods, services, and health-related information beneficial to her and her family.

Language Spoken by Latinas. Twenty-seven percent of Latino households in California are monolingual Spanish speaking, compared to 55 percent which speak both Spanish and/or English. The highest percentage of counties with monolingual Latino households are Orange (34 percent), Los Angeles (31 percent), and Ventura (26 percent) (LCHC, 1999—UC Data run, Berkeley Calif.— US Bureau of Census STF 3A, 1996). In addition, there are Latinas who although they may speak English are Spanish preferent, choosing Spanish as the language of choice or preference when listening to radio, television, or other media sources (Durazo Communications, 1998). Spanish language preference is tied to the maintenance of traditional values and norms, some of which provide cultural protection (Marin and VanOss Marin, 1991). For example, traditional norms and values tend to be associated with lower smoking rates (Marin and others, 1989; Marin, Pérez-Stable, and VanOss Marin, 1989).

High Rate of Family Formation. According to Hayes-Bautista, Baezconde-Garbanati, and Hayes-Bautista (1994), Latinas are embedded within households that are more likely to be composed of a nuclear family. The authors reveal that in 1990, 41.3 percent of Latino households were composed of a couple with children, compared to only 21.7 percent among non-Latino Whites and even fewer among African Americans (18.4 percent). Rates, however, were similar to those of Asian households, which had 39.9 percent of families living within a nuclear family arrangement. Hayes-Bautista, Baezconde-Garbanati, and Hayes-Bautista (1994) also revealed that Latinos consistently are the least likely of any group to have a household composed of a person living alone in a nonfamily situation. This points to the high value placed on family among Latinas and Latinos in general. It is also tied to income and enhancement of opportunities for survival and adaptation in the United States. Individuals with lower incomes have better possibilities of economic survival if they live together with other individuals and/or family members. Latinos who welcome newly arrived immigrant relatives into their homes also facilitate the process of adaptation into the United States and provide financial means and shared opportunities for the exchange of goods and services within nuclear and extended families.

The Health Status of Latinas

Leading Causes of Death. Based on Mexico's National Survey of Chronic Disease (Castro, Gomez-Dantés, Negrete-Sánchez, and Tapia-Conyer, 1996), the leading causes of death in Mexico in 1993 were heart disease, diabetes, and cerebrovascular disease. They represent 47 percent of all deaths among persons 65 years of age or older. In 1993, the California Department of Health Services, Death Records (Hayes-Bautista, 1997), showed that for Latinos in California, the leading causes of death were heart disease, malignant neoplasm, and unintentional injuries. Hayes-Bautista (1997) reports that the Latino crude death rate is much lower than the state's overall rate. He attributes this to the fact that the Latino population in California is much younger than the state's overall population. For this reason, it is important to "age adjust" to make appropriate data comparisons.

Life Expectancy. When one looks at life expectancy, Latinas in California have similar life expectancy to Asian women (84 years) and better than non-Latino White (79) and African American women (74) (California Department of Health Services, Planning and Data Analyses Section, 1994), and much better than that of women in Mexico (76 years) (Secretaría de Gobernación, 1996). Hayes-Bautista (1997) states that paradoxically, although Latinos have the least access to care, they exhibit longer life expectancy. However, Hayes-Bautista (1997) recognizes that the question of illnesses presents a different portrait. This suggests that longer life expectancy does not necessarily imply a better quality of life and one free of disease. An examination of areas in need of improvement for Latina health is critical so as not to mask the illness realities that do exist for this population. These data are not meant to be exhaustive and do not cover all the important factors that contribute to overall disease or wellness among Latinas. What follows is an analysis of selected diseases for which health disparities exist and that call for policy and advocacy action.

Disease-Specific Health Profile

Breast Cancer. Despite the fact that the Latina age-adjusted mortality rate for all cancers is lowest among ethnic/racial groups and despite Latinas having one of the lowest breast cancer incidence rates of all groups, they are overrepresented in terms of breast cancer mortality. This indicates that Latinas are more susceptible to death if they contract this disease. Latinas are the only group that the California Department of Health Services, Office of Women's Health (1997) found to have a higher age-adjusted death rate for breast versus lung cancer, making breast cancer the top killer among Latinas of all cancer-related diseases. The death rate in 1994 for Latinas with breast cancer was 11.8 per 100,000 versus 7.3 for lung cancer. This is due in part to lower use of early detection and follow-up to abnormal findings (Baezconde-Garbanati, Kerner, Richardson, and Cantero, 1995), delayed diagnosis, and coming in to care with late-stage disease (American Cancer Society, 1989; LCHC, 1999; McWhorter and Mayer, 1987). Late-stage disease and within-stage mortality have been attributed to poverty, fatalism, failure to receive timely diagnosis and treatment, treatment availability, acceptability of services, and/or quality of treatment and services (American Cancer Society, 1989; McWhorter, and Mayer, 1987).

Cervical Cancer. Cervical cancer is one of the cancers for which screening and early detection are most available. Latinas in all age groups have both higher incidence and mortality than their non-Latino White counterparts and, in some cases, double that of other ethnic/racial groups. For example, the LCHC (1999) reports that among women in the 45- to 64-year-old group, Latina incidence rates are 17.6 compared to 11.3 for African American and 7 for non-Latino Whites. Among the 65 and older group, these incidence rates increase dramatically, with Latinas reaching a high incidence of 21.2 compared to 6.7 among non-Latino White women and 16.8 among African American women. Mortality rates for cervical cancer are sometimes more than double those for non-Latino White women. In the 45- to 64-year-old group, the Latina mortality rate is 4.4 versus 2.2 for non-Latino White women. In the 65 and older group, mortality is 7.7 for Latinas versus 3.4 for non-Latina Whites. Younger Latinas in the 21- to 44-year-old group have a lower cervical cancer mortality than do their non-Latino White and African American counterpart.

Heart Disease. Heart disease is the leading cause of death among women in the United States. More than 500,000 women in the United States die each year, and another 2.5 million are hospitalized due to complications of heart disease (Winkleby, Kraemer, Ahn, and Varady, 1998). Although mortality is lower for Latinas when compared to other population groups, heart disease is still responsible for the second highest age-adjusted death rate (California Department of Health Services, Office of Women's Health, 1997). The problem is especially noticeable in various geographical regions of the state and for women in their middle years, among whom mortality may surpass that of other ethnic/racial groups.

In some counties in California, the heart disease mortality rate for women in the 45- to 64-year-old group is higher for Latinas than their non-Latino White counterparts (LCHC, 1999). Heart disease rates are higher for Latinas in counties such as Santa Clara (6.4 for Latinas versus 5.7 for non-Latino Whites) and Ventura (7.0 for Latinas versus 5.2 for non-Latino Whites).

However, if Latinas, especially those in more rural communities and with a high cardiac risk profile, survive the middle years, those older than age 65 have a better cardiac mortality profile, compared to other ethnic groups (LCHC, 1999). The mortality rate of 104 for Latinas is significantly lower compared to 170 for non-Latino White women and 203 for African American women. Nevertheless, some Latinas are still disadvantaged in the 65 and older group for selected rural communities, such as San Bernardino, Fresno, and Kern counties, where mortality rates for Latinas ranked at 114, 106, and 117 per 10,000, respectively (LCHC, 1999). In part, this can be explained by the lack of access to adequate and timely care for Latinas in these areas, because mortality rates for Latinas in this age group are lower in wealthier and more urban counties.

These data are more ominous when considering cardiac risk profile, which shows that Latinas are actually at higher risk than non-Latino White women (Winkleby, Kraemer, Ahn, and Varady, 1998). Winkleby, Kraemer, Ahn, and Varady (1998) found that Mexican American women had significantly higher rates of systolic blood pressure and diabetes than their non-Latino White counterparts in the same age group with similar levels of education. Other data from the CORE Program using the Behavioral Risk Factor Survey Sample (1994–1996) (Gazzaniga and others, 1998) revealed that the rate of hypertension or high blood pressure among California's Latinas (25 percent) was similar to that of non-Latina Whites (23.7 percent), although much lower than that of African American women (35 percent) and higher than for other women (21.5 percent). The prevalence of high blood pressure for Latino females varied by county in 1996. For example, Latinas in Riverside and in the Central Valley had substantially higher prevalence of high blood pressure (35 percent and 29.9 percent, respectively) than Latinas in Los Angeles and San Diego (25.1 percent and 21.6 percent, respectively) (Gazzaniga and others, 1998). This prevalence among Latinas in California (25 percent) is substantially lower than the prevalence of hypertension found in 1993 among women in Mexico who participated in the National Survey of Chronic Disease (Castro, Gomez-Dantés, Negrete-Sánchez, and Tapia-Conyer, 1996). Prevalence of hypertension among women in Mexico at the time was estimated at 38 percent (Castro, Gomez-Dantés, Negrete-Sánchez, and Tapia-Conyer, 1996). According to the LCHC (1999), women in Riverside, however, had a prevalence (35 percent) much more similar to that of women in Mexico (38 percent) than to Latinas in the more urban communities (Los Angeles, San Diego) mentioned previously.

Diabetes. Without question, diabetes morbidity and mortality for Latinas ranks the highest compared to their non-Latino White counterparts or individuals in Mexico. Data from Mexico's 1993 National Survey of Chronic Diseases (Castro, Gomez-Dantés, Negrete-Sánchez, and Tapia-Conyer, 1996) show a diabetes prevalence of 21 percent. In the United States, the U.S. Department of Health and Human Services (1997) reported that the prevalence of diabetes for the total population had increased. Increases were recorded from 28 per 1,000 in 1986 to 30 cases per 1,000 in 1994. However, the increase among Mexican Americans nationwide was much higher. Between 1986 and 1994, there was a seventeen-point increase in prevalence estimates (from 54 to 66 per 1,000 cases) among individuals of Mexican origin.

Little progress has been made in eliminating diabetes disparities in California among Latinas and other populations. Based on the California Behavioral Risk Factor Survey (Gazzaniga and others, 1998), the prevalence of diabetes among California's adults is significantly higher among Latinos when compared to non-Latino Whites. Diabetes data for Latinas by region in 1996 showed substantially higher prevalence (LCHC, 1999), especially in the Central Valley and Riverside, when compared to non-Latino White women (16.5 for Latinas versus 4.3 for non-Latino Whites in Riverside and 17.9 for Latinas versus 4.9 for non-Latino Whites in the Central Valley). Mortality rates from diabetes for Latinas are more than double those for non-Latino Whites and almost double those of the total female population in California. Rates for Latinas are 14.6 versus 7.3 for non-Latino White women and 8.9 for the total female population in California.

Again, in this disease, there is a trend for more rural communities to show higher rates of diabetes for women in the 45- to 64-year-old group than for urban areas. Higher rates of diabetes were found in San Bernardino, Fresno, and Kern counties (4.5, 5.2, and 7.6, respectively), compared to the rates of 2.3 in Los Angeles, 2.3 in Orange, and 1.0 in San Diego (Gazzaniga and others, 1998). This pattern of higher rates of diabetes in more rural communities was again evident in Latinas 65 years of age or older, for which rates in some counties were higher than both non-Latino Whites and African Americans and almost double for other Latino women in more urban communities. The female diabetes mortality rates for Latinas 65 and older in San Bernardino County were 22.5, 26.2 in Fresno, and 23.4 in Ventura, compared to 13.1 in Los Angeles, 12.4 in Orange, and 14.5 in San Diego (LCHC, 1999).

AIDS. Although the number of AIDS cases overall among Latinas is lower than for non-Latino White women in California, the number of AIDS cases is comparable to those of African American women. AIDS cases among Latinas, however, are increasing, despite availability of better drug therapy combinations and perhaps because they have less access to care. Some counties, such as Los Angeles, Fresno, and Ventura, have the highest cumulative number of AIDS cases among Latinas, and in Fresno and Ventura, this number of cases is higher than that for non-Latino Whites (LCHC, 1999).

In Los Angeles, a total of 6,536 cases of AIDS were diagnosed and reported to the Department of Health Services by September 1998 (Los Angeles County Department of Health Services, 1999a). Of these, 2,562 were among women.

This represents 13 percent of all cases in Los Angeles County. This is similar to the 13.6 percent of AIDS cases reported among women in Mexico in 1994 (Secretaría de Gobernación, 1996). However, when one looks at Latinas specifically, in Los Angeles, they have the highest percentage of cases (40 percent) compared to African Americans (37 percent), Whites (21 percent), and Asians (2 percent) (Los Angeles County Department of Health Services, 1999a).

The main mode of exposure for Latinas in California is heterosexual contact (46 percent), followed by intravenous drug use (23 percent). In contrast, in Mexico, among adult women, the main reported mode of HIV transmission is blood transfusions (56.5 percent) (Secretaría de Gobernación, 1996). With better measures in place currently for the checking of blood supply, it is possible that higher reports of exposure by blood transfusions may be tied to social stigma regarding exposure to HIV infection within more traditional populations.

Factors That Place Latinas at Risk

Considering the above illnesses for which advocacy action is needed, this section examines those factors that contribute to Latina risk.

Poverty. Latina poverty has been associated with increased risk for illnesses, but this increased risk is closely tied to lack of health care access. Poor persons generally are less able to afford the cost of insurance, whether or not premiums are subsidized (Weissman and Epstein, 1994). This link between poverty and lack of insurance occurs despite Medicaid access, a program designed to insure individuals who are poor (Weissman and Epstein, 1994). The poor are also less able to afford food purchases and have less access to health information.

The proportion of Latinas earning $14,000 or less annually for a family of four in California is slightly higher than for African American females (23 percent versus 22 percent, respectively). In addition, it is nearly three times higher than the proportion of non-Latino White females living below poverty (8 percent) and substantially higher than the 13 percent total of all females in California living below poverty (California Department of Finance, 1997). One out of every three Latinas in California living below the poverty line is 25 to 44 years of age. But the problem is worst among Latinas younger than age 17. Nearly half of all Latinas living below poverty are younger than age 17 (42.5 percent). Twenty-eight percent of young Latina girls younger than age 5 live in poverty, compared to 10 percent of non-Latino White and 34 percent of African Americans. Another 27 percent are below poverty among the 6- to 17-year-old group, compared to 29 percent among African Americans and 9 percent of non-Latino White girls. The Department of Finance 1996 data indicate that in California, the younger a Latina or African American female is, the more likely she will be living in poverty (LCHC, 1999).

Elevated High School Dropout Rates. Nearly one out of every four students in California is Limited English Proficient (LEP), with a large percentage being Spanish speaking (19.2 percent) (California Department of Education, 1995). The same data show that nearly half of all students (49 percent) enrolled in California's public high schools in grades 9 through 12 are female, and 45 percent of all dropouts in grades 9 through 12 are also female.

Dropout rates for all female groups in California have been slowly declining (LCHC, 1999). Nonetheless, Latinas are also overrepresented in the proportion of females per 1,000 students who drop out of high school, when compared to the proportion of females who actually enroll in public high schools in California. Although Latinas constitute 17 percent of female enrollment in California's public high school system, they constitute 23 percent of dropouts (California Department of Education, 1995).

Special data runs from the California Department of Education, CBEDS, Educational Demographics Unit (1995) showed that from 1995 to 1996, selected counties with the highest Latina dropout rate per 1,000 students in grades 9 through 12 were Santa Clara, Kern, Los Angeles, and Fresno, with 25.5, 24.5, 22.4, and 20.1 percent, respectively.

High dropout rates from school among Latinas imply less access to health-related information; less monitoring by school authorities of Latina engagement in alcohol, drug, or tobacco use; and potentially less access to information regarding measures to protect them from HIV, other sexually transmitted diseases, and pregnancy. Out-of-school girls are also more prone to be the victims of violence and crime. To properly evaluate the educational situation of Latinas in California, their educational attainment needs to be seen in the context of educational attainment in Mexico (Hayes-Bautista, 1990b). Although there have been great advances in the Mexican educational system, high levels of illiteracy persist. Illiteracy is especially prevalent among women in Mexico older than age 15 (15.2 percent) compared to men (9.8 percent) (Secretaría de Gobernación, 1996). Mexico's educational data reveal that about two out of every three adults who cannot read or write are women. The situation is worse among older women and those in the poorer areas of Mexico, where female illiteracy reaches 30 percent, compared to 20 percent among men. Among indigenous populations in Mexico, more than half of indigenous women 15 years of age or older cannot read or write. With immigration, especially among younger segments, education becomes open to more individuals, providing opportunities for social and economic progress and mobility.

Lack of Health Insurance. The overall proportion of uninsured Americans in California has remained relatively stable (19 percent in 1989, 20 percent in 1996) (Carrasquillo, Himmelstein, Woolhandler, and Bor, 1999). However, when one examines data for Latinos nationally, the picture is mixed. For example, among Cuban Americans nationwide, those with health insurance coverage increased, from 22 percent in 1989 to approximately 27.4 percent in 1994. Among Puerto Ricans younger than age 65, insurance coverage decreased from 22 percent in 1989 to 17.4 in 1994. Among Mexican Americans across the country, there was a two percentage point decrease, from 39 percent in 1989 to 37.2 percent in 1994. Compared to the total population, in 1994, the proportion of Latinos younger than age 65 without health insurance (32.9 percent) was almost double that of the total population (17.8 percent) (U.S. Department of Health and Human Services, 1997). In California Wyn, Leslie, Glick, and Solis (1997) reported that 2.1 million of California's women between the ages of 18 and 64 were uninsured. According to Brown, Pourat, Wyn, and Solis (1997), more than 33 percent of Latinas (1.2 million) are uninsured compared to 14 percent of non-Latino Whites, 19 percent of African Americans, and 21 percent of Asian women.

In another study, de la Torre, Friis, Hunter, and Garcia (1996) reported that health insurance coverage was greater among those who reported a family income above the poverty level. These authors also reported that more recently arrived Mexican immigrants used health care services less than those who had been in the United States for a longer period of time. They associated recency of immigration with insurance status. The Center for Health Policy Research (Brown, Pourat, Wyn, and Solis, 1997) revealed that although only 42 percent of Latinas have private insurance, a majority of African American and non-Latino White females (54 percent and 76 percent respectively) are privately insured. Among Latinas, Central and South American women were more likely to be uninsured. In 1994, nearly half of Central and South American females in California were uninsured, compared to one out of every three Mexican American females.

Other data from the Center for Health Policy Research (Brown, Wallace, Pourat, and Yu, 1998) revealed that of the 11.74 million uninsured children in California, 400,000 were eligible for a new Healthy Families program and another 668,000 are eligible for MediCal. However, many are not accessing the system because they are afraid of compromising the processing of citizenship or other immigration documentation. It is not surprising then to find data from the UCLA Center for Health Policy Research (Brown, Pourat, Wyn, and Solis, 1997) that reveal that approximately one out of every three Latinas younger than age 17 is uninsured. Thirty-seven percent of all Latinas ages 45 to 64 are uninsured. The situation worsens if Latinas are unemployed. These data also revealed that in 1994, nearly two-thirds of unemployed Latinas in California lacked insurance coverage.

Lack of health insurance is one of the leading risk factors for poor health among Latinas. Lack of health insurance is linked to failure in obtaining life-saving and timely screening services for women. Many women younger than age 65 lack health insurance coverage. Latinas, even though they may work, tend to be either uninsured or underinsured. In part, this is due to the nature of the jobs they occupy and the percentage of time they work in these jobs.

The Nature of Latino Women's Jobs. Weissman and Epstein (1994) showed that the percentage of uninsured varied by occupation, with 41 percent of those working in agriculture being uninsured, versus 31 percent of those in construction, 25 percent of those in retail, 22 percent of the self-employed, and 17 percent of individuals involved in service jobs. Although Latinas are increasingly gaining high-level positions, Latinas in California comprise the largest percentage of females in agricultural (51 percent) and manufacturing (61 percent) industries. However, only 10 percent of Latinas are in managerial positions, whereas 74 percent of female managers are non-Latino Whites. Latinas are also underrepresented in the sales industries, in contrast to their non-Latino White counterparts (17 percent and 65 percent, respectively). Latinas are disproportionately represented in the service industry when compared to non-Latino White females (87 and 6 per 1,000, respectively). Latinas who work as housekeepers and nannies, taking care of children in people's homes, cleaning houses, and caring for the elderly, often work in jobs without proper health benefits or security.

Unemployment. In 1995, the unemployment rate for Latinas was significantly higher than for non-Latino White women (11.7 versus 7.3, respectively) and higher than the unemployment rate for all females (7.9 per 1,000). The nature of women's jobs and high unemployment rates for Latinas in California are other contributing factors to Latinas' being uninsured or underinsured, which place them at higher risk for disease and mortality from these illnesses.

Overweight. Obesity is one of the leading causes of hospitalization and death among women due to its link with heart disease, stroke, cancer, and diabetes (California Department of Health Services, 1997). Data from California's Behavioral Risk Factor Survey revealed that the percentage of overweight adults in California increased from 17.9 percent in 1984 to 23.1 percent in 1992. Behavioral Risk Factor Survey (BRFS) data (Gazzaniga and others, 1998) show that both male and female Latinos tend to have a higher prevalence of overweight and obesity when compared to other groups. For Latinas in particular, the prevalence of overweight is higher (42.7) than for African Americans (40.2), non-Latino Whites (24.2), and Asian/other women (16.3). This prevalence of overweight among California's Latinas is also higher than the prevalence found in Mexico in 1993. The National Survey of Chronic Diseases found among women living in Mexico a 25 percent prevalence in overweight (Castro, Gomez-Dantés, Negrete-Sánchez, and Tapia-Conyer, 1996), although due to more liberal criteria for obesity in Mexico, numerical comparisons are problematic.

Other data (U.S. Department of Health and Human Services, 1997) have also revealed an increase nationally in the prevalence of overweight among Latinas 20 years of age or older. The Healthy People 2000 objectives target was 25 percent overweight; however, in 1993, Latinas' overweight prevalence had increased to 33 percent from 27 percent in 1985. This indicates that in this risk factor for many diseases, including high blood pressure and diabetes, Latinas are actually increasing rather than decreasing in weight, in contradiction to the goal.

Physical Inactivity. The Centers for Disease Control and California's "On the Move Physical Activities Programs" have defined physical inactivity as exercising less than 20 minutes at a time, less than three times a week (Cassidy, Jang, Tanjasiri, and Morrison, 1999). Being physically inactive or having a sedentary lifestyle has been linked to an increased risk of many chronic diseases and is particularly prevalent in minority communities (Cassidy, Jang, Tanjasiri, and Morrison, 1999). More than 250,000 deaths (approximately 12 percent of the total) each year are attributable to physical inactivity, making it the second leading cause of death after cigarette smoking (McGinnis and Foege, 1993; Powell and Blair, 1994). California's Latinos have the highest proportion of physical inactivity of any group (Gazzaniga and others, 1998). Latinas' physical inactivity inversely varies with income, with those in the higher income brackets engaging in more physical activity than those with lower incomes. Prevalence of physical inactivity among Latinas in California varies by region and is higher than for non-Latino Whites. Rates for Los Angeles County are 69.6, 64.8 for Riverside, 63.2 for Orange, and 73.7 for San Diego. In contrast, prevalence of physical inactivity among non-Latino White women is consistently lower in those same counties: Los Angeles, 52.1; Riverside, 50.4; Orange, 44.3; and San Diego, 46.3 (LCHC, 1999).

Latinas experience a series of barriers that influence their physical activity. According to Grassi, Gonzalez, Tello, and He (1999), 202 Latinas in the San Joaquin Valley of Central California reported that (1) not having a nearby location to exercise, (2) living in unsafe neighborhoods, (3) lacking transportation, (4) unaffordability of programs, (5) not knowing where to go, (6) not knowing how to start a physical activity program, (7) family responsibilities, and (8) work schedules prevented them from engaging in physical activities programs. Although all women may experience difficulties in maintaining a regular exercise regime, these data suggest that for Hispanic women, external factors (such as unsafe neighborhoods and affordability), lack of knowledge (of where to go and how to start, for example), and familial obligations are often strong barriers to participation.

Lack of Knowledge Regarding Preventative Measures. As mentioned previously, lack of knowledge regarding where to go and how to start a physical activity program prevented Latinas from participating in these life-enhancing and disease-preventing measures. Another example of this relates to a lack of knowledge among Latinas regarding the benefits of the presence of folic acid in the diet prior to and during pregnancy. A lack of folate or folic acid has been associated with neural tube defects, such as spina bifida and anencephaly, in more than 500 pregnancies each year in California (California Department of Health Services, Office of Women's Health, 1997). A consumption of 400 micrograms per day of folic acid in the diet meets 100 percent of daily value requirements.

Latinas have the highest incidence of neural tube defects of all ethnic/racial groups in California. In 1997, 4,010 women of various ethnicities were randomly selected to participate in the California Women's Health Survey (California Department of Health Services, 1998). Data reveal that only 29 percent of Latinas surveyed had ever heard or read anything about folate or folic acid, compared to 69 percent of non-Latino Whites, 48 percent of African Americans, and 54 percent of Asian/other women. Low consumption of folic acid–related foods or supplements is pervasive for all age groups of Latinas, especially those of childbearing age. With such a large group of women of childbearing age, areas such as this, for which culturally and linguistically appropriate interventions are of relative low cost, call for particular attention from researchers and women's health advocacy groups. The anticipated gains in savings of health care services are much greater than the potential costs incurred for educational interventions.

Low Prevalence of Early Prenatal Care. Concerns with folic acid, for example, can readily be alleviated among Latinas, especially if they come in early for prenatal care and through proper education programs before pregnancy. However, Latinas in California have one of the lowest percentages of women receiving early prenatal care (within the first trimester of pregnancy) that permits early identification of risks and allows for proper interventions to take place (California Department of Health Services, Office of Women's Health, 1997). Data from the Office of Women's Health (California Department of Health Services, 1997) show that Latinas had a rate of early prenatal care of 70.5 compared to African American women with a rate of 74.6, non-Latino Whites with a rate of 85.2, and Asian women with a rate of 81.9. When one looks at the rates of prenatal care by Latina subgroup, data reveal that Cuban women have rates equal to or better than those of non-Latino White women (88.1). Mexican women have one of the lowest rates of early prenatal care of all groups (69.6) compared only to the low rates found among Laotian women (65.3) and Samoan females (51.5), who lead women in California with the lowest rate of early prenatal care. For Mexican-origin women in California, this percentage (69.6) is much lower than the rate of prenatal care of women in Mexico, which in 1994 was reported as 85.3 percent (Secretaría de Gobernación, 1996).

The LCHC (1999) reports that only 68 percent of Latino women in California received first trimester care versus their non-Latino White (85 percent), African

American (73 percent), and Asian (79 percent) counterparts. Interestingly enough, despite low participation in early prenatal care, Latinas, and especially women of Mexican origin, still have excellent birth outcomes (Hayes-Bautista, 1997) in terms of low birth weight babies, high vaginal deliveries, and a low number of cesarean sections. This is consistent with the low prevalence of early prenatal care found in Mexico (Secretaría de Gobernación, 1996).

Low Levels of Participation in Screening Tests. Failure to receive a mammogram for breast cancer screening or a Pap test for cervical cancer screening can cause delayed detection of life-threatening illnesses. Data from the National Health Interview Survey (U.S. Department of Health and Human Services, 1997) indicate that although both statewide and nationally there has been an effort to provide screening services for breast cancer to all population groups, Latinas are still 10 percent away from the set targets of Healthy People 2000. Nationally in 1994, 50 percent of Latinas 50 years of age or older had received a clinical breast exam and a mammogram; this is 10 percent less than the expected Year 2000 target of 60 percent.

In addition, Latinas have the second highest prevalence of women in California between 1989 and 1994 who report never having had a Pap screening exam: 14.1 percent for Latinas versus approximately 4 percent for non-Latino Whites and African Americans, and 20.9 percent for Asian women (LCHC, 1999). This percentage among Latinas is two to three times higher than among non-Latino Whites or African Americans. This percentage is consistent with data from Mexico, which show that less than 25 percent of women between the ages of 15 and 49 in 1994 had received a Pap test. In rural areas of Mexico, only 17 percent of these women had received a screening test for cervical cancer (Secretaría de Gobernación, 1996).

Further research is needed to understand the conditions that prevent Latinas from coming in to early screening, especially in terms of cervical cancer. Cultural and religious factors are often used to explain this screening failure, but each Latina who gets cervical cancer represents a failure of the medical system to have reached these women in a timely fashion (Rodriguez-Trias, 1999).

Acculturation. Some studies on the effects of acculturation on Latina health have shown that for some indicators, such as smoking, alcohol abuse, depression, and infant mortality, immigrant Latinas fair better than their U.S.-born counterparts and better than African Americans and non-Hispanic Whites (Baezconde-Garbanati, 1994; Hayes-Bautista, 1997; Marin, Pérez-Stable, and VanOss Marin, 1989; Vega and others, 1998). In contrast, when one compares other indicators, the more educated and acculturated Latinas have a better health profile. If one compares with data from Mexico, for some health indicators, such as diabetes and hypertension, Latinas in California fare better than their Mexican counterparts. In others, such as obesity, they fare significantly worse (Castro, Gomez-Dantés, Negrete-Sánchez, and Tapia-Conyer, 1996). In a 1993 national survey of chronic conditions (Encuesta Nacional de Enfermedades Crónicas) using a sample of 1,239 60- to 69-year-olds in Mexico, Castro, Gomez-Dantés, Negrete-Sánchez, and Tapia-Conyer (1996) found a prevalence of 38 percent for hypertension, 25 percent for obesity (measured as a body mass index of 30.0 to 34.9 as obese and of 35 or more as very obese), and 21 percent for diabetes. When one compares these data to data on Latinas in California presented previously, prevalence of hypertension in the United States is lower (25 percent) than in Mexico (38 percent). Diabetes prevalence is also lower among Latinas in the United States (approximately 17 percent versus 21 percent among women in Mexico), but prevalence of obesity among Latinas in California is significantly higher (42.7 percent) than that of women in Mexico (25 percent).

With respect to psychiatric disorders, Mexican immigrants in rural and urban settings have one-half the total DSM-IIIR psychiatric disorders when compared to their more acculturated, U.S.-born counterpart (Vega and others, 1998). The pattern is again repeated among Mexican immigrant women in Los Angeles who have lower infant mortality and a low rate of low birth weight babies when compared to more acculturated Mexican, Puerto Rican, non-Hispanic White, and African American women (Hayes-Bautista, 1997; Zambrana, 1990; Zambrana, Dunkel-Schetter, and Scrimshaw, 1991). Latinas also tend to smoke and drink less than non-Hispanic Whites, with immigrants faring better than their more acculturated counterpart (Gilbert and Cervantes, 1986). They also tend to use drugs less than U.S.-born Mexican Americans, Blacks, and non-Hispanic White women (Zambrana, Dunkel-Schetter, and Scrimshaw, 1991).

The effects of acculturation on health and mental health appear to be mixed, in part, because of a possible interaction of acculturation with age. Cantero, Richardson, Baezconde-Garbanati, and Marks (forthcoming) studied the preventative behaviors of Latinas in various age groups in relation to acculturation. Study findings revealed that middle-age Latinas (45 to 64 years of age) had higher health risks associated with acculturation than Latinas 65 years of age or older. The authors also found that more acculturated middle-age Latinas engaged in less preventative health behaviors than their immigrant or older counterparts. However, acculturation did not affect the health practices of elderly Latinas (age 75 and older).

How Latinas can look healthy with respect to other ethnic groups but their actual condition be masked by immigration status, state of residence, and acculturation is more easily seen with respect to smoking rates among Latinos in California, the United States in general, and Latin America. If conclusions about Latina smoking rates were based only on comparisons among ethnic groups in California, the comparisons would indicate that Latinas are at the lowest risk for smoking. However, California has one of the lowest smoking prevalence rates of any state, especially among Latinas (Baezconde-Garbanati and others, forthcoming). Within California, Latinas overall have the lowest smoking prevalence (11.1 percent) when compared to other racial/ethnic groups, such as African American women (26. percent) and non-Latino White females (19.2 percent). This comparison is true for all age groups (Pierce and others, 1998). Although rates for Latinas vary within California, with the highest rates found in the Northern Bay Area (19.1 percent) and San Diego (16.3 percent) (Gazzaniga and others, 1998), the overall rate of 11.1 percent for California is consistent with smoking rates among women in Latin America reported in 1987. For example, smoking rates in 1987 in Costa Rica were 11 percent for women, 12 percent in El Salvador, and 11 percent in Honduras. Slightly higher rates are reported for other Latin American countries, with an 18 percent prevalence reported among women in Guatemala, 20 percent in Nicaragua, and 18 percent in Mexico (Pan American Health Organization, 1992). Although California's Latinas have lower rates than some Latin American countries, conclusions would be premature until national rates of Latino smoking were considered. For example, smoking rates nationwide were 17.4 percent for women of Mexican origin, 20.4 percent for women of Cuban origin, and 24.0 percent for women of Puerto Rican origin (Hispanic Health and Nutrition Examination Survey in Kaiser Permanente National Diversity Council, 1996; Pan American Health Organization, 1992). Thus, smoking rates for Latinos in the United States are often higher than in many Latin American countries. The low rates of smoking in California would be expected because California has one of the strongest anti-smoking programs in the world. Furthermore, the lower rates for smoking for Latina immigrants appear to be further eroded when considering the effects of acculturation.

Several authors have studied the role of acculturation on the attitudes, norms, and expectancies of Hispanic smokers (Marin and others, 1989) and on the role of acculturation and gender on the prevalence of smoking among Hispanics in San Francisco (Marin, Pérez-Stable, and VanOss Marin, 1989). These authors found that the more acculturated Hispanic men and women were, the more they tended to smoke. Thus, the longer Latinas are here in the United States, the more at risk they are for smoking-related diseases. In fact, the age-adjusted overall smoking prevalence among Hispanics 15 to 64 years of age in a 1989 sample of Latinos in San Francisco was 25.4 percent, with more men (32.4 percent) smoking than women (16.8 percent). These rates are higher than the overall smoking rates found for Latinas in California (Pierce and others, 1998) and reflect possible cohort differences and/or the rates prior to the California antismoking campaign. These 1989 California smoking rates are higher compared to the 1987 rates in some Latin American countries discussed above.

These results need to be qualified: although smoking prevalence rates in the Marin, Pérez-Stable, and VanOss Marin (1989) San Francisco study were higher among the more acculturated females (22.6 percent) versus the less acculturated females (13.6 percent), the opposite was true for males. Smoking rates were higher among the less acculturated males (37.5 percent) versus the more acculturated males (26.7 percent). Nonetheless, the more acculturated, independent of gender, smoked a greater number of cigarettes per day (Marin, Pérez-Stable, and VanOss Marin 1989).

DISCUSSION

Data presented here are limited to specific health indicators and are not meant to be exhaustive. Other data are available through the Latina Health Policy Project at the LCHC (1999). Data reviewed revealed inconsistencies in the literature and among data sets. Explanations for these inconsistencies may be found in differing sampling schemes, in variations in the conceptualization and operationalization of variables, in instrumentation complexities and statistical analyses, and lack of consideration of Latina heterogeneity. These problems make it more difficult to present a more accurate picture of Latino health. For example, often studies fail to account for Latinas' heterogeneous nature in terms of national origin, level of acculturation, generational status, and age of immigration (Castro and Baezconde-Garbanati, 1987). Comparing data sets with different measurements and varying degrees of statistical control limits the generalizability and reliability of the findings. More weight is given to results that were consistent among data sets, except where critique of design oversights is warranted, given the current state of knowledge.

In some areas, such as in diabetes and cervical cancer, the picture is clear, with Latinas having worse health outcomes than their non-Latina White counterpart. In others, such as in cardiac risk, Latinas, although they have a worse cardiac risk profile in their middle years (ages 45 to 64), if they survive, they actually have a lower mortality from heart disease than their African American and non-Latina White counterpart. Although women in this age group are in the workforce, due to the nature of the jobs they occupy, many lack health insurance. This is especially noticeable among the 45- to 64-year-old group and among rural women. Possibilities of survival tied to high cardiac risk will be strongly influenced by Latina access to health insurance, preventative lifesaving screening services, and participation in health-enhancing disease prevention programs.

This review showed that women in Mexico actually have a higher prevalence of hypertension and diabetes than Latinas in California. However, their prevalence of obesity, an important risk factor for hypertension, diabetes, and other illnesses, is substantially lower than that of California's Latinas. Although women in Mexico may appear to be less obese, these data must be interpreted with caution, due to varying standards in body mass index in the different countries.

Data examined by the coalition also revealed a high percentage of Latinas living in poverty, with elevated high school dropout rates as well as lack of health insurance and unemployment. Interestingly, the negative health outcomes of exposure to these risk-producing situations are not always present. Evidence of positive outcomes is found in less infant mortality, longer life expectancy, and lower mortality from cardiovascular disease and cancer, especially in particular age groups. Demographic and cultural protective factors may help in part explain these findings. Some factors that are currently protective, such as Latina youthfulness, could signal increased health-related problems as Latinas age.

Positive outcomes in some conditions must not mask the realities in terms of risks that can potentially jeopardize Latina health if appropriate interventions are not taken, especially among rural women and those in their middle years (ages 45 to 64). Areas in need of intervention include, but are not limited to, being overweight; physical inactivity; and the provision of health education, intervention programs, and culturally based research on those factors that affect diabetes, cardiovascular disease, access to health services, and early detection for breast and cervical cancer. In addition, better access to lifesaving and quality-of-life-enhancing new AIDS combination therapies should be made available to Latinas; education programs that focus on HIV infection prevention among adolescents are critical as well as other interventions and research that seek to understand and reduce ethnic disparities in health status.

The situation among rural Latinas requires special attention, as well as the situation among Latinas in the 45- to 64-year-old group (LCHC, 1999). Lack of health insurance is significantly higher in these two groups, which present a higher risk profile than other Latino women. It seems that Latinas are in greater jeopardy in their middle years on some selected disease categories. This is due to the presence of various risk factors, some of which are closely tied to each other (obesity and lack of exercise).

Although life expectancy is better for Latinas in California when compared to women in Mexico and to non-Latina Whites and African Americans, Latinas in their middle years may not be living as healthful lives as one would expect, especially those who are more acculturated. Life expectancy data in view of high risk is consistent with the paradoxical scenario for Latinos presented by Hayes-Bautista (1997) and Markides and Coreil's "epidemiologic paradox" (1986) of high risk and overall low mortality found among Latinos in the Southwest. In essence, if Latinas survive the middle years of high risk, the hardy ones may actually live longer than other population groups. Part of this paradox may be due to cohort differences as a function of age or immigration status. Hardier females may immigrate to the United States. Whether age interacts with self-selectivity of hardy females is not clear. However, another cohort difference may be attributable to the interaction of acculturation with age, in that acculturation has a more negative effect on middle-age versus older Latinas (Cantero, Richardson, Baezconde-Garbanati, and Marks, forthcoming).

Negative health outcomes for selected indicators appear to be buffered by the presence of protective factors among Latinas, such that risks may exercise a reduced effect in the presence of some protective factors. For example, although Latinas suffer from unemployment, poverty, and hunger, in contrast they also give birth at younger ages, have better birth outcomes in terms of low birth weight, and have fewer delivery complications. They are also embedded within strong familial networks that help to buffer negative health and mental health outcomes, alleviate the burden of poverty as families live in multigenerational and extended family households, and transmit cultural norms and values, often protective of women within the culture. These intergenerational households and family members are providers of instrumental and financial support for women and also transmit health information. Latina mothers, for example, have been found to be a major source of support among Latinos (Salgado de Snyder and Padilla, 1987). It seems that a combination of factors within the culture and demographic composition of Latinas may help buffer the impact of poverty and poor nutrition on potentially negative health outcomes.

On the other hand, some protective factors may not be enough to buffer the effects of risk. For example, Latinas had a high cardiac risk profile, especially in middle age and among those living in rural communities (Cantero, Richardson, Baezconde-Garbanati, and Marks, forthcoming; LCHC, 1999; Winkleby, Kraemer, Ahn, and Varady, 1998). Their high cardiac risk profile, along with lack of health insurance, may help explain the finding that during middle age (ages 45 to 64), Latinas are not significantly different from non-Latina Whites (8.2 versus 8.8) in terms of mortality from heart disease. At older ages (65 and older), however, even though mortality rates are higher for all women, Latinas actually have a significantly lower mortality rate (104) than non-Latina Whites (170). Health insurance coverage in middle age and in rural communities is worse for Latinas than when they are 65 years of age and older. The lack of health insurance is probably such a strong predictor for cardiovascular disease that when combined with other predictors (heredity, obesity, and physical inactivity), the negative effects on health cannot be buffered by culturally based or other protective factors. More research is needed to explore these possible explanations, to understand the role of protective factors in Latina health outcomes and their at-risk status for several diseases, and to understand the role of poverty, education, rural versus urban differences, acculturation, and age on health outcomes for Latinas in California.

If Latinas, through appropriate interventions (reducing overweight and obesity, increasing physical activity, increasing involvement in healthy practices, and greater screening for breast and cervical cancer, among others), lower their risk status, they may actually live longer than non-Latina Whites. Life expectancy for Latinas is 84 years versus 79 years for non-Latina Whites. But risk factor reduction for Latinas on cardiovascular disease, diabetes, and other illnesses is no easy task.

Programs need to be targeted in culturally appropriate ways (Zambrana, Dunkel-Schetter, and Scrimshaw, 1991) and developed in a scientifically sound manner and in response to culturally based research on disease risk at different stages of the life cycle. Levels of acculturation, language preference, low literacy, and regional differences within the state need to be taken into account. Special attention needs to be placed on addressing the particular needs of rural women versus women in more urban settings. Research on the exposure to environmental factors that may present barriers to risk reduction and health enhancement programs is also needed. Understanding and changing negative attitudes about exercise, facilitating physical activity interventions in the workplace, reducing barriers in culturally specific ways (conducting "salsa" aerobics versus regular aerobics classes; Whitehorse, Manzano, Baezconde-Garbanati, and Hahn, 1999), and creating safe spaces for these to occur are among the challenges we face.

This is a critical time for Latinas, as the population of women grows to potentially become the largest female population in California's future. Advocacy on the improvement of access to care, on the training of ethnic professionals—bilingual, bicultural, and biliterate—that can serve these communities, and on community-driven, scientifically sound, more in-depth, and culturally appropriate research is imperative. Improving Latina health requires greater involvement from not just the research community but the formation of partnerships with community-based organizations, educational, consumers, and advocacy groups, among others, working in unison for better health outcomes on all indicators for all Latinas in California.

LIMITATIONS OF THE STUDY

An important limitation of this study is that data on California's Latinas are compared to a baseline of non-Hispanic White and other ethnic women, without providing for all health indicators a baseline for women in Latin America, and Mexico in particular. As available, for comparison purposes, data from the Secretaría de Gobernación (1996), the Pan American Health Organization, and Mexico's 1993 National Survey of Chronic Diseases were presented. Some of these data revealed that Latinas in California were in better health than their counterparts in Mexico. The information on obesity is more ambiguous in that more rigorous standards are applied in U.S. studies. Nonetheless, using the same U.S. standards, there is a greater prevalence of obesity in Latinas compared to other ethnic groups. Should additional funding become available, this study should be expanded to include critical baseline information from Mexico for all health indicators presented. Findings may reveal greater gains in health for Latinas with immigration to the United States. Nevertheless, gains in health with immigration may in part be also due to the hardiness of women who immigrate to the United States through a possible self-selection process. The ideal would be the conduct of binational research that focuses on young Latinas in Mexico, follows them prospectively as they immigrate, and follows them longitudinally as they acculturate and age in the United States. This type of study would be critical for establishing trends and understanding how and what changes among Latinas in terms of basic health indicators with immigration, through the acculturation and aging process.

References

American Cancer Society. *Cancer and the Poor: A Report to the Nation.* Atlanta, Ga.: American Cancer Society, 1989.

Baezconde-Garbanati, L. A. "Do Latino Social Nets Work? The Direct and Mediating Effects of Social Resources on Stressful Life Events and Depression Among Mexican, Mexican Americans, and Non-Latino Whites." Unpublished doctoral dissertation, University of California, Los Angeles, 1994.

Baezconde-Garbanati, L. A., Kerner, J., Richardson, J., and Cantero, P. *Breast Cancer Among Latinas.* Los Angeles: COSSMHO and Norris Comprehensive Cancer Center, 1995.

Baezconde-Garbanati, L. A., and others. "Entering a New Era: Strategies of the H/LaTEN for Organizing and Mobilizing Hispanic Communities." In M. L. Frost (ed.), *Successful Tobacco Education and Prevention Programs.* San Francisco: Charles C. Thomas, forthcoming.

Brown, E. R., Pourat, N., Wyn, R., and Solis, B. *38 Percent de los Latinos de Edades 0–64 en California No Tienen Aseguranza.* Los Angeles: University of California, Los Angeles, Center for Health Policy Research, Aug. 1997.

Brown, E. R., Wallace, S., Pourta, N., and Yu, H. *New Estimates Find 400,000 Children Eligible for Healthy Families Program.* Los Angeles: University of California, Los Angeles, Center for Health Policy Research, Oct. 1998.

California Department of Education, Educational Demographic Unit. "Percent Enrollment and Drop Out Rates in California Public High Schools, Grades 9–12, 1994–1995." Sacramento: California Department of Education, 1995. Electronic data tape.

California Department of Finance. Demographics Research Unit. "1989–1996 Projected Population." Sacramento: California Department of Finance, 1993. Electronic data tape.

California Department of Finance. *Interim County Population Projections.* Sacramento: California Department of Finance, Apr. 1997. Electronic data tape.

California Department of Health Services. Office of Women's Health. *A Profile of Women's Health Status in California, 1984–1994.* Sacramento: California Department of Health Services, 1997.

California Department of Health Services. Planning and Data Analysis Section. "Death Files." Sacramento: California Department of Health Services, 1994. Electronic data tape.

California Department of Health Services. Tobacco Control Section. "California Youth Smoking Prevalence by Gender, 1990–1997, California Tobacco Survey and California Youth Tobacco Survey, 1994–1997." Sacramento: California Department of Health Services, 1998.

California Employment Development Department. "Table 12: States, Employment Status of the Civilian Non Institutional Population by Sex, Age, Race, Latino Origin and Marital Status, 1995 Annual Averages. Labor and Occupation by Industry." Sacramento: California Employment Development Department, 1995. Electronic data tape.

Cantero, P., Richardson, J., Baezconde-Garbanati, L. A., and Marks, M. "The Association Between Acculturation and Health Practices Among Middle-Aged and Elderly Latinas." *Journal of Ethnicity and Disease*, forthcoming.

Carrasquillo, O., Himmelstein, D., Woolhandler, S., and Bor, D. "Going Bare: Trends in Health Insurance Coverage. 1989 Through 1996." *American Journal of Public Health*, 1999, *89*(1), 36–42.

Cassidy, D., Jang, V., Tanjasiri, S., and Morrison, C. (1999). "California Gets 'On the Move!'" *Journal of Health Education*, 1999, *30*(2, Suppl.), 6–12.

Castro, F. G., and Baezconde-Garbanati, L. "A Schema for Greater Specificity in Sampling from Latino Populations." Paper presented at the convention of the American Public Health Association, New Orleans, 1987.

Castro, V., Gomez-Dantés, H., Negrete-Sánchez, J., and Tapia-Conyer, R. "Las enfermedades crónicas en las personas de 60–69 anos." *Salud Pública de México*, 1996, *38*, 438–447.

de la Torre, A., Friis, R., Hunter, H. R., and Garcia, L. "The Health Insurance Status of US Latina Women: A Profile from the 1982–1984 Hispanic Health and Nutrition Examination Survey (HHANES)." *American Journal of Public Health*, 1996, *86*(4), 533–537.

Durazo Communications. *Community Assessment Work Book for the Hispanic Latino Tobacco Education Network.* Los Angeles: Durazo Communications, 1998.

Gazzaniga, J. M., and others. *Cardiovascular Disease Risk Factors Among California Adults, 1984–1996.* San Francisco: CORE Program, University of California at San Francisco, Institute for Health and Aging, and California Department of Health Services, Dec. 1998.

Gilbert, M. J., and Cervantes, R. C. "Patterns and Practices of Alcohol Use Among Mexican-Americans: A Comprehensive Review." *Hispanic Journal of Behavioral Sciences*, 1986, *8*, 1–60.

Golding, J., and Baezconde-Garbanati, L. "Ethnicity, Culture and Social Resources." *Journal of Community Psychology*, 1990, *18*(3), 465–486.

Grassi, K., Gonzalez, M. G., Tello, P., and He, G. "La Vida Caminando: A Community Based Physical Activity Program Designed by and for Rural Latino Families." *Journal of Health Education*, 1999, *30*(2, Suppl.), 13–17.

Hayes-Bautista, D. E. "Latino Family Policy: An Explanatory Framework from California." Unpublished manuscript, 1990a.

Hayes-Bautista, D. E. "Latino Health Indicators and the Underclass Model: From Paradox to New Policy Models." Unpublished manuscript, 1990b.

Hayes-Bautista, D. E. *The Health Status of Latinos in California.* Los Angeles: California Endowment and California Health Care Foundation, Center for the Study of Latino Health, 1997 report.

Hayes-Bautista, D. E., Baezconde-Garbanati, L., and Hayes-Bautista, M. "Latino Health in Los Angeles." *Family Practice-An International Journal,* 1994, *11,* 318–324.

Hayes-Bautista, D. E., Baezconde-Garbanati, L. A., Schink, W., and Hayes-Bautista, M. "Latino Health in California, 1985–1990. Implications for Family Practice." *Journal of Family Medicine,* 1994, *26,* 556–562.

Kaiser Permanente National Diversity Council. *A Provider's Handbook on Culturally Competent Care: Latino Population.* Los Angeles: Kaiser Permanente National Diversity Council, 1996.

Latino Coalition for a Healthy California. *Ensuring Health Access for Latinas.* San Francisco: Latino Coalition for a Healthy California, 1999.

Los Angeles County Commission for Women. *Los Angeles County Women's Health Policy Summit.* Los Angeles: Los Angeles County Commission for Women, 1998.

Los Angeles County Department of Health Services. *Distribution of Births by Race/ Ethnicity, 1995.* Los Angeles: Department of Health Services, 1997.

Los Angeles County Department of Health Services. *An Epidemiologic Profile of HIV and AIDS in Los Angeles County.* Los Angeles: Los Angeles County Department of Health Services, 1999a.

Los Angeles County Department of Health Services. "HIV Testing and Sexual Risk Behaviors Among Adults in Los Angeles County." *L.A. Health,* 1999b, *2*(1), 1–7.

Los Angeles County Department of Health Services, HIV Epidemiology Program. *An Epidemiologic Profile of HIV and AIDS in Los Angeles County.* Los Angeles: Los Angeles County Department of Health Services, 1999c.

Marin, G., Pérez-Stable, E., and VanOss Marin, B. "Cigarette Smoking Among San Francisco Hispanics: The Role of Acculturation and Gender." *American Journal of Public Health,* 1989, *79*(2), 196–198.

Marin, G., and VanOss Marin, B. *Research with Hispanic Populations.* Thousand Oaks, Calif.: Sage, 1991.

Marin, G., and others. "The Role of Acculturation on the Attitudes, Norms and Expectancies of Hispanic Smokers." *Journal of Cross Cultural Psychology,* 1989, *20,* 478–493.

Markides, K. S., and Coréil, J. "The Health of Hispanics in the Southwestern United States: An Epidemiologic Paradox." *Public Health Report,* 1986, *101,* 253–265.

McGinnis, J. M., and Foege, W. H. "Actual Causes of Death in The United States." *Journal of the American Medical Association,* 1993, *270,* 2207–2212.

McWhorter, W., and Mayer, W. "Black/White Differences in Type of Initial Breast Cancer Treatment and Implications for Survival." *American Journal of Public Health,* 1987, *77*(12), 1515–1517.

Morrison, C., and others (eds.). "California Is 'On the Move.'" (Special issue). *Journal of Health Education,* 1999, *30*(Suppl. 2).

Pan American Health Organization. *Tobacco or Health? Status in the Americas.* Washington, D.C.: Pan American Health Organization, 1992.

Pierce, J. P., and others. *Tobacco Control in California: Who's Winning the War? An Evaluation of the Tobacco Control Program, 1989–1996.* La Jolla: University of California, San Diego, 1998.

Powell, K., and Blair, S. N. "The Public Health Burdens of Sedentary Living Habits. Theoretical but Realistic Estimates." *Medicine and Science in Sports and Exercise,* 1994, *26,* 851–856.

Rodriguez-Trias, H. "Latina Health Access." Testimony before the California Senate Health Committee for the Latino Coalition for a Healthy California, Sacramento, Jan. 1999.

Salgado de Snyder, N. V., and Padilla, A. M. "Social Support Networks: Their Availability and Effectiveness. In M. Gaviria and J. D. Arana (eds.), *Health and Behavior: Research Agenda for Hispanics.* Chicago: University of Illinois at Chicago, 1987.

Secretaría de Gobernación. *Programa Nacional de la Mujer, 1995–2000. Estados Unidos Mexicanos: Alianza Para la Igualdad, Poder Ejecutivo Federal.* [http://www.sdnp.undp.org/ww/followup/national/mexico.htm]. 1996.

U.S. Bureau of the Census. *Population Projections for States by Age, Sex, Race and Latino Origin 1995–2025.* Hyattsville, Md.: U.S. Bureau of the Census, 1996.

U.S. Department of Health and Human Services, Public Health Service. *Progress Review: Hispanic Americans. Healthy People 2000.* Hyattsville, Md.: U.S. Department of Health and Human Services, Apr. 1997.

Vega, W. A., and others. "Lifetime Prevalence of DSM-III-R Psychiatric Disorders Among Urban and Rural Mexican Americans in California." *Archives of General Psychiatry,* 1998, *55*(9), 771–778.

Weissman, J. S., and Epstein, A. *Falling Through the Safety Net. Insurance Status and Access to Health Care.* Baltimore, Md.: Johns Hopkins University Press, 1994.

Whitehorse, L. E., Manzano, R., Baezconde-Garbanati, L. A., and Hahn, G. "Culturally Tailoring a Physical Activity Program for Hispanic Women: Recruitment Successes of La Vida Buena's Salsa Aerobics." *Journal of Health Education,* 1999, *30*(Suppl. 2), S18–S24.

Winkleby, M. A., Kraemer, H. C., Ahn, D. K., and Varady, A. N. "Ethnic and Socioeconomic Differences in Cardiovascular Disease Risk Factors. Findings for Women from the Third National Health and Nutrition Examination Survey, 1988–1994." *Journal of the American Medical Association,* 1998, *280*(4), 356–362.

Wyn, R., Leslie, J., Glick, D., and Solis, B. "Low Income Women and Managed Care in California." Los Angeles: University of California, Los Angeles, Center for Health Policy Research, Aug. 1997.

Zambrana, R. "Changing Characteristics of Patient Populations in Los Angeles: The Growth of Latino Families." Paper presented at the Valley Presbyterian Hospital Conference, Van Nuys, Calif., Sept. 1990.

Zambrana, R., Dunkel-Schetter, C., and Scrimshaw, S. "Factors Which Influence the Use of Prenatal Care in Low-Income Minority Women in Los Angeles." *Journal of Community Health,* 1991, *16*(5), 283–295.

CHAPTER FOUR

The Role of Health Insurance on Latinas' Health

Estelamari Rodriguez
Olveen Carrasquillo

Although the high rate of uninsured Latinos has caught the attention of the research, policy, and provider communities, very little, if any, work has focused on the current status and impact of the situation on Latinas. This omission became apparent to the editors of this book in the search of the literature, and as a result they commissioned this chapter for the book. The chapter authors address the current status of uninsured Latinas and the implications, and they set out a suggested course of action in this important contribution to understanding the issues related to uninsured Latinas.

Latinos have the highest uninsured rates among all racial or ethnic groups in the United States. Although they comprise only 13.3 percent of the U.S. population (Ramirez and de la Cruz, 2003), Latinos accounted for 30 percent of the nation's 41 million uninsured people in 2001 (Mills, 2002). Previous studies have analyzed the health insurance patterns of the general Latino population (Brown, Ojeda, Wyn, and Leban, 2000; Carrasquillo and Barbot, 2000), but few have focused on patterns and trends of insurance utilization among women. In this chapter, we present an analysis of data from the 2001 Current Population Survey (CPS), which provides data on coverage for the year 2000. This annual Census Bureau survey samples over 130,000 persons to provide nationally representative data and is considered one of the standard sources of annual health insurance data.

In the year 2000, 29 percent of all Latinas living in the United States reported not having health insurance, compared to 17 percent of blacks and 9 percent of White women. The disparity in health insurance status between Latinas and White women remains constant at all age and income levels (see Table 4.1). For example, among families with incomes less than the federal poverty level (FPL), $17,050 a year for a family of four, 41 percent of Latinas were uninsured versus 23 percent of Whites; among families with incomes over $50,000, 23 percent of Latinas were uninsured as compared to only 7 percent of Whites (Table 4.1).

Table 4.1. Percentage of Uninsured Females in the United States

	Hispanics (n = 16.9 million)	Black (n = 18.5 million)	White (n = 98.9 million)	Mexican (n = 11.1 million)	Puerto Rican (n = 1.5 million)	Cuban (n = 625,000)	Dominican (n = 660,000)	Citizens (N = 12.4 million)	Noncitizens (N = 4.5 million)
Total uninsured	29%	17%	9%	33%	14%	14%	27%	21%	53%
Age									
Under 18	24	13	7	26	10	9	15	20	51
18–39	38	24	14	42	17		34	26	56
40–64	31	17	10	34	19	19	a	22	53
Over 64	4	1	0	7	a	a	a	2	17
Family income									
Below the federal poverty level	41	23	23	47	15	a	a	29	64
100–150% of the federal poverty level	37	24	17	38	23	a	a	28	56
Above 150% of the federal poverty level	23	14	7	25	12	15	24	16	45

Note: Baseline population according to the Current Population Survey, 2000.

aThe cell size was too small (estimated at below 200,000) to make reliable estimates.

Analysis by country of origin shows that Latinas of Mexican and Dominican origin were the least likely to have coverage, with 33 percent and 27 percent being uninsured, respectively. Women of Puerto Rican and Cuban origin had relatively better health coverage, with insurance rates of 14 percent (Table 4.1). The variation in health insurance coverage among different Latino subgroups can be explained in part by citizenship status, patterns of immigration, and the types of employment available to these subgroups. In 1998, 56 percent of Latino immigrants did not have health insurance, with recently arrived immigrant groups, encompassing those from Central America, having the highest proportion of uninsured, including 55 percent of Salvadorans, 55 percent of Mexicans, and 58 percent of Guatemalans (Carrasquillo, Carrasquillo, and Shea, 2000). Cubans, who in general have resided in the United States longer than the other groups, have higher rates of job-based coverage and public health insurance than other Hispanic subgroups (see Table 4.2). But rich or poor, recent immigrants or not, Latinas at all levels of society experience less health coverage and in turn less access to health care services than their White counterparts.

WHY DOES THE NUMBER OF LATINAS WITHOUT HEALTH INSURANCE KEEP GROWING?

If we examine trends in health insurance coverage for Latinas over the past decade, the results are disconcerting. The absolute number of uninsured Latinas grew 81 percent between 1989 and 2000, from 2.7 million in 1989 to almost 5 million in 2000 (see Table 4.3). In part due to an overall population growth and the constant gap in health insurance coverage, Latinas continue to make up a disproportionate share of the uninsured population in the United States. Latinas made up 11 percent of the U.S. female population but accounted for 29 percent of the total number of uninsured women in the year 2000 (Table 4.3).

The most cited reason for the lack of health coverage among Latinos has been the lower rate of employer-based coverage offered to Latinos (Carrasquillo, Carrasquillo, and Shea, 2000; Quinn, 2000; Seccombe, Clarke, and Coward, 1994). As shown in Table 4.2, only 44 percent of Latino women benefit from employer-provided insurance as compared to 70 percent of White women. The lower rate of employer-based coverage for Latinos is not related to unemployment. In fact, 56 percent of uninsured Latinos live in households where at least one member of the family works, a figure very similar to 55 percent for Whites (Quinn, 2000). In addition, when health insurance is offered to Latinos, they are as likely as any other group to accept coverage, with insurance take-up rates of 82 percent. Only 8 percent had declined coverage due to cost concerns, and less than 1 percent declined coverage because they did not feel it was important (Quinn, 2000).

Lack of employer insurance among Latinos is due to the types of employment they have access to. Latinos in general are more likely to work for employers that

Table 4.2. Types of Insurance Coverage Among Females

	Race and Ethnicity			Hispanic Subgroups by Ethnic Origin				Hispanic Subgroup by Citizenship Status	
	Hispanic	Black	White	Mexican	Puerto Rican	Cuban	Dominican	Citizen	Noncitizen
Employer provided[a]	44%	56%	70%	44%	52%	47%	39%	51%	30%
Government insurance	27	32	25	22	29	27	13	31	17
Medicaid[b]	20	21	8	25	29	35	40	23	14
Medicare[b]	7	12	17	6	12	27	7	9	4
Medicaid (less than 150% of the federal poverty level)	36	44	28	34	58	41	53	44	18

[a]Employer insurance and government insurance are not mutually exclusive.

[b]Medicaid and Medicare are not mutually exclusive.

Table 4.3. Trends in Number Uninsured by Race/Ethnicity (in thousands)

	1989	1992	1993[a]	1994[b]	1995	1996	1997	1998	1999[b]	2000	Absolute Increase in Number Uninsured	Percentage Increase in Number Uninsured
All females												
Hispanic	2,747	3,756	3,707	4,205	4,219	4,440	4,669	5,247	4,888	4,981	2,234	81%
Black	2,753	2,957	3,051	3,088	3,269	3,515	3,679	3,810	3,502	3,320	567	21
Non-Hispanic White	8,495	9,841	10,455	10,377	10,374	10,817	11,017	10,227	9,176	9,143	648	8

[a]Implementation of 1990 Census weights, which may account for a portion of the increase in the number of uninsured from 1992 to 1993.
[b]Health insurance questions were redesigned in 1994 and again in 1999 to reduce underreporting of private health insurance.

offer fewer benefits, such as small firms, part-time jobs, or so-called off-the books occupations (such as domestic service, garment, food, and child care service jobs) that do not offer health benefits to any of their employees. Women who are recent immigrants are at a particularly high risk due to the lack of language proficiency, lack of work skills, and restricted access to social services and education that limit their access to jobs with health insurance coverage. Their immigration status also becomes a barrier to the types of occupations available to some of these immigrants. Among Latinas who are not U.S. citizens, the uninsured rate is twice as high as that of Latina U.S. citizens (53 percent versus 21 percent) and almost six times as high as Whites (Table 4.1). Such disparities have persisted over time. Even after fifteen years of living in the United States, foreign-born Latinos are significantly more likely to be uninsured than U.S.-born Latinos: 34 percent versus 24 percent (Schur and Feldman, 2001).

Latinas are also disproportionately more likely to be represented among the poor, and such uninsured low-income women face additional challenges when it comes to health care insurance. Poor women are more likely than other women to be uninsured or to rely on Medicaid as a source of insurance. (Reinsenger, 1995). In Table 4.2 we demonstrate that government-sponsored insurance programs such as Medicaid and Medicare play a critical role in providing insurance to low-income Latinas. About 36 percent of Latinas with incomes less than 150 percent of the FPL are covered by Medicaid.

Such government-sponsored insurance programs nevertheless fail to provide a complete safety net for Latinas. In 2000, 41 percent of Latinas living below the federal poverty level were uninsured, compared to 23 percent of White women (Table 4.1). There are many reasons for this. First, in many states, nonelderly low-income women without children are not eligible for Medicaid coverage unless they are disabled. Also, pregnant women who qualify for Medicaid services lose these services at sixty days postpartum unless they qualify by other criteria. More recently, welfare reforms separating Medicaid from cash assistance and changes in Medicaid eligibility for immigrants have decreased the number of Latinas covered by Medicaid. According to the Kaiser Commission on Medicaid and the Uninsured, Medicaid coverage for Latinos between 1994 and 1997 declined from 20 percent to 16 percent (Kaiser Commission on Medicaid and the Uninsured, 2000; Garrett and Hudman 2002).

IMPLICATIONS OF LACK OF HEALTH INSURANCE COVERAGE FOR LATINAS

Among the general population, not having health insurance has been associated with difficulties accessing the health care system, having unmet medical needs, and lacking a regular source of care (Berk, Schur, and Cantor, 1995;

Kogan and others, 1995; Donelan and others, 1996; Schoen and others, 1997). The uninsured are less likely to obtain preventive services such as mammograms and Pap smears (Himmelstein and Woolhandler, 1995; Kirkman-Liff and Kronenfeld, 1992), and they have higher preventable hospitalization rates (Hadley, Steinberg, and Feder, 1991) and adjusted mortality rates (Franks, Clancy, and Gold, 1993). Two recent reviews by the Institute of Medicine and the American College of Physicians conclude that adults without health insurance coverage experience poorer health outcomes and die sooner than do adults with health insurance coverage (American College of Physicians–American Society of Internal Medicine, 2000; Institute of Medicine 2002).

The lack of health insurance is particularly important for women because they use health services more than men do (Reinsenger, 1995). The demand for medical services is greater for women in part because of their need for regular reproductive health services during their childbearing years and a higher rate of chronic illnesses in their older years. In general, women are more likely to see physicians, be hospitalized, use mental health services, and rely on prescription drugs as they age (Lambrew, 2001).

Because their need for health care services is greater, the impact of lack of health insurance on the health of Latinas is far more dramatic. They have less access to a regular source of care and a worse perception of their health. Uninsured Latinas are more likely to rate their health as fair or poor and less likely to have visited a doctor when compared to White women. In fact, one in four uninsured Latinas (24 percent) in fair to poor health went for more than one year without seeing a physician, three times the rate of those with coverage and twice the rate of uninsured White women (13 percent) (Brown, Ojeda, Wyn, and Leban, 2000).

Lack of insurance among Latinas is also related to lower rates of preventive service utilization. Uninsured Latinas are less likely to have Pap smears and mammograms (Laws and Mayo, 1998) than are insured Latinas, and not surprisingly, they tend to be younger when diagnosed with breast or cervical cancer, present with these cancers at a later stage of diagnosis, and have higher mortality rates than non-Latinas. Lack of insurance coverage and restricted access to a regular source of care are the major determinants for lower use of preventive and screening services among Latinas (American College of Physicians–American Society of Internal Medicine, 2000).

Finally, health insurance coverage affects Latinas' use of reproductive health services. Multiple studies have found that as a whole, uninsured women initiate prenatal care too late and have fewer prenatal visits when compared to women with private fee-for-service insurance (Braverman, Bennet, and Lewis, 1993). Among pregnant women, Latinas are three times more likely not to receive any prenatal care as non-Latinos. On average, 72 percent of Latinas receive prenatal care within the first trimester. Mexican Americans receive prenatal care the least, at 71 percent, Puerto Ricans at 75 percent, Cuban Americans at 85 percent, and Central and South Americans at 75 percent (American College of Physicians-American Society of Internal Medicine, 2000).

POLICY RECOMMENDATIONS

After the demise of President Clinton's plan for comprehensive health insurance reform in 1994, there has been limited legislation to address the plight of the uninsured. One piece of such legislation was the 1996 Health Insurance Portability Act, allowing workers to maintain coverage after leaving an occupation. Insurance companies, however, were permitted to charge exorbitant rates for coverage, and the act benefited only a small number of persons. In fact, the only significant initiative during the 1990s was the State Children's Health Insurance Program (SCHIP), enacted in 1997.

SCHIP provides government insurance for low-income children who are not poor enough to qualify for Medicaid, but it does not address the health insurance needs of Latino adults. As of July 2002, 3.8 million children had been enrolled. Studies have shown that enrollment in these programs dramatically improves access to quality health care (Holl and others, 2000). However, these state programs continue to face major hurdles, including lack of public awareness, and applicants face numerous enrollment obstacles (Ross and Cox, 2000). Examples of such barriers have included twenty-seven-page applications, complicated eligibility asset tests, poorly translated forms, use of non-Spanish-speaking outreach workers to target Latinos, requiring parental social security numbers (not required by federal law and a major barrier for undocumented parents), and requiring mailed monthly copayments by check (many of the poor lack checking accounts). Although some states have made headway into reducing some of these barriers, it is estimated that nearly three-quarters of uninsured children are Medicaid or SCHIP eligible but not enrolled (Ross and Cox, 2002).

Furthermore, policies that require yearly recertification documentation have proved problematic, with nearly 50 percent of children in some states being automatically disenrolled at the time of recertification (Bachrach, Belfort, and Lipson, 2000). As a consequence of welfare reform, millions of children and adult women were removed from state Medicaid rolls and became uninsured (Garrett and Hudman, 2002). Thus, despite the partial success of SCHIP in insuring near-poor children, the overall number of uninsured children has decreased only slightly in the past ten years. For Latino children in particular, the number without coverage actually increased by nearly 50 percent during the previous decade, and over one-quarter continue to lack coverage (Carrasquillo and Barbot, 2000).

There is consensus that additional policy initiatives are needed to address the plight of the uninsured in America and that universal health coverage should be the ultimate goal of health insurance reform (Kahn and Pollack, 2001). Yet the perceived political repercussions of the failed Clinton health plan have had a chilling effect on any government initiatives that rely on an overhaul of the entire health care system. Instead, most policy proposals tend to favor smaller-scale incremental approaches. Yet even such limited efforts have been stymied by major political differences concerning the role of government (expanding existing government programs such as Medicaid or CHIP) versus the private sector in providing insurance.

Most conservatives favor the private sector approach. Among these, three types of proposals are frequently discussed: tax credits, small business pooling, and medical savings accounts. The most widely touted of these are tax rebates. The major limitation of this proposal is that the proposed amounts of such a rebate fall far short of the cost of such policies. Thus, while tax credits may help make individual insurance more affordable for young, healthy, higher-income persons, they do little to make insurance affordable for low-income people (Hadley and Reschovsky, 2002).

Another set of proposals based on private sector initiatives centers on helping small businesses purchase insurance through pooling to lower the price of such policies. Although such options have shown some success among wealthier workers, small businesses employing primarily low-wage workers have not shown much enthusiasm for such employee benefits (Rosenberg, 2002). Medical savings accounts (MSAs), which allow individuals to set a certain amount of money aside on a pretax basis to use for future health care expenses, have been proposed. Unfortunately, MSAs will not work for poor and near-poor families with no surplus income to save. Even among the healthy and wealthy for whom MSAs are designed, fewer than forty thousand individuals have wanted to take the risk of giving up traditional insurance protection for an MSA (Families USA, 2002). In addition, by luring the healthiest persons out of the broader insurance pool, MSAs will drive up premium costs for those who cannot participate. Thus, it is unlikely that any of these private sector proposals will make a significant dent on the rising number of uninsured Latinas.

It is clear that if any headway is to be made in improving coverage of Latino families, expansion of government insurance programs is needed. In fact, even groups that strongly favor private sector solutions for the healthy and wealthy families agree that for poor and near-poor families, expansions of government coverage programs are the most appropriate approaches (Kahn and Pollack, 2001). The most popular of these government expansion proposals centers on the expansion of the SCHIP program to parents of SCHIP or Medicaid-eligible children. Although federal initiatives in this direction have foundered, as of January 2002 twenty states had enacted their own programs to cover parents of Medicaid or SCHIP-eligible children, and some states, such as New York, even provide coverage for poor single adults (Ross and Cox, 2002). Again, however, the major limitations of these programs will remain the onerous requirements for enrollment and yearly recertification processes. Clearly, if means testing and automatic disenrollment were eliminated, these programs would hold great promise in decreasing the number of uninsured Latinos. Although a few states have moved in this direction, state budget deficits have limited the political support for such changes.

Although attempts to overhaul the entire health care sector are widely perceived as being politically unattainable, a vast body of research has shown that the most cost-effective way to provide coverage for the entire U.S. population would be a single-payer national health insurance system (Woolhandler and Himmelstein, 2002). In the latest nonpartisan analysis of nine different proposals for the state of California, the single-payer approaches were found to be the only proposals that would both achieve universal coverage and save the state and its taxpayers nearly $4 billion annually (Spelman, 2002). Such a system would provide patients with universal access to any doctor or hospital of their choice by diverting most of the 25 percent of health expenditures associated with health administration into providing quality health care.

Such a measure is fiercely opposed by the health insurance industry and for-profit managed care corporations, which would have little, if any, role under such a system. Concerned that a single buyer may lower the price of their products, the pharmaceutical industry also adamantly opposes a single-payer plan. Although these special interests remain among the most powerful lobbying groups, the continued dramatic rise in health expenditures, the downturn in the U.S. economy, and the associated increase in the number of uninsured may signal opportunities to reconsider an overhaul of the health care system. Among the direct beneficiaries of such a system would be the 5 million Latinas who currently lack coverage.

References

American College of Physicians–American Society of Internal Medicine. *No Health Insurance? It's Enough to Make You Sick. Latino Community at Great Risk.* Philadelphia: American College of Physicians–American Society of Internal Medicine, 2000.

Bachrach, D., Belfort, R., and Lipson, K. *Closing Coverage Gaps: Improving Retention Rates in New York's Medicaid and Child Health Plus Programs.* New York: New York Community Trust, Dec. 2000.

Berk, M. L., Schur, C. L., and Cantor, J. C. "Ability to Obtain Health Care: Recent Estimates from the Robert Wood Johnson Foundation National Access to Care Survey." *Health Affairs,* 1995, *14,* 139–146.

Braverman, P., Bennet, T., and Lewis, C. "Access to Prenatal Care Following Major Medicaid Eligibility Expansions." *Journal of the American Medical Association,* 1993, *269*(10), 1258–1259.

Brown, R. E., Ojeda, V. D., Wyn, R., and Leban, R. *Racial and Ethnic Disparities in Access to Health Insurance and Health Care.* Los Angeles: UCLA Center for Health Policy Research/Henry J. Kaiser Family Foundation, 2000.

Carrasquillo, O., and Barbot, O. "The Uninsured: A Call to Action for All Latinos." *Harvard Journal of Hispanic Policy,* 2000, *12,* 33–46.

Carrasquillo, O., Carrasquillo, A. I., and Shea, S. "Health Insurance Coverage of Immigrants Living in the United States: Differences by Citizenship Status and Country of Origin." *American Journal of Public Health,* 2000, *90*(6), 917–923.

Donelan, K., and others. "Whatever Happened to the Health Insurance Crisis in the Untied States? Voices from a National Survey." *Journal of the American Medical Association,* 1996, *276*(16), 1346–1350.

Families USA. "Medical Savings Accounts Fact Sheet." [http://www.familiesusa.org/media/factsheets/msa.htm]. Aug. 14, 2002.

Fennelly, K. "Barriers to Prenatal Care Among Low-Income Women in New York City." *Family Planning Perspectives, 22*(5), 215–218, 231.

Franks, P., Clancy, C. M., and Gold, M. R. "Health Insurance and Mortality: Evidence from a National Cohort." *Journal of the American Medical Association,* 1993, *270,* 737–741.

Garrett, B., and Hudman, J. A. *Women Who Left Welfare: Health Care Coverage, Access, and Use of Health Services.* Menlo Park, Calif.: Kaiser Commission on Medicaid and the Uninsured, 2002.

Hadley, J., and Reschovsky, J. D. *Tax Credits and the Affordability of Individual Health Insurance.* Washington, D.C.: Center for Studying Health System Change, 2002.

Hadley, J. U., Steinberg, E. P., and Feder, J. "Comparison of Uninsured and Privately Insured Hospital Patients: Condition on Admission, Resource Use, and Outcome." *Journal of the American Medical Association,* Jan. 16, 1991, pp. 374–379.

Himmelstein, D. U., and Woolhandler, S. "Care Denied: US Residents Who Are Unable to Obtain Needed Medical Services." *American Journal of Public Health,* 1995, *85,* 341–344.

Holl, J. L., and others. "Evaluation of New York State's Child Health Plus: Access, Utilization, Quality of Health Care, and Health Status." *Pediatrics,* 2000, *105*(3 Suppl., E), 711–718.

Institute of Medicine. *Care Without Coverage: Too Little, Too Late.* Washington, D.C.: National Academy Press, May 2002.

Kahn, C. N., and Pollack, R. F. "Building a Consensus for Expanding Health Coverage." *Health Affairs,* 2001, *20*(1), 40–48.

Kaiser Commission on Medicaid and the Uninsured. *Health Insurance Coverage and Access to Care Among Latinos.* Washington, D.C.: Henry J. Kaiser Family Foundation, June 2000.

Kirkman-Liff, B. L., and Kronenfeld, J. J. "Access to Cancer Screening Services for Women." *American Journal of Public Health,* 1992, *82*(5), 733–735.

Kogan, M. D., and others. "The Effect of Gaps in Health Insurance on Continuity of a Regular Source of Care Among Preschool-Aged Children in the United States." *Journal of the American Medical Association,* 1995, *274*(18), 1429–1435.

Lambrew, J. M. "Diagnosing Disparities in Health Insurance for Women: A Prescription for Change." The Commonwealth Fund, Aug. 2001.

Laws, M. B., and Mayo, S. J. "The Latina Breast Cancer Control Study, Year One: Factors Predicting Screening Mammography Utilization by Urban Latina Women in Massachusetts." *Journal of Community Health,* 1998, *23*(4), 251–267.

Mills, R. J. "Health Insurance Coverage 2001." *Current Population Reports.* Washington, D.C.: Department of Commerce, Economics and Statistics Administration, 2002.

Quinn, K. "Working Without Benefits: The Health Insurance Crisis Confronting Hispanic Americans." New York: Commonwealth Fund, 2000.

Ramirez, R. R., and de la Cruz, G. P. "The Hispanic Population in the United States: March 2002." *Current Population Reports.* Washington, D.C.: Department of Commerce, Economics and Statistics Administration, 2003.

Reinsenger, A. L. *Health Insurance and Access to Care: Issues for Women.* New York: Commonwealth Fund, Jan. 1995.

Rosenberg, S. N. *Lessons from a Small Business Health Insurance Demonstration Project.* New York: Commonwealth Fund, 2002.

Ross, D. C., and Cox, L. *Making It Simple: Medicaid for Children and CHIP Income Eligibility Guidelines and Enrollment Procedures—Findings from a Fifty-State Survey.* Washington, D.C.: Kaiser Commission on Medicaid and the Uninsured, Oct. 2000.

Ross, D. C., and Cox, L. *The Promise of Doing More: A Report on a National Survey of Enrollment and Renewal Procedures in Medicaid and SCHIP.* Washington, D.C.: Kaiser Commission on Medicaid and the Uninsured, June 2002.

Schoen, C., and others. "Insurance Matters for Low-Income Adults: Results from a Five-State Survey." *Health Affairs,* 1997, *16,* 163–171.

Schur, C., and Feldman, J. *Running in Place: How Job Characteristics, Immigrant Status, and Family Structure Keep Hispanics Uninsured.* New York: Commonwealth Fund, May 2001.

Seccombe, K., Clarke, L. L., and Coward, R. T. "Discrepancies in Employer-Sponsored Health Insurance Among Hispanics, Blacks, and Whites: The Effects of Sociodemographic and Employment Factors." *Inquiry,* 1994, *31*(2), 221–229.

Spelman, J. *Calcare: A Single Payer Health Plan for California.* SB 480/Health Care Options Project, 2002.

Woolhandler, S., and Himmelstein, D. U. "National Health Insurance: Liberal Benefits, Conservative Spending." *Archives of Internal Medicine,* 2002, *162*(9), 973–975.

PART THREE

SEXUAL AND REPRODUCTIVE HEALTH ISSUES

CHAPTER FIVE

The Reproductive Years

The Health of Latinas

Aida L. Giachello

*This chapter represents the most recent and comprehensive review
of Latina reproductive health and related health issues. It both
contains what is known in the literature and provides context.*

Despite the rapid growth of the Latino population in the United States and
the large percentage of Latinas in this population, data about the health
and social well-being and the quality of health care being delivered to
Latinas are still limited. Review of recent research and available data document
their poor health as well as the barriers to their health care, which are due to
financial, institutional, and cultural factors. It has been argued (Giachello,
1994a) that socioeconomic factors (for example, health insurance) appear to be
the strongest determinants of Latino women's ability to enter the formal medical care system. Once they enter the medical care system, they experience
linguistic, sociocultural, and systemic barriers. They encounter health care services that are often unresponsive to women's health needs. Many health care
providers are biased against women in general and have stereotypical views of
women of color in particular; moreover, they often have limited knowledge,
understanding, or skills to meet the needs of populations who may have
illnesses with which they are inexperienced and cultural practices or languages
different from their own. These factors affect the quality of health services delivered to Latino women of all age groups, their adherence to medical treatment,
and often their health outcomes and general well-being.

This chapter provides an overview of the health of Latino women, with
emphasis on issues related to women in their reproductive years (ages fifteen
to forty-four years). Specifically, the chapter (1) identifies the major factors
affecting Latino women's health; (2) describes selected sociodemographic and

economic factors affecting Latino women's health; (3) discusses some of the major health disparities, selected lifestyle practices, and medical risk factors of Latino women; (4) describes the use of selected health services related to pregnancy, delivery, and family planning, including abortion; (5) discusses some findings on selected pregnancy outcomes and infant health; and (6) concludes with program, policy, and future research recommendations.

SOCIODEMOGRAPHIC CHARACTERISTICS

Latinas comprise 51.5 percent of the total Latino population in the United States (Hajat, Lucas, and Kington, 2000). The sex distribution varies by Latinos of different national origins, with Puerto Rican women substantially outnumbering Puerto Rican men in the United States (54.3 percent versus 45.7 percent) (U.S. Bureau of the Census, 2000; Hajat, Lucas, and Kington, 2000) (see Table 5.1). Latinos are one of the youngest population groups in the United States. Differences in median age by gender indicate that currently, Latino women are slightly older as a group than Latino men but are mostly concentrated in much younger age groups than are White men and women. Latino women tend to be concentrated in two age groups: either they are extremely young (twenty-one years or younger) or they are in the prime age workers' group (twenty-two to fifty-five years). Very few of them are currently of retirement age. This situation is expected to change by 2025, when 18 percent of the Latino population will be sixty-five years of age and over (Kaiser Family Foundation, 1999).

Most Latino women are concentrated in low-paying occupations (for example, factories, restaurants, or clerical work). They experience twice the rate of unemployment compared to that of Whites and suffer from multiple social and economic disadvantages, such as low levels of education, low income, single parenting, and high levels of poverty, all of which have an impact on their health and social well-being and limit their access to and utilization of health services.

LIFE EXPECTANCY AND LEADING CAUSES OF DEATH

Latino women's life expectancy in 1995 was higher (77.1 years) compared to that of Latino men (69.6 years), slightly lower than that of White women (79.6 years), but higher than that of African American women (74.4 years) (National Institutes of Health, 1998). These actuarial projections need to be interpreted with caution, however, considering (1) the trends and patterns of certain diseases affecting Latino women, such as diabetes, HIV/AIDS, and cervical cancer; (2) the higher rates of women in the labor force and now entering nontraditional (more stressful) occupations, which might lead to an increase of

Table 5.1. Selected Characteristics of Latinos by Gender and National Origin Compared to Those of Whites, March 1999

Characteristics	Total Latino			Mexican			Puerto Rican			Cuban			Central and South American[a]			White		
	Male	Female	Total	Male	Female	Total	Male	Female	Total	Male	Female	Total	Male	Female	Total	Male	Female	Total
Sex distribution	48.5	51.5	—	49.6	50.4	—	45.7	54.3	—	50.3	49.7	—	—	—	—	31.7	28.2	29.9
Not U.S. born	b	—	48.9	—	—	47.5	—	—	3.0	—	—	72.1	—	—	63.0	—	—	4.7
Age distribution																		
Under 15 years	31.1	30.1	30.6	32.6	33.1	32.8	31.7	26.3	28.9	15.8	16.6	16.2	27.7	24.7	26.2	20.5	18.7	19.6
15–19 years	8.5	9.4	8.9	7.8	9.0	8.5	9.0	10.2	9.6	6.8	5.0	5.9	7.5	6.7	7.0	7.0	6.5	6.7
20–24 years	8.9	8.3	8.6	9.6	8.8	9.2	8.3	7.1	7.7	3.4	5.1	4.3	8.6	8.8	8.7	6.3	6.0	6.1
25–29 years	8.7	8.4	8.5	9.4	9.0	9.2	7.9	7.1	7.5	5.3	6.0	6.0	8.5	10.4	8.3	6.4	6.3	6.4
30–34 years	9.2	8.7	8.9	8.9	8.5	8.7	7.3	9.1	8.3	9.2	7.7	8.4	12.0	11.3	11.3	7.0	6.9	6.9
35–44 years	14.5	14.7	14.6	13.6	13.9	13.7	14.0	15.2	14.6	15.7	13.7	14.7	19.0	16.5	18.5	17.2	16.5	16.9
45–54 years	8.7	9.3	9.0	7.9	8.0	8.0	10.5	10.9	10.7	13.0	12.2	12.6	11.3	7.2	10.5	14.1	13.9	14.0
55–64 years	4.8	6.0	5.4	4.2	5.0	4.6	5.8	6.6	6.2	14.1	14.3	14.2	7.2	3.5	5.4	9.3	9.4	9.4
65–74 years	3.1	3.8	3.4	2.6	3.1	2.9	3.6	5.0	4.3	11.5	8.2	10.2	2.6	3.5	3.0	7.0	8.1	7.6
75 years and older	1.6	2.3	1.9	1.4	1.6	1.5	1.8	2.5	2.2	5.1	9.8	7.6	1.1	1.3	1.2	5.2	7.8	6.4

(Continued)

Table 5.1. Selected Characteristics of Latinos by Gender and National Origin Compared to Those of Whites, March 1999 (Continued)

Characteristics	Total Latino			Mexican			Puerto Rican			Cuban			Central and South American[a]			White		
	Male	Female	Total	Male	Female	Total	Male	Female	Total	Male	Female	Total	Male	Female	Total	Male	Female	Total
Median age			26.6															38.4
Education (pop. 25 years and older)																		
Less than 9 years	28.1	27.4	27.1	33.2	32.2	32.7	17.4	17.3	17.4	19.2	21.6	20.4	24.3	22.8	23.5	4.5	4.4	4.5
9–12 (no diploma)	15.9	16.3	16.1	16.9	18.2	17.6	19.6	18.1	18.8	10.5	8.2	9.3	12.7	12.3	12.5	7.8	7.8	7.8
High school graduate	27.2	26.6	26.9	26.6	25.9	26.2	31.4	29.1	30.1	28.2	28.1	28.2	24.2	26.7	25.5	32.1	36.3	34.3
Some college or associate degree	18.1	18.7	18.4	16.2	16.6	16.4	21.2	23.2	22.6	14.4	17.3	17.4	20.4	20.5	20.4	25.0	26.3	25.7
Bachelor's degree	7.4	8.2	7.8	5.2	5.4	5.3	7.4	8.4	8.0	14.7	17.8	16.3	12.5	13.3	12.9	19.8	17.3	18.5
Four years of advanced degree	3.3	2.8	3.1	1.9	1.7	1.8	3.1	3.3	3.2	10.1	7.0	8.5	5.9	4.3	5.1	10.8	7.6	9.1
Marital status (pop. 15 years and older)																		
Married, spouse present	54.7	51.0	52.8	46.3	51.0	49.6	45.5	35.9	40.3	61.3	54.0	57.5	45.7	47.6	46.7	54.7	51.0	52.8
Married, spouse absent	1.3	1.1	1.2	4.6	2.0	3.3	1.6	2.7	2.2	1.3	0.4	0.8	5.6	2.3	3.9	1.3	1.1	1.2
Widowed	2.5	10.0	6.4	1.4	5.6	3.5	0.8	6.0	3.6	1.5	10.8	6.3	1.1	5.3	3.3	2.5	10.0	6.4
Divorced	8.4	10.2	9.3	4.9	6.8	5.8	8.5	11.0	9.9	10.4	10.6	10.5	4.6	8.9	6.9	8.4	10.2	9.3

Separated	1.8	2.7	2.3	2.4	5.2	3.7	3.8	6.5	5.3	3.7	4.0	3.8	3.4	5.3	4.4	1.8	2.7	2.3
Never married	31.3	25.1	28.1	38.4	29.4	34.0	39.8	38.0	38.8	21.7	20.3	21.0	39.6	30.6	4.8	31.3	25.1	28.1
Type of family																		
Married couple	—	—	15.7	—	—	18.8	—	—	12.5	—	—	7.7	—	—	14.4	—	—	3.8
Female householder	—	—	43.7	—	—	46.9	—	—	48.0	—	—	25.3	—	—	31.6	—	—	20.7
Male householder, nonspouse	—	—	19.6	—	—	20.8	—	—	28.2	—	—	14.3	—	—	13.7	—	—	7.8
Labor force participation	78.4	55.8	67.0	80.4	55.2	68.1	66.3	52.6	58.8	73.4	49.2	60.8	80.8	61.8	70.7	74.3	60.3	67.1
Percentage unemployment (pop. 16 years and older)	6.0	7.6	6.7	5.9	8.6	7.0	7.4	7.3	7.3	4.7	5.3	4.9	6.4	5.3	5.9	3.8	3.3	3.6
Type of occupation																		
Executive, administrative/ managerial	14.9	14.3	14.6	5.2	8.1	6.3	8.8	11.5	10.1	15.5	10.1	13.2	8.9	7.1	8.1	6.9	8.8	7.7
Professional	13.4	17.8	15.5	3.7	7.5	5.2	6.6	11.9	9.2	9.8	13.7	11.4	6.5	9.2	7.8	4.9	9.0	6.6
Technical	2.9	3.4	3.1	1.2	2.1	1.5	2.2	2.5	2.4	1.9	6.5	3.9	2.7	2.1	2.4	1.6	2.3	1.9

(Continued)

Table 5.1. Selected Characteristics of Latinos by Gender and National Origin Compared to Those of Whites, March 1999 (Continued)

Characteristics	Total Latino			Mexican			Puerto Rican			Cuban			Central and South American[a]			White		
	Male	Female	Total	Male	Female	Total	Male	Female	Total	Male	Female	Total	Male	Female	Total	Male	Female	Total
Sales	11.7	12.8	12.2	6.7	13.2	9.2	9.6	11.1	10.3	14.4	10.9	12.9	8.1	11.6	9.8	7.9	12.7	9.9
Administrative support	5.5	23.7	14.1	4.9	22.0	11.5	9.4	27.5	18.3	6.5	31.6	17.0	5.5	19.5	12.1	5.7	22.6	12.7
Precision production, crafts, and repairs	18.6	2.1	10.9	21.9	3.0	14.6	18.1	2.9	10.6	15.0	4.0	10.4	20.4	1.1	11.7	20.6	2.8	13.2
Transportation	6.8	4.4	5.7	7.3	1.1	4.9	9.4	9.4	9.4	8.2	5.4	7.0	9.6	9.3	9.5	10.3	9.1	9.8
Handlers, equipment cleaners, laborers	6.7	0.9	4.0	11.7	2.8	8.2	7.5	0.5	4.0	8.9	0.6	5.4	6.9	0.5	3.9	7.3	0.8	4.6
Workers, private household	6.0	1.6	4.0	0.1	3.3	1.3	8.2	2.7	5.5	9.8	1.6	6.4	10.5	3.5	9.2	10.8	2.8	9.5
Workers, except private household	0.1	1.3	0.6	15.6	24.8	19.1	—	—	—	—	0.9	0.4	0.2	10.5	5.0	0.1	4.0	1.7
Farming, forestry, fishing	10.0	16.7	13.1	10.9	2.3	7.6	17.6	19.7	18.6	8.9	14.6	11.3	17.0	24.5	20.6	15.7	23.6	19.0
Machine operators, assemblers, inspectors	3.5	1.0	2.3	11.1	9.8	10.6	2.5	0.4	1.5	1.3	—	0.7	3.5	0.6	2.1	8.1	1.5	5.4

Persons with
money earnings

Less than $10,000	24.4	46.4	34.7	24.8	47.2	34.6	28.7	48.8	39.7	25.5	49.0	37.2	17.8	40.4	29.0	16.0	35.5	25.9
$10,000–24,999	25.6	35.7	39.5	45.2	37.7	41.9	31.7	30.3	30.9	31.7	26.7	29.2	47.3	40.0	43.7	26.2	33.3	29.8
$25,000 and over	29.8	16.9	23.8	27.8	14.3	22.3	46.3	19.5	27.0	35.6	23.7	29.6	31.3	18.6	25.2	47.2	28.7	37.8
Median income	$17,252	$10,862	—	—	—	—	—	—	—	—	—	—	—	—	—	$29,862	$15,217	—
Poverty level, 1998																		
Families below poverty level	—	—	10.0	—	—	24.4	—	26.7	—	—	—	11.0	—	—	18.5	—	—	6.1
Married couple below poverty level	—	—	5.3	—	—	18.0	—	12.5	—	—	—	7.7	—	—	14.4	—	—	3.8
Family headed by female	—	—	29.9	—	—	46.9	—	48.0	—	—	—	25.3	—	—	31.6	—	—	20.7

aIncludes Central and South Americans and other and unknown Latinos.

bData not available, February 2000.

Sources: U.S. Bureau of the Census. (1999, Mar.). The Hispanic population in the United States. *Current Population Reports*, pp. 20–527. United States Bureau of the Census, Ramirez (1999, Dec.); *Advance Data*, No. 3 (Feb. 25, 2000), Table 2; U.S. Bureau of the Census, The Hispanic population in the United States. *Current Population Reports* (2000, Mar.). United States Bureau of the Census, Historical income tables: People (Mar.); *Current Population Survey* (1999, Nov. 1999).

heart disease and strokes; and (3) the poor health and quality of life of women who live longer, as they are most likely to experience acute symptoms of illnesses, chronic conditions, and short- and long-term disabilities (National Institutes of Health, 1992).

The leading causes of death of Latino women are heart disease, cancer, injuries, cerebrovascular diseases, diabetes mellitus, homicide, pneumonia and influenza, liver diseases, pulmonary respiratory problems, and HIV/AIDS (see Tables 5.2 and 5.3 and Figure 5.1) (Hoyert, Kochanek, and Murphy, 1999).

Latino women, compared to Latino men, are more likely to die of cerebrovascular diseases and diabetes. The age-specific mortality data shown in Tables 5.2 and 5.3 indicate that cancer (for instance, cervical, breast, or lung cancers) for women aged 25 to 44 emerged as the leading cause of death in 1997 (19.8 per 100,000) (Hoyert, Kochanek, and Murphy, 1999). Increased smoking among women in the United States, Latin America, and Spain has been the result of heavy marketing by the tobacco industry (Centers for Disease Control and Prevention, 1999c). This may explain the increase in cancer rates for lung and other pulmonary conditions. Infection with human papillomavirus (HPV), a sexually transmitted disease (STD), may well explain the high incidence of cervical cancer and mortality due to it among Latino women (Centers for Disease Control and Prevention, 1998b; Napoles-Springer and Pérez-Stable, 1996).

Latino women aged 25 to 44 are also more likely to die of injuries, representing the second leading cause of death (12.5 per 100,000); injuries are the number one cause of death among young women between the ages of 15 and 24 (14.9 per 100,000) (Hoyert, Kochanek, and Murphy, 1999). Motor vehicle accidents accounted in 1997 for most of these types of deaths (see Tables 5.2 and 5.3). Homicide emerged as the second cause of death among young Latino women (15 to 24 years). HIV/AIDS emerged as the third leading cause of death for Latino women between the ages of 25 and 44, despite the fact that this condition has been declining in the past five years or so for the population as a whole (Centers for Disease Control and Prevention, 1998b). Due to the long period of infection, this means that women of reproductive age become infected in their late teens and early twenties.

CHARACTERISTICS OF LATINO MOTHERS

Latino women have the highest fertility rates and birth percentages in the United States (Ventura and others, 2000) (see Table 5.4). About 18.6 percent of the total U.S. births in 1998 were to Latino women. Most of the Latino births were to Mexican American mothers, representing 70.2 percent of the total Latino births. In 1998, the estimated birthrate (number of live births per 1,000 population) for the total Latino population was 24.3, compared to 12.1 for the White

Table 5.2. Age-Specific Leading Causes of Death by Total Latino Men and Women and by Latino Women's Age Groups Compared to Those of Whites, 1997 (rates per 100,000)

Causes of Death	Total Latino			Latino Women's Age Groups						White		
	Female	Male	Total	1–4	5–14	15–24	25–44	45–64	65 and Over	Total Female	Total Male	Total
Diseases of the heart	78.3	83.9	81.2	NA[a]	NA	1.2	5.2	68.6	975.2	292.5	295.3	293.8
Cancer	61.4	65.4	63.5	2.2	2.9	3.5	19.8	128.9	513.7	203.4	233.2	217.9
Cerebrovascular diseases	19.6	16.7	18.1	NA		NA	3.0	20.1	228.4	76.9	51.6	64.6
Diabetes mellitus	17.2	13.8	15.5				1.6	28.6	184.0	26.1	22.4	24.3
Injury or accidents	13.7	39.7	27.0	10.4	4.9	14.9	12.5	15.5	41.0	26.0	47.9	36.6
Pneumonia and influenza	10.6	10.7	10.6	NA	NA	NA	1.2	6.5	129.3	37.2	32.3	34.8
Chronic obstructive pulmonary diseases	7.8		8.4	NA	NA	NA		7.2	94.1	42.3	46.9	44.6
Conditions related to the perinatal period	5.8			NA	NA							
Liver diseases and cirrhosis	5.5	13.3	9.5				2.4	13.7	40.0		12.2	9.3
Congenital anomalies	5.3			3.1	1.4	NA						
Alzheimer's disease									31.1	12.3		
Kidney failure								4.1	35.7	10.4		10.2
Septicemia				NA						10.0		
Homicide and legal intervention		18.6	11.1	2.3	NA	4.8	4.5				10.8	
Suicide		9.8		NA	NA	NA	2.2				19.7	12.0
Benign neoplasms and carcinoma in situ				NA	NA	NA						
Human immunodeficiency virus infection		12.3	7.8	NA	NA	NA	6.7	5.3				

[a]Rates are not available.

Source: National Center for Health Statistics (1999, Table 9).

Table 5.3. Age-Specific Leading Causes of Death by Total Latino and by Latino Women's Age Groups Compared to Those of Whites, 1997 (rates per 100,000)

Causes of Death	Total Latino	Latino Women's Age						White		
		1–4	5–14	15–24	25–44	45–64	65 and Over	Total Female	Total Male	Total
Diseases of the heart	81.2	NA[a]	NA	1.2	5.2	68.6	975.2	292.5	295.3	293.8
Cancer	63.5	2.2	2.9	3.5	19.8	128.9	513.7	203.4	233.2	217.9
Cerebrovascular diseases	18.1	NA	NA	NA	3.0	20.1	228.4	76.9	51.6	64.6
Diabetes mellitus	15.5				1.6	28.6	184.0	26.1	22.4	24.3
Injury or accidents	27.0	10.4	4.9	14.9	12.5	15.5	41.0	26.0	47.9	36.6
Pneumonia and influenza	10.6	NA	NA	NA	1.2	6.5	129.3	37.2	32.3	34.8
Chronic obstructive pulmonary diseases	8.4	NA	NA	NA		7.2	94.1	42.3	46.9	44.6
Conditions related to the perinatal period		NA	NA							
Liver diseases and cirrhosis	9.5	3.1	1.4	NA	2.4	13.7	40.0		12.2	9.3
Congenital anomalies										
Alzheimer's disease							31.1	12.3		
Kidney failure						4.1	35.7	10.4		10.2
Septicemia		NA						10.0		
Homicide and legal intervention	11.1	2.3	NA	4.8	4.5				10.8	
Suicide			NA	NA	2.2				19.7	12.0
Benign neoplasms and carcinoma in situ			NA	NA						
Human immunodeficiency virus infection	7.8	NA	NA	NA	6.7	5.3				

[a]Rates are not available.

Source: National Center for Health Statistics (1999, Table 9).

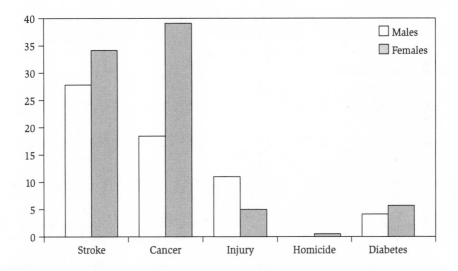

Figure 5.1. Leading Causes of Death of U.S. Latinos, 1997 Rates

Source: Hoyert, Kochanek, and Murphy (1999).

population (Ventura and others, 2000) (see Table 5.4). Birthrates by Latino origin were as follows: 26.4 for Mexican Americans, 19.0 for Puerto Ricans, 10.0 for Cubans, and 23.2 for Central and South American women in the United States (see Figure 5.2). The birthrate for Mexican Americans has increased slightly (from 25.7 in 1989 to 26.4 in 1998), while it dropped for Puerto Ricans (from 23.7 to 19.0) and for women of Central and South American origins and for other unidentified Latino women in the United States (from 28.3 to 23.2) (Ventura and others, 2000; Hoyert, Kochanek, and Murphy, 1999).

Data on age-specific fertility rates (number of births per 1,000 women aged 15 to 44) indicate that Mexican American mothers between the ages of 20 and 24 in 1998 had the highest fertility rate (197.6) among all women, regardless of race or ethnicity. The fertility rate for this age group is more than twice the rate of White women (90.7). In 1998, Cuban women had the lowest fertility rate (50.1) of all racial and ethnic groups in the United States. Cuban women are also most likely to have their children between the ages of 25 and 29 (data not shown). This can be partly explained by their older median age (see Table 5.1) (Ventura and others, 2000).

In examining selected characteristics of Latino women giving birth in the United States in 1998, we find that Latino mothers were considerably less likely to have completed twelve or more years of education (50.7 percent) than were White and African American mothers (87.2 percent and 73.3 percent, respectively) (Ventura and others, 2000) (see Table 5.4). Specifically, Mexican American mothers had the lowest levels of schooling of all racial and ethnic

Table 5.4. Total Birthrates and Percentage of Births by Selected Demographic Characteristics, Latino Origin of Mothers, Non-Latino Mothers, and Place of Birth of Mothers: United States, 1998

Characteristics	All Origins[a]	Latino						Non-Latino		
		Total Latino	Mexican American	Puerto Rican	Cuban	Central and South American	Other	Total Non-Latino[b]	White	African American
Births	3,941,553	734,661	516,011	57,349	13,226	98,226	49,849	3,158,975	2,361,462	593,127
Rate										
Birthrate[c]	14.6	24.3	26.4	19.0	10.0	23.2		13.2	12.1	18.1
Fertility rate[d]	65.6	101.1	112.1	75.5	50.1	90.2		59.8	56.7	72.6
Total fertility rate[e]	2,058.5	2,947.5	3,198.0	2,268.0	1,560.0	2,719.0[g]		1,919.5	1,837.0	2,235.5
Sex ratio[f]	1,047	1,040	1,037	1,044	1,105	1,042	1,050	1,049	1,052	1,034
All births										
Percentage										
Births to mothers under 20 years	12.5	16.9	17.5	21.9	6.9	10.3	20.2	11.6	9.4	21.6
Fourth and higher-order births	10.5	13.6	14.7	12.3	5.7	11.1	11.0	9.8	8.5	15.0
Unmarried mothers	32.8	41.6	39.6	59.5	24.8	42.0	45.3	30.9	21.9	69.3
Mothers completed 12 years or more of school	78.1	50.7	44.8	64.1	87.0	61.5	66.4	84.4	87.2	73.3
Mothers born in the United States	80.5	39.9	39.7	63.8	39.7	10.1	73.3	89.9	94.9	90.3

Mothers born in the United States				Percentage					
Births to mothers under 20 years	13.6	25.4	26.4	23.7	12.1	21.8	24.0	12.4	9.7	23.3
Fourth and higher-order births	9.9	11.2	11.8	11.1	4.9	5.0	10.8	9.8	8.4	15.1
Unmarried mothers	33.8	48.0	46.3	61.8	25.5	45.8	47.5	32.4	22.5	72.3
Mothers completed 12 years or more of school	82.2	64.5	62.7	64.3	86.1	78.4	67.9	84.0	87.0	72.2
Mothers born outside the United States				**Percentage**					
Births to mother under 20 years	8.1	11.2	11.6	18.7	3.5	9.0	9.8	3.9	3.5	6.3
Fourth and higher-order births	12.8	15.2	16.6	14.5	6.2	11.8	11.5	9.5	9.7	13.7
Unmarried mothers	28.5	37.2	35.1	55.2	24.4	41.6	37.3	16.6	10.7	40.7
Mothers completed 12 years or more of school	61.0	41.4	32.7	63.6	87.6	59.5	62.2	87.6	90.2	83.5

Note: Race and Latino origin are reported separately on birth certificates. Persons of Latino origin may be of any race. In this table, Latino women are classified only by place of origin; non-Latino women are classified by race.

[a] Includes "origin not stated."

[b] Includes races other than White and African American.

[c] Rate per 1,000 population.

[d] Rate per 1,000 women aged 15 to 44 years.

[e] Rates are sums of birthrates for five-year age groups multiplied by five.

[f] Male live births per 1,000 female live births.

[g] Includes Central and South American women and other and unknown Latinas.

Source: National Center for Health Statistics. (2000, Mar. 28). *National Vital Statistics Report, 48, 3,* Table 14.

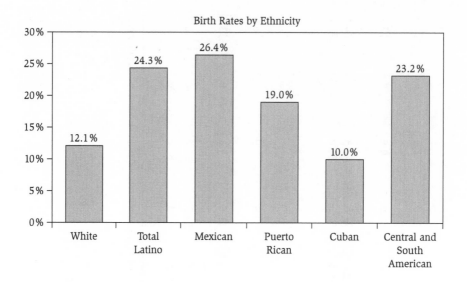

Figure 5.2. Latino Birthrates, 1998

Source: Ventura and others (2000).

groups, with only 44.8 percent reporting twelve or more years of school completed. In 1998, the percentage of Cuban mothers who completed twelve or more years of schooling (87 percent) was the highest, compared to Latino mothers of other nationalities (see Table 5.4) and to African American mothers (73.3 percent). This percentage was similar to that of White women (87.2 percent).

Data by place of birth of mothers shown in Figure 5.3 indicate that Latino women born outside the fifty states and the District of Columbia who gave birth in 1998 were least likely to complete twelve or more years of education (41.4 percent). This was true for women born in Mexico (32.7 percent) and for those born in Central or South America (59.5 percent). No clear pattern emerged in reference to Puerto Rican and Cuban mothers born on either island (see Table 5.4).

The age distribution of Latino women who gave birth in the United States in 1998 indicates that they begin having children at a young age and continue until their older years, with variations by national origin (Ventura and others, 2000). In addition, Latino mothers were more likely than White mothers to give birth to their fourth- or higher-order child (13.6 percent versus 8.5 percent) (see Table 5.4) (Ventura and others, 2000). Mexican American and African American mothers were most likely to have larger families (based on their percentages of fourth- and higher-order births: 14.7 percent and 15 percent, respectively; see Table 5.4). The percentages of fourth- and higher-order births for other Latino groups were as follows: Puerto Ricans, 12.3 percent; Cuban Americans,

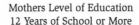

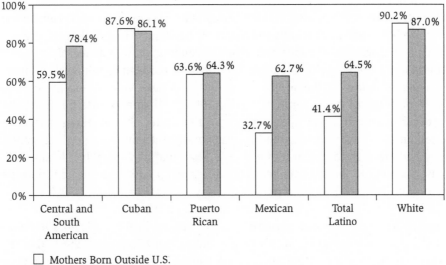

Mothers Level of Education
12 Years of School or More

☐ Mothers Born Outside U.S.
▨ Mothers Born in U.S.

Figure 5.3. Latino Mothers' Levels of Education by Place of Birth, 1998

Source: Ventura and others (2000).

5.7 percent; Central or South Americans, 11.1 percent; and "other and unknown Latinas," 9.8 percent (Ventura and others, 2000).

An area of social concern is the increased number of births to unmarried women. Regardless of ethnicity, the proportion of births to unmarried women has been rising steadily in the United States in recent years (Ventura and others, 2000). Data on marital status shown in Table 5.4 indicate that in 1998, approximately one-third (32.8 percent) of all Latino infants had an unmarried mother, compared to one-fifth (21.9 percent) of White infants and more than two-thirds (69.3 percent) of African American infants (Ventura and others, 2000). African American and Puerto Rican mothers were the groups most likely to give birth out of wedlock (69.3 percent and 59.5 percent, respectively), and Cuban mothers were least likely to do so (24.8 percent). The percentages of births to unmarried women for other Latino groups were as follows: Mexican American mothers, 39.6 percent; Central or South Americans, 42 percent; and "other and unknown Latinas," 45.3 percent (Ventura and others, 2000). Having children out of wedlock leads to sustained poverty not only for women but also for their children and a stressful life often due to limited financial support of the family from the children's father(s), with consequent severe financial problems and strained family relations (Sherraden and Barrera, 1996; Zambrana, Scrimshaw, and Dunkel, 1996).

IMPACT OF ACCULTURATION

Acculturation is the process of incorporating aspects of the mainstream (host) culture into each individual's repertoire of behaviors. External acculturation such as changing food habits and styles of clothing, as well as learning and/or adapting to the majority language, tend to take place first, followed by internal acculturation, or the adoption of cultural beliefs, values, and more complex patterns of behavior (Giachello, 1995). All immigrants confront the process of acculturation upon arriving in the United States. Initial studies in the mid-1980s showed that the Mexican immigrant population, which generally had lower socioeconomic status (SES) than that of Whites, had health indicators similar to those of Whites. This relationship has been referred to in the literature as the "Hispanic paradox" (Hayes-Bautista, 1992; Markides and Coreil, 1986; Scribner, 1996). Further research on the Mexican immigrant population has demonstrated that the effect of SES on health indicators is modified by the acculturation status of the individual (Scribner, 1996). English language fluency and place of birth are usually used as principal markers of acculturation. Other indicators often used are length of time in the community, age at time of immigration, language spoken at home and in the community, celebration of certain cultural events (for instance, *Cinco de Mayo*), and contact with ethnic groups and institutions. Acculturation and its measurement are poorly understood (Zambrana and Ellis, 1995). It has often been said that acculturation or adopting behaviors of the mainstream White culture may lead to negative health outcomes among Latinos (Scribner and Dwyer, 1989; Balcazar and Krull, 1999) and, most recently, among other racial and ethnic groups (for example, Asian immigrants) (Ventura and others, 2000). It has been argued that health status for Latino women deteriorates over time with increasing acculturation to high-risk behaviors such as smoking, alcohol and substance abuse, poor nutrition, and the increased stress of living in U.S. communities (Black and Markides, 1993; Guendelman and Abrams, 1994; Wolff and Portis, 1996).

Lamberty (1994) has summarized some of the "cultural" or "acculturation" explanations in the research literature about the beneficial effect of foreign-born status in reference to Latino pregnancy outcomes:

- Persons with low levels of acculturation maintain indigenous cultural dietary practices, which lead to better nutrition (less sodium, less fat, more fruits and vegetables, and so on).

- Value systems of the indigenous culture promote healthy lifestyles. For example, migrants bring with them or join extended family support networks that buffer the stress generated by the host culture.

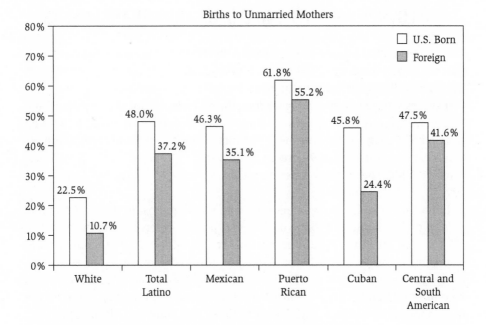

Figure 5.4. Births to Unmarried Mothers by Place of Birth, 1998

Source: Ventura and others (2000).

Apparently, the longer the migrants live in the United States, the more their family and social support networks appear to weaken. Newcomers tend to be healthier, as are their young children (although this may not necessarily be the case for those Latino immigrant groups who have come to the United States as refugees, escaping from violence and political persecution).

The effect of acculturation, measured by place of birth, is clearly seen by the percentage of mothers who give birth out of wedlock (see Figure 5.4). Women, regardless of ethnicity, born in the United States (not including Puerto Rico) were considerably more likely to give birth out of wedlock. The percentages doubled for Whites and almost doubled for African Americans when we examined those born in the United States as opposed to those born in the their countries of origin (Whites, 22.5 percent versus 10.7 percent; African Americans, 72.3 percent versus 40.7 percent; see Table 5.4). This pattern is similar for mothers of other racial groups (for example, various Asian and Pacific islanders (Ventura and others, 2000). Similar patterns emerged regarding adolescent pregnancy and having births of low birth weight, as we will see in the next section.

EMPLOYMENT STATUS AND CHILD CARE ARRANGEMENTS

The 1995 National Survey of Family Growth (NSFG) (Abma and others, 1997) found that 57.8 percent of Latino women aged 15 to 44 were not employed at the time of their most recent childbirth.

This percentage was much higher than the 44.7 percent for White women and 53.5 percent for African American women. Latino women aged 22 to 44 who were employed at the time of the pregnancy were also most likely not to have taken maternity leave (28.9 percent), compared to 39.6 percent and 34.5 percent for White and African American women, respectively (Abma and others, 1997).

In the NSFG, of Latino women who were working most of the time and had at least one child under 5 years of age, 37.3 percent received help in child care from one of the child's grandparents or from another relative, compared to 28.6 percent and 36.3 percent for White and African American mothers, respectively (Abma and others, 1997). This pattern also emerged for Latino women who had children between 5 and 12 years old (Abma and others, 1997), except that White and African American mothers with older children relied less (18.9 percent and 27.9 percent, respectively) on grandparents' support than did Latino women (32.6 percent). Regardless of children's age, Latino mothers depend less on day care centers or preschool (Abma and others, 1997).

In summary, Latino mothers—particularly the Mexican cohort—constitute the most prolific ethnic group in the United States. In 1998, they had the highest birth and fertility rates of all racial and ethnic groups. This was particularly true for women born outside the United States. Latino women were also most likely to have the lowest level of education and to have given birth to four or more children. The impact of acculturation, measured by mothers' place of birth, indicates that Latino women born in the United States are most likely to have children out of wedlock and high levels of adolescent pregnancy, as we will see in the following section.

ADOLESCENT PREGNANCY

Almost 17 percent of the total live births to Latino mothers were to adolescents under the age of 20, which is almost twice as high as those of White teen mothers (9.4 percent) but lower than those of African American teen mothers (21.6 percent; see Table 5.4 and Figure 5.5) (Ventura and others, 2000). Puerto Ricans had the highest teen births (21.9 percent) of all racial or ethnic groups. Teen births were also quite high among mothers of "other and unknown" Latino origins (20.2 percent).

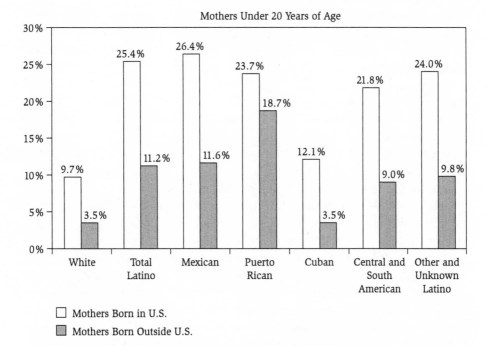

Figure 5.5. Latino Teen Births by Place of Birth and Nationality, 1998

Source: Ventura and others (2000).

Most of the literature indicates that adolescent pregnancy is related to increased sexual activity at an earlier age. Fifty percent of Latino women between the ages of 15 and 17 are sexually active, compared to 34.9 percent and 48.2 percent for White and African American teens, respectively (Abma and others, 1997), and engage in unprotected sex. Other factors that are related to adolescent pregnancy among Latinas are low use of contraceptives (U.S. Department of Health and Human Services, 1999; Piccinino and Mosher, 1998; Abma and others, 1997; Darroch-Forrest and Frost, 1996) and low knowledge about sexuality issues and birth control methods (Abma and others, 1997). Latino women, including teens, are less likely to have received formal health education (35.2 percent) on birth control methods, STDs, or how to say no to sex, compared to 26 percent and 36 percent for White and African American women, respectively. Others are subjected to involuntary sexual intercourse (including rape) that may result in unwanted pregnancy. Approximately 18 percent of Latino women under the age of 16 reported that their first intercourse was not voluntary, compared to 15 percent for Whites and African Americans of the same age group. Another factor that influences adolescent pregnancy rates is the lower abortion rates (Alan Guttmacher Institute, 1999). The Alan Guttmacher Institute (AGI) estimated that the abortion ratio (abortions per

100 pregnancies of Latino women aged 15 to 19) for Latina teens was 27.5 percent. This is lower than the abortion ratio for White adolescents (32 percent) and considerably lower that the abortion ratio for African American teens (40.8 percent) (AGI, 1999). Obviously, differences prevail by levels of acculturation and assimilation of Latino youth into the mainstream culture or place of origin (for example, urban versus rural) if those teenagers were born outside the United States (Figure 5.5). More acculturated adolescents are most likely to be at risk for unwanted pregnancies and to become single mothers. This may be due to conflicts between the value system of the mainstream culture and that of the parents' country of origin or to barriers to accessing the medical care system for contraceptive services and education.

Giachello (1994a) suggests that the high rate of teen pregnancy among Latino women is also related to the fact that Latino adolescents are least likely to use family planning services (Abma and others, 1997). Often teens have no financial resources or health insurance coverage to pay for family planning services or feel embarrassed to approach health clinics for family planning services or to go to the drugstore to purchase contraceptives that do not require prescriptions (for instance, condoms). In addition, family planning services may not be accessible to teens because of distance, inconvenience of clinic hours, and the high cost of care. When teens visit a clinic, they have to complete complicated intake forms, and often there are long waiting periods before they are seen. Awkwardness in using the English language as well as low literacy are additional barriers for many Spanish-speaking teens who may have limited formal education and go to clinics where there are no bilingual or bicultural staffs. If the clinic is in their neighborhood, teens may be worried that community workers or other patients may recognize them and find out the purpose of their visits.

Teen pregnancy is associated with a series of negative social and economic consequences to the mother and her child. Teen pregnancy is the most reported cause of school dropouts among young women. Early childbearing leads to overall lower levels of education, as teen mothers have fewer opportunities to return to school and limited opportunities to enroll in training programs or to go to college (U.S. Department of Health and Human Services, 1999). For married young Latino women, the possibility of going back to school is even lower than for single parents. Married women have the responsibility of both raising a child and taking care of a home and a husband or partner (Giachello, 1994a) or going to work. Those adolescents who marry or live with the father of their child are also more likely to become pregnant again, resulting in larger family size with close spacing of children. This leads to the phenomenon that often is called "excess fertility." Teenaged mothers are also least likely to marry or stay married, resulting in a higher incidence of female-headed households and an increase of what sociologists often call the "feminization of poverty." They are more likely to need public assistance than their peers who are not mothers (U.S. Department of Health and Human Services, 1999). Again, caution is needed, as this pattern may vary depending on adolescents' levels of acculturation, parents' emotional and financial support and involvement, and youth academic or career aspirations and goals.

With regard to the medical consequences of teen pregnancy, studies on the entire population indicate that such pregnancy may lead to complications during both gestation and delivery. Their age is a medical risk factor. Young women's bodies are not prepared for prolonged labor and safe delivery (Giachello, 1994a). The literature on adolescent pregnancy medical risk factors states that dietary and nutritional patterns of teens before and during the pregnancy (for example, adequacy of the diet, amount of folic acid intake, anemia, obesity, or anorexia), social and cultural factors (notably, support from the family and from the baby's father) (Sherraden and Barrera, 1996), and the use of prenatal care are highly important determinants of complications during and after the pregnancy. In reference to nutrition, Gutierrez (1999) found that the most powerful factors contributing to good food practices among pregnant Mexican immigrant teens were maternal concern about the well-being of the offspring and the role of motherhood, as well as family support. For U.S.-born Mexican teens, these concerns were not as strong (Gutierrez, 1999).

Studies also indicate that teen pregnancy, especially of mothers under the age of 15, is associated with low birth weight, neonatal death, high infant mortality, and sudden infant death syndrome (SIDS) (U.S. Department of Health and Human Services, 1999). Some of these consequences are related to a teen's low SES and behaviors before and during the pregnancy. Again, they include poor nutrition; lack of knowledge of proper health care during pregnancy; poor personal health habits or lifestyle practices such as smoking and use of alcohol and illicit drugs (Ventura and others, 2000; U.S. Department of Health and Human Services, 1999; Abma and others, 1997; Substance Abuse and Mental Health Services Administration, 1998); young women's or parents' financial problems; and delays in obtaining prenatal care or not getting medical care at all. Furthermore, the infants may be at greater risk of child abuse, neglect, and behavioral and educational problems at later stages (U.S. Department of Health and Human Services, 1999).

SMOKING BEHAVIOR

Scientific evidence indicates that women who smoke during pregnancy have a higher risk of miscarriages, stillbirths, and premature and low-birth-weight babies than do nonsmokers (Giachello, 2000; Floyd, Zahniser, Gunter, and

Kendrick, 1991; Center for the Future of Children, 1991). On average, in 1998, 4 percent of Latino mothers reported smoking during the pregnancy, compared with 16.2 percent of White mothers and 9 percent of African American mothers (Ventura and others, 2000). Within the Latino population, tobacco use during pregnancy was especially high for Puerto Rican mothers (10.3 percent), particularly those between the ages of 18 and 24 (11.2 percent), and considerably lower for mothers of Central or South American origins (1.5 percent), followed by mothers of Mexican (3.8 percent) and Cuban origins (3.7 percent) (see Table 5.5). Differences by place of birth of the mother (as a marker of acculturation) shown in Table 5.5 indicate that mothers born outside the United States and Puerto Rico reported considerably less smoking behavior during the pregnancy, regardless of race or ethnicity (Ventura and others, 2000).

Studies indicate that regardless of race or ethnicity, pregnant women reduce their smoking behavior during pregnancy but resume it after the birth of the child (Substance Abuse and Mental Health Services Administration, 1998). This means that more aggressive interventions should be implemented to assist and support mothers to abstain from smoking after they have given birth as well as during pregnancy.

ALCOHOL USE

Alcohol use during pregnancy can cause a series of adverse effects such as fetal alcohol syndrome (FAS), which is characterized by growth retardation, facial malformations, and dysfunctions of the central nervous system, including mental retardation and low birth weight (Center for the Future of Children, 1991). Data available on FAS indicate that Latino infants' rates of FAS are comparable to those of Whites (0.8 and 0.9 per 10,000 total births, respectively). The 1997 National Household Survey on Drug Abuse (Substance Abuse and Mental Health Services Administration, 1998) found that 14.1 percent of all pregnant women in childbearing years (15 to 44 years) at the time of the survey reported having used alcohol in the past month. In this age group, those most likely to report this behavior were Whites (15.5 percent) and African Americans (16.7 percent), compared to Latino pregnant women (7.1 percent). Binge drinking in the past month during the pregnancy was low for all women: Whites (1.3 percent), African Americans (1.5 percent), and Latino women (1.0 percent) (Substance Abuse and Mental Health Services Administration, 1998). Furthermore, 0.6 percent of pregnant Latino women reported heavy drinking during pregnancy in the past month, compared to 0.3 percent for the total sample (Substance Abuse and Mental Health Services Administration,

Table 5.5. Percentage of Births with Selected Medical or Health Characteristics by Latino Origin of Mothers, Race for Mothers of Non-Latino Origin, and Place of Birth of Mothers: United States, 1998

Characteristics of Mothers	Latino						Non-Latino		
	Total	Mexican American	Puerto Rican	Cuban	Central and South American	Other	Total[a]	White	African American
All births									
Prenatal care beginning in the first trimester	74.3	72.8	76.9	91.8	78.0	74.8	84.8	87.9	73.3
Late or no prenatal care	6.3	6.8	5.1	1.2	4.9	6.0	3.4	2.4	7.0
Smoker[b]	4.0	2.8	10.7	3.7	1.5	8.0	14.4	16.2	9.6
Drinker[c]	0.0	0.5	0.9	0.5	0.4	1.3	1.2	1.1	1.4
Weight gain of less than 16 pounds[d]	13.4	14.7	12.7	7.8	11.1	12.0	11.0	9.6	16.8
Median weight gain[d]	30.0	28.6	30.5	32.2	30.3	30.4	30.6	30.8	29.8
Cesarean delivery rate	20.6	20.0	21.1	31.0	22.2	18.8	21.3	21.2	22.4
Births to mothers born in the United States									
Prenatal care beginning in the first trimester	76.4	76.0	76.8	91.5	81.7	75.0	85.0	88.1	73.0
Late or no prenatal care	5.1	5.2	5.0	1.4	3.5	5.9	3.3	2.3	7.0
Smoker[b]	7.1	5.4	12.1	5.1	4.7	10.0	15.5	16.7	10.4
Drinker[c]	1.0	0.9	0.9	0.7	0.7	1.6	1.2	1.1	1.5
Weight gain of less than 16 pounds[d]	12.4	12.9	12.1	7.8	8.2	12.3	11.0	9.6	17.1
Median weight gain[d]	30.0	28.6	30.5	32.2	30.3	30.4	30.6	30.8	29.8
Cesarean delivery rate	20.7	20.7	20.8	27.0	20.5	19.6	21.4	21.3	22.2

(Continued)

Table 5.5. Percentage of Births with Selected Medical or Health Characteristics by Latino Origin of Mothers, Race for Mothers of Non-Latino Origin, and Place of Birth of Mothers: United States, 1998 (Continued)

Characteristics of Mothers	Latino						Non-Latino		
	Total	Mexican American	Puerto Rican	Cuban	Central and South American	Other	Total[a]	White	African American
Births to mothers born outside the United States									
Prenatal care beginning in the first trimester	77.1	72.9	77.2	92.0	77.6	74.7	83.0	85.5	76.6
Late or no prenatal care[b]	5.8	7.0	5.1	1.2	5.0	5.9	4.0	3.5	6.4
Smoker[b]	2.6	1.6	8.3	2.8	1.2	1.9	3.8	6.9	1.6
Drinker[c]	0.5	0.3	0.9	0.3	0.3	0.5	0.6	1.0	0.4
Weight gain of less than 16 pounds[d]	12.2	14.3	13.7	7.8	11.5	11.0	10.1	8.5	13.9
Median weight gain[d]	30.0	28.5	30.2	32.2	30.2	30.2	30.3	30.7	29.8
Cesarean delivery rate	20.6	20.5	21.8	33.7	22.4	20.5	20.7	19.7	24.6

Note: Race and Latino origin are reported separately on birth certificates. Persons of Latino origin may be of any race. In this table, Latino women are classified only by place of origin; non-Latino women are classified by race.

[a]Includes races other than White and African American.

[b]Excludes data for California, Indiana, New York State (except for New York City), and South Dakota, which did not report mother's tobacco use on the birth certificate.

[c]Excludes data for California and South Dakota, which did not report mother's alcohol use on the birth certificate.

[d]Excludes data for California, which did not report weight gain on the birth certificate. Median weight gain is shown in pounds.

Source: National Center for Health Statistics. (2000, Mar. 28).

1998). No data were available for White or African American pregnant women or for Latino women of different national origins.

Drinking behavior during pregnancy seems to be associated with marital status and with cultural and social factors. One study examined the alcohol behaviors of White, African American, and Latino women and found that women who are most likely to be heavier drinkers before, during, or after the pregnancy were those who were never married, divorced, or separated (Stroup, Trevino, and Trevino, 1988; Zambrana and Scrimshaw, 1997). Cultural factors (such as Latino women's self-sacrificing role), multiple and conflicting roles, and other psychosocial stressors (unplanned pregnancy, not having the partner's financial or emotional support, not living with the newborn's father) may lead to higher levels of stress and subsequent heavier drinking (Stroup, Trevino, and Trevino, 1988).

Based on the 1998 national birth data, alcohol consumption during the pregnancy was considerably lower for all women. About 1.1 percent of White mothers and 1.4 percent of African American mothers giving birth in that year reported alcohol use during pregnancy (Ventura and others, 2000) (see Table 5.5). The percentage for Latino mothers was even lower (0.6 percent) (Ventura and others, 2000). This behavior increased slightly to 1.3 percent among "other and unknown" Latino women (Ventura and others, 2000). This behavior was slightly less for all women born outside the fifty states and the District of Columbia. Alcohol consumption during the pregnancy is either substantially underreported on the birth certificates for all women, or alcohol use is declining among women during pregnancy. The underreporting of alcohol use might be the result of stigma associated with alcohol consumption, especially during pregnancy, or the potential negative consequences (such as removal of the infant from the mother's home if reported to a child welfare agency). Another explanation for the low percentage of reported alcohol use on the birth certificate might be related to the fact that the national birth data exclude California (a state in which one-third of its population is Latino) (Ventura and others, 2000). The National Household Survey on Drug Abuse (Substance Abuse and Mental Health Services Administration, 1998) found that 16.7 percent of women between 15 and 44 years of age drank alcohol in the previous month of the survey. However, the percentage that reported alcohol consumption during the pregnancy dropped to 1.3 percent, which is consistent with the 1998 national birth data (Ventura and others, 2000). The Substance Abuse and Mental Health Services Administration (SAMHSA) survey also found that the percentage of women of childbearing age who reported binge drinking in the past month and who had a child under the age of 2 was 9.2 percent. This could mean that women resume their alcohol use after the birth of the child (Substance Abuse and Mental Health Services

Administration, 1998) or that they increase their drinking due to the additional tension of raising a child.

NUTRITION AND MATERNAL WEIGHT GAIN DURING PREGNANCY

Overweight is more common in minority populations, particularly women. Combined findings from the 1988–1994 Third National Health and Nutrition Examination Survey (NHANES III) for adults aged 20 to 74 indicate that African American women have the highest prevalence of overweight (53 percent), followed closely by Mexican American women (51.8 percent), compared to 33.9 percent for White women (American Heart Association, 1999). Overweight varies by levels of education and family income, with those having the lowest levels of education and poor or near-poor family income reporting the highest percentages of overweight. This is particularly true among Latinos, regardless of gender. The lack of sustained physical exercise is the main factor for increased overweight among the entire U.S. population, including communities of color. For example, 1988–1991 data from NHANES III indicate that Latino women were least likely to report engaging in physical activity for leisure (43.9 percent), compared to African American women (38.1 percent) or White women (23.1 percent) (American Heart Association, 1999).

Research in the area of pregnancy and nutrition is limited. The number of pregnant women included in most national sample surveys of the general U.S. population is usually too small for analyses that take into account the nutrition-related physiological changes that occur over the nine months of pregnancy (U.S. Department of Health and Human Services, 1999). Maternal weight gain during the pregnancy is one of the key components in the complex relationship between lifestyle characteristics of the mother and the development of the fetus (Chomitz, Cheung, and Lieberman, 1995). In 1990, the National Academy of Science published weight gain guidelines that varied according to the mother's body mass index (BMI) calculated from women's prepregnancy weight and height. The guidelines recommend that women who are underweight (low BMI) gain twenty-eight to forty pounds during pregnancy; those who are of normal weight should gain twenty-five to thirty-five pounds; those who are overweight (25 percent and above BMI) should gain fifteen to twenty-five pounds; and obese women should gain no more than fifteen pounds (Committee on Nutritional Status During Pregnancy and Lactation, Institute of Medicine, 1990). The data in Table 5.5 indicate that Puerto Rican women were most likely among Latino mothers to have gained less weight during pregnancy. The relatively low maternal weight gained by Puerto Rican mothers was associated with having infants of low birth weight (see the section to follow on birth weight) (Ventura and others, 2000).

USE OF PRENATAL CARE

In 1998, 74.3 percent of Latino mothers of all ages who gave birth began prenatal care in their first three months of pregnancy (see Table 5.5). This percentage was considerably lower than that of White mothers (87.9 percent) but similar to that of African American mothers (73.3 percent) (Ventura and others, 2000). Among Latinas by nationalities, Mexican mothers reported the lowest use of early prenatal care (72.8 percent), whereas Cuban mothers reported higher use than White mothers during their first trimester (91.8 percent). In the past ten years, there has been a remarkable increase of use of prenatal services by Latino women (see Figure 5.6) (Ventura and others, 2000).

The effects of prenatal care are difficult to measure (Huntington and Connell, 1994; Fiscella, 1995). Early competent care, however, can promote healthier pregnancies by detecting and managing preexisting medical conditions, providing medical advice, and assessing the risk of poor pregnancy outcome. It can, according to Ventura and others (2000), be vital to maternal health and can serve as a gateway into the health care system, especially for socially disadvantaged women.

In 1998, about 6.3 percent of all Latino mothers had late or no prenatal care at all, compared to 2.4 percent and 7 percent of White and African American mothers, respectively. Within the Latino population, Mexican American mothers

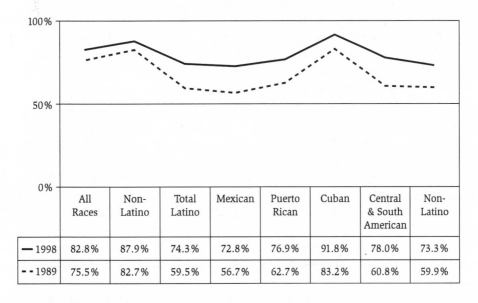

	All Races	Non-Latino	Total Latino	Mexican	Puerto Rican	Cuban	Central & South American	Non-Latino
—— 1998	82.8%	87.9%	74.3%	72.8%	76.9%	91.8%	78.0%	73.3%
- - 1989	75.5%	82.7%	59.5%	56.7%	62.7%	83.2%	60.8%	59.9%

Figure 5.6. First Trimester Prenatal Care: Ten-Year Trend

Source: Ventura and others (2000).

(6.8 percent), those from Central and South America (4.9 percent), and Puerto Ricans (5.1 percent) were most likely to delay or not to go for prenatal care at all (Ventura and others, 2000). The percentage for Cuban mothers was the lowest of any other racial and ethnic group (1.2 percent) (Ventura and others, 2000). The 1998 birth data shown in Table 5.5 indicate that the percentage of prenatal care received varies by mother's place of birth. Latino mothers born in the United States were more likely to go for prenatal care in their first trimester (76.4 percent) than Latino women born outside the fifty states or the District of Columbia (72.9 percent). The only exception is the Puerto Rican mothers. Those born on the island of Puerto Rico were slightly more likely to go for prenatal care in the first trimester of pregnancy (77.2 percent) than those born on the mainland (76.8 percent) (Ventura and others, 2000).

Barriers to Accessing Prenatal Care and Other Services

Latino women confront a series of problems in accessing the health care system for preventive and maintenance health care or for the treatment of illness (Giachello, 1994b, 1995). The high cost of care and the lack of health insurance make it difficult for Latino women to have access to a broad array of preventive health services, including prenatal care. In the 1995 National Survey of Family Growth (NSFG) (Abma and others, 1997), 21 percent of Latino women aged 15 to 44 reported no health insurance coverage, compared to 7.5 percent for Whites and 9.3 percent for African Americans of that age group. Latino women were less likely to be covered by their employers (31.5 percent) or by their husbands' employment insurance (28.3 percent), compared to Whites (38.9 percent and 49.9 percent, respectively) and African American women (42.3 percent and 41.1 percent, respectively) (Abma and others, 1997). The same survey found that the most often used method of payment for recent delivery for Latino women aged 15 to 44 was Medicaid (56.3 percent). The percentage for Medicaid coverage for recent delivery for White women was 23 percent and for African American women 62 percent (Abma and others, 1997). However, having health insurance coverage does not ensure equal access to prenatal care for Latino women, because of inequalities in benefits packages, providers' discretion in deciding which health insurance company to accept, increased search costs due to private cost-containment efforts (for example, deductibles and copayments), and poor quality of care (Raube, Handler, and Giachello, 1995; Oakley, 1990).

Other factors affecting prenatal care use among Latino women are the levels of satisfaction that Latino women experience during such care (Handler, Raube, Kelley, and Giachello, 1996; Brown and Lumley, 1993). In Chicago, Latino women mentioned not minding waiting longer periods of time to see the doctor if their physicians devoted their complete attention to them and answered all the questions they might have about the pregnancy (Handler, Raube, Kelley, and Giachello, 1996).

ANEMIA

Anemia is a condition that occurs often during pregnancy, representing the third most frequently reported complication with a rate in 1998 of 21.8 per 1,000 for all mothers (Ventura and others, 2000). Anemia is more common among mothers under age 20 (30.6 per 1,000), compared with 17.6 for mothers 40 years of age and over (Ventura and others, 2000). In 1998, the rate of anemia per 1,000 live births for Latino mothers was 21.7, compared to 18.4 for Whites. The rate was the highest among African American women (34.6). Among Latino mothers, the rate was almost three times higher among Latino mothers of the "other and unknown" category (44.4), followed by Puerto Rican mothers (32.2), while only 13.9 per 1,000 Cuban mothers reported anemia (see Table 5.6).

GESTATIONAL DIABETES MELLITUS

Gestational diabetes mellitus (GDM) is a condition of insulin resistance that develops during pregnancy or is first recognized during pregnancy; it may lead to respiratory distress syndrome, congenital abnormalities, infant mortality, and heavier birth-weight babies (a condition known as macrosomia or abnormal largeness: birth weight more than 4,000 grams) (American Diabetes Association, 2000; Pierce, Hayworth, Warburton, Keen, and Bradley, 1999; Illinois Diabetes Control Program, 1999; Glasgow and Eakin, 1998; Smits, Paulk, and Kee, 1995; U.S. Department of Health and Human Services, 1998). Having large babies may result in early delivery or harm to the baby or mother during delivery. GDM may also lead to increased incidence of preeclampsia, cesarean delivery, and a longer length of maternal hospitalization. Fetal and perinatal deaths are three to eight times greater in pregnancies of mothers with diabetes than in pregnancies of nondiabetic mothers, as well as congenital malformations in children (American Diabetes Association, 2000). The infant may be born with glycemia or hypoglycemia (high or low levels of glucose in the blood) and may be at higher risk of becoming obese and developing diabetes as a child or during adolescence, particularly in children or youth who do not have proper nutrition and do not engage in regular exercise. Latinos have twice the risk of developing diabetes than do Whites. Puerto Rican women have the highest rate of GDM (34.7 per 1,000), compared to Mexicans (25.4), African Americans (24.9), and Whites (25.6) (American Diabetes Association, 2000) (see Table 5.6). High-risk women are those over the age of 25 who are overweight; have family histories of

Table 5.6. Number and Rate of Live Births to Mothers with Selected Medical Risk Factors, Complications of Labor, and Obstetric Procedures, by Latino Origin of Mothers and by Race of Mothers of Non-Latino Origin: United States, 1998 (×1,000 Live Births)

Medical Risk Factor, Complication, and Obstetric Procedure	Total	Latino						Non-Latino	
		Mexican American	Puerto Rican	Cuban	Central and South American	Other	Total[a]	White	African American
Medical risk factors									
Anemia	22	20	32	14	15	44	22	18	35
Diabetes	27	25	35	21	29	28	27	26	25
Hypertension, pregnancy associated	28	27	32	29	28	37	40	41	41
Uterine bleeding[b]	5	4	7	4	5	5	7	8	5
Complications of labor and/or delivery									
Meconium, moderate to heavy	57	55	62	37	65	58	55	49	77
Premature rupture of membrane	19	17	30	21	20	29	28	28	31
Dysfunctional labor	22	18	34	41	28	36	28	29	26
Breech/malpresentation	30	28	36	38	32	37	41	44	30

Cephalopelvic disproportion	15	15	14	14	15	16	21	22	15
Fetal distress[b]	32	30	41	24	34	38	41	39	52
Obstetric procedures									
Amniocentesis	13	9	23	28	24	22	32	36	16
Electronic fetal monitoring	791	773	877	887	799	831	852	859	840
Induction of labor	129	122	154	182	122	178	207	226	151
Ultrasound	549	527	651	582	559	636	673	699	592
Simulation of labor	163	156	212	166	171	174	181	187	161

Note: Race and Latino origin are reported separately on birth certificates. Persons of Latino origin may be of any race. In this table, Latino women are classified only by place of origin; non-Latino women are classified by race.

[a]Includes races other than White and African American.

[b]Texas does not report this risk factor or complications on the birth certificate.

Source: National Center for Health Statistics (2000, March 28). *National Vital Statistics Report, 48*, 3.

diabetes and/or are Latinas, African Americans, Native Americans, or Asian Americans (American Diabetes Association, 2000; Illinois Diabetes Control Program, 1999); and have a sedentary lifestyle. Latino women who experience diabetes complications during pregnancy are at much higher risk of developing type 2 diabetes within five years after the pregnancy.

HYPERTENSION

Hypertension during pregnancy is self-reported in the birth certificates and is usually classified as chronic or pregnancy-related hypertension (Ventura and others, 2000). Hypertension can lead to preeclampsia or eclampsia complications, a condition during the pregnancy marked by high blood pressure, proteinuria (presence of protein in the urine), and edema (retention of body fluid). If seizures occur, the condition is known as eclampsia or toxemia, which can be fatal for the mother and/or the offspring. Most recent research is associating maternal hypertension and low birth weight among racial and ethnic groups (Fang, Madhavan, and Alderman, 1999).

In 1998, the prevalence of chronic hypertension among mothers of all races was 7.1 per 1,000 live births. This rate doubles among women between the ages of 35 and 39 (13.6) and triples among women between the ages of 40 and 45 (24.8) (see Table 5.6) (Ventura and others, 2000). The rate of pregnancy-associated hypertension in 1998 was considerably higher for mothers of all groups, with a rate of 37.6 per 1,000 live births and increasing to 43.4 for women under age 20 and to 48.0 for women between ages 40 and 54 (Ventura and others, 2000).

The rate was lower for Latino mothers as a whole (27.7), compared to White mothers (41.0) and African American mothers (40.8) (see Table 5.6). The rate was the highest among "other and unknown" Latinas (36.6), followed by Puerto Ricans (31.9). For all women, the rate of eclampsia was considerably lower (3.2), increasing slightly among women under age 20 (4.4) and among older women between 40 and 54 (4.3). No data on the rate of eclampsia were available for Latino women (see Table 5.6) (Ventura and others, 2000).

ASTHMA

Asthma is one of the most common illnesses that complicates pregnancy. Approximately 4 percent of pregnancies are complicated by bronchial asthma (National Heart, Lung, and Blood Institute, 1992). The exact incidence of asthma varies by region. For example, among pregnant Latino women in East Boston, Massachusetts, the prevalence of chronic wheeze syndromes was lower in Latino women than in White women. The asthma condition in this study appears to be strongly associated with women who are active smokers and have a parental history of asthma. Little research, however, has been conducted among pregnant Latino women with asthma to understand its causes and its impact on women and fetuses during pregnancy.

DYSFUNCTIONAL LABOR

This situation occurs when women in active labor suddenly stop making progress without any clear reason or explanation. It can also occur when the head of the newborn is too big in proportion to the mother's cervix. This often occurs when the mother has GDM, as discussed previously. In 1998, Latino mothers as a whole and Mexican American mothers in particular were less likely to have had a dysfunctional labor (22.3 and 18.1 per 1,000) compared to White (29.1) and African American mothers (25.8) (Ventura and others, 2000). However, Puerto Rican and Cuban mothers were considerably more likely to have had a dysfunctional labor (34.4 and 41.4, respectively) (Ventura and others, 2000). This can be explained by the fact that Puerto Rican women usually have poorer health prior to pregnancy and a higher tendency to develop GDM, and Cuban women tend to experience higher pregnancy-related complications because of age and/or genetics. More research is needed in this area to understand ethnic differences better.

Cesarean Section

The rate of primary cesarean section has declined over the past decade from 16.1 per 1,000 to 14.9 per 1,000 (Ventura and others, 2000). Vaginal births after previous cesarean delivery rates have increased from 18.9 per 1,000 to 26.3 per 1,000 (Ventura and others, 2000). In 1998, 20.6 percent of Latino mothers' live births were by cesarean delivery. This rate is slightly lower than those for White and African American mothers (21.2 and 22.4, respectively) (see Table 5.5). However, the rate of cesarean procedures was the highest among Cuban mothers (31.0), regardless of place of birth of the mother, although Cuban mothers born outside the United States had relatively lower rates (27.0) than did Cuban mothers born in the United States (33.7) (Ventura and others, 2000). Older age places Cuban women at higher risk for pregnancy-related complications and therefore for the need to have this procedure done. In addition, in Cuba, cesarean section was fashionable among upper-class Cubans. Also, area variation studies (Goldfard, 1984) have found an association between cesarean procedures performed and mothers having health insurance coverage.

LATINO INFANTS' OVERALL PHYSICAL HEALTH AT BIRTH

The Apgar score is a measure used to evaluate the newborn infant's overall phys-ical condition at birth. This measure consists of five factors: infant heart rate, res-piratory effort, muscle tone, irritability, and color. Each component is assigned a value, which ranges from 0 to 2. The overall score is the sum of the five values, with the score of 10 being optimum (Ventura and other, 2000). Scores are reported at one and five minutes after birth. Data for Latino mothers based on this mea-sure for 1998 indicate that the percentage of Latino babies evaluated as low (a score of less than 7) in the five-minute Apgar score was close to those for White mothers (1.2 and 1.3, respectively), compared to 2.4 for African American mothers. No clear difference emerged regarding the Apgar score and the mother's place of birth (see Table 5.7). The five-minute Apgar score is considered to have better long-term predictive value concerning the infant's health status and survival chances.

Birth Weight

This is considered to be one of the most critical measures of pregnancy out-comes. There is a well-established association between low birth weight and a greatly elevated risk of infant mortality, congenital malformation, mental retar-dation, and other physical and neurological impairments. The birth certificate collects data on very low birth weight (VLBW; those infants born weighing less than 1,500 grams or 3 pounds, 4 ounces) and low birth weight (LBW; those infants born weighing 2,500 grams, or 5 pounds, 8 ounces or less). These measures are generally used as proxies for the adjective *premature*. Latino mothers have rates of VLBW and LBW comparable to those of White mothers (VLBW, 1.1 for each group; Latinos' LBW, 6.4, and Whites' LBW, 6.6). VLBW for Latino mothers slightly increased for those born in the United States, with a rate of 1.3, compared to 1.0 for foreign-born Latino mothers. Puerto Rican mothers, in both Puerto Rico and on the U.S. mainland, were most likely to have higher rates of VLBW babies (1.9 for mainland-born mothers versus 1.8 for those born on the island; see Table 5.7).

Puerto Rican mothers also were most likely to have LBW infants (9.7), as compared to 6.0 for Mexican mothers. LBW is associated with maternal weight gained during the pregnancy. Puerto Rican women were most likely among Latino mothers to have gained less mean weight during the pregnancy. The rate of LBW varies by the mother's place of birth, with Latino mothers born in the United States having a slightly higher rate of LBW (6.4 versus 5.9). Again, regardless of place of birth, Puerto Rican mothers were most likely to have babies of LBW (mainland born, 9.7; island born, 9.6; see Table 5.7) (Ventura and others, 2000).

Table 5.7. Infant Health, Percentage of Selected Medical or Health Characteristics, by Latino Origin of Mothers, Race of Mothers of Non-Latino Origin, and Place of Birth of Mothers: United States, 1998

Medical Risk Factor, Complication, and Obstetric Procedure	Latino						Non-Latino		
	Total	Mexican American	Puerto Rican	Cuban	Central and South American	Other	Total[a]	White	African American
Infant health/all births									
Preterm births[b]	11.4	11.0	13.9	11.4	11.6	12.1	11.6	10.2	17.6
Birth weight									
Very low birth weight[c]	1.1	1.0	1.9	1.3	1.2	1.4	1.5	1.1	3.1
Low birth weight[d]	6.4	6.0	9.7	6.5	6.5	7.6	7.8	6.6	13.2
4,000 grams or more[e]	9.0	9.3	7.1	10.0	9.1	7.7	10.3	11.8	5.3
Five-minute Apgar score of less than 7[f]	1.2	1.2	1.4	0.7	1.0	1.2	1.5	1.3	2.4
Infant health/births to mothers born in the United States									
Preterm births[b]	12.1	11.7	13.6	11.3	11.4	12.6	11.7	10.3	17.9
Birth weight									
Very low birth weight[c]	1.3	1.2	1.8	1.3	1.4	1.4	1.5	1.1	3.1
Low birth weight[d]	7.2	6.7	9.7	7.0	7.1	8.1	7.9	6.6	13.5
4,000 grams or more[e]	8.1	8.4	7.2	8.9	8.4	7.1	10.5	11.9	5.0
Five-minute Apgar score of less than 7[f]	1.3	1.2	1.4	0.8	1.1	1.3	1.5	1.3	2.4

(Continued)

Table 5.7. Infant Health, Percentage of Selected Medical or Health Characteristics, by Latino Origin of Mothers, Race of Mothers of Non-Latino Origin, and Place of Birth of Mothers: United States, 1998 (Continued)

Medical Risk Factor, Complication, and Obstetric Procedure	Latino							Non-Latino		
	Total	Mexican American	Puerto Rican	Cuban	Central and South American	Other	Total[a]	White	African American
Infant health/mothers born outside the United States										
Preterm births[b]	11.0	10.6	14.5	11.5	11.7	10.3	10.5	9.2	14.2
Birth weight										
Very low birth weight[c]	1.0	0.9	1.9	1.3	1.2	1.0	1.4	1.1	2.8
Low birth weight[d]	5.9	5.5	9.6	6.1	6.4	5.9	7.3	6.0	9.9
4,000 grams or more[e]	9.7	10.0	6.9	10.8	9.2	9.4	8.1	11.2	8.2
Five-minute Apgar score of less than 7[f]	1.1	1.1	1.5	0.7	1.0	0.8	1.2	1.0	2.0

Note: Race and Latino origin are reported separately on birth certificates. Persons of Latino origin may be of any race. In this table, Latino women are classified only by place of origin; non-Latino women are classified by race.

[a]Includes races other than White and African American.

[b]Born prior to thirty-seven completed weeks of gestation.

[c]Birth weight of less than 1,500 grams (3 pounds, 4 ounces).

[d]Birth weight of less than 2,500 grams (5 pounds, 8 ounces).

[e]Equivalent to 8 pounds, 14 ounces.

[f]Excludes data for California and Texas, which did not report five-minute Apgar score on the birth certificate.

Source: National Center for Health Statistics (2000, Mar. 28). *National Vital Statistics Report, 48,* 3.

In 1998, 9 percent of all infants born to Latino mothers weighed 4,000 grams (8 pounds, 14 ounces or more), compared to 11.8 percent for White mothers. The percentage for African American mothers was the lowest (5.3 percent). This percentage varies by Latino mothers of different origins, with Cuban mothers experiencing the highest percentage (10 percent) and Puerto Rican mothers the lowest (7.1 percent). This percentage slightly increased for Latino mothers born outside the United States (9.7 percent versus 9 percent), with the exception of mothers born in Puerto Rico. For Latino mothers born in the United States, the difference is most pronounced among Mexican mothers (U.S. born, 8.4 percent; Mexico born, 10 percent) and Cuban mothers (U.S. born, 8.9 percent; Cuba born, 10.8 percent) (Ventura and others, 2000). A number of studies (Zambrana, Scrimshaw, and Dunkel, 1996; Hayes-Bautista, 1992; Guendelman, Gould, Hudes, and Eskenazi, 1990; Sherraden and Barrera, 1996, among others) have demonstrated reduced rates of LBW infants among less acculturated Mexican American women. While LBW rates among Latinos as a group are not among the highest, second-generation Mexican American women are almost twice as likely to experience an LBW outcome than first-generation Mexican immigrants. Zambrana, Scrimshaw, Collins, and Dunkel-Schetter (1997), in a comparative study of Mexican Americans and Mexican-born women, found that Mexican Americans were at higher medical risk during pregnancy but found no significant differences between the two groups in infant gestational age and birth weight. However, the same study did provide evidence that higher acculturation was associated with higher prenatal stress, which was correlated with preterm delivery, substance use, and low social support.

Babies born with LBW vary by the mother's age. In 1998, 6.4 percent of all Latino births were babies born weighing 2,500 grams (5 pounds, 8 ounces) or less. This percentage of LBW infants was close to the percentage of LBW babies born to White mothers (6.6 percent) but considerably less than LBW babies born to African American women (13.2 percent; see Table 5.7) (Ventura and others, 2000). The percentage of Latino LBW babies was highest among older Latino mothers aged 45 to 54 (17.4 percent) and among Latino mothers under the age of 15 (10.5 percent; data not shown on the table) (Ventura and others, 2000). Latino mothers between the ages of 25 and 29 were the least likely to have had LBW babies (5.7 percent) (Ventura and others, 2000). Again, infants born to U.S.-born Latino mothers were at the highest risk.

BREAST-FEEDING

There are numerous advantages to breast-feeding children, including reduced illness in both the mother and the child after birth and a more rapid postpartum recuperation period. According to the American Academy of

Pediatrics (AAP), breast-feeding (Pickering and others, 1998) provides the child with numerous advantages, among them protection against infections, iron deficiency, asthma and other respiratory illnesses, ear infections, bacterial and intestinal disorders, juvenile onset diabetes, and childhood cancer (Wright and others, 1998; Davis, Savitz, and Graubard, 1998). It also reduces the risk of sudden infant death syndrome (SIDS) and Hodgkin's disease and contributes to decreased infant mortality rates (McKenna, Mosko, and Richard, 1997).

Although Latinas are viewed as coming from a breast-feeding culture, nursing rates begin to decline when immigrants settle in the United States. By the third generation, Latinas breast-feed at the same rate as other women in the same socioeconomic group. However, according to the 1995 NSFG (Abma and others, 1997), of the Latino babies born in the combined years of 1990–1993, some 62.2 percent were breast-fed by their Latino mothers, compared to 59.1 percent of babies breastfed by White mothers. Slightly more White women breast-fed their infants for five or more months than Latino mothers (53.3 percent and 50.2 percent, respectively). African American babies were the least likely of the three groups to be breast-fed by their mothers (25.1 percent); when they were, the duration of breast-feeding was relatively short (Abma and others, 1997). Factors that may have an impact on the likelihood of breast-feeding include the mother's age, education, marital status, level of acculturation, employment, perceived benefits of bottle-feeding as opposed to breast-feeding for both the mother's and the child's health, the nature of the interaction with the physician, and the structural characteristics of the health delivery system (Wright and others, 1988; Stern and Giachello, 1977).

Another important factor that affects breast-feeding rates among Latino women is the successful penetration of the baby formula industry into the markets of developing countries such as those in Latin America. Bottle-feeding campaigns attempted to convey the message that using baby formula is healthier for infants than breast-feeding, without consideration of sanitation measures such as access to potable water and proper education regarding the preparation and use of the formula. This trend, in conjunction with a series of myths regarding mothers' inadequacies in their physiological capacity to breast-feed, may explain the decline in breast-feeding rates in Puerto Rico and among groups of Latinas in the United States (Giachello, 1994b). Other factors that affect breast-feeding behaviors are the following: (1) myths such as that it will cause cancer or that thin women and those with small breasts do not produce enough milk to satisfy the new infant; (2) the increased participation of mothers in the labor force; and (3) women's concerns with physical appearance.

INFANT MORTALITY

The infant mortality rate is generally considered a good index of the standard of living of any population group: the lower the infant mortality rate, the better is the standard of living. The rate of infant mortality is also a good indicator of the general health status prevailing in a population.

The infant mortality rate (per 1,000 live births) for Latinos in 1997 was lower than that for non-Latinos (6.0 versus 7.5) (Hoyert, Kochanek, and Murphy, 1999); the rate for African Americans was twice as high (14.2). Among Latino women by nationalities, the infant mortality rate was the lowest among the Mexican American population and the highest among Puerto Ricans. The ten major causes of infant mortality in 1997 for Latino infants as a whole per 100,000 live births were as follows: congenital anomalies (161.3); disorders relating to short gestation and unspecified LBW (73.7); SIDS (47.6); respiratory distress syndrome (26.5); the newborn affected by maternal complications of pregnancy (20.6); the newborn affected by complications of the placenta, cord, and membranes (17.8); injuries and accidents (17.5); infections specific to the perinatal period (16.6); pneumonia and influenza (10.7); and intrauterine hypoxia and birth asphyxia (8.3) (Hoyert, Kochanek, and Murphy, 1999). Studies indicate that infant mortality rates tend to be higher for infants whose mothers began prenatal care after the first trimester, were adolescents or older than age 40, did not complete a high school degree, were unmarried, or smoked during pregnancy (MacDorman and Atkinson, 1998). Infant mortality also has been found to be higher among male infants, multiple births, and infants born preterm or of LBW (Hoyert, Kochanek, and Murphy, 1999). In addition, studies document that infant mortality increases by mother's levels of acculturation, with U.S.-born mothers most likely to have an infant death compared to those born outside the United States. Also, Puerto Rican mothers (both born on the U.S. mainland and in Puerto Rico) are most likely to experience an infant death (Becerra, Hague, Atrash, and Perez, 1991).

MATERNAL DEATHS

In 1997, Latino women experienced higher maternal deaths than did Whites. The crude rate of Latino maternal mortality due to complications of pregnancy, childbirth, and the puerperium for all age groups was higher, 8.0 per 100,000, than that of White women (5.8). The age-adjusted rate of maternal mortality for Latino women was less (7.6), but still almost twice as high as that for White women (4.4) (National Center for Health Statistics, unpublished data for 1997).

African American women have a substantially higher risk of maternal death than do Latinas or Whites; the crude rate for 1997 was 20.8 per 100,000 live births (Hoyert, Kochanek, and Murphy, 1999).

In summary, Latino mothers' pregnancy outcomes are overall quite similar to that of Whites or have outcomes that are in between those obtained by White mothers and African American mothers. Pregnancy outcomes overall were more positive for Mexican mothers and relatively less positive for Puerto Rican women. The impact of acculturation, measured by place of birth, indicates that pregnancy outcomes deteriorate among U.S.-born Latino mothers.

ROLE OF FAMILY PLANNING SERVICES

About three-fourths (74.4 percent) of young Latino women between the ages of 15 and 24 reported receiving help from a family planning service at some point in their lives; this compares to 79.9 percent of White women and 83.1 percent of African American women (Abma and others, 1997). More than one-third of Latinas (36.9 percent) had their family planning visit at a clinic, and an additional 30 percent had it at a private doctor or health maintenance organization (HMO) (Abma and others, 1997). All young women reported receiving help with a birth control method, birth control counseling, or a birth control checkup. Consistently, Latino women were least likely to have received any of those services (Abma and others, 1997).

In 1995, about one-third (32.7 percent) of Latino women (as well as White and African American women) between the ages of 15 and 44 reported receiving family planning services from a medical provider in the twelve-month period prior to the survey (Abma and others, 1997). About one-fourth of Latino women received a birth control method, 15 percent received birth control counseling, 20 percent received a birth control checkup or test, and 3.9 percent received sterilization counseling. The percentages of types of services received by White and African American women were quite close to those of Latinas.

In another national survey among 1,852 women whose incomes were below 200 percent of the poverty level and who were sexually active and between the ages of 18 and 34, Darroch-Forrest and Frost (1996) found that Latino women reported that what they liked the most in their previous gynecological visit were the cleanliness of the facility, respectful and courteous treatment by staff, and the good quality of care. However, the vast majority of Spanish-speaking Latino women (96 percent) in the survey would have liked to have received their services in Spanish (Darroch-Forrest and Frost, 1996).

In the 1995 NSFG, 59 percent of Latino women between the ages of 22 and 44 reported using a method of contraception at the time of the study. This percentage was lower than that of White (66.1 percent) and African American women (62.1) (Abma and others, 1997). The methods that these women most often reported using were female sterilization (Latino women, 36.6 percent; Whites, 24.6 percent, and African Americans, 40.1 percent), the pill (Latino and White women, 23 percent; African Americans, 28.5 percent), and a condom (about 20 percent each) (Abma and others, 1997). The most common form of sterilization reported by all women was tubal ligation, ranging from 20.9 percent among Latinas, 16.3 percent among Whites, and 24.6 percent among African Americans (Abma and others, 1997). Married women of all racial and ethnic backgrounds reported much higher percentages of sterilization. The percentages were higher among White and African American married women (42 percent and 46.2 percent, respectively), compared to Latino women (36.7 percent) (Abma and others, 1997). Also, African American married women reported a much higher percentage of hysterectomies (11.3 percent) than Latino and White women (5 percent and 6.8 percent, respectively) (Abma and others, 1997).

Another study conducted by the Alan Guttmacher Institute (1999), which examined trend data on contraceptive use by women between the ages of 15 and 44 from the National Survey of Family Growth, found that the percentage of Latino women relying on female sterilization increased from 23 percent in 1982 to 37 percent in 1995 (see Table 5.8). There also was a drastic reduction in the use of the IUD (intrauterine device) and the pill. There was also an increase in male condom use, reflecting an acceptance of this method as a result

Table 5.8. Percentage of Distribution of Contraceptive Users Aged 15–44, by Current Method, According to Race and Ethnicity, 1995

Method	Latino	White	African American
Female sterilization	37	25	40
Male sterilization	4	14	2
Pill	23	29	24
Implant	2	1	2
Injectable	5	2	5
IUD	2	1	1
Diaphragm	1	2	1
Male condom	21	20	20
Other	6	7	5
Total	100	100	100
Number (in thousands)	3,957	28,120	5,098

Source: Henshaw (1998).

of the increased awareness of HIV/AIDS and other sexually transmitted diseases (see Table 5.8).

Finally, about 13 percent of Latino and African American women between the ages of 15 and 44 reported in 1995 receiving infertility services to help them get pregnant or to prevent a miscarriage, compared to 16.3 percent for Whites (Alan Guttmacher Institute, 1999). The services most often received were advice (with percentages for all women ranging between 4 percent and 7 percent) or tests on women or men (percentages ranging between 2 percent and 5 percent) (Alan Guttmacher Institute, 1999).

Unintended Pregnancy and Abortion

Data from the 1982, 1988, and 1995 cycles of the National Survey of Family Growth, as well as other supplementary data sets, were used to estimate the 1994 unintended births and abortions among the U.S. population (Henshaw, 1998). The study found that 49 percent of all the pregnancies reported in these surveys in the United States were unintended and that 54 percent of these unintended pregnancies ended in abortion. Among Latino women, the study found that about half of all pregnancies were also unintended, that is, that the women did not want to have a child at that time or wanted no more births. Of the total unwanted pregnancies, about half (26 percent) ended in abortion.

The acceptance of abortion seems to be increasing among Latino women, particularly younger ones, with higher levels of acculturation. A mail survey conducted by the National Latino Institute for Reproductive Health (NLIRH) (1999) found that 37 percent of the respondents said that women should have unrestricted access to abortion, and another 31 percent stated that access to abortion should be granted under almost all circumstances. Furthermore, 55 percent of the mail respondents identified themselves as "prochoice," and a majority (68 percent) said women should have easy access to abortion. Most of the Latino women who supported a prochoice view were Mexican Americans or women of South American origins, were between the ages of 36 and 50, and spoke English fluently. In addition, most of them relied on doctors, Planned Parenthood, and community health clinics for information about birth control. Most of those Latinas who were not prochoice or did not strongly support the prochoice movement were Puerto Ricans, Central Americans, or Cubans; persons whose language was primarily Spanish; or persons between the ages of 16 and 25 (National Latino Institute for Reproductive Health, 1999). Few Latinas said that they rely on the church or school advisers for birth control information, but dependence on the church, according to the NLIRH survey, increased with age (1999). Surprisingly, reliance on family and on friends was relatively low in this study.

HIV/AIDS AND OTHER SEXUALLY TRANSMITTED DISEASES

Through December 1998, women as a group represented 19.1 percent (or 131,446) of all the U.S. adult or adolescent accumulated AIDS cases (688,200) (Centers for Disease Control and Prevention, 1999a, 1999b). Latinas represented 20.2 percent of the total AIDS cases among women. The main modes of transmission for Latino women are heterosexual contact (47 percent) and the use of infected needles (41 percent) during intravenous drug use (IVDU) (Centers for Disease Control and Prevention, 1999a). Prior to the use of a combination of drug therapies to treat HIV infections, AIDS incidence was increasing at rates of 15 to 30 percent each year among African American and Latino women (National Institutes of Health, 1998). Despite a decline of HIV/AIDS among the U.S. population as a whole, the number of new infections continues to increase among women of color. African American and Latino women represent less than one-fourth of the total U.S. female population, but they account for more than three-fourths (82 percent) of new infections between 1995 and 1998 among all infected women (African American women, 64 percent; Latino women, 18 percent) (Centers for Disease Control and Prevention, 1998b; see also Chapter Seven).

Most of the public response in reference to women has been on how to prevent pregnancies among infected women and, if the woman is pregnant, on how to minimize the risk of perinatal transmission and its potential impact on the newborn. Among all the pediatric AIDS cases recorded until December 1998, Latino children under the age of 13 represented 11.5 percent. Perinatal transmission was the main mode of infection for this population (Centers for Disease Control and Prevention, 1999a). In 1994, research showed that zidovudine (called AZT in the United States) therapy given to HIV-infected pregnant women from the fourteenth to thirty-fourth week, continuing throughout the pregnancy and during labor and delivery, and then administered to the child for six weeks after birth could significantly reduce perinatal HIV transmission (Centers for Disease Control and Prevention, 1999a). Antiretroviral therapy has helped to reduce the number of U.S. infants who acquire HIV by 73 percent from 1992 through 1998 (Centers for Disease Control and Prevention, 1999a).

Unfortunately, lack of access to medical care due to financial, cultural, and institutional barriers and lack of knowledge about HIV/AIDS prevention— combined with cultural norms and gender roles, fear of deportation (among undocumented women), and lack of culturally and linguistically competent HIV/AIDS counseling services—are some of the major obstacles that confront poor Latino women who need HIV counseling, testing, and therapy (Kaiser Family Foundation, 1998).

There are more than twenty diseases (including chlamydia, gonorrhea, syphilis, genital herpes [HSV-2], human papillomavirus infection [HPV], hepatitis B, trichomoniasis, bacterial vaginosis, chancroid, and others) that are sexually transmitted, and the trend for each disease varies considerably (Centers for Disease Control and Prevention, 1998b). The latest estimate indicates that there are 15 million new cases of STDs in the United States each year, and while syphilis and gonorrhea have been brought to all-time lows, others, such as herpes and chlamydia, continue to spread widely throughout the population (Centers for Disease Control and Prevention, 1998a, 1998b).

By far, women bear the greatest burden of STDs. The most serious STDs among women are chlamydia (with one out of ten young women infected), followed by gonorrhea and HPV. The prevalence of chlamydia in 1998 was higher among African American, White, and Mexican American women (7 percent, 5 percent, and 2 percent, respectively) than men (6 percent, 2 percent, and 1 percent, respectively). Among teen women aged 15 to 19, the prevalence was more than 12 percent for African Americans, 6 percent for Mexican Americans, and close to 4 percent for Whites (Centers for Disease Control and Prevention, 1999). The prevalence in Puerto Rico in 1997 was much higher, ranging from 5 percent to 10 percent. No data are available for other Latino groups.

The rate of gonorrhea among all women in 1998 was 119.3 per 100,000 (Centers for Disease Control and Prevention, 1998b). It remained almost three times greater for Latinas (69.4 per 100,000) than for Whites (26.0 per 100,000) of all age groups (Centers for Disease Control and Prevention, 1998b); the rate is substantially higher among African Americans (807.9 per 100,000). This condition dramatically affects teen women and young adult women, reaching the rate of 327 per 100,000 among Latino women between the ages of 15 and 19 and 251.6 per 100,000 among Latino women between the ages of 20 and 25. Untreated, both chlamydia and gonorrhea can lead to infertility, potentially fatal ectopic pregnancies, and chronic pelvic pain and scarring; they can also increase an individual's risk of becoming infected with HIV if exposed. Women who are not diagnosed and treated in time during pregnancy are at risk for spontaneous abortion and stillbirth; moreover, gonorrhea and chlamydia can result in serious health problems for newborn infants. For example, chlamydia can cause conjunctivitis in infants born to infected mothers. In general, infants born to mothers with certain STDs are at risk of blindness, mental retardation, and death.

The rate of congenital syphilis is nine times higher among Latino infants than among White infants. Syphilis elimination efforts are critical to improving infant health, slowing the spread of HIV infection, and reducing racial disparities in health. Untreated syphilis during pregnancy can result in infant death in up to 40 percent of cases (Centers for Disease Control and Prevention, 1998b). Syphilis can be a major cause of cardiovascular disease, neurological disease, and blindness for the mother (Centers for Disease Control and Prevention, 1998b). The incidence is higher among men than women, although the rates of primary and secondary syphilis among Latino women is twice the rate of non-Latino women (Centers for Disease Control and Prevention, 1998b).

Human papilloma virus (HPV) infection is the most common STD, affecting 75 percent of the reproductive-age population (Koutsky, 1997). The prevalence among all Mexican Americans is 5.4 per 100,000, and it triples to 14.8 for Mexican Americans between the ages of 20 and 29 (Koutsky, 1997). The rates for African Americans of the same categories are 8.8 and 33.3 per 100,000, respectively; and for Whites, 4.5 and 14.7 per 100,000 (Koutsky, 1997). Herpes is more common among women than men, affecting one out of four women (Centers for Disease Control and Prevention, 1998b).

In summary, health disparities exist among Latinas reflected in the highest rates of HIV/AIDS, chlamydia, gonorrhea, and HPV (Centers for Disease Control and Prevention, 1999b), among other types of STDs. Although most of these conditions have declined for the U.S. population as a whole and for the White population, they have either remained stable for African Americans and Latinos or have increased in the past decade. A Centers for Disease Control and Prevention study (1999b) demonstrates that many young people at risk lack even basic information about how to protect themselves from infection with STDs. Anecdotal information from health providers suggests that Latinos deny the possibility of having any of the STD conditions and that they are not likely to seek health care for STDs unless symptoms are noticeable or are accompanied by pain. However, perhaps the lack of STD knowledge, lack of basic knowledge about how to protect themselves from infection, combined with lack of health insurance and cultural and linguistic barriers to accessing the health care system, might be better explanations for the lack of early screening, diagnosis, and treatment of STDs.

MENTAL HEALTH AND STRESSFUL LIFE EVENTS

In a 1993 national survey, more than one-half of Latino women (53 percent) reported severe chronic depression, compared to Whites (37 percent) and African Americans (47 percent) (Louis Harris and Associates, 1993). This study found that Mexican American women between the ages of 20 and 74 were more than twice as likely as Mexican American men to exhibit high levels of depressive symptoms (18.7 percent versus 8.0 percent). It has been argued that Latino women are exposed to a number of psychosocial and environmental stressors that may lead them to mental illness. These include high poverty, stress associated with single parenting, gender roles, low educational achievement, the effects of migration, the process associated with acculturation and adaptation, domestic violence, and social discrimination (see Chapter Seventeen for more information).

A study investigating the psychosocial factors related to pre- and postnatal anxiety among primiparous Mexican American women in Los Angeles found that high prenatal anxiety was significantly associated with high postnatal anxiety. High postnatal anxiety, in turn, may negatively affect parenting behavior (Engle, Scrimshaw, Zambrana, and Dunkel-Schetter, 1990). High prenatal anxiety was also associated with a lower desire for an active role during labor, lower assertiveness, higher pain expectation, and a lack of support from family members other than the husband. This study, however, did not find any significant correlations of the baby's condition or of complications in labor and delivery with prenatal anxiety (Engle, Scrimshaw, Zambrana, and Dunkel-Schetter, 1990).

USE OF ILLICIT DRUGS

The 1997 National Household Survey on Drug Abuse (Substance Abuse and Mental Health Services Administration, 1998) found that Latinos are less likely than Whites or African Americans to report ever having tried illicit drugs, although they were most likely to report being current users of diverse substances (for example, heroin, cocaine, crack, PCP [phencyclidnine, or "angel dust"], sedatives, tranquilizers, stimulants, or analgesics). These types of drugs are usually associated with physical addiction, excess mortality, and other negative social consequences for the individual, his or her family, and the community. These problems are expected to increase as the percentage of Latinos reporting ever having used cocaine increases, particularly among young adults of both sexes between the ages of 18 and 25 (Substance Abuse and Mental Health Services Administration, 1998). It has been suggested in the literature that Whites may be more likely to experiment with illicit drugs, whereas African Americans and Latinos are more likely to use them regularly (National Council of La Raza, 1990). A series of legal and ethical controversies have emerged regarding substance use during pregnancy. The National Association for Perinatal Addiction Research and Education (1991) found that an increased number of women have been charged nationwide with felony crimes ranging from delivery of a drug to a minor to use or possession of a controlled substance, based on their prenatal drug use. It has been argued that criminalization of prenatal drug use may lead pregnant drug users to either delay their entry into the medical care system or not to use the medical system at all for prenatal care because of fears of prosecution. This may have particularly negative consequences for Latino women who already delay seeing a health care provider for prenatal care or do not see one at all (Giachello, 1991). The patterns of illicit drug use among Latino women require attention and monitoring because pregnant addicted women require special intervention and attention. Despite recent increases in drug treatment rehabilitation programs for women, as yet few have the capacity to treat pregnant women with addiction.

SUMMARY AND CONCLUSIONS

This chapter has summarized current knowledge of reproductive health, maternal risk factors and behaviors, and complications regarding pregnancy, labor, and delivery, as well as health problems and illnesses that affect them the most. Most of the information described indicates that Latino women continue having the highest birth and fertility rates of any other racial and ethnic minority group in the United States. The incidence of teen births and births out of wedlock continues to increase among the Latino groups, particularly to those mothers who have been born in the United States. Latino mothers as a group are least likely to benefit from state-of-the-art medical techniques during prenatal care (such as ultrasound diagnosis) and labor (fetal monitoring). Although most Latinas are not likely to experience complications during delivery, a substantial number may develop gestational diabetes with its associated risks (such as large babies requiring delivery by cesarean section). Finally, the health of Latino infants is comparable to those of White infants, although exceptions in Puerto Rican babies occur (like low birth weight). A series of challenges remain, and they must be addressed to improve the health and well-being of Latino mothers and children.

RECOMMENDATIONS

- *Diversity of Latino women.* Currently, we know very little about the health and social needs of women from Central or South America. We know little about posttraumatic stress disorders that many of them might be experiencing as a result of their personal and family experiences related to political persecution or wars in their countries of origin. Also, we know little about the diverse health beliefs and behaviors of Mexican American and Puerto Rican populations. From the research perspective and for effective program development and planning, we need to examine such differences as they reflect specific places of origin (for example, rural villages versus small towns versus big cities).
- *Financial investment in public health.* About 70 percent of premature deaths and illnesses are preventable. They are related to environmental health factors and to individual behaviors and lifestyles. However, 90 percent of U.S. health care resources go to cover medical treatment of conditions once they have occurred. This must change.
- *Race and sex bias.* There is a need to reduce institutional racism and sexism, which deprive Latino communities of socioeconomic opportunities, have

a negative impact on the quality of life of communities by producing low self-esteem, and cause a series of psychosocial stresses that increase the risk factors for a number of health and mental illnesses. A recent study on race, ethnicity, and medical care commissioned by the Kaiser Family Foundation (1999) found that 13 percent of Latinos reported that either they themselves had directly experienced unfair treatment in seeking medical care or a family member had done so (25 percent) or a friend or someone else they knew (25 percent).

• *Increase access to health and medical care.* Recent research and data indicate that 35 percent of Latinos are not linked to a regular source of health care (Kaiser Family Foundation, 1999) and about 35.3 percent do not have health insurance (Giachello, 2000). The lack of health insurance goes up to 44 percent for poor Latinos, compared to 28.5 percent for poor Whites (U.S. Bureau of the Census, 1999). Furthermore, half of the poor foreign residents in the United States and half of those who are not citizens do not have health insurance (53.3 percent and 58.6 percent, respectively). Therefore, strong policies need to be developed at the national level that clearly convey the message that access to health care is a fundamental human right and not a privilege. Sooner or later, the United States must recognize this essential self-evident truth: that without health, "we the people" cannot work, take care of our families, or be productive members of society.

• *Culturally appropriate programs.* There must be a strong commitment to developing, implementing, and institutionalizing culturally appropriate programs and approaches in the delivery of health care, as well as in reducing linguistic barriers to medical services.

• *Monitor accessibility to health and medical services under managed care.* A number of concerns have been raised about marketing strategies of HMOs directed to Latinos and other communities and the poor quality of care provided to individuals and families enrolled in these plans. The mainstream media, through cases that have come to public attention or to the courts, have documented the barriers to accessing specialists and hospitals or even emergency rooms; the limited support and follow-up services that these HMOs have in place; and the consequences in terms of premature deaths and serious disabilities. There is a need to scrutinize these practices as well as the types of incentives provided by HMOs to health care providers to limit services to patients, including the amount of time spent with each patient, and other possible violations of patients' rights.

• *Improve the quality of health and medical care.* Studies have documented variations in the quality of medical care in relation to certain medical procedures used (such as cesareans) and certain patient characteristics (notably having or not having health insurance) (see Lawlor and Raube, 1995). Part of the problem is that physicians and other health care providers have limited familiarity with clinical guidelines and appropriate protocols for the management and treatment of certain conditions such as asthma, diabetes, and cancer (McDermott, Silva, Giachello, and Rydman, 1996; Lipton, Losey, and Giachello, 1996; Raube, Handler, and Giachello, 1995).

• *Innovative interventions.* The federal government's Racial and Ethnic Approaches to Community Health (REACH) 2010 initiative to eliminate health disparities is a clear example of needed interventions in communities of color. This initiative is aimed at the community as a whole by creating coalitions with health and human services organizations aimed at changing community norms, as well as the development of culturally appropriate and gender-appropriate interventions and the supportive environment for sustaining behavioral changes. Part of this effort is to study the impact of Medicaid and Medicare managed care plans: how they have been implemented, how they have been accepted by poor communities of color and by elderly Latinos, and what the quality of care is that Latinos enrolled in those plans are receiving from them. There is also a need to get managed care organizations to collect data on demographic and socioeconomic characteristics of enrollees to determine the impact of these systems on the health of Latinos in general and of Latino women in particular.

• *Improve data systems.* Tremendous progress has occurred in the past decade in generating more and better data and research on Latinos (including Latinas), yet more progress is needed in collecting information pertaining to diverse Latino groups. For example, the fastest-growing Latino populations are those coming from Central and South America, but data on them are categorized (that is, grouped together) as "Central and South American," and details are practically nonexistent. This category does not provide the needed information that would enable us to understand the health profile of each population in particular and to develop the necessary individual interventions. Local data are very limited even for the larger Latino populations such as recent Mexican immigrants and Mexican Americans. Many public health departments do not have the financial resources or staffing to develop or support an infrastructure for the gathering, analyses, and dissemination of data, or the data systems do not have the ethnic identifiers to produce detailed information. At the national level, there are also a number of deficiencies: the National Health and Nutritional Examination Survey includes samples of Mexican Americans, yet no information is included for Puerto Ricans or for any other Latino groups, and the national data system does not include the data from the island of Puerto Rico, making it difficult to assess the health of Puerto Ricans who come back and forth from the island. This information could be valuable in understanding the health problems and patterns of health services utilization, as well as risk factors.

• *Assessment of public policy impact.* There is a great need to investigate the performance and impact of public policies such as welfare reform, immigration reform, Medicaid and Medicare managed care plans, child care legislation, and health insurance for children on the life of Latino men, women, and children.

- *Increase the number of Latinos in health professions and workforce.* To increase the representation of Latinos in the health fields in proportion to their total U.S. population, an additional 225,000 Latinos are needed (Gray and Puente, 1996). To accomplish this goal at present seems almost impossible, as Latinos are increasingly going to public or private segregated schools located in areas where those schools have limited financial resources to provide them with the technology for top scientific education and with the resources (financial and human) to teach them well. Moreover, nationally it is estimated that only 3 percent of teachers are Latinos; therefore, the lack of mentorship and role models makes it more difficult to encourage Latino students to enter and finish courses of study at health professional school.

Specific Recommendations for Latino Women's Health

1. There is a need to educate and support immigrants' families about their daughters (born or raised in the United States) and about their increased risks of unwanted pregnancies, injuries, homicide, HIV/AIDS and other STDs, and tobacco, alcohol, and other drug use.

2. There is a need to study effective ways to engage Latino communities in risk reduction behaviors to delay the development of diabetes and other chronic conditions before, during, and after pregnancy, such as supporting exercise, healthy eating, and developing or maintaining other healthy behaviors.

3. There is a need to study biological, behavioral, environmental, and social processes, including community norms, that determine the physical, emotional, and cognitive growth of Latinas from the moment of inception and through transitions of infancy, childhood, and adolescence, which set the foundation for conditions, diseases, and behaviors that have an impact on human reproduction and ultimately lead to health disparities.

4. There is a need to study the quality of prenatal care and Latino women's access to available and new technology during labor and delivery. The information provided in this chapter indicates that Latino women are least likely to receive the benefits of the available technology in the area of perinatal health.

5. There is little or no research in the area of eating disorders (for example, obesity and anorexia) or estimates about the prevalence of eating disorders in Latino communities.

References

Abma, J., and others. "Fertility, Family Planning and Women's Health: New Data from the 1995 National Survey of Family Growth. National Center for Health Statistics." *Vital and Health Statistics,* 1997, *23,* 19.

Alan Guttmacher Institute. *Teenage Pregnancy: Overall Trends and State-by-State Information.* Washington, D.C.: Alan Guttmacher Institute, 1999.

American Diabetes Association. *Clinical Guidelines on Diabetes Care.* Washington, D.C.: American Diabetes Association, 2000.

American Heart Association. *2000 Heart and Stroke Statistical Update.* Dallas: American Heart Association, 1999.

Balcazar, H., and Krull, J. "Determinants of Birth-Weight Outcomes Among Mexican-American Women: Examining Conflicting Results About Acculturation." *Ethnicity and Disease,* 1999, *9*(3), 410–422.

Becerra, J. E., Hague, C. J., Atrash, H., and Perez, N. "Infant Mortality Among Hispanics: Portrait of Heterogeneity." *Journal of the American Medical Association,* 1991, *265,* 217–221.

Black, S. A., and Markides, K. S. "Acculturation and Alcohol Consumption in Puerto Rican, Cuban-American, and Mexican-American Women in the United States." *American Journal of Public Health,* 1993, *83,* 6, 890–893.

Brown, S., and Lumley, J. "Antenatal Care: A Case of the Inverse Care Law?" *American Journal of Public Health,* 1993, *17,* 19–103.

Center for the Future of Children. *The Future of Children: Drug-Exposed Infants.* Los Altos, Calif.: David and Lucile Packard Foundation, 1991.

Centers for Disease Control and Prevention. *National STD Prevention in the New Millennium Conference.* Dallas, Dec. 6–9, 1998a.

Centers for Disease Control and Prevention. *Tracking the Hidden Epidemics Trends in STDs in the United States.* Atlanta, Ga.: Centers for Disease Control and Prevention, 1998b.

Centers for Disease Control and Prevention. *HIV/AIDS Surveillance Report: U.S. HIV/AIDS Cases Reported Through December 1998.* Atlanta, Ga.: Centers for Disease Control and Prevention, 1999a.

Centers for Disease Control and Prevention. *National HIV Seroprevalence Surveys: Summary of Results. Data from Serosurveillance Activities Through 1998.* Atlanta, Ga.: Centers for Disease Control and Prevention, 1999b.

Centers for Disease Control and Prevention. *Tobacco Use in the U.S.: Report from the U.S. Surgeon General.* Washington, D.C.: Government Printing Office, 1999c.

Chomitz, V. R., Cheung, L.W.Y., and Lieberman, E. "The Role of the Lifestyle in Preventing Low Birth Weight." *Future of the Children: Low Birth Weight,* 1995, *5*(1).

Committee on Nutritional Status During Pregnancy and Lactation, Institute of Medicine. *Nutrition During Pregnancy: Part I: Weight Gain, Part II: Nutrient Supplements.* Washington, D.C.: National Academy Press, 1990.

Darroch-Forrest, J., and Frost, J. "The Family Planning Attitudes and Experiences of Low-Income Women." *Family Planning Perspectives,* 1996, *28,* 246–255, 277.

Davis, M. K., Savitz, D. A., and Graubard, B. "Infant Feeding and Childhood Cancer." *Lancet,* 1998, *2*(8607), 365–368.

Engle, P., Scrimshaw, S., Zambrana, R. E., and Dunkel-Schetter, C. "Prenatal and Post-natal Anxiety in Mexican Women Giving Birth in Los Angeles." *Health Psychology,* 1990, *9*(3), 285–299.

Fang, J., Madhavan, S., and Alderman, M. H. "The Influence of Maternal Hypertension on Low Birth Weight: Differences Among Ethnic Populations. *Ethnicity and Disease,* 1999, *9*(3), 369–376.

Fiscella, K. "Does Prenatal Care Improve Birth Outcomes? A Critical Review." *Obstetrical and Gynecology,* 1995, *85*(3), 46–79.

Floyd, R. L., Zahniser, S. C., Gunter, E. P., and Kendrick, J. S. "Smoking During Pregnancy: Prevalence, Effects, and Intervention Strategies." *Birth,* 1991, *18*(1), 48–53.

Giachello, A. L. "Issues of Substance Abuse and AIDS Among Women, Infants and Children." In *Common Ground: HIV/AIDS, Alcoholism and Illicit Drug Use.* Chicago: Illinois Prevention Resource Center, 1991.

Giachello, A. L. "Issues of Access and Use." In C. W. Molina and M. Aguirre-Molina (eds.), *Latino Health in the U.S.: A Growing Challenge.* Washington, D.C.: American Public Health Association, 1994a.

Giachello, A. L. "Maternal/Perinatal Health Issues." In C. W. Molina and M. Aguirre-Molina (eds.), *Latino Health in the U.S.: A Growing Challenge.* Washington, D.C.: American Public Health Association, 1994b.

Giachello, A. L. "Cultural Diversity and Institutional Inequality." In D. L. Adams (ed.), *Health Issues for Women of Color: Cultural Diversity Perspective.* Thousand Oaks, Calif.: Sage, 1995.

Giachello, A. L. "Issues and Challenges in Eliminating Health Disparities Among Hispanics/Latinos in the U.S." Presentation at a televised meeting, Chapel Hill School of Public Health, Chapel Hill, N.C., 2000.

Glasgow, R. E., and Eakin, E. G. "Issues in Diabetes Self-Management. In S. A. Schumaker and others (eds.), *The Handbook of Health Behavior Change.* New York: Springer, 1998.

Goldfard, M. G. *Who Receives Cesareans: Patient and Hospital Characteristics.* Washington, D.C.: National Center for Health Services Research, 1984.

Gray, J., and Puente, S. "Overview of Hispanic/Latinos." *Journal of Medical Systems,* 1996, *20*(5), 229–233.

Guendelman, S., and Abrams, B. "Dietary, Alcohol and Tobacco Intake Among Mexican-American Women of Childbearing Age: Results from NHANES Data." *American Journal of Health Promotion,* 1994, *8*(5), 363–372.

Guendelman, S., Gould, J. B., Hudes, M., and Eskenazi, B. "Generational Differences in Prenatal Health Among the Mexican American Population: Findings from NHANES, 1982–1984." *American Journal of Public Health,* 1990, *80*(Suppl.), 761–765.

Gutierrez, Y. M. "Cultural Factors Affecting Diet and Pregnancy Outcome of Mexican American Adolescents." *Journal of Adolescent Health,* 1999, *25*(3), 227–237.

Hajat, A., Lucas, J., and Kington, R. "Health Outcomes Among Hispanic Subgroups: Data from the National Health Interview Survey, 1992–95." Atlanta, Ga.: Centers for Disease Control and Prevention, Feb. 25, 2000.

Handler, A., Raube, K., Kelley, M., and Giachello, A. "Women's Satisfaction with Prenatal Care Settings: A Focus Group Study." *Birth,* 1996, *23*(1), 31–37.

Hayes-Bautista, D. E. "Latino Health Indicators and the Underclass Model: From Paradox to New Policy Models." In A. Furino (ed.), *Health Policy and the Hispanic.* Boulder, Colo.: Westview Press, 1992.

Henshaw, S. "Unintended Pregnancy in the United States." *Family Planning Perspectives,* 1998, *30*(1), 24–29, 46.

Hoyert, D. L., Kochanek, K. D., and Murphy, S. L. *Deaths: Final Data for 1997.* Hyattsville, Md.: National Center for Health Statistics, 1999.

Huntington, J., and Connell, F. A. "For Every Dollar Spent: The Cost-Savings Arguments for Prenatal Care." *New England Journal of Medicine,* 1994, *331*(19), 1303–1307.

Illinois Diabetes Control Program. *Diabetes Clinical Practice Recommendations.* Springfield: Illinois Department of Health and Human Services, 1999.

Kaiser Family Foundation. *National Survey of Latinos on HIV/AIDS.* Menlo Park, Calif.: Kaiser Family Foundation, Spring 1998.

Kaiser Family Foundation. *Medicare and Minorities.* Menlo Park, Calif.: Kaiser Family Foundation, 1999.

Koutsky, J. L. "Epidemiology of Genital Human Papillomavirus Infection." *American Journal of Medicine,* 1997, *102*(5A), 3–8.

Lamberty, G. "Infant Mortality: Experience of Hispanics." Paper presented to the 1994 National Advisory Committee on Infant Mortality, Washington, D.C., 1994.

Lawlor, E., and Raube, K. "Social Interventions and Outcomes in Medical Effectiveness Research." *Social Science Review,* 1995, *69,* 383–403.

Lipton, R., Losey, L., and Giachello, A. "Factors Affecting Diabetes Treatment and Patient Education Among Latinos: Results of a Preliminary Study in Chicago." *Journal of Medical Systems,* 1996, *20*(5), 267–276.

Louis Harris and Associates. *The Commonwealth Fund Study of Women's Health.* New York: Commonwealth Fund, 1993.

MacDorman, M. F., and Atkinson, J. O. "Infant Mortality Statistics from the 1996 Period Linked Birth/Infant Death Data Set." *Monthly Vital Statistics Report,* 1998, *46*(12, Suppl.).

Markides, K. S., and Coreil, J. "The Health of Hispanics in the Southwestern United States: An Epidemiologic Paradox." *Public Health Reports,* 1986, *101*(3), 253–265.

McDermott, M., Silva, J., Giachello, A. L., and Rydman, R. "Practice Variations in Treating Urban Minority Asthmatics in Chicago." *Journal of Medical Systems,* 1996, *20*(5), 255–266.

McKenna, J. J., Mosko, S. S., and Richard, C. A. "Bedsharing Promotes Breast Feeding." *Pediatrics,* 1997, *100,* 214–219.

Napoles-Springer, A., and Pérez-Stable, E. "Risk Factors for Invasive Cervical Cancer in Latino Women." *Journal of Medical Systems,* 1996, *20*(5), 277–294.

National Association for Perinatal Addiction Research and Education. *Criminalization of Prenatal Drug Use: Punitive Measures Will Be Counterproductive.* Chicago: National Association for Perinatal Addiction Research and Education, 1991.

National Council of La Raza. *Hispanic Consultation on Alcohol and Substance Abuse: A Community Network Response.* Washington, D.C.: National Council of La Raza, Nov. 17–20, 1990.

National Heart, Lung, and Blood Institute. *Executive Summary: Management of Asthma During Pregnancy: Report of the Working Group on Asthma and Pregnancy.* Bethesda, Md.: National Institutes of Health, 1992.

National Institutes of Health. Office of Women's Health Research. *Summary Report of Women's Health.* Bethesda, Md.: National Institutes of Health, 1992.

National Institutes of Health. Office of Women's Health Research. *Women of Color Health Data Book.* Bethesda, Md.: National Institutes of Health, 1998.

National Latino Institute for Reproductive Health. Latina Abortion Survey. *Instantes.* Winter, 1999.

Oakley, A. "Using Medical Care: The Views and Experiences of High-Risk Mothers." *Health Services Research,* 1990, *26*(5), 651–669.

Piccinino, L. J., and Mosher, W. D. "Trends in Contraceptive Use in the United States: 1982–1995." *Family Planning Perspectives,* 1998, *30*(1), 4–10, 46.

Pickering, L., and others. "Modulation of the Immune System by Human Milk and Infant Formula Containing Nucleotides." *Pediatrics,* 1998, *101,* 242–249.

Pierce, M., Hayworth, J., Warburton, F., Keen, H., and Bradley, C. "Diabetes Mellitus in the Family: Perceptions of Offspring's Risk." *Diabetics Medicine,* 1999, *16*(5), 431–436.

Raube, K., Handler, A., and Giachello, A. L. "Quality of Prenatal Care of Latinas in the Midwest." Paper presented at the 123rd American Public Health Association annual meeting, Washington, D.C, 1995.

Scribner, R. "Paradox as Paradigm: The Health Outcomes of Mexican Americans." *American Journal of Public Health,* 1996, *86*(3), 303–305.

Scribner, R., and Dwyer, J. "Acculturation and Low Birthweight Among Latinos in the Hispanic HANES." *American Journal of Public Health,* 1989, *79*(9), 1263–1267.

Sherraden, M., and Barrera, R. "Prenatal Care Experiences and Birth Weight Among Mexican Immigrant Women." *Journal of Medical Systems,* 1996, *20*(5), 329–350.

Smits, W., Paulk, T., and Kee, C. "Assessing the Impact of an Outpatient Education Program for Patients with Gestational Diabetes." *Diabetes Educator,* 1995, *21*(2), 129–134.

Stern, G., and Giachello, A. L. "Applied Research: The Latino Mother-Infant Project." Paper presented at the annual meeting of the American Anthropology Association, New York, 1977.

Stroup, M., Trevino, F. M., and Trevino, D. "Alcohol Consumption Patterns Among Mexican-American Mothers and Children from Single- and Dual-Headed Households." *American Journal of Public Health*, 1988, *80*(Suppl.), 36–41.

Substance Abuse and Mental Health Services Administration. *Preliminary Results from the 1997 National Household Survey on Drug Abuse.* Bethesda, Md.: Substance Abuse and Mental Health Services Administration, 1998.

U.S. Bureau of the Census. *The Hispanic Population in the United States, Population Characteristics, March 1998.* Washington, D.C.: U.S. Department of Commerce, Dec. 1999.

U.S. Bureau of the Census. *The Hispanic Population in the United States: March, 1999.* Washington, D.C.: U.S. Government Printing Office, Feb. 2000.

U.S. Department of Health and Human Services. *Healthy People 2010—Conference Edition.* Washington, D.C.: U.S. Government Printing Office, 1999.

U.S. Department of Health and Human Services. *Tobacco Use Among U.S. Racial/ Ethnic Minority Groups: A Report of the Surgeon General.* Washington, D.C.: U.S. Government Printing Office, 1998.

Ventura, S. J., and others. *Births: Final Data for 1998.* Hyattsville, Md.: National Center for Health Statistics, 2000.

Wolff, C. B., and Portis, M. "Smoking, Acculturation, and Pregnancy Outcome Among Mexican Americans." *Health Care for Women International*, 1996, *17*(6), 563–573.

Wright, A. L., and others. "Infant Feeding Practices Among Middle-Class Anglos and Hispanics (Pt. 2)." *Pediatrics*, 1988, *82*, 496–503.

Wright, A. L., and others. "Increasing Breastfeeding Rates to Reduce Infant Illness at the Community Level." *Pediatrics*, 1998, *101*, 837–844.

Zambrana, R. E., and Ellis, B. K. "Contemporary Research Issues in Hispanic/Latino Women's Health." In D. Adams (ed.), *Health Issues for Women of Color: A Cultural Diversity Perspective.* Thousand Oaks, Calif.: Sage, 1995.

Zambrana, R. E., and Scrimshaw, S. C. "Maternal Psychosocial Factors Associated with Substance Use in Mexican-Origin and African-American Low-Income Pregnant Women." *Pediatric Nursing*, 1997, *23*(3), 253–259.

Zambrana, R. E., Scrimshaw, S., Collins, N., and Dunkel-Schetter, C. "Prenatal Health Behaviors and Psychosocial Risk Factors in Pregnant Women of Mexican Origin: The Role of Acculturation." *American Journal of Public Health*, 1997, *87*(6), 1022–1026.

Zambrana, R. E., Scrimshaw, S., and Dunkel, C. "Prenatal Care and Medical Risk in Low-Income, Primiparous, Mexican-Origin and African American Women." *Families, Systems and Health*, 1996, *14*(3), 349–359.

CHAPTER SIX

Agency and Constraint

Sterilization and Reproductive Freedom Among Puerto Rican Women in New York City

Iris Lopez

This chapter examines the historical and current factors that influence the use of sterilization as a birth control method among Puerto Rican women in New York City and in Puerto Rico. The historical and structural backgrounds provide important insights into the political and social evolution of the factors that resulted in the unprecedented sterilization guidelines for informed consent adopted in the United States—guidelines that have affected the lives of all poor women and women of color in the United States. As noted in the dedication of this book, Dr. Helen Rodriguez-Trias was instrumental in the passage of the guidelines.

This chapter focuses on the social, historical, and personal conditions that shape, influence, and constrain Puerto Rican women's fertility decisions with respect to sterilization.[1] It examines the reasons that Puerto Rican women have one of the highest documented rates of sterilization in the world by concentrating on the interplay between resistance and constraints and by teasing out some of the contradictions in their reproductive decisions about sterilization.[2] It also highlights the diversity of experiences that sterilized Puerto Rican women have with *la operación,* the colloquial term used to refer to sterilization among Puerto Rican women.

With the exception of cases of sterilization abuse, this ethnographic study demonstrates that Puerto Rican women make decisions about sterilization that are limited by their sociopolitical conditions. Their reproductive decisions are based on a lack of options circumscribed by a myriad of personal, social, and

I thank my good friends Alice Colon and Caridad Souza for reading and discussing my chapter and for their insightful and editorial recommendations.

historical forces that operate simultaneously to shape and constrain Puerto Rican women's fertility options. Presenting women as active agents of their reproductive decisions does not suggest that they are exercising free will or that they are not oppressed but that they make decisions within the limits of their constraints. As their oral histories reveal, women do actively seek to transform and improve their lives, and controlling their reproduction is one of the primary means of which they avail themselves to do so. Yet as their oral histories also show, the constraints of their lives play an equally significant role in shaping their reproductive decisions and experiences. Consequently, this study takes into account the role that class, race, and gender play in determining the range of options that individuals have available and how much control they have over them. While it is undeniable that all women have had their fertility options limited by the types of contraceptives developed and because they have had to bear much of the burden of population control, it is imperative to recognize that poor women are even more constrained.

It is also important to note that while the social and economic forces that limit Puerto Rican women's fertility options are not more or less constraining for them than they are for other lower-income people, particularly poor women of color, the historical antecedents that have led to the high rate of sterilization among Puerto Rican women are unique. In exploring the reasons for the high rate of sterilization among Puerto Rican women, I reformulate the binary model between submission and agency as well as withstand the temptation to use the term *resistance* in a monolithic way in the context of this study. I found that there are "elements of resistance" in their attempts to forge a social space for themselves on a personal level. Some women use sterilization as an "element of resistance" against the constraints of patriarchy/female subordination that subject them to double standards and make them primarily responsible for their fertility, child rearing, and domestic work. Other personal difficulties related to female subordination such as abusive relationships that involve substance abuse also play an important role in some women's decisions to become sterilized. However, these "elements of resistance" do not make their decisions entirely defiant and conscious acts of resistance or a complete break with the social conditions that have perpetuated high rates of sterilization.

In contrast to most of the studies on Puerto Rican women's reproductive experiences, I diverge from an exclusively cultural perspective that focuses on the women themselves as the principal unit of analysis and consider women within the wider structural and historical contexts that gave rise to and continue to perpetuate the high rate of sterilization. This aspect of Puerto Rican women's reproductive experience is as much a political as a cultural phenomenon and ultimately speaks to wider issues of reproductive control and women doing the best that they can with their lives within the parameters of their sociopolitical oppression.[3]

MIGRATION AND STERILIZATION: TWO SIDES OF THE POPULATION COIN

In order to understand the reasons that Puerto Rican women in Puerto Rico as well as in the United States have such a high rate of sterilization, it is essential to examine the sociopolitical and ideological framework in which sterilization developed in the island. Puerto Rico became a colony of the United States in 1898. As early as 1901, government officials attributed Puerto Rico's poverty and underdevelopment to an "overpopulation problem." Though the "problem of overpopulation" in Puerto Rico was more the result of U.S. capitalist, policy, and legislative interests than of uncontrollable growth in population, an ideology of population was developed and implemented as a rationale for encouraging the migration of Puerto Ricans along with the sterilization of over one-third of all Puerto Rican women (Bonilla and Campos, 1983).[4] As a result of this ideology, migration was used as a temporary escape valve to the "overpopulation problem," while they experimented with more lasting and efficacious solutions, such as sterilization and diverse methods of fertility control.[5]

In New York City, sterilization became available for "birth control" purposes in the decade of the sixties. Puerto Rican women migrating to New York City in the fifties were already familiar with *la operación* because of its extensive use in Puerto Rico. By the decade of the seventies, sterilization abuse in New York City had become a pervasive theme among, though not exclusively, poor women of color (Committee for Abortion Rights and Against Sterilization Abuse, 1979; Rodriguez-Trias, 1978; Velez, 1978; Davis, 1981). Sterilization abuse takes place when an individual submits to a tubal ligation or vasectomy without their knowledge or consent or because they are blatantly pressured to accept sterilization. In the seventies, many judicial cases were documented of poor women who had been threatened with having their welfare rights taken away if they did not accept sterilization, were not given consent forms at all, or were provided with consent forms to sign while they were in labor (Rodriguez-Trias, 1978). In this study, I found a few cases of women who were interned in a hospital for a different kind of surgery and were sterilized without their knowledge or consent, and many cases of women who were sterilized but were not aware of the permanent nature of a tubal ligation. In 1975, after a long and harrowing struggle undertaken by women's groups and health and community activists, sterilization guidelines were implemented in New York City to protect women and men against sterilization abuse.[6]

One of the questions my work raises is how do we then talk about agency and freedom of reproductive choice among Puerto Rican women in the context of the historical legacy of coercion and sterilization abuse? Although sterilization abuse is an important part of Puerto Rican women's experiences, on the island as well as in the United States, it is important to keep in mind that not all Puerto Rican women who have undergone the operation perceived themselves as having been coerced. Therefore, in examining Puerto Rican women's reproductive decisions, I take into account the diversity of their reproductive circumstances by considering the variation of their experiences, which range from sterilization abuse to those women who suggest that they have voluntarily made the decision to be sterilized. Rather than pose these experiences in opposition to each other, I contend that all decisions are socially constrained and mediated when individuals confront them as active social agents.

THE SETTING AND METHODOLOGY

The high rate of sterilization among Puerto Rican women on the island has been reproduced in the United States, where Puerto Ricans in New York City have one of the highest documented rates of sterilization. In the context of New York City as a changing metropolis, in one of the inner city's oldest and poorest neighborhoods, I set out in 1981 to learn more about the individual and social conditions that shape the reproductive decisions of Puerto Rican women with respect to sterilization on a daily basis.[7] The neighborhood where these women live is located between Williamsburg and Bushwick in Brooklyn, New York. This is one of Brooklyn's oldest garment districts. It is also the home of one of the largest Puerto Rican communities in New York City. Of the households with one or more Puerto Rican women over age 20, 47 percent included one or more sterilized women. Ninety-three percent of the sterilized women were born in the island, but they were sterilized between the ages of 17 and 21, after they migrated to New York.

The ethnographic methods used to collect the data for this study are participant observation, oral histories, and an in-depth survey of a selected sample of Puerto Rican women. Intensive interviews were conducted with 128 Puerto Rican women, 85 of whom were sterilized. After spending two months in the field doing participant observation, I developed an extensive questionnaire that contained open-ended and closed questions. This questionnaire was administered by three women from the neighborhood and myself. After completing the survey, I continued doing participant observation and collecting oral histories from a select number of women who represented different situations that led women to either accept or opt for sterilization. I collected oral histories from seven families, which consisted of a total of twenty mothers, daughters, and grandmothers. This intergenerational perspective is important because it enables me to compare the perceptions and experiences of women from different generations within the same families. Through the collection of oral histories, I explored the different ways that Puerto Rican women use sterilization, the constraints that they face in making reproductive decisions, and how they resist these constraints. Many use sterilization to help them solve the immediate problem of unwanted pregnancies.[8]

REVISITING THE IDEOLOGY OF CHOICE

The ideology of choice is paramount in a discussion of sterilization among Puerto Rican women. At the heart of this research lies the question of what constitutes a "choice" and what the concept of "voluntary" means in the context of the lives of Puerto Rican women. The "ideology of choice" is based on the assumption that people have options, that we live in a "free" society and have infinite alternatives from which to choose. As individual agents, we are purportedly capable of making decisions through envisioning appropriate goals in order to increase our options implicitly; the higher the social and class status, the greater the options. Striving toward the middle or upper class is, in part, a striving toward a "freedom" of expanded choice, which is part of the reward of upward mobility. By focusing on individual choice, we overlook the fact that choices are primed by larger institutional structures and ideological messages.

The discrepancy and contradictions between agency and constraints led me to reconceptualize the ideology of choice in order to develop and refine a new language that enables us to think in a more dialectical way about Puerto Rican women's fertility behavior. In this formulation of individual choice, a distinction needs to be made between a decision that is based on a lack of alternatives versus one that is based on reproductive freedom. A decision is said to be more voluntary when it is based on a greater space of viable alternatives and the conditions that make this possible. Moreover, it is not simply a matter of the alternatives that women have available to them but also the perceptions or knowledge women have about the various alternatives that are available to them. For example, a large number of women in this study did not know about the diaphragm.

Even though today's contraceptive technology is limited for all women, the options presented to these women were constrained by their lack of knowledge about the different forms of birth control technology as a result of limited resources and staff in the clinics and hospitals available to them. Therefore, reproductive freedom not only requires the ability to choose from a series of safe, effective, convenient, and affordable methods of birth control developed for men and women, but also a context of equitable social, political, and economic conditions that allows women to decide whether to have children, how many, and when (Colon and others, 1992; Hartman, 1987; Petchesky, 1984). Consequently, I have deliberately avoided framing the fertility decisions of Puerto Rican women within a paradigm of choice because it obfuscates the reality of their fertility histories and experiences as colonial and neocolonial women.

BIRTH CONTROL VERSUS POPULATION CONTROL

Although sterilization is technically considered birth control, a distinction needs to be made between sterilization and birth control on an analytical level as a result of the way it is used and its consequences for women's lives. For my purposes, birth control is defined as the ability to space children, while sterilization entirely eliminates the management of birth control. In fact, it renders the need to control fertility irrelevant. In most cases, sterilization marks the end of a woman's ability to reproduce. It is a method of population control that I have termed "fertility control" rather than "conception control." The important distinction is between population control as a state imposition and birth control as a personal right. It is not between sterilization and other forms of controlling births. Population control may be achieved through other methods: Norplant and abortion, for example, are considered. Population control is when a population policy imposes the control of fertility, as opposed to the individual right to control one's own fertility, and even be sterilized if that is the desire. Fertility control can be defined as a population policy that imposes the curtailment of population growth on women, eliminating the individual's right to control her own fertility.

In addition to the technical differences between sterilization and birth control, sterilization also functions as fertility control when population policy is defined and implemented by health care providers to curtail the rate of population growth among a particular class or ethnic group because they are considered, in eugenic terms, a social burden and therefore should not procreate (Hartman, 1987). Consequently, the important issue here is not sterilization technology per se, but the way population policy is defined, translated, and implemented.

On the national and international levels, health care policy plays an important role in narrowing women's fertility choices. Whereas federal funding initially covered the cost of abortion, the Hyde Amendment of 1977 changed this policy by denying women on Medicaid funding for abortions except in restricted cases or special circumstances. The refusal of the state to provide public funds for abortion services, except in narrowly defined therapeutic cases, while making sterilization readily available suggests a definite predilection for sterilization over temporary methods of birth control and abortion (Committee for Abortion Rights and Against Sterilization Abuse, 1979). This reflects the goals of the director of U.S. Agency for International Development who stated in 1987 that by 1995, he wanted to sterilize one-quarter of the world's female population (Hartman, 1987).

I depart from a political economic analysis of sterilization as population control in order to consider the diversity of women's experiences and the different levels of resistance they engage in. I seek to establish a much needed new paradigm of reproductive choice that explores, interrogates, and expands on what consent, choice, and coercion really mean within the context of these women's lives. In doing this, I hope to broaden the concept of what constitutes coercive sterilization by showing the variety of factors that lead women to sterilization, including the active participation of women in sterilization and the elements of resistance they engage in. It is then possible to distinguish between birth control and population control.[9]

DIVERSITY OF EXPERIENCES

In addition to becoming sterilized for a series of reasons, Puerto Rican women experience sterilization in a host of different ways. For example, while sterilization may give one woman a great deal of freedom, it may be oppressive to another. Moreover, at one point, a woman may perceive sterilization as independence, yet at a different point in her life, she may perceive it as oppressive. For example, a woman who is glad she is sterilized may regret it later if her child dies or if she remarries and is not able to have any more children. Sometimes resistance and oppression occupy different spaces, and other times they occupy the same space because different realities can, and often do, coexist within a particular context. For example, a Puerto Rican woman may decide to get sterilized because she does not want any more children. This is a vital decision for her because it gives her more control over her body, therefore giving her more self-determination over her life. In contrast, the state's motivation for encouraging her sterilization is due to her dependency on welfare, where she is considered a burden on the state. By attempting to control her fertility, motivated by considerations of economy and politics, the state imposes its double standard of "choice" and "freedom," which is potent oppression. Consequently, women and the state's interests intersect on the level that there is consensus between the woman and the state to control her fertility.

Sterilization becomes simultaneously oppressive while it offers elements of empowerment, because both the state and women's motivation for wanting to limit their own fertility are at once synchronized as well as diametrically opposed. Therefore, on this level, there is consensus as well as conflict and oppression (Lopez, forthcoming).

Another way that women experience sterilization differently is based on their life situations. Often, there are conflicting conditions in women's lives where resisting one set of circumstances subjects them to another, potentially oppressive set. Thus, a woman may get sterilized as a way of resisting forced maternity, submitting as well to a health practitioner's recommendation or state policy on sterilization (Colon and others, 1992).

Finally, it is also important to consider that voluntary sterilization must be available as a means of "birth control" for women to exert their reproductive freedom. Some women seek sterilization because they have achieved their desired family ties and they either decide independently or with their companion/husband that they do not desire, or cannot afford, to have any more children. Those women tend to use sterilization as fertility control because of their social and historical predisposition toward this technology and due to the lack of viable options. Given a women's conditions, in some cases, sterilization may be the most reasonable decision they can make. There is also the possibility that even if these women had viable alternatives and their conditions were different, they still might elect sterilization. However, for the majority of women in this study, this is not the case.

WOMEN'S PERCEPTIONS OF THEIR BODIES AND AGENCY

In unraveling the complicated subject of the interplay between women's resistance, constraints, and agency, I begin with an examination of the ways that women exert agency. This is best illustrated through women's perceptions of their bodies and their decision to become sterilized. Forty-four percent felt that if their economic conditions had been better, they would not have undergone surgery.

With the exceptions of those who were openly victims of sterilization abuse, most women in this neighborhood adamantly shared the view that sterilization was their decision because it was their body and they would do with it as they pleased. Consequently, most women did not feel that they had to ask the men in their lives for permission to get sterilized. Concurrent with this attitude, men rarely objected to a woman's decision to become sterilized unless the couple disagreed about the number and gender of the children desired. This was the case because most couples in this study agreed that it was difficult to raise and provide for more than three children.

It is important to remember that the perception that sterilization was their decision and the fact that they felt they had no other viable options appear to them as two separate issues. When I asked the question: "Who influenced your decision to get sterilized?" only 1 out of 96 women responded that her husband directly influenced her. This does not mean that women do not consult their husbands/companions about their sterilization decision. In most cases, they did. What it means is that regardless of the man's view, most women felt they had the right to ultimately make the final decision about sterilization, because they were the ones who were going to have the baby and would be the primary caretakers. These data demonstrate the ways that women assert agency and the ways that agency and constraints sometimes intersect. It also illustrates that what may appear at first glance to be an "individual" or "cultural" factor may actually be socially or economically intermeshed. In addition to attitudes about who should control their bodies and their perceptions that they have been sterilized "voluntarily," population policy, class, and poverty play a critical role in limiting the fertility options of Puerto Rican women.

SOCIOECONOMIC CONSIDERATIONS

While most lower-income women experience difficult socioeconomic situations, households headed by female single parents fare even worse. Sixty-six percent of the women in this study are heads of households. Almost all of the women in this study stated that they had been married at least once, though 53.1 percent said that they were separated, widowed, or divorced. Almost three-quarters (70 percent) received either supplementary or full assistance from Aid to Dependent Children. The mean annual income in 1981 was $7,000 or less. This income supports a mean of 3.4 children and two adults. With this money, women support themselves and their children, buy food and clothing, and also pay the rent.[10]

The employed Puerto Rican women in this neighborhood are low-wage workers with little job stability, generally working in tedious jobs and often under difficult conditions. Eighty percent of the women in this study claimed that their economic circumstances directly or indirectly strongly influenced their decisions to become sterilized. Forty-four percent felt that if their economic conditions had been better, they would not have undergone surgery. As one woman stated:

> If I had the necessary money to raise more children, I would not have been steril-
> ized. When you can't afford it, you just can't afford it. Girl, I wish that I could
> have lived in a house where each of them had their own room, nice clothing,
> enough food, and everything else that they needed. But what's the sense of hav-
> ing a whole bunch of kids if when dinnertime rolls around all you can serve them
> is soup made of milk or codfish because there is nothing else. Or when you are
> going to take them out, one wears a new pair of shoes while the other one has to
> wear hand-me-downs because you could only afford one pair of shoes. That's
> depressing. If I had another child, we would not have been able to survive.

Although their socioeconomic position permeates every aspect of these women's lives, many of them did not reduce their reasons for becoming sterilized to strictly economic considerations because this was not how most of them expressed their views about sterilization and their lives. Instead they talked about the burglaries, the lack of hot water in the winter, and the dilapidated environment in which they live. Additionally, mothers are constantly worried about the adverse effect that the environment might have on their children. Their neighborhoods are poor, with high rates of visible crime and substance abuse. Often women claimed that they were sterilized because they could not tolerate having children in such an adverse environment or because they simply could not handle more children than they already had under the conditions in which they lived. However, rarely did anyone say that they were sterilized because their annual income was only $7,000. They mostly talked indirectly about the conditions that led them to get sterilized.

LACK OF ACCESS TO QUALITY HEALTH CARE SERVICES

On a local level, a person's resources profoundly affect the type of health care services an individual has access to, as well as their knowledge of their options. On a microlevel, the quality of care and information that middle-class women receive in private hospitals broadens their choices by enabling them to make informed decisions within the limits of the contraceptive technology that is available. Conversely, the inadequate quality of care that poor women receive diminishes their ability to make informed reproductive decisions and in this way further restricts their already limited options. For instance, because public hospitals have fewer health providers, facilities, and time to spend with their patients, poor women are not always informed about all of the contraceptives that are available. This is particularly true about the diaphragm.

There is a prevalent belief among health care providers that Puerto Rican women reject the diaphragm because of a cultural aversion to the manual manipulation involved in its use. While this may be true for some Puerto Rican women, there are other equally compelling reasons that a large number of low-income Puerto Rican women do not use the diaphragm. Some of the women in this study did not use the diaphragm because they had never heard of it. This is true primarily because it is not frequently recommended to poor women, since in order to prescribe it, the health provider must show the woman how to use it properly. This requires a minimum of ten to fifteen minutes of the health provider's individual time, as well as a private space. Time and space are premium commodities in municipal hospitals. Moreover, if the health providers believe that the diaphragm is a culturally unacceptable method of birth control for the poor, chances are that they are not going to recommend it. Finally, there is also the attitude among health care providers that it is better to recommend mechanical and surgical forms of fertility control to the poor because they do not have sufficient initiative or responsibility for controlling their fertility.

PROBLEMS WITH BIRTH CONTROL

The quality of health care services a woman has access to significantly influences her knowledge of contraceptives and attitudes about them. The lack of safe and effective temporary methods of birth control prompted many women in this sample to get sterilized. Although 76 percent of the women used temporary methods of birth control before getting sterilized, they expressed dissatisfaction with the contraceptives available, especially the pill and the IUD. As one woman stated:

> The pill made me swell up. After three years, I had an IUD inserted. It made me bleed a lot so I had it removed. I was sterilized at the age of twenty-five because I couldn't use the pill or the IUD. I tried using Norforms and the withdrawal method before I was sterilized but neither method worked very well.

Thus, because women are cognizant of the constraints that their economic resources, domestic responsibilities, and problems with contraceptives place on their fertility options, many of them feel that sterilization is the only feasible "choice." In addition to the combination of social and historical factors previously mentioned that limit and constrain Puerto Rican women's fertility decisions, such as socioeconomic considerations, these women's fear to allow their children to play outdoors because of the high rate of crime in their neighborhood, their lack of access to quality health care services, and many of the domestic difficulties that stem from poverty, personal, and familial issues also influence their fertility decisions.

WOMEN MARRY YOUNG AND ARE PRIMARILY RESPONSIBLE FOR THEIR FERTILITY AND CHILD REARING

The tendency to either marry or have their children while they are still relatively young precipitates their decision to get sterilized at a younger age: 66 percent of these women were sterilized between the ages of 25 and 29 as compared to Euro-American and Afro-American women at the age ranges of 30 to 34 (New York City Health and Hospital Corporation, 1982). Moreover, most of the women in this study married and had their children before the age of 25.

Therefore, by their mid-twenties, they had already achieved their desired family size but still had approximately twenty years of fecundity left. Since the most effective method available to curtail fertility is sterilization, their "choice" was to accept it or continue using temporary methods of birth control for the next twenty years.

The average woman in this study had between two and three children, their perception of the ideal family size. More than half (56.7 percent) claimed that they were completely responsible for their fertility and child rearing. While this may appear as an issue of individual choice, it is part and parcel of the construction of the nuclear family in a patriarchal society in which the brunt of the responsibility of child rearing and birth control is relegated to women. This is accomplished by providing birth control mainly to women and few, if any, contraceptives for men.

WOMEN'S RELIGIOUS VIEWS AND FAMILIARITY WITH *LA OPERACIÓN*

Although Puerto Rico is a Catholic country, Catholicism does not appear to have a direct effect on most women's decisions to be sterilized. Eighty-seven percent of the women in this sample were raised as Catholics. Of these women, only 32 percent felt that sterilization goes against their religious beliefs. In contrast, however, women's familiarity with *la operación* has had a profound affect on predisposing them toward sterilization.

The prolonged use of tubal ligation has transformed it into part of the cultural repertoire for a large segment of the Puerto Rican population. Women's perceptions about *la operación* are also strongly influenced by the large number of females within their own families who have been sterilized. The effect that almost six decades of exposure to this operation has had on predisposing Puerto Rican women to sterilization cannot be underestimated.

To acknowledge that sterilization has a cultural dimension to it does not, however, make the decision to become sterilized one based on free will since free will does not exist in a vacuum. Nor does such a decision suggest that it originates from women's "folk" culture, as some scholars have implied through the language that they have used to describe this phenomenon (Presser, 1973).[11]

Although the cultural beliefs of Puerto Rican women play an important role in their fertility decisions, particularly because of their misinformation about this procedure, this approach, like the culture of poverty thesis, blames the individual (Lewis, 1968). For Puerto Rican women, sterilization became part of their cultural repertoire because of the political, social, and economic conditions that favored it, creating the conditions for their predisposition toward sterilization through the use of population control policies and initiatives.

MISINFORMATION AND REGRET

Puerto Rican women have a very high rate of misinformation about the permanency of sterilization. Eighty-two percent of the women in this study make a distinction between the "tying" and the "cutting" of the fallopian tubes, a differentiation that does not exist. In one woman's words, "I feel that if a woman is not sure if she wants any more kids, then she should have her tubes tied. If a woman has decided she absolutely does not want to have more children, then she should have her tubes 'cut.'"

The importance of the high rate of misinformation about sterilization is that it is one of the main factors that maintains and perpetuates the high rate of sterilization.

The simplistic language used to discuss sterilization in hospitals such as "Band-aid sterilization" and the "bikini cut" is another factor that contributes to Puerto Rican women's confusion about the permanency of this operation. This issue is complicated because in some cases, women have these beliefs and do not communicate them to health providers. In other cases, health providers do not tell women about the permanent nature of *la operación,* or they talk to them in a language that deemphasizes the permanency of this surgery, thus making the situation worse. This leads to a high rate of regret among the women in this study.[12]

Of the ninety-six sterilized women, a third (33 percent) regretted that they were sterilized. Twenty percent do not regret their decision. The others (46 percent) fall somewhere in the middle. That is, they did not regret their decision, but they were not happy with it either, although they felt they made the best decision they could under their given conditions. Women tend to regret their decisions because they remarry and would like to have a child with their new spouse, their socioeconomic situation improves, or because one of their children dies.

CONCLUSION

In order to accentuate the interplay between elements of resistance and constraints/oppression, this study has highlighted the complex, contradictory, and multidimensional nature of Puerto Rican women's experiences with sterilization. The issue of sterilization among Puerto Rican women is a complicated one indeed. With the exception of victims of sterilization abuse, the majority of Puerto Rican women suggest that they made a decision between getting sterilized or continuing to have children under adverse conditions. Because of the limited nature of this "choice," however, many women feel they had no other viable alternative but to opt for, or to accept, sterilization.

In the conceptualization of my work, I have deliberately rejected the language of choice. Such language invokes ideas of free will based on individual freedom, part of the liberal ideology of choice that promotes a binary framework of choice/no choice, voluntary/nonvoluntary decision making, and obscures the interplay between social constraints and human activity. Moreover, all human decisions are socially mediated, but some people have more social space to make decisions than others.

In attempting to exercise control over their lives, Puerto Rican women may use sterilization as an element of resistance to forge some social space for themselves by refusing to have more children than they desire or by attempting to exert some control over their socioeconomic situation, female subordination, or problematic relationships. This forces us to reevaluate the culture of poverty thesis of Puerto Rican complacency, passivity, and lack of planning.

At the same time, it is necessary to frame their reproductive decisions within the context of the constraints that they face. Despite women's desire to plan their lives, in addition to having children there are other forces operating simultaneously to shape, frame, and limit their fertility choices. Puerto Rican women's "individual choice" has been substantively circumscribed by the United States/Puerto Rican colonial population policy as well as by women's poverty, race, and gender oppression. The problem with sterilization is, of course, not the technology itself but the way it has been used to solve Puerto Rico's economic problem of underdevelopment and poverty by sterilizing Puerto Rican women. Then, moreover, given the social and economic constraints discussed, sterilization appears to them as the only viable alternative.

After four decades of residence in the United States, Puerto Rican women are still living in poverty, and they are still faced with the same dilemma of how to control their fertility. Although there are certainly more contraceptives today than there were in the past, after using and experiencing health problems with the pill and IUD, a large number of Puerto Rican women turn to sterilization, a method of fertility control they have now been practicing for approximately six decades. Aside from their predisposition to *la operación,* sterilization is also frequently recommended to them in municipal hospitals. Although public attention in New York City is not directed at an overpopulation problem, as it is in Puerto Rico, the "welfare problem" is an item of considerable debate since it is the poor who are considered to have too many children.

In addition to the historical antecedents, there are a host of individual and societal forces that maintain, condition, and perpetuate the fertility decisions of Puerto Rican women in New York City. Women's familiarity with *la operación,* combined with the high rate of misinformation among Puerto Rican women about sterilization procedures, poverty, and lack of access to quality health care, further circumscribes women's fertility decisions by limiting their knowledge about their options. Moreover, the lack of access to safe, effective, convenient, and affordable birth control, in conjunction with the goals of sterilization policy to control the rate of population growth among the poor, play an equally important role in constraining women's reproductive options.

By not offering women alternatives such as quality health care services, safe and effective temporary methods of birth control for both men and women, abortion services, quality and affordable day care centers, and opportunities for a better standard of living (Hartman, 1987), women's fertility options have been effectively narrowed, at times making sterilization the only viable alternative. Until Puerto Rican women achieve a more equitable status in society and are able to improve their socioeconomic situation, they will continue to have one of the highest documented rates of sterilization in the world. Reproductive freedom means having all the alternatives and the conditions in order to decide whether or not to have children. As long as women continue to have children under these inequitable conditions we cannot talk about reproductive freedom.

Notes

1. Sterilization consists of cutting and suturing the fallopian tubes in the female to permanently block the flow of the sperm to the egg cell and to prevent the egg cell from entering the uterus. In its broadest meaning, sterilization includes hysterectomies and vasectomies. The latter is the method used to sterilize men. Female sterilization is also referred to as tubal ligation.

2. In 1982, a study by a Puerto Rican demographer, Vazquez-Calzada, showed that 39 percent of Puerto Rico's female population between the ages of 15 and 45 were surgically sterilized (Vazquez-Calzada, 1982). A similar situation can be found for Puerto Rican women and other minorities in the United States. In New York City, where this research took place, Latinas have a rate of sterilization seven times greater than that of Euro-American women and almost twice that of Afro-American women (New York City Health and Hospital Corporation, 1982). Although information is scarce for most cities, my study of Puerto Rican women in one neighborhood in New York found that in 47 percent of the households, one or more Puerto Rican women over age 20 were surgically sterilized. Moreover, another study reveals that in Hartford, Connecticut, 51 percent of Puerto Rican females of reproductive age were sterilized (Gangalez, Barrera, Guanaccia, and Schensul, 1980).

3. Contending views of Puerto Rican women's reproductive decisions are paradoxical because they have been posed in binary terms. Puerto Rican women are either presented as victims of population policy (Mass, 1976) or free agents making voluntary decisions about their reproductive lives (Stycos, Hill, and Back, 1959; Presser, 1973). There are numerous problems with this logic. The argument that the high rate of sterilization is based on reproductive freedom glosses over the importance of power dynamics in relation to Puerto Rican women as colonial and neocolonial subjects of population programs in Puerto Rico. In contrast, the view that state-initiated Puerto Rican women are victims of sterilization abuse makes them appear passive and does not take into account the range of their diversity or the complexity of their experiences.

4. After World War II, Puerto Rico became a model for the strategy of development known as Operation Bootstrap and a testing laboratory for the pill, IUD, EMKO contraceptive cream, and the development of sterilization technology. By 1937, sterilization was implemented in Puerto Rico as a method of "birth control." The legislation grew out of the eugenics movement that developed in the United States to sterilize people considered socially or intellectually inferior. Finally, it is also important to keep in mind that for thirty-one years in Puerto Rico, sterilization was systematically available while temporary methods of birth control were only haphazardly available. For a complete history of Puerto Rico's birth control movement see Ramirez de Arellano and Scheipp (1983).

5. Interestingly, sterilization was never official government policy in Puerto Rico (Presser, 1973; Henderson, 1976; Ramirez de Arellano and Sheipp, 1993). It took place unofficially and became a common practice condoned by the Puerto Rican government and many of its health officials, frequently filling the gap for the systematic lack of temporary methods of birth control. Albeit many birth control clinics opened and closed throughout Puerto Rico's history, it was not until 1968 that federally funded contraceptives were made available throughout the island. It is within this context of a policy prompting population control, particularly for poor women, that decisions regarding sterilization must be analyzed.

6. This legislation mandated that a thirty-day period of time be observed between the time an individual signs a consent form to the day she is operated on. It also stipulated that women under the age of 21 could not be sterilized with federal funds and that a consent form must be provided in a person's native language and administered in written and oral form.

7. Although this research originally took place in 1981, in 1993 I collected more oral histories from some of these women in order to update my ethnographic material.

8. An article on the conceptualization and methods used to collect the data for this research are explored in "Negotiating Two Worlds: The Experiences of Puerto Rican Anthropologists in Brooklyn, New York," in Capello and Souza (1994).

9. Time and space do not allow me to elaborate further on the distinction between sterilization and population control and on the different levels that the women in this study resist. This will be the focus of my upcoming book on this topic.

10. In 1981, more than three-quarters of the women in this study were not working outside the home, although 12.5 percent were actively looking for jobs. Of the women who have spouses, 31.3 percent had husbands who were employed and 15.6 percent had husbands who were not working at the time this study took place.

11. The language that Presser used to describe this phenomenon is problematic. In reference to sterilization she states: "Its widespread practice represents a 'grass roots' response among Puerto Rican women who sought an effective means of limiting their family size" (Presser, 1973, p. 1). The difficulty is not with the acknowledgment that there is a cultural dimension to sterilization but that she disassociates culture from the social, political, and historical context.

12. Although minority and poor women are likely to be misinformed about the permanent nature of sterilization, a study found that regardless of ethnic group or class, most women are likely to be misinformed (Carlson and Vickers, 1982).

References

Bonilla, F., and Campos, R. "Evolving Patterns of Puerto Rican Migration." In S. Sanderson (ed.), *The Americas in the New International Division of Labor.* New York: Holmes and Meier, 1983.

Capello, D. C., and Souza, C. (eds.). *U.S. Puerto Rican Women: Creative Resistance.* Berkeley, Calif.: Third Woman Press, 1994.

Carlson, J., and Vickers, G. *Voluntary Sterilization and Informed Consent: Are Guidelines Necessary?* New York: Women's Division of the United Methodist Church, 1982.

Colon, A. "Salud y Derechos Reproductivos." Paper presented at the third meeting of researchers supported by the City University of New York–University of Puerto Rico Exchange Project, 1992.

Committee for Abortion Rights and Against Sterilization Abuse. *Women Under Attack: Abortion, Sterilization Abuse, and Reproductive Freedom.* New York: Committee Against Sterilization Abuse, 1979.

Davis, A. *Women, Race, and Class.* New York: Random House, 1981.

Gangalez, M., Barrera, V., Guanaccia, P., and Schensul, S. "The Impact of Sterilization on Puerto Rican Women, the Family, and the Community." Unpublished report. Connecticut: Hispanic Health Council, 1980.

Hartman, B. *Reproductive Rights and Wrongs: The Global Politics of Population Control and Contraceptive Choice.* New York: HarperCollins, 1987.

Henderson, P. "Population Policy, Social Structure, and the Health System in Puerto Rico: The Case of Female Sterilization." Unpublished doctoral dissertation, University of Connecticut, 1976.

Lewis, O. *La Vida: A Puerto Rican Family in the Culture of Poverty—San Juan and New York.* New York: Random House, 1968.

Lopez, I. *A Question of Choice: An Ethnographic Study of the Reproduction of Sterilization Among Puerto Rican Women,* forthcoming.

Mass, B. "Emigration and Sterilization in Puerto Rico." In B. Mass (ed.), *Political Target: The Political Economy of Population in Latin America.* Ontario: Charters, 1976.

New York City Health and Hospital Corporation. "Sterilizations Reported in New York City." Unpublished data. New York: New York City Health and Hospital Corporation, Department of Biostatistics, 1982.

Petchesky, R. *Abortion and Woman's Choice: The State, Sexuality, and Reproductive Freedom.* New York: Longman, 1984.

Presser, H. *Sterilization and Fertility Decline in Puerto Rico.* Berkeley: University of California Press, 1973.

Ramirez de Arellano, A., and Scheipp, C. *Colonialism, Catholicism, and Contraception: A History of Birth Control in Puerto Rico.* Chapel Hill: University of North Carolina Press, 1983.

Rodriguez-Trias, H. *Women and the Health Care System: Committee Against Sterilization Abuse.* New York: Barnard College, 1978.

Stycos, M., Hill, R., and Back, K. *The Family and Population Control: A Puerto Rican Experiment in Social Change.* Chapel Hill: University of North Carolina Press, 1959.

Vazquez-Calzada, J. *La Población de Puerto Rico Y Su Trajectoria Historica.* Rio Piédras: University of Puerto Rico, School of Public Health, Medical Sciences Campus, 1982.

Velez, C. "Se Me Acabo la Canción." Paper presented at the International Congress of Anthropological and Ethnological Sciences, New Delhi, India, Dec. 1978.

CHAPTER SEVEN

Subverting Culture

Promoting HIV/AIDS Prevention Among Puerto Rican and Dominican Women

Blanca Ortiz-Torres
Irma Serrano-García
Nélida Torres-Burgos

The authors present original findings and discuss reports from the literature that provide valuable insights into the cultural factors that have application to Puerto Rican and Dominican women, the primary subgroup of Latinas discussed in this chapter, and many other Latina groups with similar immigration experiences and acculturation levels. Their attention to Puerto Rican and Dominican women makes a substantive contribution to the literature. Although much has been made of the role of traditional sex roles, cultural beliefs, and values as they affect HIV/AIDS among Latinas, rarely are such commentaries and research accompanied by substantive recommendations for prevention and intervention within a Latina feminist construct.

One of the crucial challenges faced by researchers and interventionists in the HIV/AIDS prevention field is how to promote change in social norms and normative beliefs that promote HIV/AIDS risk-related behaviors in specific cultural contexts. Once we acknowledge the importance of variables such as cognition, emotion, and culture in facilitating or impeding preventive behaviors, we face the dilemma of how to intervene with variables that seem more resistant to change than knowledge and information (Auerbach, Wypijewska, and Brodie, 1994). Our goal in this chapter is to increase our understanding of those aspects of culture that might promote or impede HIV/AIDS prevention with Puerto Rican (living in Puerto Rico and New York) and Dominican women (living in New York), an issue that becomes particularly important when we consider the sizable impact of the epidemic on Latinos and

149

Latinas. We intend to accomplish this goal through the review of extant literature and of research conducted by the authors.

Although Latinos and Latinas make up 11 percent of the U.S. population (U.S.
Census Bureau, 1997), they represent 20 percent of HIV/AIDS cases (Centers
for Disease Control, 1998). The situation in Puerto Rico and the Caribbean
is also alarming. In Puerto Rico as of November 1998, more than 20,000 AIDS
cases had been reported, of which 64 percent have died. Since 1990, AIDS has
become the leading cause of death for males and females 25 to 29 years of age
in Puerto Rico. Of the total number of AIDS cases on the island, 21 percent are
women, of whom 58 percent report having been infected through heterosexual
contact (PASET, 1998). A similar situation is found in other Caribbean countries. As of December 1997, the World Health Organization reported that some
1.3 million people are believed to be living with HIV in Latin America and the
Caribbean. By 1993, 8 percent of pregnant women in Haiti were infected
with the virus, and the same prevalence was reported from one surveillance site
in the Dominican Republic.

In this chapter, we attempt to shed light through the review of research that
focused on the role of culture in HIV/AIDS prevention with Puerto Rican
and Dominican women by (1) analyzing the sociohistorical context of some cultural beliefs, (2) illustrating the tension between risk-related and protective
cultural beliefs within our research with Puerto Rican and Dominican women
living in New York and Puerto Rico, (3) presenting the challenge this analysis
poses for community psychology, and (4) proposing that promoting changes in
sex-related social norms and normative beliefs might be constructed as a subversive act. Initially, an analysis of the way culture interacts with the social construction of gender and may foster unequal power relationships is presented.

HIV/AIDS PREVENTION: THE INTERPLAY
OF CULTURE, GENDER, AND POWER

One of the most cherished values in community psychology is that of cultural
diversity. Diversity has become central to the discipline stemming from an ecological perspective that promotes goals of individual and collective empowerment (Serrano-García and Bond, 1994; Trickett, Watts, and Birman, 1994).
Because U.S. society has become increasingly multicultural and multiethnic as
well as sociodemographically varied, a diversity perspective allows us to better
understand behavior and to better interpret our findings regarding individuals
and groups. This improved understanding of ethnic and cultural groups that are
usually in oppressed and underserved positions can also lead us to improve our
interventions in the direction of greater social justice (Alarcón and Foulks, 1995;
Lonner, 1994). To support this kind of analysis, Watts (1994) has identified

four paradigms relevant to a psychology of human diversity, which include population-specific psychologies, cross-cultural psychology, sociopolitical psychology, and intergroup theory.

Within the perspective that Watts defines as cross-cultural, the notion of culture is emphasized. "Culture" has been defined in many ways (Comas-Díaz, Griffith, Pinderhughes, and Wyche, 1995). According to Lonner (1994), existing definitions have various characteristics in common. They establish culture (1) as an abstract, human-made idea; (2) as a context or setting within which behavior occurs, is shaped, and transformed; (3) as containing values, beliefs, attitudes, and languages that have emerged as adaptations; and (4) as important enough to be passed on to others. Stemming from these considerations, it is reasonable to assert that culture affects constructions of gender, power, and sexuality; defines possibilities and conditions for action; and influences conceptualizations of health and sickness (Amaro, 1988, 1995; Miles, 1997).

The population-specific paradigm focuses on understanding a single population. HIV/AIDS researchers and interveners have most often incorporated this paradigm into their analyses of HIV/AIDS-related behaviors (Becker, Rankin, and Rickel, 1998), focusing their studies on gay men (Hays and Peterson, 1994; Kelly, 1994), African American youth (Jemmott, 1996), or drug users (Leukefeld, Battjes, and Amsel, 1990), to mention a few. Various authors have indicated that those who adopt a population-specific perspective ignore differences within groups, and when they do incorporate cultural components, they focus their analysis on stereotyped or unproven assumptions about the groups' culture (Fernández, 1995; VanOss Marin, Gómez, Tschann, and Gregorech, 1997). In summarizing findings from a research effort in thirteen countries, Gupta and Weiss (1995) identified "social beliefs and norms that constrain women's ability to protect themselves from HIV" as part of "the most immediate barriers that women face in adopting risk reduction behaviors" (p. 261).

In the HIV/AIDS literature, cultural variables are most often framed as barriers to risk-reduction behaviors (Fernández, 1995; Marín, 1996). This is especially true about Latinas. In this case, certain beliefs and values such as *machismo, marianismo,* and *familismo* have been typically associated only with risky behaviors such as unprotected sex and drug use (Marín, 1996; Peragallo, Talashek, Norr, and Dancy, 1998). Certainly, these can be barriers to HIV prevention, but it is also true that little is known about the potential protective dimensions of these same values. The tensions between protective and risk-related cultural beliefs that are explored in this chapter need to be better understood to enable us to tailor preventive interventions for Latinas.

Due in good part to the influence of feminist theories, gender can be conceived as a relational, rather than a "natural," variable that is influenced by sociohistorical and cultural forces and dynamics (Tiefer, 1997). Gender is considered relational because expectations, scripts, and behaviors defining what is feminine and masculine are manifest in the context of social relations and transactions, rather than being exclusively determined by biological or intrapsychic factors. A relational theory of gender recognizes that the behavior of actors is not only restricted by, but simultaneously influences and shapes, the social context (Ferrand and Snijders, 1997).

This relational and sociohistoric model also applies to sexual behaviors. The norms that surround this conduct come into play within the context not only of romantic and sexual interactions, but also within the context of power relationships between the genders. These power relationships are rooted in the belief in the superiority of men, who are expected to be strong and in control, and the inferiority or subservience of women, who are expected to be delicate and submissive to men's needs and demands (Miles, 1997).

Because of the importance we attribute to the relational and socially constructed nature of gender and sexuality, and the norms and beliefs that surround these concepts within many Latino cultures, we thought it necessary to describe them and to present briefly their sociohistorical roots in the Spanish Caribbean, where both the Puerto Rico and Dominican Republic are located. Although we acknowledge the cultural differences between Puerto Rico and the Dominican Republic, we build our arguments on the common sociohistorical grounds shared by both countries, colonized by Spain and located in the same geographical region. By doing this, we clarify the cultural content of the norms we are suggesting be questioned, as well as changed in the following sections.

VALUES, BELIEFS, AND NORMS ASSOCIATED WITH RISKY BEHAVIORS

Values, beliefs, and norms are part of the many cultural constructs that influence sexual behaviors. Despite this knowledge, previous research has focused almost exclusively on *marianismo, machismo,* and *familismo* as those beliefs most central to Latinos' and Latinas' sexuality. In Latino culture, *marianismo* has been characterized as the complement of *machismo* (Stevens, 1973). *Marianismo* defines the role of the ideal woman, modeled after the Virgin Mary, as based on chastity, abnegation, and sacredness, while reinforcing obedience and virginity (Gil and Inoa-Vázquez, 1996). *Machismo* characterizes the male gender role in Latino society (De la Cancela, 1986). It stresses virility, independence, physical strength, and sexual prowess (Ramírez, 1993). According to De la Cancela (1986), Puerto Rican *machismo* is an ideology that tends to alienate men from themselves and their families. Both *marianismo* and *machismo* are socially constructed and promote and reinforce a particular set of behaviors.

The concept of *familismo* was first used by Stycos (1952) to describe a high degree of interpersonal bonding within the Puerto Rican family, resulting in greater identification with the group and dependence on the family. Recent studies also have demonstrated the importance of the nuclear and extended family as a source of social support. Research also illustrates how Latinos and Latinas "adopt" close friends as "compadres" and family members in the absence of blood ties. This redefinition of friends as family legitimizes their supportive roles (Bravo, 1989; Delgado and Humm-Delgado, 1982; Salgado de Snyder and Padilla, 1987; Vega and Kolody, 1985).

Sociohistorical Context

Understanding the sociohistorical context that contributed to the formation and maintenance of these beliefs allows us to understand their origins and why they are so deeply ingrained in Latinos and Latinas' constructions of gender. This in turn allows us to understand the difficulties encountered in changing these ideas.

As part of Latin America's colonization process, the Catholic monarchy that ruled Spain utilized Catholicism as an effective strategy to dominate and conquer the indigenous population in Cuba, the Dominican Republic, and Puerto Rico (Picó and Rivera-Izcoa, 1991). However, by the turn of the nineteenth century, missionary Protestantism arrived in Puerto Rico and other Spanish-speaking countries as a result of the expansion of an emerging power, the United States of America (Silva-Gotay, 1996). Both Catholicism and Protestantism played a major role in disseminating ideal female images such as the Virgin Mary and other biblical women (such as Ruth, Elizabeth, and Sarah).

The Judeo-Christian tradition was immersed in a patriarchal society that legitimized men's rule over the Israel tribes. Religious traditions incorporated the subordination of women by men in the central role played by the male deity (Yahweh) and in the restricted role of women in ecclesiastical structures (Aquino, 1993; González, 1996; Farley, 1990). In present times, the hierarchy of the Catholic church, which continues to be dominant in Puerto Rico and the Dominican Republic, and some fundamentalist leaders of the Protestant church, are instrumental in reinforcing *marianismo, machismo,* and *familismo,* particularly as regards sexual matters (for example, "only sex for reproduction is moral"; "only women must remain faithful to their husbands").

The fact that until recently both Puerto Rico and the Dominican Republic were agrarian societies (Williams, 1970) also helped in the promotion and reinforcement of the values and beliefs we have been discussing. In the case of Puerto Rico, coffee production (under Spanish rule) and sugar plantations (under U.S. control) were labor-intensive activities; therefore, large families were needed in order to maximize work capacity. Values that promoted reproduction were well suited for the economic survival of the family and society. In agrarian societies, the transmission of wealth from one generation to the next depended on clear paternal linkages (Fox, 1967), which in turn relied on women's virginity until marriage (legal or consensual) and in their fidelity during marriage (Mair, 1965).

As shown, patriarchy in Catholic and colonial societies provided the background for the social construction of gender roles in Puerto Rico and in the Dominican Republic. However, gender roles, as well as values, are continually evolving as a result of diverse social influences, such as the ones we will now discuss.

Current Influences on Gender Roles and Sexuality

When industrialization, urbanism, and migration became strong forces in Puerto Rico and the Dominican Republic, gender roles, values, and beliefs were tested, and some were transformed. As a result of these processes, there is some indication of change toward a more liberal attitude among Latinas regarding women's roles (Mantell, Rapkin, Tross, and Ortiz-Torres, 1992). In a study conducted in Puerto Rico by McCann-Erickson (1990) with a sample of 800 women, only 33 percent of surveyed women agreed that men must initiate sex relations and courtship. In this same survey, 21 percent endorsed the right to abortion, 63 percent endorsed the use of contraceptive pills, and 25 percent agreed that today's sexual liberty is positive.

One of the social transformations that has led to changes is the massive incursion of women into the industrialized labor force. Their increased participation has brought about changes in family and work relations as well as in community life (Carnivalli, 1993; Colón-Warren, 1997). Many women are now single heads of families, and when this is not the case, men and women are increasingly sharing financial responsibilities at home. Both situations promote changes in gender roles. Access to financial resources strengthens women's sense of independence and control over their lives, opens new and more diverse options for them, and leads to increased participation in private and public decision-making processes. Women's roles have changed rapidly with their integration into the public sphere. In order to compete and survive in the industrialized labor market, women must develop assertiveness, public leadership, and entrepreneurship. These new requirements frequently clash with traditional ones, creating a double bind for women (Colberg-Luciano and Ramos-Marcano, 1997).

Another major transformation that has been greatly influential is migration to the United States and the encounter with the Anglo-Saxon culture that this move entails. Women who have migrated to the United States have been exposed to gender role transformations (Gil and Inoa-Vázquez, 1996). Research with Latinas in the United States has demonstrated that the acculturation process is most often characterized by the adoption of less traditional beliefs and values (Comas-Díaz and Duncan, 1985; Ortiz-Torres, Rapkin, Mantell, and Tross, 1992; Soto and Shaver, 1982).

The impact of women's movements in many parts of the world, including Puerto Rico, has also been extremely important in the articulation and promotion of alternative values such as the right of women to control their sexuality, affirmative actions for the recruitment of women in nontraditional jobs, and protection against sexual harassment at the workplace. Women's movements have been crucial in the adoption of public policies related to women's reproductive and health rights (Miles, 1997; Tiefer, 1997).

Finally, and most recently, the HIV/AIDS epidemic has not only increased the tension between traditional (or conservative) and "new" (or progressive) social norms, but has projected what were considered individual- or private-level issues into the public realm. Confronted with the increasing number of deaths associated with AIDS-related diseases, the increasing number of infected women, and the increasing number of pediatric cases, public authorities can no longer ignore the fact that heterosexual sex is one of the principal modes of HIV transmission. Thus, they realize, probably for the first time, that they must talk about sex in prevention campaigns. However, in Puerto Rico, even prevention campaigns are timid and scarce and influenced by the social norm that "you don't talk openly about sex" (notwithstanding the marked sexual content of many TV shows and commercials). Just recently, while several nongovernmental organizations and women's groups in Puerto Rico aggressively lobbied for the approval of a public policy expanding adolescents' reproductive rights, a journalist strongly opposed sex education in the schools, by emphasizing "the beauty of virginity and marriage" (Soltero, 1997).

In conclusion, industrialization, migration, and women's movements have generated conditions that facilitate challenging traditional religious and patriarchal values that hinder women's well-being. It is within this dynamic context that HIV/AIDS research and preventive interventions with and for Puerto Rican and Dominican women have been taking place. The next section will illustrate the tensions we have alluded to and the challenging, sometimes defiant, ways in which we have attempted to address them. It includes examples of our research and interventions conducted both in Puerto Rico and New York with Puerto Rican and Dominican women.

HIV/AIDS PREVENTION RESEARCH WITH PUERTO RICAN AND DOMINICAN WOMEN: THE TENSION BETWEEN RISK-RELATED AND PROTECTIVE CULTURAL NORMS AND BELIEFS

Factors Influencing Sexual Negotiation and the Practice of Safer Sex

To explore the relationship between the social construction of sexuality and gender roles as it relates to sexual practices and negotiation, we have conducted research with samples of Puerto Rican female and male college students on the island (Ortiz-Torres and others, 1996a). Ortiz-Torres and others (1996a) used discussions within five focus groups ($n = 66$) and in-depth interviews (still in progress) to test and refine a model in which these social constructions would be linked to social transactions with microsystems such as family, church, peers, school, and media. Preliminary findings from the focus groups and findings from three prior surveys administered to this population (Cunningham and Cunningham, 1992) generated similar results. Many participants described a conflict between the guilt and fear of rejection they face if they challenge the social prescription of virginity and their desire to engage in sexual intercourse. Female college students expressed fear of rejection by their parents whom they respect and feel that they must obey (*familismo*) and by future partners, who value virginity in their potential wife (*marianismo*). The fact that these participants are college educated does not seem to be enough to transform these complex beliefs and norms.

Serrano-García and her colleagues have been involved in an intervention/ research project entitled "Our VOICES against HIV/AIDS" (VOCES in Spanish). The project involves the development, implementation, and evaluation of an empowering intervention to prevent HIV/AIDS among young heterosexual Puerto Rican women (Serrano-García, Torres-Burgos, and Galarza, forthcoming). The goals of the VOCES' intervention (Serrano-García, 1994; Torres-Burgos and Serrano-García, 1997) are the reduction of risky sexual practices among participants, an increase in awareness of their power relations with their partners, and an increase in their conflict resolution and negotiation skills. The intervention consists of a three-day workshop and follow-up support group meetings with cognitive, behavioral, and social support components. A participatory methodology integrating elements of *Teatro del Oprimido* (participatory theater) developed by Boal (1980) in Brazil is incorporated in order to increase participants' involvement and motivation.

The intervention has as its theoretical underpinning a social constructionist framework that emphasizes the analysis of the impact of the power relationships between the genders as a major contributor to the practice of risky sexual behaviors. The influence of *machismo* and *marianismo* on sexuality and gender roles leads to the exaltation of penetrative sexual behavior and to women's ignorance about their bodies and about sexuality. These values in turn support and reinforce a social context characterized by unequal power gender relationships. Research informs us that women are oppressed, have little control over the power relationships in which they participate, and have fewer options for conflict resolution than men (Cantera, 1992; Patton, 1990; Santos-Ortiz, 1991). This inequality also has a direct impact on the possibilities of HIV infection particularly in regard to women's difficulty negotiating safer-sex practices (Bennet, 1990; Cochran, 1989). Thus, the design of the intervention has taken into consideration some of the previously discussed cultural prescriptions that lead to the practice of high-risk sexual behaviors among women, which are themselves embedded in the social construction of gender differences in general, and of sexuality in particular. The intervention attempts to promote a process of deconstruction of those cultural prescriptions.

The research project has been developed with female college students in Puerto Rico. It combines both qualitative and quantitative methods. To evaluate the intervention's impact, a pre–posttest design with various measures was undertaken (Noboa, Serrano-García, and Torres-Burgos, 1997; Serrano-García and others, 1996; Toro-Alfonso and others, 1997). To further understand the cultural prescriptions and norms, the researchers have used qualitative methods such as focus groups regarding sexuality and sexual negotiation, open-ended interviews about morality and sexuality, and content analyses of videotaped sexual negotiation simulations.

A summary of the research related to morality follows. This is particularly relevant since behaviors that are normatively rejected are labeled as immoral, while those that are fostered are considered moral.

Morality

The qualitative studies that VOCES undertook have been particularly helpful in providing information about the cultural context of HIV/AIDS prevention. Cruz and Serrano-García (1997) have reported on open-ended interviews with twenty college women regarding the relationship between morality and sex. The researchers identified several social norms and normative beliefs that may hinder safer sex, including what follows: (1) "women should not speak about sexuality, particularly with strangers or in large groups"; (2) "sexual practices linked to reproduction are moral while those that are engaged in solely for pleasure are immoral"; (3) "pleasurable and complete sexual relations require penetration"; and (4) "women should please their partners during sexual intercourse."

Safer sex is further impeded, according to their data, by women's perception of safer-sex behaviors as dirty or immoral and their perception of unprotected vaginal penetration as moral. Women also reported that they felt ashamed, guilty, and sad when they chose to please their partners by engaging in immoral behaviors. Participants linked their "duty" to please their partner not only to the passive sexual role that is assigned to a wife or a decent woman, but also to women's fear of communicating what they feel or want. *Machismo* was also evident in their acceptance of "good" sex as penetrative and with ejaculation and central to their male partners. However, the protective nature of *marianismo* was also present in the following norms and beliefs that the women identified that may facilitate HIV/AIDS protection: (1) the belief in abstinence or virginity, (2) women's need to care for themselves so they can care for others, and (3) women's need to be perceived as chaste, pure, and moral rather than promiscuous, loose, or immoral.

In summary, we can see that women's expressions vividly demonstrated the preeminence of the male role (*machismo*), the morality of sex linked to reproduction, the construction of decent women as chaste and pure (*marianismo*), and women's subservience to men's desires despite their feelings (*marianismo/machismo*). They also identified values that although immersed in the dominant constructions of sexuality and gender, facilitate their protection from HIV infection. Emotions are an essential component of human behavior; normative and moral behavior usually feels "good" or "right," while nonnormative practices, such as sexual negotiation, feel "bad" or "wrong" (Markus and Kitayama, 1994). Because of their importance on women's capacity for sexual negotiation, another study within the VOCES project focused on this topic.

Emotions

Tensions between protective and risk-related norms are clearly evident when women have to face the task of sexual negotiation. The HIV/AIDS epidemic has created the need for explicit sexual negotiation because few female-controlled methods exist that protect them against HIV/AIDS infection. Thus, women must speak out about sex and confront the exclusivity of penetrative sexuality, tasks that are quite formidable within the cultural and oppressive context in which they find themselves.

These tensions became evident in a study that explored the emotions that surround sexual negotiation (Feliciano-Torres, Badillo-Cordero, and Serrano-García, 1997). A focus group of Puerto Rican college women ($n = 15$) discussed their emotions at three moments: when initiating negotiation, upon being rejected by their partner, and when the negotiation was completed and successful. Emotions most frequently linked to initiation included fear, insecurity, and anxiety. Participants stated that when they were rejected, they felt anxious, frustrated, and hurt, and when they were successful, they felt happy, understood, and satisfied. When asked which emotions they felt were barriers to the negotiation process, women mentioned fear, insecurity, and love, and in response to which emotions facilitated negotiating they included security, enthusiasm, and fulfillment.

Barriers and facilitators of sexual negotiation were also explored with a content analysis of videotaped sexual negotiation simulations (Galarza and Serrano-García, 1997). In the simulations, two women role-played a heterosexual couple negotiating safer sex. One woman played the male role and was instructed to reject the other woman's request for condom use. The other participant, in the female role, had to use all available strategies to persuade "him" to use a condom. These simulations were part of the VOCES intervention and were used both to develop a Video Tape Rating Scale of Sexual Negotiation (Galarza and others, 1996) as well as to develop and measure change in participants' negotiation skills. There was much resistance both to the simulations and to the videotaping; therefore, data refer to a small group of eleven women.

In the videotapes, Galarza and others (1996) identified personal, social, and material resources that women used to facilitate their negotiations. Individual resources referred to women's personal attributes, as well as to their attitudes, cognitions, and emotions. Social resources included information or sources of support and material resources related to objects that could facilitate protection, such as condoms. Sources of resistance to protection that women identified in the "men" or in their own internal processes were also examined.

Results demonstrated that women relied mostly on their personal resources in the negotiation process. Those most frequently used were their experiences with safer-sex practices and identifying weaknesses in the partner's arguments or in characteristics of the relationship, particularly if it was short-lived. However, the argument most used to negotiate safer-sex practices, particularly condom use, was pregnancy prevention rather than prevention of sexually transmitted diseases or HIV/AIDS. The only social resource mentioned was the information obtained in VOCES workshops, and the only available material resource in the simulation, a condom, was not used. When asked about barriers, they identified those stemming from their partners much more frequently than those within themselves. The former included his multiple reasons for not using a condom, use of verbal aggression, indicating that she was responsible for "spoiling" the moment with her demands, chastising her for doubting him, and questioning her faithfulness. Barriers that stemmed from the women related to their limited knowledge of alternative and safer-sexual behaviors and to their own doubts about condom use.

Which cultural values emerge anew in these data? Negative emotions related to the initiation of the negotiation process can be linked to the unacceptability of speaking openly about sex and to constructions that indicate that women are not supposed to know about sex or enjoy it. They are also supposed to engage in sex with the goal of pleasing their partners instead of themselves. Since sexuality has been constructed as such an intimate area, it is of no surprise that women rely mostly on personal resources to negotiate a sexual encounter. However, in women's eyes, men depend mostly on arguments based on the prevailing social constructions and on their social and physical dominance to control the relationship. One important note of optimism is the identification of sexual education experiences as the main social resource used by women. If they can use the knowledge and skills obtained from education in their negotiation process, then there is some indication that preventive efforts can be successful.

Before concluding the presentation of these studies, we would like to draw attention to a particular issue identified in this research. A notion that emerged and that VOCES has yet to further explore is the link between constructions of romantic love and sexual behaviors. It is fascinating to note that women identify love as one of the feelings that serve as barriers to negotiation. "Men's" arguments related to faithfulness and trust are also related to this broader issue. A profound look at gendered constructions of love and trust, as well as to how these concepts contribute to women's domination, seems necessary at this point.

The studies described thus far suggest that there are some aspects of Puerto Rican culture that promote HIV/AIDS-related risk behaviors and that Puerto Rican women may still hold conservative beliefs, attitudes, and social norms about sexuality, some of which can be protective. There are other findings from recent prevention research, however, that suggest different ways of explaining these complex patterns of beliefs and behaviors. As we suggested earlier, these notions and beliefs do not escape the fluid social and material conditions present in the contexts in which they are manifested. One of the important factors to consider within women's social contexts are social networks.

Social Networks

Social networks can become a barrier or a facilitator to HIV/AIDS prevention depending on the social norms they convey and endorse (Fisher, 1988; Ickovics and Rodin, 1992). Their influence has been examined by members of the Cultural Network Project (CNP; Mantell, Rapkin, Tross, and Ortiz-Torres, 1992), of which Ortiz-Torres was a member. The CNP carried out a repeated measures study ($n = 1,922$) assessing promoters and barriers to HIV counseling and testing and risk-reduction behavior among inner-city African American women and Latinas in New York City.

The CNP study provides information regarding the importance of preventive role models within women's social network. Having a greater proportion of network members endorsing safer-sex practices predicts condom use by a woman's main male partner, and if he also supports prevention, condom use is more likely to increase in their most recent sexual encounter (Gillespie and others, n.d.) These authors also found that women who receive support for prevention from a larger proportion of their social network are more likely to be concerned about prevention and more likely to have been tested for HIV. It also seemed that less acculturated Latinas in the sample were members of social networks that provided less support for prevention. This complicates an already difficult situation for these women who are already at high risk of HIV infection due to these and other factors.

An additional look at the role of women's networks in facilitating or impeding the negotiation and practice of safer sex was undertaken by Ortiz-Torres and others (1996b) in a project entitled *Rompiendo el Silencio* (Breaking the Silence). They piloted an intervention targeting Latinas ($n = 116$; predominantly Dominican) in New York City to assess the effectiveness of preventive messages delivered in an AIDS education video through women's social networks. Their findings reiterate that social networks cannot only sustain existing social norms but could also become vehicles for change. This is supported by data that showed that participating in a group discussion with network members after viewing the educational video led the women (1) to favor safer-sex practices, (2) to reject the notion that being married protects you from HIV/AIDS infection, and (3) to increase their willingness to talk about condoms with potential partners and to ask them to use condoms to prevent HIV. The study will be replicated in Puerto Rico to assess similarities and differences in a Puerto Rican sample. For Latinas who have migrated to the United States, adopting to, or resisting immersion within, the Anglo culture becomes a day-to-day issue. Thus, acculturation and biculturalism have been studied as processes that influence diverse types of behaviors. We present transculturation as a more comprehensive concept and relate it to our HIV/AIDS concerns.

Transculturation

"Transculturation" is defined as a multidimensional construct involving social relationships, language and media use, participation in rituals, and group identification. We distinguish this construct from term *biculturalism*, which means that people share two cultures. Instead, the person has one culture, or identifies with one culture, but incorporates some behaviors from another. The transculturation process is characterized by simultaneous behaviors, perception, and cognitions that could have different, even contradictory, manifestations as people interact with the dominant culture (Ortiz-Torres, Rapkin, Mantell, and Tross, 1992). It does not assume that people strive to be assimilated into the host culture; rather, it is sensitive to the fact that some people choose not to be absorbed. Transculturation, however, is not an all-or-none process: people can choose to adopt certain patterns and practices of the dominant culture, while retaining others from their culture of origin.

Transculturation is also dynamic and dialectical. It suggests an individual who is actively engaged not only in adapting to but in influencing the dominant culture as she or he interacts with it. Evidence of the dynamic nature of this process was apparent in the Ortiz-Torres, Rapkin, Mantell, and Tross (1992) study. They conducted a cluster analysis on the data obtained from the sample of immigrant Latinas and found seven patterns of transactions with the host (North American) culture. Findings from the CNP have reiterated the complexity of the dynamics between culture and sex-related beliefs and behaviors and point to the importance of further examining the impact of transculturation. Immigrant Latinas in their sample (predominantly Puerto Rican) (1) rejected the notion that there is nothing wrong with their men having other partners, (2) believed that bringing up a condom on a date means they are loose, and (3) tended to link condom use to a lack of trust in their partners (Ortiz-Torres, 1995). These women perceived men as the main initiators of sexual activity, and 46 percent considered themselves as total or partial initiators of the most recent sexual activity. Participants also reported more openness within their sexual relationships and higher rates of communication with their partners regarding what they want or do not want and what they prefer sexually than typically expected of Latina women. They also reported refusing to participate in sexual activities that they dislike. These results exhibit a mix of traditional norms (for example, suggesting condom use means being loose) and "new" ones (for example, rejecting infidelity, speaking up about sex).

As has been noted earlier, samples of the studies conducted in Puerto Rico are composed of college students, while participants in the New York studies are community-based samples with participants who are older and, on the average, less educated than the Puerto Rican samples. These sociodemographic characteristics could account for some of the differences in research findings, but this does not seem to be the case.

Given their exposure to alternative belief systems, we would have expected the more educated and younger women to be less influenced by traditional values and beliefs than others. This is not what was found. One possible interpretation is that immigrant Latinas in New York are in a different, more diverse context, which results in a tendency to endorse less traditional beliefs. Ortiz-Torres, Rapkin, Mantell, and Tross (1992) have found that Latinas who have a proactive relationship with the dominant culture (they speak both English and Spanish, have a heterogeneous network, actively let other people know about their culture of origin), and thus do not fall into the typical "acculturated" category, engage more often in safer-sex practices than the traditionally acculturated Latinas.

Overall, both the existing literature and our research efforts present the pervasive role of cultural norms and beliefs on women's individual and social behaviors, which can in turn facilitate or hinder HIV/AIDS infection and prevention. Although traditional views of gender and sexuality still appear to be dominant, sociohistorical forces, particularly migration, and some intervention efforts (such as VOCES and *Rompiendo el Silencio*), open spaces for women to question and change these norms. This happens when they receive ample and pertinent information or training, or when they receive support from their social networks. How community psychologists deal with the challenges posed by these results is the subject the next section.

CHALLENGES POSED TO COMMUNITY PSYCHOLOGY

Community psychology has always been at the forefront of the discussion of the pertinence of values in all its endeavors (Prilleltensky, 1994; Trickett, 1996). Not only is this part of a broadening epistemological posture that includes constructionist and critical analysis, it is also part of the empowering and collaborative ideals that we have espoused. Thus, when faced with issues that

challenge our definitions of morality and of right and wrong, we have been prepared to face the challenge and to validate it, even if we have not always been
ready to produce immediate solutions.

Within this disciplinary tradition, the HIV/AIDS prevention research and
interventions we have presented pose a diversity of challenges to community
psychologists who are constantly considering what behaviors, norms, and
beliefs should be promoted. The focus on more individual-level issues such as
morality and emotion, and on broader issues such as social networks and acculturation, has definite implications for community psychology's values. It also
questions the applicability of community psychology's methods to changes in
cultural and normative beliefs.

The Role of Values

If we intend to prevent HIV/AIDS, the obvious conclusion could be to work at
discouraging cultural norms that hinder risk-protective behaviors while facilitating those that promote protective behaviors. This is not, however, that simple.
Some prevalent cultural norms we have discussed are contradictory. Two examples come to mind. On the one hand, if a woman is urged to remain a virgin, she
will have difficulty pleasing a partner with "uncontrollable urges," both norms
encountered within *machismo.* On the other, the norm that women must care for
themselves so as to protect others is in contradiction with the one that ascertains
that they cannot talk about their bodies or about sexuality, both norms espoused
by *marianismo.*

To complicate matters further, if we decide to promote norms that facilitate
protection, we may find that many of them are inconsistent with our values as
feminist community psychologists. A few examples include whether (1) to promote abstinence or virginity or the use of various safer-sex behaviors, (2) to
support women's care of themselves as a means to care for others or stress
healthy behaviors for their own wellness, and (3) to accept the construction of
penetrative sex as "good" sexuality and focus interventions on condom use or
foster alternative definitions that would lead us to promote the use of condoms
and of other nonpenetrative sexual behaviors.

The challenges just described can be faced only if a relational theory of sexuality is adopted. Such a theory underscores the importance of interactions,
which include not only the players but also the context in which sexual interactions are played out (Ferrand and Snijders, 1997). The context is determined by
variables such as culture, space, time, and the nature of partners' involvement
(Van Campenhoudt and Cohen, 1997).

When sexuality is considered a part not only of the private but also of the
public realm (Foucault, 1993), the individual level of intervention can be tran-
scended in favor of interventions that would facilitate the transformation of
sexual interactions (Ferrand and Snijders, 1997). These social interactions are

clearly multidimensional, incorporating gender, power, and political aspects that go beyond changes in individual sex-related behaviors.

The Applicability of Our Methods

In consonance with our discipline's values, various authors in our discipline have stressed the importance of multilevel analysis, intervention, and research (Perkins, 1995; Rappaport, 1977; Trickett, 1991). This is particularly pertinent to the issues we have presented that include emotions, cognitions, and behaviors at the individual level, social interactions within couples, support group and network norms, as well as the broader sociopolitical and cultural context.

The literature on empowerment is particularly relevant. Although the field focused on psychological empowerment until recently (Ortiz-Torres, forthcoming; Prilleltensky, 1994; Serrano-García and Bond, 1994), current efforts have broadened the analysis of empowering behaviors, interventions, and research to the group, organization, community and policy levels. Perkins and Zimmerman (1995) state,

> Empowerment theory, research and intervention link individual well being with the larger social and political environment. It compels us to think of wellness versus illness, competence versus deficit and strength versus weakness. Similarly, empowerment research focuses on identifying capabilities instead of cataloguing risk factors. . . . Empowerment oriented interventions enhance wellness . . . , provide opportunities for participants to develop knowledge and skills, and engage professionals as collaborators [pp. 569–570].

With these ideas in mind, we propose some ideas for interventions for Spanish Caribbean women, after considering the issues we have presented in this chapter.

Interventions

Individual-level interventions that have proven effective in HIV/AIDS research with other populations (Kalichman, 1998) are usually interactive and labor intensive. They focus on strategies such as workshops, small group interactions, and counseling. These strategies can be used with Puerto Rican and Dominican women if the content of the intervention places strong emphasis on examining and questioning cultural norms and beliefs. Activities should facilitate women's awareness of the socially constructed nature of these norms, of the link between the norms and their health, and of their capacity to change them, if they so desire.

It seems that certain groups of Latinas perceive they have the capability to practice safer sex if they wanted to. This perceived self-efficacy should be translated into behaviors (Ortiz-Torres, 1995). The barrier that should be dealt with is the gap between cognitions and behaviors that is created when faced with conflicting cultural norms: on the one hand, women feel strong and determined; on the other, they should please their partners. To deal with this barrier, the discussion of culturally specific issues previously mentioned could focus on the false relationship between trust and condoms and between ignorance about sexual matters and purity.

Interventions at the level of social networks or support groups is one of the most common vehicles for empowerment (Fawcett and others, 1994; Perkins, 1995). Gottlieb (1982) has identified two types of preventive interventions at this level: (1) those that attempt to improve the quality of support within the prevailing normative belief structure and (2) those that foster different norms and behaviors by incorporating new members into old networks or creating alternate networks. Fostering the importance of networks in Latinas' lives, with either one of these strategies, does not conflict with our values as feminists or as community psychologists.

An example of interventions that strengthen existing networks can be rooted in the belief that women should take care of themselves so as to take care of others, a belief that could be construed as a competency and a strength if it leads to empowering outcomes. This could be carried out through interactions with network members, such as diffusing safer-sex messages in group meetings, mobilizing women and the members of their networks to attend health clinics, and fostering discussions of factors that create obstacles to their health care. Thus, taking care of others will be positive as long as it goes along with self-protection and control of women's sexuality. The value of *familismo* might be relevant in this context, particularly if a close relationship with relatives allows women to request their help or endorsement to achieve changes in the direction of improving their health. Examples of this could be providing child care so they can attend the clinics, being mediators between family members who see things differently, and providing support when faced with obstacles.

Intervention geared at new values may require new networks. Changes that facilitate practicing safer sex or negotiating safer practices may require the creation of peer support groups or the availability of community spaces (health centers, women's groups) that allow for the discussion of these issues. Gillespie and others, n.d.) have pointed out that it is particularly important to include male partners in these efforts. The preventive strategies could promote network members' endorsement of safer sex and the modification of the belief that it is inappropriate to talk about sex with friends.

At the community level, our discipline has consistently promoted the importance of community partnerships when designing interventions (Fernández, 1995). HIV/AIDS interventions are particularly suited for this type of collaboration, since most of the creative and daring interventions in this area have been performed by nongovernmental community-based organizations. Examples of these include the following: (1) peer education efforts; (2) mass media campaigns through comic books, rap concerts, "novelas," and murals (Marín, 1990); and (3) counseling in case management sessions. Community psychologists can collaborate in strengthening these efforts through our increased awareness of the influence of cultural factors, research consultation, and research training, as well as information as to how to make their educational messages more behaviorally specific. These community partnerships can provide the opportunity for reciprocal learning as well as generating challenges to psychologists, who should respond to the urgent and ever changing needs within this constantly evolving field.

With these contributions from the field and the challenges posed by our context, culture, cognitions, and emotions, the proposal for interventions at the level of social norms and beliefs could indeed be construed as subversive (Bayer, 1994). It can be thought of as subversive because we abandon the conservative nationalist point of view that would suggest that to preserve each country's culture, it should be idealized, perpetuated, and transmitted as intact as possible to future generations. We believe that for a culture to grow and regenerate, it should fight for the elimination of double standards and inequality based on gender, class, sexual orientation, or any other categorization. Culture, we believe, cannot become a haven for oppression, but must instead be a space where respect for diversity and participation in the development of new values leads all of us closer to health, dignity, and freedom.

References

Alarcón, R., and Foulks, E. "Personality Disorders and Culture: Contemporary Clinical Views." *Cultural Diversity and Mental Health,* 1995, *1*(1), 3–17.

Amaro, H. "Considerations for Prevention of HIV Infection Among Hispanic Women." *Psychology of Women Quarterly,* 1988, *12,* 429–443.

Amaro, H. "Love, Sex and Power: Considering Women's Realities in HIV Prevention." *American Psychologist,* 1995, *50,* 437–447.

Aquino, M. *Our Cry for Life: Feminist Theology from Latin America.* New York: Orbis Books, 1993.

Auerbach, J., Wypijewska, C., and Brodie, K. (eds.). *AIDS and Behavior: An Integrated Approach.* Washington, D.C.: National Academy Press, 1994.

Bayer, R. "AIDS Prevention and Cultural Sensitivity: Are They Compatible?" *American Journal of Public Health,* 1994, *84*(6), 895–898.

Becker, E., Rankin, E., and Rickel, A. *High-Risk Sexual Behavior: Interventions with Vulnerable Populations.* New York: Plenum, 1998.

Bennet, O. (ed.). *Triple Jeopardy: Women and AIDS.* London: Pannos Institute, 1990.

Boal, A. *Teatro del oprimido: Teoría y práctica.* Mexico City: Editorial Nueva Imagen, 1980.

Bravo, M. "Las redes de apoyo social y las situaciones de desastre: Estudio de la población adulta en P.R." Unpublished doctoral dissertation, University of Puerto Rico, 1989.

Cantera, L. "Sexualidad y relaciones de poder entre los géneros: Análisis de las experiencias de un grupo de puertorriqueños/as." Unpublished doctoral dissertation, University of Puerto Rico, 1992.

Carnivalli, J. "Perfil sociodemográfico de la población femenina en Puerto Rico en cifras." Paper presented at the First Conference on Women and AIDS, San Juan, P.R., Apr. 1993.

Centers for Disease Control. *The HIV/AIDS Epidemic in the United States, 1997–1998. Directory.* [cdc.gov/nchstp/hiv_aids/pubs/facts/hivrepfs.htm]. 1998.

Cochran, S. "Women and HIV Infection: Issues in Prevention." In V. Mays, G. Albee, and S. Schneider. (eds.), *Primary Prevention of AIDS: Psychological Approaches.* Thousand Oaks, Calif.: Sage, 1989.

Colberg-Luciano, E., and Ramos-Marcano, E. "Work and Family Situations of Women in Top Management in Puerto Rico." In J. Frankee (ed.), *Families of Employed Mothers: An International Perspective.* New York: Garland, 1997.

Colón-Warren, A. "Reestructuración industrial, empleo y pobreza en Puerto Rico y el Atlántico Medio de los Estados Unidos: La situación de las mujeres puertorriqueñas." *Revista de Ciencias Sociales,* 1997, *3,* 35–188.

Comas-Díaz, L., and Duncan, J. W. "The Cultural Factor in Assertiveness Training with Mainland Puerto Rican Women." *Psychology of Women Quarterly,* 1985, *9,* 463–476.

Comas-Díaz, L., Griffith, E., Pinderhughes, E., and Wyche, K. "Coming of Age: Cultural Diversity and Mental Health." *Cultural Diversity and Mental Health,* 1995, *1*(1), 1–2.

Cruz, D., and Serrano-García, I. "La relación entre la percepción de moralidad y las prácticas sexuales de alto riesgo en mujeres puertorriqueñas." Paper presented at the Interamerican Congress of Psychology, Sao Paulo, Brasil, July 1997.

Cunningham, I., and Cunningham, E. "The Metaphor of AIDS in Puerto Rico: Reporting an Epidemic." In I. Cunningham, C. Ramos, and R. Ortiz (eds.), *El SIDA en Puerto Rico: Acercamientos multidisciplinarios.* Rio Piedras, P.R.: Editorial Universitaria, 1992.

De la Cancela, V. "A Critical Analysis of Puerto Rican *Machismo*: Implications for Clinical Practice." *Psychotherapy,* 1986, *23*(2), 291–296.

Delgado, M., and Humm-Delgado, D. "Natural Support Systems: Source of Strength in Hispanic Communities." *Social Work,* 1982, *1,* 83–88.

Farley, M. "Feminist Theology and Bioethics." In A. Loades (ed.), *Feminist Theology: A Reader.* Louisville, Ky.: John Knox Press, 1990.

Fawcett, S., and others. "A Contextual-Behavioral Model of Empowerment: Case Studies Involving People with Physical Disabilities." *American Journal of Community Psychology,* 1994, *22*(4), 471–496.

Feliciano-Torres, Y., Badillo-Cordero, E., and Serrano-García, I. "Las emociones relacionadas a la negociación de sexo seguro: Consideraciones para la prevención del VIH/SIDA." Paper presented at the Twenty-Sixth Interamerican Congress of Psychology, Sao Paulo, Brasil, July 1997.

Fernández, M. I. "Latinas and AIDS: Challenges to HIV Prevention Efforts." In A. O'Leary and L. Jemmot (eds.), *Women at Risk: Issues in the Primary Prevention of AIDS.* New York: Plenum, 1995.

Ferrand, A., and Snijders, T. "Social Networks and Normative Tensions." In L. V. Campenhoudt, M. Cohen, G. Guizzardi, and D. Hausser (eds.), *Sexual Interactions and HIV Risk: New Conceptual Perspectives in European Research.* London: Taylor and Francis, 1997.

Fisher, J. "Possible Effects of Reference Group-Based Social Influence on AIDS Risk Behavior and AIDS Prevention." *American Psychologist,* 1988, *43*(11), 914–919.

Foucault, M. *Historia de la sexualidad.* Mexico, DF, Mexico: Siglo XXI, 1993.

Fox, R. *Kinship and Marriage.* Middlesex, England: Penguin Books, 1967.

Galarza, M., and Serrano-García, I. "Hacia la negociación del sexo más seguro: Barreras y recursos de un grupo de mujeres puertorriqueñas." Paper presented at the Twenty-Sixth Interamerican Congress of Psychology in Sao Paulo, Brasil, 1997.

Galarza, M., and others. *Escala de Análisis de Vídeo para el Manejo de Conflicto.* San Juan, P.R.: Centro Universitario de Servicios y Estudios Psicológicos, University of Puerto Rico, 1996.

Gil, R. M., and Inoa-Vázquez, C. *The María Paradox: How Latinas Can Merge Old World Traditions with New World Self-Esteem.* New York: G. P. Putnam, 1996.

Gillespie, C., and others. "Social Network Influence and HIV Prevention Among Inner-City African American and Latina Women." Unpublished manuscript, n.d.

González, S. "Discurso y práctica feminista en el protestantismo en Puerto Rico." Unpublished master's thesis, Seminario Evangelico de Puerto Rico, 1996.

Gottlieb, B. "Preventive Interventions Involving Social Networks and Social Support." In B. Gottlieb (ed.), *Social Networks and Social Support.* Thousand Oaks, Calif.: Sage, 1982.

Gupta, G., and Weiss, E. "Women's Lives and Sex." In R. Parker and J. Gagnon (eds.), *Conceiving Sexuality: Approaches to Sex Research in a Postmodern World.* New York: Routledge, 1995.

Hays, R., and Peterson, J. "HIV Prevention for Gay and Bisexual Men in Metropolitan Cities." In R. DiClemente and J. Peterson (eds.), *Preventing AIDS: Theories and Methods of Behavioral Interventions.* New York: Plenum, 1994.

Ickovics, J., and Rodin, J. "Women and AIDS in the U.S.: Epidemiology, Natural History and Mediating Mechanisms." *Health Psychology,* 1992, *11,* 1–16.

Jemmott, J. "Social Psychological Influences on HIV Risk-Behaviors Among African-American Youths." In S. Oskamp and S. Thompson (eds.), *Understanding and Preventing HIV Risk Behavior: Safer Sex and Drug Use.* Thousand Oaks, Calif.: Sage, 1996.

Kalichman, S. C. "Post-Exposure Prophylaxis for HIV Infection in Gay and Bisexual Men: Implications for the Future of HIV Prevention." *American Journal of Preventive Medicine,* 1998, *15*(2), 120–127.

Kelly, J. "HIV Prevention Among Gay and Bisexual Men in Small Cities." In R. DiClemente and J. Peterson (eds.), *Preventing AIDS: Theories and Methods of Behavioral Interventions.* New York: Plenum, 1994.

Leukefeld, C. G., Battjes, R. J., and Amsel, Z. *AIDS and Intravenous Drug Use: Community Intervention and Prevention.* New York: Hemisphere, 1990.

Lonner, W. "Culture and Human Diversity." In E. Tricket, R. Watts, and D. Birman (eds.), *Human Diversity: Perspectives on People in Context*. San Francisco: Jossey-Bass, 1994.

Mair, L. *Introducción a la antropología social*. Madrid, Spain: Alianza Editorial S.A., 1965.

Mantell, J., Rapkin, B., Tross, S., and Ortiz-Torres, B. *Cultural Network Project*. New York: Medical Health and Research Association, 1992.

Marín, B. "AIDS Prevention for Non-Puerto Rican Hispanics." In C. G. Leukefeld, R. J. Battjes, and Z. Amsel (eds.), *AIDS and Intravenous Drug Use: Community Intervention and Prevention*. New York: Hemisphere, 1990.

Marín, B. "Traditional Gender Roles Beliefs Increase Coercion and Lower Condom Use in Latino Men." Poster session presented at the Eleventh International Conference on AIDS, Vancouver, B.C., Canada, July 1996.

Markus, H., and Kitayama, S. "The Cultural Construction of Self and Emotion: Implications for Social Behavior." In S. Kitayama and H. Markus (eds.), *Emotion and Culture*. Washington, D.C.: APA, 1994.

McCann-Erickson, X. *Estudio psicográfico de la mujer puertorriqueña: Una mujer, mil caras*. San Juan: Ramallo Brothers, 1990.

Miles, L. "Women, AIDS and Power in Heterosexual Sex: A Discourse Analysis." In M. Gergen and S. Davis (eds.), *Toward a New Psychology of Gender: A Reader*. New York: Routledge, 1997.

Noboa, P., Serrano-García, I., and Torres-Burgos, N. *Escala de autoeficacia para la negociación sexual*. San Juan, P.R.: Centro Universitario de Servicios y Estudios Psicológicos, University of Puerto Rico, 1997.

Ortiz-Torres, B. "Mistaken Assumptions About Women: The Case of Culture." Paper presented at the Annual Convention of the American Psychological Association, New York, Aug. 1995.

Ortiz-Torres, B. "El 'empowerment' como alternativa teórica en América Latina." *Interamerican Journal of Psychology*, forthcoming.

Ortiz-Torres, B., Rapkin, B., Mantell, J., and Tross, S. "Is Transculturation Related to Sexual Risk Behavior Among Latinas?" Paper presented at the Eighth International Conference on AIDS/III STD World Congress, Amsterdam, The Netherlands, July 1992.

Ortiz-Torres, B., and others. "La construcción social de la sexualidad y los roles de género en estudiantes universitarios y su relación con la conducta de riesgo para contraer VIH/SIDA." Paper presented at Psicosalud '96, Habana, Cuba, Oct. 1996a.

Ortiz-Torres, B., and others. "Rompiendo el Silencio: Un modelo de difusión de innovación para la prevención del VIH/SIDA en mujeres heterosexuales." Paper presented at Psicosalud '96, Habana, Cuba, Oct. 1996b.

PASET. *Surveillance Report*. San Juan, P.R., 1998.

Patton, C. *Inventing AIDS*. New York: Routledge, 1990.

Peragallo, N., Talashek, M., Norr, K., and Dancy, B. "Culturally Specific AIDS Prevention Needs of Mexican and Puerto Rican Inner-City Women." Poster session presented at the Twelfth World AIDS Conference, Geneva, Switzerland, June 1998.

Perkins, D. "Speaking Truth to Power: Empowerment Ideology as Social Intervention and Policy." *American Journal of Community Psychology,* 1995, *23*(5), 765–794.

Perkins, D., and Zimmerman, M. "Empowerment Theory, Research and Application." *American Journal of Community Psychology,* 1995, *23*(5), 569–580.

Picó, F., and Rivera-Izcoa, C. *Puerto Rico: Tierra adentro y mar afuera.* Rio Piedras: Ediciones Huracán, 1991.

Prilleltensky, I. *The Morals and Politics of Psychology: Psychological Discourse and the Status Quo.* New York: State University of New York Press, 1994.

Ramírez, R. L. *Dime capitán: Reflexiones sobre la masculinidad.* Río Piedras, P.R.: Ediciones Huracán, 1993.

Rappaport, J. *Community Psychology: Values, Research and Action.* New York: Holt, 1977.

Salgado de Snyder, N. V., and Padilla, A. M. "Social Support Networks: Their Availability and Effectiveness." In M. Gaviria and J. Arana (eds.), *Health and Behavior: Research Agenda for Hispanics.* Chicago: University of Illinois at Chicago, 1987.

Santos-Ortiz, M. "El SIDA y las relaciones heterosexuales." In I. Cunningham, C. Ramos, and R. Ortiz (eds.), *El SIDA en Puerto Rico: Aspectos multidisciplinario.* Rio Piedras, P.R.: Editorial Universitaria, 1991.

Serrano-García, I. "Empowerment and HIV/AIDS: A Prevention Project for Young, Heterosexual, Puerto Rican Women." NIMH Grant No. 2R24MH49368–04, 1994.

Serrano-García, I. "Tensions Between Research Methods and Values: Evaluating an HIV/AIDS Prevention Project for Puerto Rican Women." Paper presented at the Public Health in the Twenty-First Century Conference, Atlanta, May 1998.

Serrano-García, I., and Bond, M. "Empowering the Silent Ranks: Introduction." *American Journal of Community Psychology,* 1994, *22*(4), 433–445.

Serrano-García, I., Torres-Burgos, N., and Galarza, M. "Las relaciones de poder y la prevención del VIH/SIDA: Una Intervención/investigación entre mujeres puertorriqueñas." In F. Balcázar, M. Montero, and S. Fuks (eds.), *Community Health Promotion in the Americas.* Washington, D.C.: PAHO, forthcoming.

Serrano-García, I., and others. *Escala de relaciones de poder.* San Juan, P.R.: Centro Universitario de Servicios y Estudios Psicológicos, University of Puerto Rico, 1996.

Silva-Gotay, S. *Protestantismo y política en Puerto Rico 1898–1930: Hacia una historia del protestantismo evangélico en Puerto Rico.* San Juan. P.R.: Editorial de la Universidad de Puerto Rico, 1996.

Soltero, S. "Sex Education Belongs to the Parents." *San Juan Star,* Nov. 23, 1997, p. 22.

Soto, E., and Shaver, P. "Sex Role Traditionalism, Assertiveness and Symptoms of Puerto Rican Women Living in the United States." *Hispanic Journal of Behavioral Sciences,* 1982, *4*, 1–19.

Stevens, E. P. "Machismo and Marianismo." *Transaction/Society*, 1973, *10*(6), 57–63.

Stycos, J. M. "Family and Fertility in Puerto Rico." In F. Cordasco and E. Bucchioni (eds.), *The Puerto Rican Community and Its Children on the Mainland: A Source Book for Teachers, Social Workers and Other Professionals*. Metuchen, N.J.: Scarecrow Press, 1952.

Tiefer, L. "Sexual Biology and the Symbolism of the Natural." In M. Gergen and S. Davis (eds.), *Toward a New Psychology of Gender: A Reader*. New York: Routledge, 1997.

Toro-Alfonso, J., and others. *Inventario de conducta sexual para mujeres*. San Juan, P.R.: Centro Universitario de Servicios y Estudios Psicológicos, University of Puerto Rico, 1997.

Torres-Burgos, N., and Serrano-García, I. "Empowerment and HIV/AIDS: A Prevention Project for Young Heterosexual Puerto Rican Women." In M. Montero (ed.), *Memorias de Psicología Comunitaria del XXV Congreso Interamericano de Psicología*. Caracas, Venezuela, 1997.

Trickett, E. *Living an Idea: Empowerment and the Evolution of an Inner City Alternative High School*. Cambridge, Mass.: Brookline Books, 1991.

Trickett, E. "A Future for Community Psychology: The Contexts of Diversity and the Diversity of Contexts." *American Journal of Community Psychology*, 1996, *24*(2), 209–234.

Trickett, E., Watts, R., and Birman, D. (eds.). *Human Diversity: Perspectives on People in Context*. San Francisco: Jossey-Bass, 1994.

U.S. Census Bureau. *Current Population Reports: The Hispanic Population in the United States*. [blue.census.gov/prod/3/98pubs/p20–511.pdf]. 1997.

Van Campenhoudt, L., and Cohen, M. "Interaction and Risk-Related Behaviour: Theoretical and Heuristic Landmarks." In L. Van Campenhoudt, M. Cohen, C. Guizzardi, and D. Haussen (eds.), *Sexual Interactions and HIV Risk: New Conceptual Perspectives in European Research*. London: Taylor and Francis, 1997.

VanOss Marin, B., Gómez, C., Tschann, J., and Gregorech, S. (in process). Condom Use in Unmarried Adult Latino Men: A Test of Cultural Constructs." *Health Psychology*, 1997, *16*(5), 458–467.

Vega, W. A., and Kolody, B. "The Meaning of Social Support and the Mediation of Stress Across Cultures." In W. A. Vega and M. R. Miranda (eds.), *Stress and Hispanic Mental Health: Relating Research to Service Delivery* (pp. 48–75). Rockville, Md.: National Institute of Mental Health, 1985.

Watts, R. "Paradigms of Diversity." In E. Trickett, R. Watts, and D. Birman (eds.), *Human Diversity: Perspectives on People in Context*. San Francisco: Jossey-Bass, 1994.

Williams, E. *From Columbus to Castro: The History of the Caribbean*. New York: Vintage Books, 1970.

World Health Organization. *World Report on HIV/AIDS*. Geneva, Switzerland: World Health Organization, 1998.

PART FOUR

CHRONIC CONDITIONS

Heart Disease, Cancer,
and Diabetes

Mortality from Coronary Heart Disease and Cardiovascular Disease Among Adult U.S. Hispanics

Findings from the National Health Interview Survey (1986 to 1994)

Youlian Liao
Richard S. Cooper
Guichan Cao
Jay S. Kaufman
Andrew E. Long
Daniel L. McGee

This chapter address chronic conditions for which there is little, if any, literature that specifically focuses on Latinas. It reports the findings for Latinos (males and females) from the National Health Interview Survey (1986–1994), with African American and White comparisons. Of special value are the tables, which contain specific data on Latinas, offering important information that is not readily available for this group of women.

The Hispanic population, which numbers 22.4 million people in the continental United States, is the second largest minority group and is increasing at a rate five times that of the rest of the United States (*U.S. Department of Commerce News*, 1991). It has been estimated that Hispanics will become the largest minority group early in the twenty-first century (American Medical Association, 1991). However, a comprehensive description of the mortality experience

From the Department of Preventive Medicine and Epidemiology, Loyola University Stritch School of Medicine, Maywood, Illinois. This work was supported by a cooperative agreement (U83/CCU512480) from the Centers for Disease Control, Atlanta, Georgia.

Abbreviations and acronyms: CHD, coronary heart disease; CI, confidence interval; CVD, cardiovascular disease; NHIS, National Health Interview.

of Hispanics is still lacking. Vital statistics data show that cardiovascular mortality has been lower in Hispanic men (Buechley and others, 1979; Bradshaw and Fonner, 1978; Schoen and Nelson, 1981; Stern and others, 1987; Goff, Ramsey, Labarthe, and Nichaman, 1993) and in both men and women (Becker, Wiggins, Key, and Samet, 1988; National Center for Health Statistics, 1993; Wild, and others, 1995) than in non-Hispanic whites. Follow-up data on coronary heart disease (CHD) mortality from cohort studies are scarce (Sorlie, Backlund, Johnson, and Rogot, 1993; Wei, Mitchell, Haffner, and Stern, 1996). This chapter used multiple cause of death data from the National Health Interview Survey (NHIS) (1986–1994), including approximately 15,000 Hispanics, approximately 250,000 non-Hispanic whites, and approximately 38,000 blacks 45 years or older. The primary purpose of the analysis was to estimate and compare the CHD and cardiovascular disease (CVD) mortality experience of U.S. Hispanics, blacks and whites.

METHODS

NHIS

As one of the major data collection programs of the National Center for Health Statistics, NHIS is a principal source of information on the health of the resident, civilian, noninstitutionalized population of the United States (Massey, Moore, Parsons, and Tadros, 1989). This nationwide survey has been conducted continuously since 1957 and is based on a multistage area probability sample through personal household interview. Most households chosen are contacted by mail before the interviewers arrive. Interviewers make repeated trips to households when respondents have not been available. Data are collected for all family members. Proxy responses are used for children and adults who are not available or are unable to respond for themselves. The average annual sample consists of approximately 45,000 households, including 120,000 persons (86,000 who are 18 years or older). The response rate was 96 to 98 percent over the years analyzed. Race and Hispanic origin were determined according to the participant's choice of the ethnic designation that best represented his or her race: Aleut, Eskimo, or American Indian; Asian or Pacific Islander; black, white, or other. Then he or she was asked whether his or her national origin or ancestry was any of the following: Puerto Rican, Cuban, Mexican/Mexicano, Mexican American, Chicano, other Latin American, or other Spanish. Those who responded as having any of the above national origins were considered Hispanic. This chapter focuses on persons 45 years or older only. Because the numbers were small for persons other than the three primary groups of interest, they were omitted from this report ($n = 7,568$ [2.4 percent]). The term *white* was used to represent non-Hispanic whites.

Family income was determined by asking which category best represented the total combined family income during the past twelve months from wages, salaries, and all other sources. The twenty-seven income categories ranged from below $1,000 (including loss) to $50,000 and up, with $1,000 increments for each category up to $20,000 and $5,000 increments thereafter to $49,999. Data on annual family income were available for 81 percent of the respondents in the study.

Mortality Follow-Up

Beginning with survey year 1986, vital status of the NHIS respondents 18 years and older is matched with files in the National Death Index system (Patterson and Bilgrad, 1985). The system is a computer database of all deaths in the United States since 1979 and has been shown (Stampfer, and others, 1984) to provide a high level of death ascertainment. To date, multiple cause of death data are available for NHIS survey years 1986 to 1994, with follow-up to include all deaths that occurred through December 31, 1995. The matching methodology used in linking to the National Death Index is a modification of the probabilistic approaches (Rogot, Sorlie, and Johnson, 1986). We used the algorithm provided by the National Center for Health Statistics (1986–1994) to determine which potential matches should be classified as deaths. Sufficient information to permit linkage with the National Death Index was unavailable in 10,524 persons (3.4 percent), and these persons were excluded from the analysis.

Causes of death were coded using the Ninth Revision of the International Classification of Diseases. Codes 410 to 414 and 429.2 were defined as CHD; codes 430 to 438 as cerebrovascular disease; codes 390 to 448 as CVD; codes 140 to 208 as cancers; and all other codes as other causes. Both underlying cause and multiple cause (any mention) of death were considered in the analyses.

Data Analysis

Death rates were calculated for each gender and race group by dividing the number of deaths during 1986 to 1995 by the total number of person-years of follow-up. The 95 percent confidence intervals for the black/white and Hispanic/white mortality ratios were estimated by the delta method (Miller, 1981). Age standardization was accomplished by the direct method for ten-year intervals using the entire cohort as the reference. The Cox proportional hazards model was used to estimate the relative risk of mortality for blacks and Hispanics compared with whites, adjusted for age (years) and family income. Family income for different survey years was standardized to the equivalent 1990 dollar value. The software program SUDAAN (Shah, Barnwell, and Bieler, 1995) was used to account for the complex sampling design of the study. Analyses were first performed for participants from survey years 1986 to 1989 and 1990 to 1994 separately. The results of racial comparisons were comparable for the two analytic cohorts with lower statistical power. The final report was presented with combined data of 1986 to 1994.

RESULTS

Source of Participants

During the years 1986 to 1994, the NHIS sampled approximately 300,000 persons 45 years and older from the U.S. population, of whom 246,239 were whites, 38,042 were blacks, and 14,965 were of Hispanic origin (Table 8.1). Among both men and women, Hispanics were younger than either whites or blacks; thus, all analyses were performed with age adjustment. The mortality follow-up period ranged from one to ten years (mean 5), with 27,702 white (11 percent), 4,976 black (13 percent), and 1,061 Hispanic deaths (7 percent).

All-Cause and Cause-Specific Mortality

All-cause and specific underlying cause of deaths, age-adjusted mortality rates (per 100,000 person-years), rate ratios, using whites as the reference, and their 95 percent confidence intervals are shown in Table 8.2. Compared with whites, the total mortality was greater in blacks and lower in Hispanics for both men and women. The 95 percent confidence intervals of the rate ratios were all

Table 8.1. Number of Respondents at Baseline and Deaths During Follow-Up by Gender, Race, and Age Groups

Age Group (years)	Whites		Blacks		Hispanics	
	Number (%) at Baseline	Number of Deaths	Number (%) at Baseline	Number of Deaths	Number (%) at Baseline	Number of Deaths
			Men			
45–54	39,159 (35)	1,275	5,541 (36)	354	3,058 (46)	95
55–64	32,032 (29)	2,886	4,676 (30)	621	2,048 (31)	156
65–74	26,715 (24)	5,112	3,444 (22)	828	1,096 (16)	161
75 and older	14,357 (13)	5,367	1,765 (11)	701	514 (8)	162
Total	112,263 (100)	14,640	15,426 (100)	2,504	6,716 (100)	574
			Women			
45–54	40,771 (30)	887	7,900 (35)	305	3,509 (43)	56
55–64	35,406 (26)	1,891	6,522 (29)	557	2,405 (29)	109
65–74	33,749 (25)	3,960	5,033 (22)	721	1,538 (19)	142
75 and older	24,050 (18)	6,324	3,161 (14)	889	797 (10)	180
Total	133,976 (100)	13,062	22,616 (100)	2,472	8,249 (100)	487

Table 8.2. Age-Adjusted All-Cause and Cause-Specific Mortality by Gender and Race: National Health Interview Survey, 1986–1994

Mortality	Men			Women		
	Number of Deaths	Rate[a]	Rate Ratio (95% CI)	Number of Deaths	Rate[a]	Rate Ratio (95% CI)
All causes						
Whites	14,640	3,089	1.00	13,062	1,897	1.00
Blacks	2,504	3,895	1.26 (1.20–1.33)	2,472	2,339	1.23 (1.17–1.29)
Hispanics	574	2,466	0.80 (0.73–0.88)	487	1,581	0.83 (0.76–0.92)
Coronary heart disease						
Whites	4,326	928	1.00	3,390	490	1.00
Blacks	604	951	1.02 (0.93–1.13)	616	605	1.23 (1.12–1.36)
Hispanics	153	717	0.77 (0.64–0.93)	113	401	0.82 (0.66–1.01)
Cerebrovascular accident						
Whites	807	178	1.00	1,043	149	1.00
Blacks	138	218	1.22 (0.99–1.50)	191	191	1.28 (1.07–1.53)
Hispanics	45	198	1.11 (0.78–1.58)	39	131	0.88 (0.63–1.22)
Cardiovascular disease						
Whites	6,500	1,398	1.00	5,880	844	1.00
Blacks	1,063	1,680	1.20 (1.12–1.29)	1,167	1,144	1.36 (1.26–1.46)
Hispanics	243	1,101	0.79 (0.68–0.91)	193	682	0.80 (0.69–0.94)

[a]Age-adjusted rate/100,000 person-years. CI 5 confidence interval.

significantly different from 1.0. The specific causes with a significantly greater rate ratio for blacks included CHD and CVD in women and CVD in both men and women. In general, Hispanics had about 20 percent lower CHD and CVD mortality than did whites. The rate ratios were significantly lower than 1.0, except for CHD among women. The confidence intervals of the Hispanic/white ratio for cerebrovascular disease were wide as the result of the small number of deaths among Hispanics.

When mortality rates for CHD and CVD were estimated using any mention of them on the death certificates, the Hispanic/white rate ratios were essentially unchanged among men (CHD: 0.77, 95 percent confidence interval [CI] 0.65 to 0.92, CVD: 0.81, 95 percent CI 0.72 to 0.91). Among women, the ratio increased to 0.93 (95 percent CI 0.78 to 1.10) for CHD and 0.93 (95 percent CI 0.83 to 1.04) for CVD, respectively.

Components of Causes of Death

The age-adjusted proportion of total deaths due to various causes in Hispanics and whites are presented in Figure 8.1 for men and Figure 8.2 for women. These data provide an indication of the relative importance of various causes of death in each subpopulation. There was no apparent racial difference in the proportion of death due to CHD among both men (28.1 percent versus 29.7 percent,

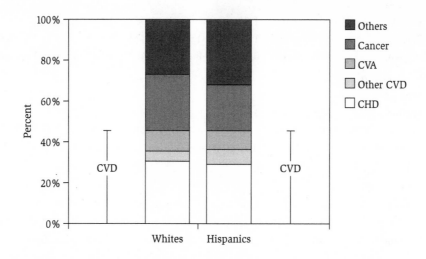

Figure 8.1. Proportional Mortality in White and Hispanic Men, 45 Years and Older: NHIS, 1986–1994

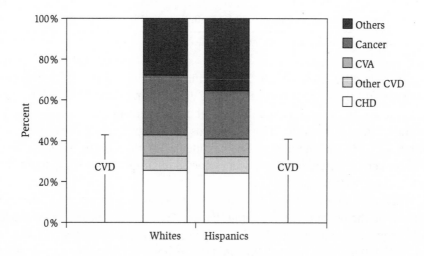

Figure 8.2. Proportional Mortality in White and Hispanic Women, 45 Years and Older: NHIS, 1986–1994

Hispanics versus whites) and women (24.1 percent versus 24.9 percent). Likewise, similar proportions due to CVD were found (44.3 percent versus 44.7 percent for men, 41.0 percent versus 43.2 percent for women, respectively). The proportion of deaths due to cancer was smaller in Hispanics than in whites for both men (23.7 percent versus 28.4 percent, Hispanics versus whites) and women (23.8 percent versus 29.6 percent) but greater for other causes (32.1 percent versus 26.8 percent for men, 35.2 percent versus 27.2 percent for women, respectively).

Effect of Income Difference

The standardized mean annual family income was, respectively, $35,800 and $30,400 among white men and women, $25,200 and $20,500 among blacks, and $28,700 and $25,800 among Hispanics. Lower income was significantly associated with increased all-cause and cause-specific mortality in each group (data not shown). Adjustment for income, in addition to age, narrowed the gap of mortality from CHD and CVD between blacks and whites (Table 8.3). As expected, the relative risk for Hispanics compared with whites was reduced, to a smaller degree, however, after the differences in income distribution were considered.

Table 8.3. Adjusted Risk of Death from Coronary Heart and Cardiovascular Disease: Blacks and Hispanics Versus Whites

Adjustment	CHD [RR (95% CI)]	CVD [RR (95% CI)]
Men		
Black versus white		
Age	1.07 (0.96–1.20)	1.29 (1.18–1.41)
Age and income	0.92 (0.82–1.03)	1.12 (1.03–1.23)
Hispanic versus white		
Age	0.75 (0.61–0.93)	0.79 (0.67– 0.94)
Age and income	0.68 (0.55–0.84)	0.72 (0.62–0.85)
Women		
Black versus white		
Age	1.28 (1.13–1.44)	1.42 (1.30–1.54)
Age and income	1.14 (1.01–1.29)	1.29 (1.19–1.40)
Hispanic versus white		
Age	0.83 (0.66–1.04)	0.85 (0.72–1.01)
Age and income	0.80 (0.63–1.00)	0.83 (0.70–0.98)

Note: RR = relative risk.

DISCUSSION

Vital Statistics

Until recently, our knowledge about CVD mortality in Hispanic populations in the United States was limited mostly to data from vital statistics. Before the early 1980s, vital statistics from New Mexico (Buechley and others 1979; Becker, Wiggins, Key, and Samet, 1988), Texas (Bradshaw and Fonner, 1978; Stern and others, 1987), and California (Schoen and Nelson, 1981) indicated lower CHD and CVD among Hispanic American men than non-Hispanic men, but less clearly so in Hispanic American women. Recent reports (Bradshaw and Fonner, 1978; Wild, and others, 1995) extended the findings to the subsequent decade. There was no evidence to indicate that the mortality gap between Mexican American and non-Hispanic white men was closing. A specific item about Hispanic origin was included in the death certificate in fifteen states after 1980 and was gradually extended to forty-nine states and the District of Columbia by 1993. At the national level, Hispanics experienced about two-thirds the heart disease mortality of non-Hispanic whites for both men and women (National Center for Health Statistics, 1993). The major weaknesses of using vital statistics to estimate mortality in Hispanics are misclassification (that is, incorrectly assigning race to decedents) and underregistration (Hahn, 1992). Most misclassified decedents are falsely reported to be white, understating Hispanic mortality. Comparing the information on death certificates and the National Mortality Followback Survey demonstrated that 19.6 percent more Hispanic decedents were reported on the questionnaire than on the death certificate (Poe and others, 1993). In contrast, the 1980 census undercounted Hispanics by as much as 8 percent, blacks by 6 percent, and white and others by 1 percent (Fay, Passel, Robinson, and Gowan, 1988). The aggregate effect of these errors is not precisely known.

Cohort Studies

To date, two cohort studies (Sorlie, Backlund, Johnson, and Rogot, 1993; Wei, Mitchell, Haffner, and Stern, 1996) have reported mortality from CVD among the Hispanic population. The National Longitudinal Mortality Study (Sorlie, Backlund, Johnson, and Rogot, 1993) followed up approximately 700,000 respondents, including 40,000 Hispanics, from 1979 to 1987. Hispanics (25 years and older) had significantly lower CVD mortality than did whites (standardized rate ratios: 0.65 for men, 0.80 for women) (Sorlie, Backlund, Johnson, and Rogot, 1993). The recent eight-year follow-up of the San Antonio Heart Study (Wei, Mitchell, Haffner, and Stern, 1996) reported that the death rate from CVD was nonsignificantly higher (rate ratio 1.3) in Mexican Americans than non-Hispanic whites. The number of deaths for all cohorts was only 137; hence, the analysis was performed with men and women combined.

Coronary Heart Disease in Hispanics

A less favorable cardiovascular risk factor profile has been documented in Hispanics than in non-Hispanic whites. On average, Hispanics have higher body mass indexes (Mitchell and others, 1990), more central obesity (Mitchell and others, 1990; Burchfiel and others, 1990), and lower high density lipoprotein cholesterol and higher triglycerides levels (Mitchell and others, 1990). Cigarette smoking (Mitchell and others, 1990; Haynes and others, 1990) and diabetes (Mitchell and others, 1990; Flegal, and others, 1991; Baxter and others, 1993) are more prevalent in Hispanics, and the prevalence of hypertension is similar to that in whites (Caralis, 1990). Overall, Hispanics have higher risk scores for CHD than non-Hispanic whites (Mitchell and others, 1990), and the impact of the major risk factors is similar to that of whites (Wei, Mitchell, Haffner, and Stern, 1996). Hispanics also have lower levels of socioeconomic status and health insurance coverage and utilize fewer preventive services than non-Hispanic whites (Andersen and others, 1981; Trevino, Moyer, Valdez, and Stroup-Benham, 1991; Mitchell and others, 1991). All these factors would imply higher CHD morbidity and mortality in Hispanics. Morbidity data were scarce, mainly from local areas and based on a small number of events. The prevalence of CHD in Hispanics was found to be lower than (Mitchell and others, 1991) or similar to (Rewers and others, 1993) that in non-Hispanic whites. CHD incidence has been reported (Rewers and others, 1993) to be similar among nondiabetic Hispanics and non-Hispanic whites but lower in diabetic Hispanics. The Corpus Christi Heart Project (Nichaman, Wear, Goff, and Labarthe, 1993) found that the rate of admission to coronary care units was higher in Mexican Americans than in non-Hispanic whites, and case fatality after myocardial infarction was greater (Goff, Ramsey, Labarthe, and Nichaman, 1994). Published data on sudden cardiac death and out-of-hospital CHD deaths in Hispanics are unavailable. Overall, a description of CHD in Hispanics is still incomplete. Lower-than-expected CVD mortality in Hispanics has led some investigators to formulate the concept of the "Hispanic paradox" (Markides and Coreil, 1986). Several hypotheses have been invoked, including the "healthy migrant" effect—a diet that includes more fruits and vegetables, less chronic disease risk exposure before leaving the country of birth, and health-preserving cultural and psychosocial effects (Mitchell and others 1991; Markides and Coreil, 1986). However, the findings of the present study cannot be used to support the claim that Hispanics are specifically immune to CHD. Although absolute mortality rates from CHD were lower, the proportion of deaths due to this cause was similar between Hispanics and whites. Unlike cancer and other causes of death, the extent of a lower Hispanic/white ratio of death from CHD was only parallel to that of total mortality.

Limitations and Unanswered Questions

The overall response rate is very high in NHIS (96 percent to 98 percent), but a racial difference in the response may exist. The response rate was somewhat lower in the Hispanic Health and Nutrition Examination Survey (1982 to 1984) than that in the other National Health and Nutrition Examination Surveys (Rowland and Forthofer, 1993). However, nonresponse to the present survey has been much smaller than nonresponse to the Health and Nutrition Examination Surveys. This result is due primarily to the NHIS practice of allowing proxy response to medical history questions. Hence, ill and elderly persons are more likely to be included in this study.

The present study used the National Death Index as the source for mortality follow-up data. In a validation study (National Center for Health Statistics, 1986–1994), the recommended cutoff matching scores to determine vital status correctly classified .97 percent of the true matches and .97 percent of the false matches for all race/ethnic groups combined. The correct classification rates for known decedents who are nonwhites dropped to 86 percent, whereas the rate for living persons remained high at approximately 97 percent. Misclassification of vital status could be introduced by the reliance on matching by the social security number. Hispanics may be less likely to have a social security number or one that is accurate (Herrera, Stern, Goff, and Villagomez, 1994). In the 1990 NHIS, 66.6 percent of non-Hispanic whites, 63.2 percent of blacks, and 59.3 percent of Hispanics provided their social security number (unpublished data, National Center for Health Statistics). Other potential difficulties associated with using computer matching of personal identifiers for Hispanics include the Spanish surname. For hyphenated last names, the present study submitted both portions, as well as the hyphenated form.

It has been suggested (Herrera, Stern, Goff, and Villagomez, 1994; Reyes, 1997) that some Hispanics may return to their country of birth when they retire or have a potentially fatal illness, especially those with a lower education, lower wages, and fewer employment experiences. Selective out-migration would obviously lead to underestimates of mortality with the National Death Index. The follow-up period of this cohort is relatively short, which may result in less bias because fewer persons would be expected to return to their home countries.

There are limitations in using the death certificate to classify cause of death. It has been shown (Lee, Borhani, and Kuller, 1990; Kuller, 1995) that blacks have a higher out-of-hospital death rate than whites, and the coding of CHD on death certificates is less specific for blacks than for whites. The cause of death for out-of-hospital deaths is often based on minimal to nonexistent information and is often signed as due to CHD because of a lack of better diagnoses. In contrast, death from CHD may be attributed to other causes because many physicians may believe that this disease is rare in blacks. Whether a similar ethnic bias in the coding of death certificates also exists in Hispanics deserves further study. In this study, when any mentioned cause instead of underlying cause of death on the death certificate was used, the gap of CHD mortality between Hispanic women and white women reduced sizably. Although drawn from a large survey, there is a relatively small number of events for Hispanic women and insufficient statistical power to detect the racial difference.

CONCLUSIONS

These data from a large national random sample demonstrate that mortality from CHD and CVD is lower in adult Hispanics than that observed among whites in the United States. However, the proportion of total deaths due to these two diseases is similar between the two racial groups. More data on the prevalence, incidence, and case fatality of CHD as well as descriptive information from vital statistics and cohort studies of the Hispanic population, will need to be accumulated so as to have a complete picture of CHD in this increasing portion of our population.

References

American Medical Association. Council on Scientific Affairs. "Hispanic Health in the United States." *JAMA*, 1991, *265*, 248–252.

Andersen, R. M., and others. "Access to Medical Care Among the Hispanic Population of the Southwestern United States." *Journal of Health and Social Behavior,* 1981, *22*, 78–89.

Baxter, J., and others. "Excess Incidence of Known Non-Insulin-Dependent Diabetes Mellitus (NIDDM) in Hispanics Compared with Non-Hispanic Whites in the San Luis Valley, Colorado." *Ethnicity and Disease,* 1993, *3*, 11–21.

Becker, T. M., Wiggins, C., Key, C. R., and Samet, J. M. "Ischemic Heart Disease Mortality in Hispanics, American Indians, and Non-Hispanic Whites in New Mexico, 1958–1982." *Circulation,* 1988, *78*, 302–309.

Bradshaw, B. S., and Fonner, E., Jr. "The Mortality of Spanish-Surname Persons in Texas, 1969–71." In F. D. Bean and W. P. Frisbie (eds.), *The Demography of Racial and Ethnic Groups.* Orlando, Fla.: Academic Press, 1978.

Buechley, R. W., and others. "Altitude and Ischemic Heart Disease in Tricultural New Mexico: An Example of Confounding." *American Journal of Epidemiology,* 1979, *109*, 663–666.

Burchfiel, C. M., and others. "Cardiovascular Risk Factors and Impaired Glucose Tolerance: The San Luis Valley Diabetes Study." *American Journal of Epidemiology,* 1990, *131*, 57–70.

Caralis, P. V. "Hypertension in the Hispanic-American Population." *American Journal of Medicine,* 1990, *88*(Suppl. 3B), 9–16.

Fay, R. E., Passel, J. S., Robinson, G. J., and Gowan, C. D. *The Coverage of the Population in the 1980 Census.* Washington, D.C.: Bureau of the Census, 1988.

Flegal, K. M., and others. "Prevalence of Diabetes in Mexican Americans, Cubans, and Puerto Ricans for the Hispanic Health and Nutrition Examination Survey, 1982–1984." *Diabetes Care*, 1991, *14*(Suppl. 3), 628–638.

Ginzberg, E. "Access to Health Care for Hispanics." *JAMA*, 1991, *265*, 238–241.

Goff, D. C., Jr., Ramsey, D. J., Labarthe, D. R., and Nichaman, M. Z. "Acute Myocardial Infarction and Coronary Heart Disease Mortality Among Mexican Americans and Non-Hispanic Whites in Texas, 1980 Through 1989." *Ethnicity and Disease*, 1993, *3*, 64–99.

Goff, D. C., Jr., Ramsey, D. J., Labarthe, D. R., and Nichaman, M. Z. "Greater Case-Fatality After Myocardial Infarction Among Mexican Americans and Women Than Among Non-Hispanic Whites and Men: The Corpus Christi Heart Project." *American Journal of Epidemiology*, 1994, *139*, 474–483.

Hahn, R. A. "The State of Federal Health Statistics on Racial and Ethnic Groups." *JAMA*, 1992, *267*, 268–271.

Haynes, S. G., and others. "Patterns of Cigarette Smoking Among Hispanics in the United States: Results from HHANES 1982–1984." *American Journal of Public Health*, 1990, *80*(Suppl.), 47–54.

Herrera, C. R., Stern, M. P., Goff, D., and Villagomez, E. "Mortality Among Hispanics." *JAMA*, 1994, *271*, 1237.

Kuller, L. H. "Commentary on Coronary Heart Disease in Blacks." *Public Health Report*, 1995, *110*, 570–572.

Lee, M. H., Borhani, N. O., and Kuller, L. H. "Validation of Reported Myocardial Infarction Mortality in Blacks and Whites: A Report from the Community Cardiovascular Surveillance Program." *Annals of Epidemiology*, 1990, *1*, 1–12.

Markides, K. S., and Coreil, J. "The Health of Hispanics in the Southwestern United States: An Epidemiologic Paradox." *Public Health Report*, 1986, *101*, 253–265.

Massey, J. T., Moore, T. F., Parsons, V. L., and Tadros, W. "Design and Estimation for the National Health Interview Survey, 1985–94: National Center for Health Statistics." *Vital Health Statistics*, 1989, *110*, 1–33.

Miller, R. G., Jr. *Survival Analysis*. New York: Wiley, 1981.

Mitchell, B. D, and others. "Risk Factors for Cardiovascular Mortality in Mexican-Americans and Non-Hispanic Whites: The San Antonio Heart Study." *American Journal of Epidemiology*, 1990, *131*, 423–433.

Mitchell, B. D., and others. "Myocardial Infarction in Mexican-Americans and Non-Hispanic Whites." *Circulation*, 1991, *83*, 45–51.

National Center for Health Statistics. "National Health Interview Survey Multiple Cause of Death, 1986–1994." Public Use Data File Documentation.

National Center for Health Statistics. *Health, United States, 1992 and Healthy People 2000 Review*. Hyattsville, Md.: Public Health Service, 1993.

Nichaman, M. Z., Wear, M. L., Goff, D. C. Jr., and Labarthe, D. R. "Hospitalization Rates for Myocardial Infarction Among Mexican-Americans and Non-Hispanic

Whites: The Corpus Christi Heart Project." *Annals of Epidemiology,* 1993, *3,* 42–48.

Patterson, J. E., and Bilgrad, R. "The National Death Index Experience: 1981–1985." In *Proceedings of the Workshop on Exact Matching Methodologies, May 9–10, 1985.* Washington, D.C.: Statistics of Income Division, Internal Revenue Service, 1985.

Poe, G. S., and others. "Comparability of the Death Certificate and the 1986 National Mortality Followback Survey." *Vital Health Statistics,* 1993, *118,* 1–53.

Rewers, M., and others. "Is the Risk of Coronary Heart Disease Lower in Hispanics Than in Non-Hispanic Whites? The San Luis Valley Diabetes Study." *Ethnicity and Disease,* 1993, *3,* 44–54.

Reyes, B. *Dynamics of Immigration: Return Migration to Western Mexico.* San Francisco: Public Policy Institute of California, 1997.

Rogot, E., Sorlie, P., and Johnson, N. J. "Probabilistic Methods in Matching Census Samples to the National Death Index." *Journal of Chronic Diseases,* 1986, *39,* 719–734.

Rowland, M. L., and Forthofer, R. N. "Investigation of Nonresponse Bias: Hispanic Health and Nutrition Examination Survey (National Center for Health Statistics)." *Vital Health Statistics,* 1993, *119,* 1–75.

Schoen, R., and Nelson, V. E. "Mortality by Cause Among Spanish Surnamed Californians, 1969–71." *Social Science Quarterly,* 1981, *62,* 259–273.

Shah, B. V., Barnwell, B. G., and Bieler, G. S. *SUDAAN User's Manual: Software for Analysis of Correlated Data, Release 6.40.* Research Triangle Park, N.C.: Research Triangle Institute, 1995.

Sorlie, P. D., Backlund, E., Johnson, N. J., and Rogot, E. "Mortality by Hispanic Status in the United States." *JAMA,* 1993, *270,* 2464–2468.

Stampfer, M. J., and others. "Test of the National Death Index." *American Journal of Epidemiology,* 1984, *119,* 837–839.

Stern, M. P., and others. "Secular Decline in Death Rates Due to Ischemic Heart Disease in Mexican Americans and Non-Hispanic Whites in Texas, 1970–1980." *Circulation,* 1987, *76,* 1245–1250.

Trevino, F. M., Moyer, M. E., Valdez, R. B., and Stroup-Benham, C. A. "Health Insurance Coverage and Utilization of Health Services by Mexican Americans, Mainland Puerto Ricans, and Cuban Americans." *JAMA,* 1991, *265,* 233–237.

U.S. Department of Commerce News, June 13, 1991, pp. CB91–221.

Wei, M., Mitchell, B. D., Haffner, S. M., and Stern, M. P. "Effects of Cigarette Smoking, Diabetes, High Cholesterol, and Hypertension on All-Cause Mortality and Cardiovascular Disease Mortality in Mexican Americans: The San Antonio Heart Study." *American Journal of Epidemiology,* 1996, *144,* 1058–1065.

Wild, S. H., and others. "Mortality from Coronary Heart Disease and Stroke for Six Ethnic Groups in California, 1985 to 1990." *Annals of Epidemiology,* 1995, *5,* 432–439.

CHAPTER NINE

Use of Cancer Screening Practices by Hispanic Women

Analyses by Subgroup

Ruth E. Zambrana
Nancy Breen
Sarah A. Fox
Mary Lou Gutierrez-Mohamed

Using National Health Interview Survey data (1990–1992), the authors provide important and unique data on cancer screening (Pap smear, mammogram, and clinical breast examination) among five Latina subgroups in an effort to determine the factors that influence the utilization of these screening services. The study and findings represent one of the very few efforts to study Latinas by subgroup with regard to their cancer screening behaviors and to identify the factors beyond cultural beliefs that affect these behaviors.

Early detection of breast and cervical cancer is consistent with national objectives to promote cancer screening behaviors (American Cancer Society, 1991, 1997). *The Healthy People 2000 Objectives* (Office of Disease Prevention and Health Promotion, 1993) for Hispanic women are to increase to 60 percent those women aged 50 and older who have received a clinical breast examination (CBE) and a mammogram within the past one to two years and to increase to at least 95 percent the proportion of women aged 18 and older who have ever received a Pap smear.[1]

In 1987, 13 percent of Hispanic women reported having a mammogram in the past year compared with 18 percent of non-Hispanic white women (Breen and Kessler, 1994). By 1992, rates for every group had doubled, and Hispanic women were as likely as other groups to have had a mammogram in the previous year. Despite increased screening among all women, low-income women,

We gratefully acknowledge Rich Snyder and James Cucinelli for programming assistance and Barry Graubard, Ph.D., for statistical consultation.

women over 65, and Hispanic women still remain at the greatest risk of not being screened (Siegel and others, 1993).

Hispanics, who constitute nearly 11 percent of the U.S. population, represent regional and socioeconomically distinct subgroups (Montgomery, 1994; Schur, Bernstein, and Berk, 1987; Campell, 1994; Massey, 1993; Vega and Amaro, 1994).[2] In 1990, the Hispanic population consisted of Mexican-origin (63 percent), Puerto Rican (11 percent), Cuban (5 percent), Central and South American (14 percent), and Other Hispanics (8 percent).[3] Hispanics are geographically concentrated in five states: California (34 percent), Texas (19 percent), Florida (7 percent), New York (10 percent), and Illinois (4 percent) (Campell, 1994). Hispanic women currently represent more than 9 percent of the total female U.S. population, and are expected to increase to more than 15 percent by the year 2020 (Montgomery, 1994). Hispanic women are younger, have lower median annual earnings, and are more likely to be unemployed or employed in low-wage service-sector jobs than Hispanic men or non-Hispanic women (Campell, 1994; Perez, 1996). Data on 1993 family income by Hispanic subgroup reveal that 37 percent of Puerto Ricans, 30 percent of Mexican-Americans, 18 percent of Cubans, and approximately 23 percent of Other Hispanic families were below the poverty level compared with 7.6 percent of non-Hispanic white families (U.S. Department of Commerce, 1995). The rationale for examining Hispanics by subgroups is strongly argued by several authors (Schur, Bernstein, and Berk, 1987; Campell, 1994; Massey, 1993; Vega and Amaro, 1994; Perez, 1996). For example, Massey (1993) states, "Hispanics do not comprise a single coherent community. Rather, they are a disparate collection of national origin groups with heterogeneous experiences of settlement, immigration, political participation, and economic incorporation into the United States" (p. 454). In this chapter, we compare five subgroups of Hispanic women on their use of three cancer screening procedures (Pap smear, mammogram, and CBE) and test for significant predictors of screening practices.

Hispanic women tend to be younger when diagnosed with breast or cervical cancer, present with these cancers at later stages of diagnosis, and have higher mortality rates than non-Hispanic white women (Ramirez-Gutierrez and others, 1994; Ramirez, Villareal, Suarez, and Flores, 1995; Trapido and others, 1995; Valdez, Delgado, Cervantes, and Bowler, 1993). Hispanic women are less likely to have visited a physician in the last past year, to have had a mammogram and a Pap smear, and to know cancer warning signs (Balcazar, Castro, and Krull, 1995). The underlying factors that place Hispanic women at risk are low-income status, lack of access to health care, and institutional barriers (Miller and Champion, 1997; Lewin-Epstein, 1991; Wolfgang, Semeiks, and Burnett, 1991; Makuc, Freid, and Parsons, 1994; Fulton, Rakowski, and Jones, 1995; National Center for Health Statistics, 1996; Tortolero-Luna and others, 1995; Calle, Flanders, Thun, and Martin, 1993; Stein, Fox, and Murata, 1991; de la Torre,

Friis, Hunter, and Garcia, 1995; Schur, Leigh, and Berk, 1995; Richardson and others, 1987; Zapka and Estabrook, 1995).

Screening is positively associated with younger age, higher income, greater educational level, being married, health insurance, having a usual source of care, and knowledge and use of prior cancer screening tests (Miller and Champion, 1997; Lewin-Epstein, 1991; Wolfgang, Semeiks, and Burnett, 1991; Makuc, Freid, and Parsons, 1994; National Center for Health Statistics, 1996; Tortolero-Luna and others, 1995; Calle, Flanders, Thun, and Martin, 1993). Among U.S. women, Pap smear screening rates decline with increasing age. Higher levels of education are associated with more mammography screening (National Center for Health Statistics, 1996; Tortolero-Luna and others, 1995). These patterns are similar for Hispanic women. Hispanic women who are older than 65 years of age, less educated, or poor are less likely to use mammography (Calle, Flanders, Thun, and Martin, 1993). Stein, Fox, and Murata (1991) found that for Hispanic women, financial indicators, primarily lack of insurance, reduced use of mammography more than cultural differences. A recent study on access to health care found that health insurance coverage was higher for English-speaking women of Mexican origin who reported a family income above the poverty level, had higher levels of education, were employed, and were younger, as compared with Spanish-speaking Mexican-origin women (de la Torre, Friis, Hunter, and Garcia, 1995). Puerto Rican and Mexican-origin women, aged 50 to 64, had the lowest percentage of health insurance coverage. While 95.8 percent of all women aged 65 and older report having Medicare coverage, only 88.1 percent of Mexican-American women, 86.5 percent of Cuban women, and 77.4 percent of Puerto Rican women have Medicare coverage (National Center for Health Statistics, 1996).[4]

Although the preponderance of evidence shows that low socioeconomic status is an important predictor of cancer screening practices among Hispanic women (Fulton, Rakowski, and Jones, 1995; National Center for Health Statistics, 1996; Tortolero-Luna and others, 1995; Calle, Flanders, Thun, and Martin, 1993; Stein, Fox, and Murata, 1991; de la Torre, Friis, Hunter, and Garcia, 1995; Schur, Leigh, and Berk, 1995; Richardson and others, 1987; Zapka and Estabrook, 1995), screening is most strongly associated with knowledge of screening, prior screening, and physician recommendation for a screening (Brown and others, 1995; Fox and Roetzheim, 1994; Suarez, Weiss, Rainbolt, and Pulley, 1994; Morgan, Park, and Cortes, 1995; Fox and Stein, 1991; Goldman and Simpson, 1994; Stein and Fox, 1990; Vernon and others, 1992; Potvin, Camirand, and Beland, 1995; Rakowski, Rimer, and Bryant, 1993). Hispanic women 40 years of age and older are less likely to have knowledge of mammography (31.6 percent) or CBE (13.4 percent) than non-Hispanic white women (12.2 and 7.9 percent, respectively) (American Cancer Society, 1991). Analyses of 1992 National Health Interview Survey (NHIS) data found that women 50 years and older who had received other preventive services from their providers, such as CBE and mammogram, were more likely to have had a Pap smear in the past 3 three years (Gutierrez-Mohamed, 1995). Physicians not recommending a Pap smear or mammogram due to cost of tests, women's lack of knowledge about screening tests, or lack of health insurance are strong determinants of cancer screening underutilization by elderly women, low-income women, and Hispanic women (Goldman and Simpson, 1994; Stein and Fox, 1990; Vernon and others, 1992; Potvin, Camirand, and Beland, 1995; Rakowski, Rimer, and Bryant, 1993).

For Hispanic women, acculturation, income, and education are three interrelated factors associated with health behaviors (Vega and Amaro, 1994; Balcazar, Castro, and Krull, 1995; Solis, Marks, Garcia, and Sheldon, 1990; Molina, Zambrana, and Aguirre-Molina, 1994; Rogler, Cortes, and Malgady, 1991; Cobas and others, 1996; Scribner, 1996; Suarez, 1994). Although there is limited consensus on how to measure acculturation in public health, agreement exists on two points: English language use is a principal marker of acculturation, and it is associated with country of birth, completed years of education, and number of years in the United States (Suarez, 1994). Less acculturated Hispanics are often characterized by limited education, low literacy levels, and use of Spanish language, compared with their more acculturated counterparts. These attributes are, in turn, linked to decreased access to health services, lower levels of health knowledge, less communication with providers (Schur, Leigh, and Berk, 1995; Suarez, 1994; Zambrana and Ellis, 1995; Giachello, 1994; Elder and others, 1991), and less likelihood to use preventive and primary care services, to have annual Pap smears, and, for those over 50 years of age, to report ever having had a mammogram (Coe and others, 1994; Pérez-Stable, Sabogal, and Otero-Sabogal, 1995; Gonzalez, 1989; Adler and others, 1993).

Based on factors associated with cancer screening practices for Hispanic women reported in the literature, four questions were posed: (1) Are Hispanic women with more education, a usual source of care, and who speak English more likely to be screened than less educated women, without a usual a source of care, and who are not English speaking? (2) Are Hispanic women with prior screening more likely to have had more recent screening procedures than Hispanic women without prior screening? (3) Are Mexican women, who have the least education and lowest income, least likely of all Hispanic groups to have had recent screening procedures? (4) Are Cuban women, who have more education and higher income, most likely to be screened of all subgroups?

To analyze cancer screening practices among subgroups of Hispanic women, we employ a social inequality model. This paradigm proposes that low-income individuals are more exposed to risk factors and experience more barriers in the health care system than higher-income individuals (Williams, 1990; Adler and others, 1993). For Hispanic women, the model posits that socioeconomic characteristics, including income, education, and literacy levels, reduce both knowledge of health practices and access to health care services, which, in turn, makes cancer screening less likely. Acculturation, measured by language use, place of birth, and length of time in the United States, mediates the relationship between socioeconomic status and screening practices. In contrast to standard models of health care utilization that focus on individual behaviors exclusive of socioenvironmental constraints, the social inequality model takes into account how social, cultural, and economic context shape Hispanic women's use of cancer screening (Leclere, Jenseen, and Biddlecom, 1994).

We pooled two years of nationally representative population samples from the NHIS. This afforded us a unique opportunity to examine the use of preventive cancer screening practices for total Hispanic women and by subgroup. In this chapter, we present the first national estimates of cancer screening rates and sociodemographic access and other health behavior variables for total Hispanic women and by subgroup. We believe that these new estimates will be useful in formulating more effective targeted objectives for Hispanic subgroups for the Year 2010 Healthy People Objectives.

METHOD

Data from the 1990 and 1992 NHISs were pooled to increase the statistical power to analyze the five subgroups. These data included comparable questions and showed similar screening rates for all women. Because the 1990 sample constituted 70 percent of the total pooled sample and the 1992 sample constituted 30 percent of the total pooled sample (1,667 in 1990 and 724 in 1992), we adjusted the sample weights in the combined analysis by multiplying them by the factors 0.7 and 0.3 in 1990 and 1992, respectively.

The NHIS is a continuing annual nationwide survey of approximately 49,000 households of the civilian noninstitutionalized population of the United States. Questions on cancer screening practices were included in the Health Promotion and Disease Prevention Supplement of the 1992 survey. The study sample includes 2,391 adult female Hispanic respondents, 18 years of age and older. Hispanics were grouped according to self-reported ethnic identification into precoded categories: Mexican American (668), Mexican (537), Puerto Rican (332), Cuban (143), and Other Hispanic (711).

Measures and Analyses

Dependent variables were three cancer screening practices: Pap smear, mammogram, and CBE. Women 18 years of age and older were asked questions regarding Pap smears and women 35 years of age and older were asked questions regarding mammogram and CBE. We constructed dichotomous dependent variables for screening: a woman was either screened three years prior to the interview or she was not. This yielded comparable variables for the three screening practices.

Independent variables are grouped into measures of socioeconomic status; access to health services; health perceptions, behavior, and knowledge; and acculturation. Socioeconomic variables include age (18–34, 35–49, and 50 and over), education level (less than twelve years, twelve years completed, and thirteen or more years), annual household income (less than $20,000 and $20,000 or more), labor force status (employed versus other), and marital status (married or living together versus not married). Access variables were health insurance status (private, public, government only [Medicaid, Medicare, or both], and none) and usual source of care (yes/no). Health perceptions, behavior, and knowledge include six variables. Respondent-assessed health status was measured using a five-point Likert-type scale. Respondents were asked to rate their health from 1 to 5 (1 = excellent, 5 = poor). These data were recoded into three groups: 0 = very good or excellent health, 1 = good, 2 = fair (or poor). Five self-reported items, with yes/no response options, measured smoking status, knowledge of BSE, and frequency of CBE, mammogram, and Pap smear. Acculturation proxy variables were language of interview, country of birth, and number of years living in the United States. Three variables were coded based on published evidence of differences in screening practices among Hispanic women by country of birth and length of residence (Leclere, Jenseen, and Biddlecom, 1994; Stephen, Foote, Hendershot, and Schoenborn, 1994). Language of interview was used as a trichotomous variable: English, Spanish, and both. The variables for country of birth and number of years in the United States were recoded in three categories: (1) women born in United States, (2) women not born in the United States and residing in the United States for ten years or longer, and (3) women not born in the United States and residing in the United States for less than ten years.

The SUDAAN program (1993) was used to compute population estimates for the pooled sample, including proportions and design-appropriate confidence intervals and tests for significance. The pooled sample is weighted to the total population of the United States and thus is representative of each Hispanic subgroup (within the limitations of cluster sampling). SUDAAN logistic regression was used to test group differences using regression models for each screening practice.

Several limitations of the data warrant caution in the interpretation of the findings. The sample size for the Cuban group is small, and therefore its generalizability may be limited. Other Hispanic group ($n = 711$) contains a heterogeneous mix of Hispanics from Central and South America and others who self-identified in this category. Inferences cannot be drawn for this heterogeneous group as they can for groups that represent a single nationality. Other possible limitations include whether responses are accurate, given that some respondents may not know about or understand the procedures about which they were asked, and the quality of on-site translation for the Spanish interviews (D'Onofrio and Pasick, 1997; Americanaro, 1993).

RESULTS

Characteristics of the Sample

Table 9.1 displays data on sociodemographics; access to services; health behaviors, perceptions, and knowledge; and acculturation variables for all Hispanic women aged 18 or older in the pooled NHIS sample. Data are ordered in Table 9.1 by their proportion in the Hispanic population: Mexican Americans (28 percent), Mexicans (22 percent), Puerto Ricans (14 percent), Cubans (6 percent), and all Other Hispanics (30 percent). Table 9.1 presents the data from which Figure 9.1 is derived.

Figure 9.1 provides a visual comparison of the characteristics of each Hispanic subgroup and the total Hispanic group. Demographic similarities among the five subgroups were employment status, perceived health, and smoking behavior. About half (52 percent) of all Hispanic women are in the workforce, with Mexican women least likely (46 percent) and Mexican American (54 percent) and other Hispanic women (55 percent) equally likely to be employed. Cuban women are the least likely (49 percent) to perceive their health as excellent or very good, whereas 54 percent of Mexican and Puerto Rican women perceive this level of health. Only 17 percent of the total sample are current smokers, and Mexican American women are the least likely to smoke (11 percent).

Hispanic women as a group are younger than the total U.S. population (Perez, 1996; U.S. Department of Commerce, 1995). Characteristics that vary by subgroups include age, education, and marital status. About half (51 percent) of Hispanic women are between ages 18 and 34, and less than a fourth are older than 50. Cuban women are older as a group, with half older than age 50 and about one-third between ages 18 and 34. Mexican women are both the youngest (with 55 percent aged 18 to 34) and the least educated (with more than three-fourths not completing high school). In terms of annual household income (below $20,000), Mexican women (60 percent) are the poorest, and Cuban (42 percent) and Other Hispanic women (40 percent) are the least likely to be poor. Mexican (70 percent) and Cuban (62 percent) women are the most likely to be married, whereas Puerto Rican women are least likely (52 percent) to be married.

When examining health insurance coverage, Puerto Rican women are the most likely to be insured (83 percent) and Mexican women the least likely to be insured (58 percent). Noteworthy, although only 58 percent of Mexican women report having health insurance, 65 percent report a usual source of care. Not unexpectedly, Cuban women are most likely (67 percent) to have private insurance and to have a usual source of health care (83 percent).

Additional support for disaggregating Hispanics by subgroup is gleaned by analyzing the considerable variability on language of interview and birthplace

Table 9.1. Percentage and Confidence Intervals on Selected Sociodemographics; Access to Services; Health Behaviors, Perceptions, and Knowledge; and Acculturation of Hispanic Women Aged 18 and Older by Subgroup

Characteristic	Total[a] N = 2,391	Mexican American[b] n = 668 (28%)	Mexican n = 537 (22%)	Puerto Rican n = 332 (14%)	Cuban n = 143 (6%)	Other Hispanic n = 711 (30%)
Sociodemographics						
Age						
18–34 years	51 (49–53)	54 (49–58)	55 (52–59)	51 (44–57)	32 (23–40)	48 (44–51)
35–49 years	27 (25–28)	23 (20–27)	28 (25–31)	31 (26–36)	18 (12–25)	28 (24–32)
50 years or more	23 (21–25)	23 (19–27)	16 (13–20)	18 (14–23)	50 (44–56)	24 (21–28)
Educational attainment						
Less than 12 years	58 (56–61)	58 (52–63)	77 (72–82)	55 (48–62)	48 (43–53)	48 (43–53)
High school graduate only	22 (20–24)	28 (24–32)	13 (9–16)	24 (17–32)	24 (19–29)	22 (18–26)
More than high school	20 (18–22)	15 (11–18)	10 (8–13)	21 (16–26)	28 (26–35)	30 (26–35)
Annual household income						
Less than $20,000	48 (45–51)	44 (39–50)	60 (56–64)	53 (43–62)	42 (33–50)	40 (35–45)
$20,000 or more	52 (49–55)	56 (50–61)	40 (36–44)	47 (38–57)	59 (50–66)	60 (55–65)
Labor force status						
Employed	52 (49–54)	54 (49–58)	46 (40–52)	52 (46–58)	50 (42–58)	55 (51–58)
Other	48 (46–51)	46 (42–51)	54 (48–60)	48 (43–54)	50 (42–58)	45 (42–49)
Marital status						
Married/live as married	61 (58–63)	58 (53–64)	70 (66–74)	52 (46–57)	62 (54–71)	58 (54–63)
Not married	39 (37–42)	42 (36–47)	30 (26–34)	48 (43–54)	38 (29–46)	42 (37–46)

(Continued)

Table 9.1. Percentage and Confidence Intervals on Selected Sociodemographics; Access to Services; Health Behaviors, Perceptions, and Knowledge; and Acculturation of Hispanic Women Aged 18 and Older by Subgroup (Continued)

Characteristic	Total[a] N = 2,391	Mexican American[b] n = 668 (28%)	Mexican n = 537 (22%)	Puerto Rican n = 332 (14%)	Cuban n = 143 (6%)	Other Hispanic n = 711 (30%)
Access to Services						
Health insurance						
Private	57 (53–60)	62 (55–70)	44 (39–49)	52 (44–60)	67 (61–73)	61 (56–66)
Public	16 (14–18)	16 (12–21)	14 (10–18)	31 (25–36)	16 (12–20)	12 (9–16)
None	27 (24–30)	21 (16–26)	43 (37–48)	17 (13–21)	17 (12–23)	27 (23–30)
Usual source of care						
Has usual source	74 (72–76)	77 (72–81)	65 (61–70)	77 (72–82)	83 (72–93)	76 (72–79)
No usual source	26 (24–28)	23 (20–27)	35 (30–39)	23 (18–29)	17 (7–28)	24 (21–28)
Health Behaviors, Perceptions, and Knowledge						
Respondent-assessed health status						
Excellent, very good	54 (51–58)	51 (45–57)	54 (47–61)	54 (44–63)	49 (42–55)	59 (54–64)
Good	30 (28–33)	35 (31–40)	29 (25–33)	27 (20–33)	32 (24–39)	28 (24–33)
Fair, poor	15 (13–17)	13 (10–17)	17 (12–22)	19 (14–25)	20 (14–26)	13 (10–15)
Smoking status						
Current	17 (15–20)	21 (17–25)	11 (7–15)	19 (15–24)	16 (11–22)	19 (15–22)
Other	83 (80–85)	79 (75–83)	89 (85–93)	81 (76–85)	84 (78–89)	81 (78–85)

Acculturation

Language of interview						
English	65 (62–69)	86 (80–93)	39 (32–46)	69 (61–77)	44 (35–52)	70 (65–74)
Spanish	21 (17–23)	5 (2–9)	40 (36–44)	15 (9–21)	46 (37–55)	19 (15–22)
English and Spanish	13 (11–16)	8 (5–12)	21 (16–26)	16 (11–21)	10 (5–15)	12 (9–15)
Nativity and length of stay						
Born in United States (1)	48 (44–53)	92 (90–95)	13 (10–15)	40 (34–46)	27 (19–35)	41 (34–48)
10 years or more	17 (15–19)	1 (0–2)	32 (27–38)	11 (6–15)	10 (6–14)	25 (20–29)
Less than 10 years	35 (32–38)	7 (5–9)	55 (50–60)	49 (43–55)	63 (54–73)	34 (29–40)

[a]Includes only the fifty states and the District of Columbia.

[b]Mexican Americans are the referent group.

Source: Pooled NHIS data from 1990 and 1992.

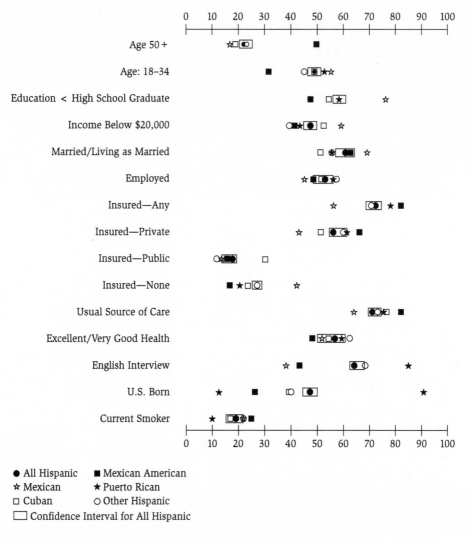

Figure 9.1. Percentage Distribution of Sociodemographic and Access Characteristics, by Total Hispanic (with Confidence Interval) and Hispanic Subgroups

(see Table 9.1). As a group, 65 percent of Hispanic women took the interview in English and 48 percent were born in the United States. A majority of Mexican American women took the interview in English (86 percent). In contrast, 39 percent of Mexican and 44 percent of Cuban women took the interview in Spanish. The majority of Mexican American women (92 percent) were born in the United States, whereas few Mexicans (13 percent) or Cubans (27 percent) were born in the United States.

Screening Practices by Hispanic Subgroup and Age

Overall and age-specific screening rates are presented in Table 9.2 for each of the procedures: Pap smear, CBE, and mammography. For this study, we analyzed women aged 18 and older for Pap screening, women 30 and older for CBE, women 35 and older for mammography use, and Mexican women were least likely to be screened for any of the three procedures. Cuban women younger than 50 years of age reported the highest screening rates of Pap smear and CBE. Cuban women 50 years and older ranked fourth in screening rates for all three procedures. Mexican American women had the highest rates of Pap smear screening (72 percent) among those 50 years and older, whereas Puerto Rican women of the same age had the highest rates of CBE (83 percent). In terms of mammography screening, Other Hispanic women, across age groups, were the most likely to be screened overall, followed by Cuban women 35 to 49 years old and Mexican American women 50 years and older.

Logistic Regression Findings

Separate logistic regression models were run for each screening modality. To avoid problems associated with missing data, the Pap regression included all women 18 years of age or older. The CBE and the mammography regression equations included Hispanic women 35 years and older, so that mammography and CBE could be used as independent variables in their respective equations. Whether a woman had a Pap smear, mammogram, or CBE in the three years prior to the interview was regressed on the variables shown in Table 9.1.

Table 9.3 displays the results from the logistic regression analyses, including the odds ratios and their corresponding confidence intervals. Although Mexican women were less likely to report being screened as displayed in Table 9.2, the multivariate analysis indicates that factors other than ethnicity may account for this result. Instead, being married, having a usual source of care, and knowledge of how to do BSE all predicted higher Pap smear screening, while older age predicted lower screening. Reported use of mammography in the past three years was associated with having insurance (public or private), having a usual source of care, and ever having had a Pap smear and a CBE. Younger age, having a usual source of care, knowledge of BSE, ever having had a Pap smear or a mammogram, and not smoking all predicted having a CBE. The most consistent predictors of use of all three cancer screening tests were use of other preventive services and having a usual source of care.

Additional analyses were conducted to examine the potential confounding effects of use of other preventive services and access variables with our acculturation proxy variables. Logistic regression models were run for each screening procedure excluding use of other preventive service variables, access to health care variables, and both of these variables. The results of these

Table 9.2. Percentage and Confidence Intervals of Hispanic Women Screened with Pap Smear, Clinical Breast Examination, and Mammography Within Three Years Prior to Interview by Subgroup

	Total[a]	Mexican American[b]	Mexican	Puerto Rican	Cuban	Other Hispanic
Pap (18 years or older)	N = 2,288	n = 640	n = 507	n = 317	n = 141	n = 683
Total	77 [74–79]	80 [75–84]	72 [69–75]	77 [71–83]	73 [65–82]	78 [74–82]
18–34 years	78 [75–82]	81 [74–87]	71 [65–76]	81 [75–88]	78 [69–88]	81 [76–87]
35–49 years	82 [77–87]	83 [72–94]	82 [76–88]	74 [61–88]	91 [78–103]	83 [77–89]
50 years or older	67 [63–71]	72 [63–81]	59 [51–67]	70 [59–80]	63 [49–78]	67 [60–75]
Clinical breast examination (30 years or older)	N = 1,560	n = 408	n = 338	n = 205	n = 121	n = 488
Total	79 [77–82]	80 [78–87]	74 [69–78]	83 [76–90]	77 [69–84]	80 [75–86]
30–49 years	83 [80–86]	84 [76–91]	78 [73–83]	83 [76–91]	86 [82–91]	85 [81–89]
50 years or older	73 [69–77]	74 [66–82]	62 [50–73]	83 [72–93]	70 [60–81]	77 [69–85]
Mammography (35 years or older)	N = 1,218	n = 315	n = 245	n = 161	n = 100	n = 397
Total	46 [42–49]	54 [48–60]	35 [28–42]	43 [36–49]	41 [28–55]	47 [40–54]
35–49 years	44 [39–49]	43 [34–52]	37 [29–45]	39 [31–47]	43 [29–57]	54 [46–62]
50 years or older	44 [39–49]	51 [42–61]	31 [19–42]	49 [38–61]	40 [21–60]	55 [46–63]

[a]Includes only the fifty states and the District of Columbia.

[b]Mexican Americans are the referent group.

Source: Pooled NHIS data for 1990 and 1992.

Table 9.3. Multiple Logistic Regression Analysis of Predictors of Having Had a Cancer Screening Test in the Past Three Years ($n = 2,391$)

	Had a Pap Smear		Had a Mammogram		Had Clinical Breast Examination	
	OR	95% CI	OR	95% CI	OR	95% CI
Sociodemographics						
Hispanic subgroup						
Mexican	1.13	0.58–2.19	0.75	0.41–1.37	0.88	0.39–1.98
Puerto Rican	0.96	0.56–1.64	0.89	0.49–1.61	1.34	0.49–3.70
Cuban	0.81	0.40–1.63	0.64	0.28–1.45	0.59	0.24–1.44
Other Hispanic	1.14	0.69–1.89	1.27	0.82–1.95	0.81	0.40–1.66
Mexican American	1.00		1.00		1.00	
Age						
50 years or older	0.43*	0.29–0.65	1.30	0.96–1.77	0.61*	0.41–0.91
18–34 years	1.19	0.77–1.83				
35–49 years	1.00		1.00		1.00	
Educational attainment						
Less than 12 years	1.00	0.70–1.45	1.43	1.01–2.03	0.55	0.31–1.99
13 years or more	1.04	0.64–1.69	1.19	0.73–1.94	1.04	0.44–2.42
High school graduate only	1.00		1.00		1.00	
Labor force status						
Other	0.70	0.49–1.00	0.78	0.51–1.20	1.12	0.66–1.90
Employed	1.00		1.00		1.00	
Marital status						
Not married	0.46*	0.32–0.65	1.02	0.75–1.38	0.98	0.59–1.63
Married/living as married	1.00		1.00		1.00	
Annual household income						
Less than $20,000	1.22	0.81–1.84	0.73	0.51–1.05	1.25	0.77–2.05
$20,000 or more	1.00		1.00		1.00	
Access to Services						
Health insurance						
None	0.76	0.50–1.15	0.60*	0.38–0.92	1.17	0.66–2.08
Public	0.77	0.47–1.27	0.83	0.46–1.48	0.69	0.34–1.41
Private	1.00		1.00		1.00	

(Continued)

Table 9.3. Multiple Logistic Regression Analysis of Predictors of Having Had a Cancer Screening Test in the Past Three Years ($n = 2,391$) (Continued)

	Had a Pap Smear		Had a Mammogram		Had Clinical Breast Examination	
	OR	95% CI	OR	95% CI	OR	95% CI
Usual source of care						
No usual source	0.29*	0.21–0.40	0.48*	0.34–0.68	0.36*	0.23–1.56
Has a usual source	1.00		1.00		1.00	
Health Behaviors, Perceptions, and Knowledge (Respondent Assessed)						
Health status						
Fair, poor	0.82	0.56–1.18	1.03	0.62–1.72	0.66	0.43–1.01
Good	0.91	0.63–1.32	1.24	0.87–1.78	1.03	0.67–1.58
Excellent, very good	1.00		1.00		1.00	
Smoking status						
Current	1.02	0.69–1.51	0.76	0.52–1.11	0.55	0.34–0.89*
Other	1.00		1.00		1.00	
Other preventive tests						
Knows how to do BSE	1.05	1.76–3.73	1.26	0.89–1.78	1.99*	1.14–3.47
Ever had CBE	2.56*	—	4.38*	1.76–10.94		
Ever had Pap smear	—	—	2.77*	1.15–6.65	6.58*	2.57–16.85
Ever had mammogram	—	—	—	—	3.44*	2.08–5.70
Acculturation						
Language of interview						
English and Spanish	0.77	0.45–1.32	0.66	0.38–1.14	2.07	1.16–3.70
Spanish	0.73	0.45–1.18	1.03	0.65–1.64	1.26	0.78–2.03
English	1.00		1.00		1.00	
Nativity and length of stay						
Less than 10 years	1.05	0.58–1.92	1.09	0.54–2.19	0.90	0.38–2.14
10 years or more	1.24	0.73–2.11	1.22	0.75–1.97	1.07	0.58–1.95
Born in United States	1.00		1.00		1.00	

*Significance: $p < 0.05$.

Note: The 1.00 are the referent group.

Source: Pooled NHIS data in 1990 and 1992.

analyses were not significantly different from our main analysis with two exceptions: (1) when access to health care was excluded in the model of predictors of having had a mammography, women over age 50 who received a mammogram were less likely to receive a Pap screening and CBE, and (2) for the three screening procedures, if access to health care is available, language appears to assume a secondary role and is not a barrier to cancer screening.

DISCUSSION

This study explored intergroup variation among Hispanic women in their use of three cancer screening practices and tested for significant predictors of each screening practice. Consistent with other studies (Fox and Stein, 1991; Goldman and Simpson, 1994; Stein and Fox, 1990; Vernon and others, 1992; Potvin, Camirand, and Beland, 1995; Rakowski, Rimer, and Bryant, 1993; Gutierrez-Mohamed, 1995), we found that usual source of care and prior screening predicted current screening practices for all subgroups of Hispanic women. The women who reported a mammogram in the past three years were almost one and one-half times more likely to know how to do a BSE and more than four times more likely to have ever had a CBE. Also, the women who reported having had a CBE were twice as likely to know how to do a BSE and six and one-half times more likely to ever have had a Pap smear. Our data confirm that like all other women, Hispanic women with access to health care are more likely to engage in more preventive health behaviors than are women without access to health care (Richardson and others, 1987; Rakowski, Rimer, and Bryant, 1993). A new finding in our analysis showed that many more women over age 50 received a mammogram than a Pap smear or CBE. Important appropriateness of care questions surface regarding whether these women are obtaining the full range of primary care services in a physician's office in addition to regular screening or whether they are simply receiving a mammogram. The extent to which Hispanic women are receiving segmented care merits further research.

Contrary to our expectations and evidence from other studies (Balcazar, Castro, and Krull, 1995; Stein and Fox, 1990; Suarez, 1994; Zambrana and Ellis, 1995; Giachello, 1994; Elder and others, 1991; Coe and others, 1994; Pérez-Stable, Sabogal, and Otero-Sabogal, 1995; Gonzalez, 1989), increased education, English language use, and Cuban subgroup did not predict use of screening. Screening rates for Mexican women, especially those older than age 50, were lower than for other subgroups in the bivariate analyses. However, the multivariate analysis demonstrated that they underscreened due to factors other than ethnicity and language. In addition, we found that Cuban women, who like Mexican women, interviewed mostly in Spanish, reported higher rates of mammography screening than Mexican women. While higher education levels, longer residence in the United States, and greater access to insurance may promote increased adherence to screening practices (Vega and Amaro, 1994; Perez, 1996; U.S. Department of Commerce, 1995; Ramirez-Gutierrez and others, 1994), our small sample of Cuban women may not provide adequate power to show the expected association between more education or more income and higher screening rates.

Our findings offer additional evidence that Hispanic women confront increased socioeconomic barriers to access and health knowledge as posited in the social inequality model (Williams, 1990; Adler and others, 1993). We found a shared set of attributes among all subgroups, including high percentages of women who did not complete high school (ranges from 48 to 77 percent), had incomes less than $20,000 (ranges from 40 to 60 percent), and did not have health insurance (ranges from 17 to 43 percent), suggesting that these socioeconomic factors may contribute to less knowledge about and access to health care that makes cancer screening less likely (American Cancer Society, 1991, 1997; Office of Disease Prevention and Health Promotion, 1993; Breen and Kessler, 1994; Siegel and others, 1993; Schur, Leigh, and Berk, 1995; Suarez, 1994; Zambrana and Ellis, 1995; Giachello, 1994; Elder and others, 1991; National Cancer Institute, Breast Cancer Screening Consortium, 1990; Pasick, D'Onofrio, and Otero-Sabogal, 1996; Brown, 1996; National Coalition of Hispanic Health and Human Services Organizations, 1995). In a recent study, Vernez and Abrahamse (1996, p. 152) found that "low income had a larger negative effect on Hispanics than on other racial/ethnic groups with respect to high school graduation, college-going and college-continuity." Accordingly, acculturation proxy variables that have been shown in previous studies to be highly associated with education and income for Hispanic groups were not significant mediators of screening practices among low-income Hispanic women in our study (Vega and Amaro, 1994; Balcazar, Castro, and Krull, 1995; Solis, Marks, Garcia, and Sheldon, 1990; Molina, Zambrana, and Aguirre-Molina, 1994; Rogler, Cortes, and Malgady, 1991; Cobas, and others, 1996; Scribner, 1996; Suarez, 1994). In fact, our analyses showed that language is not a major barrier to screening if access to care is available. Consistent with other studies (Lewin-Epstein, 1991; Schur, Leigh, and Berk, 1995; Richardson and others, 1987), we conclude that access factors and prior screening are more strongly associated with current screening than are language and ethnic factors. Our data confirm that a disproportionate percentage of Hispanic women are low income and at risk of being underscreened (Perez, 1996; Trapido and others, 1995; Valdez, Delgado, Cervantes, and Bowler, 1993). Experiential accounts and case studies suggest that additional barriers to screening and lower screening rates exist in many low-income Hispanic communities (Goldman and Simpson, 1994; Gonzalez, 1989; Brown, 1996; National Coalition of Hispanic Health and Human Services Organizations, 1995).

Since screening rates are higher than might be expected among our Hispanic sample, we can only infer that recent intervention strategies, including increased public education and community outreach, have been effective in promoting cancer screening behaviors of Hispanic women (Breen and Kessler, 1994; Valdez, Delgado, Cervantes, and Bowler, 1993; "Cancer Research in Hispanic Populations," 1995; Pérez-Stable, Otero-Sabogal, Sabogal, and Napoles-Springer, 1996; Fox, Murata, and Stein, 1991; Fox, Siu, and Stein, 1994; National Cancer

Institute, Breast Cancer Screening Consortium, 1990; Pasick, D'Onofrio, and Otero-Sabogal, 1996; Brown, 1996). Our findings have implications for provider practices, targeted health promotion activities, and future research directions. For Hispanic women, particularly Mexican women, not having a usual source of care lessens the likelihood of obtaining a screening recommendation from a physician (National Cancer Institute, Breast Cancer Screening Consortium, 1990; Flack and others, 1995). In fact, physicians may not be aware of the lack of prior screening among their low-income patients or, as other researchers have found, do not make screening recommendations due to cost concerns (Fox and Stein, 1991; Goldman and Simpson, 1994). Although physicians have been encouraged to take advantage of every clinical opportunity to promote regular screening, physician recommendation patterns vary, especially when women are culturally different from providers and low income (Fox, Murata, and Stein, 1991; Fox, Siu, and Stein, 1994; National Cancer Institute, Breast Cancer Screening Consortium, 1990; Flack and others, 1995; Auerbach and Figert, 1995; Lavizzo-Mourey and Mackenzie, 1996). If all physicians were to inform their Hispanic patients of preventive screening practices, recommend they screen according to clinical guidelines, and refer them to appropriate facilities, we would expect a considerable increase in the use of preventive screening services in Hispanic communities (Brown, 1996; National Coalition of Hispanic Health and Human Services Organizations, 1995; Flack and others, 1995).

Community-based health promotion activities, particularly patient education regarding cancer risks, have been shown to increase cancer screening practices among Hispanic women ("Cancer Research in Hispanic Populations," 1995; Pérez-Stable, Otero-Sabogal, Sabogal, and Napoles-Springer, 1996; Pasick, D'Onofrio, and Otero-Sabogal, 1996; National Coalition of Hispanic Health and Human Services Organizations, 1995). Successful interventions in different regions of the country include involving Hispanic community members (community health workers and health providers) in health education and outreach efforts; use of Spanish-language media, especially public radio announcements on health prevention; and use of existing community networks, such as churches, to promote cancer screening practices (Pérez-Stable, Otero-Sabogal, Sabogal, and Napoles-Springer, 1996; Fox and others, 1998). Pasick, D'Onofrio, and Otero-Sabogal (1996) suggest that tailoring interventions at the community level can move us beyond simple race and ethnic categories to social factors that directly influence behavior and health, such as living environment, opportunities and barriers that affect health beliefs, and ethnic-specific behaviors. Programs tailored to communities in which Hispanic women are concentrated should take into account not only level of health knowledge, language preference, and life circumstances but also available community health resources (Breen and Kessler, 1994; Ramirez, Villareal, Suarez, and Flores, 1995; Pasick, D'Onofrio, and Otero-Sabogal, 1996; National Coalition of Hispanic Health and

Human Services Organizations, 1995). In this study, despite using a pooled sample from two nationally representative surveys, we did not find any statistically significant effect on ethnicity using conventional measures. Thus, we concur with Pasick, D'Onofrio, and Otero-Sabogal (1996), who suggest that social factors, such as poverty, rather than ethnicity alone, should serve as the indicator of who needs health services, and that ethnicity (defined as a shared dynamic cultural identity) should be used to inform providers on what services to deliver and guide how services are delivered.

To continue to monitor Hispanic intergroup variation in cancer screening, we recommend that measures of health-specific sociocultural behaviors that may influence screening practices be included in future surveys conducted at the regional and local levels (Pérez-Stable, Otero-Sabogal, Sabogal, and Napoles-Springer, 1996). Patient–provider communication items, such as physician recommendation and doctor–patient race and ethnic concordance (Gray and Stoddard, 1997), should be included in future surveys, since communication with a provider has been shown to be strongly associated with increased screening for women of all ages and racial and ethnic groups (Pérez-Stable, Otero-Sabogal, Sabogal, and Napoles-Springer, 1996; Fox, Murata, and Stein, 1991; Fox, Siu, and Stein, 1994; National Cancer Institute, Breast Cancer Screening Consortium, 1990; Pasick, D'Onofrio, and Otero-Sabogal, 1996; Brown, 1996). Sample sizes of Hispanic subgroups and geographic coverage in national surveys should be increased, as should administration of surveys in language of preference, Spanish or English, by bilingual and ethnic-specific interviewers. We also recommend the development and use of measures of literacy so that the association between literacy, knowledge levels, and screening can be tested (D'Onofrio and Pasick, 1997).

In conclusion, community-based programs targeted to ethnic-specific groups appear to have been effective in increasing screening practices in various geographic regions and should be expanded, particularly for women of Mexican origin, to help meet the objectives for Hispanic women for 2000 and beyond.

Notes

1. *Hispanic women and Latino women* are used to refer to women of Hispanic origin from Mexico, Puerto Rico, Cuba, and Central and South America. The designation *Hispanic* is a federal designation, and is used in national and state reporting systems. *Latino* is a self-designated term by members of different groups. *Hispanic* is used in this chapter without preference or prejudice.

2. *Subgroup* is used throughout the chapter to refer to individuals who self-report Hispanic ethnicity and identify with a particular national origin such as Mexican American or Puerto Rican.

3. The Census Bureau definition of persons of Other Hispanic origin are those whose origins are Spain, the Spanish-speaking countries of Central and South America,

or the Dominican Republic, or persons identifying themselves generally as Spanish, Spanish-American, Hispanic, Hispano, or Latino.

4. To receive Medicare and Social Security entitlement, individuals must work a total of five years in a job where contributions are made to the government. The lower rates of Medicare coverage among Hispanic women are a reflection of immigration at later ages and less likelihood of participation in the above-ground economy.

References

Adler, N. E., and others. "Socioeconomic Inequalities in Health." *JAMA,* 1993, *269,* 3140–3145.

American Cancer Society. *Cancer Facts and Figures for Minority Americans 1991.* Atlanta, Ga.: American Cancer Society, 1991.

American Cancer Society. *Cancer Facts and Figures 1997.* Atlanta, Ga.: American Cancer Society, 1997.

Americanaro, H. "Using National Health Data Systems to Inform Hispanic Women's Health." Paper presented at the National Center for Health Statistics, Public Health Conference on Records and Statistics, Washington, D.C., July 19–21, 1993.

Auerbach, J. D., and Figert, A. E. "Women's Health Research: Public Policy and Sociology." *Journal of Health and Social Behavior,* 1995, *35,* 115–131.

Balcazar, H., Castro, F. G., and Krull, J. L. "Cancer Risk Reduction in Mexican American Women: The Role of Acculturation, Education, and Health Risk Factors." *Health Education Quarterly,* 1995, *22,* 61–84.

Breen, N., and Kessler, L. "Changes in the Use of Screening Mammography: Evidence from the 1987 and 1990 National Health Interview Surveys." *American Journal of Public Health,* 1994, *84,* 62–67.

Brown, C. L. "Screening Patterns for Cervical Cancer: How Best to Reach the Unscreened Population." *Journal of the National Cancer Institute,* 1996, *21,* 7–11.

Brown, E. R., and others. *Women's Health-Related Behaviors and Use of Clinical Preventive Services.* Los Angeles: UCLA Center for Health Policy Research, 1995.

Calle, E. E., Flanders, W. D., Thun, M. J., and Martin, L. M. "Demographic Predictors of Mammography and Pap Smear Screening in US Women." *American Journal of Public Health,* 1993, *83,* 53–60.

Campell, P. *Population Projections for States by Age, Race and Sex: 1993–2020.* Washington, D.C.: U.S. Government Printing Office, 1994.

"Cancer Research in Hispanic Populations in the United States." *Journal of the National Cancer Institute,* 1995, *18,* 1–169.

Cantor, J. C., Miles, E. L., Baker, L. C., and Barker, D. C. "Physician Service to the Underserved: Implications for Affirmative Action in Medical Education." *Inquiry,* 1996, *33,* 167–180.

Cobas, J. A., and others. "Acculturation and Low Birthweight Infants Among Latino Women: A Reanalysis of HHANES Data with Structural Equation Models." *American Journal of Public Health,* 1996, *86,* 394–396.

Coe, K., and others. "Breast Self-Examination: Knowledge and Practices of Hispanic Women in Two Southwestern Metropolitan Areas." *Journal of Community Health,* 1994, *19,* 433–448.

D'Onofrio, C. N., and Pasick, R. J. "Improving Health Surveys for Multiethnic Populations: Final Report of Grant Award Number U83/CCU908697-01." Union City: Northern California Cancer Center, Jan. 14, 1997.

de la Torre, A., Friis, R., Hunter, H. R., and Garcia, L. "The Health Insurance Status of US Latino Women: A Profile from the 1982–1984 HHANES." *American Journal of Public Health,* 1995, *86,* 533–537.

Elder, J. P., and others. "Differences in Cancer-Risk-Related Behaviors in Latino and Anglo Adults." *Preventive Medicine,* 1991, *20,* 751–763.

Flack, J. M., and others. "Epidemiology of Minority Health." *Health Psychologist,* 1995, *14,* 592–600.

Fox, S. A., Murata, P. J., and Stein, J. A. "The Impact of Physician Compliance on Screening Mammography for Older Women." *Archives of Internal Medicine,* 1991, *151,* 50–56.

Fox, S. A., and Roetzheim, R. "Screening Mammography and Older Hispanic Women: Current Status and Issues." *Cancer,* 1994, 1, *74*(7 Suppl.), 2028–2033.

Fox, S. A., and Stein, J. A. "The Effect of Physician-Patient Communication on Mammography Utilization by Different Ethnic Groups." *Medical Care,* 1991, *29,* 1065–1082.

Fox, S. A., Siu, A. L., and Stein, J. A. "The Importance of Physician Communication on Breast Cancer Screening of Older Women." *Archives of Internal Medicine,* 1994, *154,* 2058–2068.

Fox, S. A., and others. "A Trial to Increase Mammography Utilization Among Los Angeles Hispanics." *Journal of Health Care for the Poor and Underserved,* 1998, *9*(3), 309–321.

Fulton, J. P., Rakowski, W., and Jones, A. C. "Determinants of Breast Cancer Screening Among Inner-City Hispanic Women in Comparison with Other Inner-City Women." *Public Health Reports,* 1995, *110,* 476–482.

Giachello, A. "Issues of Access and Use." In C. Molina and M. Aguirre-Molina (eds.), *Latino Health in the US: A Growing Challenge.* Washington, D.C.: American Public Health Association, 1994.

Goldman, D. A., and Simpson, D. M. "Survey of El Paso Physician's Breast and Cervical Cancer Screening Attitudes and Practices." *Journal of Community Health,* 1994, *19,* 75–85.

Gonzalez, M. O. "Cancer of the Cervix in the Rio Grande Valley of South Texas." In L. A. Jones (ed.), *Minorities and Cancer.* New York: Springer-Verlag, 1989.

Gray, B., and Stoddard, J. J. "Patient–Physician Pairing: Does Racial and Ethnic Congruity Influence Selection of a Regular Physician?" *Journal of Community Health,* 1997, *22*(4), 247–259.

Gutierrez-Mohamed, M. L. "The Effect of Age on Differences in Use of Pap Smear Screening." Unpublished doctoral dissertation, Johns Hopkins University, 1995.

Harlan, L. C., Bernstein, A. B., and Kessler, L. G. "Cervical Cancer Screening: Who Is Not Screened and Why?" American Journal of Public Health, 1991, *81*, 885–890.

Komaromy, M., and others. "The Role of Black and Hispanic Physicians in Providing Health Care for Underserved Populations." *New England Journal of Medicine, 1996, 20,* 1305–1310.

Lavizzo-Mourey, R., and Mackenzie, E. R. "Cultural Competence: Essential Measurements of Quality for Managed Care Organizations." *Annals of Internal Medicine,* 1996, *10,* 919–920.

Leclere, F. B., Jenseen, L., and Biddlecom, A. E. "Health Care Utilization, Family Context, and Adaption Among Immigrants to the United States." *Journal of Health and Social Behavior,* 1994, *35,* 370–384.

Lewin-Epstein, N. "Determinants of Regular Source of Health Care in Black, Mexican, Puerto Rican, and Non-Hispanic White Populations." *Medical Care,* 1991, *29,* 543–557.

Makuc, D., Freid, V. M., and Parsons, P. E. *Health Insurance and Cancer Screening Among Women.* Hyattsville, Md.: National Center for Health Statistics, 1994.

Massey, D. "Latinos, Poverty, and the Underclass: A New Agenda for Research." *Hispanic Journal of Behavioral Science,* 1993, *15,* 449–475.

Miller, A. M., and Champion, V. L. "Attitudes About Breast Cancer and Mammography: Racial, Income and Educational Differences." *Women Health,* 1997, *26*(1), 41–63.

Molina, C., Zambrana, R. E., and Aguirre-Molina, M. "The Influence of Culture, Class and Environment on Health Care." In C. Molina and M. Aguirre-Molina (eds.), *Latino Health in the US: A Growing Challenge.* Washington, D.C.: American Public Health Association, 1994.

Montgomery, P. A. *The Hispanic Population in the United States.* Washington, D.C.: U.S. Government Printing Office, 1994.

Morgan, C., Park, E., and Cortes, D. E. "Beliefs, Knowledge, and Behavior About Cancer Among Urban Hispanic Women." *Journal of the National Cancer Institute,* 1995, *18,* 57–63.

National Cancer Institute, Breast Cancer Screening Consortium. "Screening Mammography: A Missed Clinical Opportunity?" *JAMA,* 1990, *264,* 54–58.

National Center for Health Statistics. *Health, United States, 1995.* Hyattsville, Md.: Public Health Service, 1996.

National Coalition of Hispanic Health and Human Services Organizations. "Meeting the Health Promotion Needs of Hispanic Communities." *American Journal of Health Promotion,* 1995, *9*(4), 300–311.

Office of Disease Prevention and Health Promotion. *Healthy People 2000 Progress Report for Hispanic Americans.* Washington, D.C.: Office of Disease Prevention and Health Promotion, 1993.

Pasick, R. J., D'Onofrio, C., and Otero-Sabogal, R. "Similarities and Differences Across Cultures: Questions To Inform a Third Generation for Health Promotion Research." *Health Education Quarterly,* 1996, *23*(suppl.), S142–61.

Perez, S. M. *Untapped Potential: A Look at Hispanic Women in the US.* Washington, D.C.: National Council of La Raza, 1996.

Pérez-Stable, E. J., Otero-Sabogal, R., Sabogal, F., Napoles-Springer, A. "Pathway to Early Cancer Detection for Latinas: En Acción Contra el Cancer." *Health Education Quarterly,* 1996, *23*(Suppl.), 541–559.

Pérez-Stable, E. J., Sabogal, F., and Otero-Sabogal, R. "Use of Cancer-Screening Test in the San Francisco Bay Area: Comparison of Latinos and Anglos." *Journal of the National Cancer Institute Monographs,* 1995, *18,* 147–153.

Potvin, L., Camirand, J., and Beland, F. "Patterns of Health Services Utilization and Mammography Use Among Women Aged 50–59 Years in the Quebec Medicare System." *Medical Care,* 1995, *33,* 515–530.

Rakowski, W., Rimer, B. K., and Bryant, S. A. "Integrating Behavior and Intention Regarding Mammography by Respondents in the 1990 National Health Interview Survey of Health Promotion and Disease Prevention. *Public Health Reports,* 1993, *108,* 605–624.

Ramirez, A. G., Villareal, R., Suarez, L., and Flores, E. T. "The Emerging Hispanic Population: A Foundation for Cancer Prevention and Control." *Journal of the National Cancer Institute Monographs,* 1995, *18,* 1–9.

Ramirez-Gutierrez, A., and others (eds.). *Latino Health in the US: A Growing Challenge.* Washington, D.C.: American Public Health Association, 1994.

Richardson, J. L., and others. "Frequency and Adequacy of Breast Cancer Screening Among Elderly Hispanic Women." *Preventive Medicine,* 1987, *16,* 761–774.

Rogler, L. H., Cortes, D. E., and Malgady, R. G. "Acculturation and Mental Health Status Among Hispanics." *American Psychologist,* 1991, *46,* 585–597.

Schur, C. L., Bernstein, A. B., and Berk, M. L. "The Importance of Distinguishing Hispanic Subpopulations in the Use of Medical Care." *Medical Care,* 1987, *25,* 627–641.

Schur, C. L., Leigh, L. A., and Berk, M. L. "Health Care Use by Hispanic Adults: Financial vs. Non-Financial Determinants." *Health Care Financing Review,* 1995, *17*(2), 71–88.

Scribner, R. "Paradox as Paradigm: The Health Outcomes of Mexican Americans." *American Journal of Public Health,* 1996, *86,* 303–304.

Siegel, P. Z., and others. "Behavioral Risk Factor Surveillance, 1991: Monitoring Progress Toward the Nation's Year 2000 Health Objectives." *Morbidity and Mortality Weekly Report,* 1993, 42.

Solis, J. M., Marks, G., Garcia, M., and Sheldon, A. "Acculturation, Access to Care, and Use of Preventive Services: Findings from HHANE'S 1982–84." *American Journal of Public Health,* 1990, *80*(Suppl.), 11–19.

Stein, J. A., and Fox, S. A. "Language Preference as an Indicator of Mammography Use Among Hispanic Women." *Journal of the National Cancer Institute,* 1990, *82,* 1715–1716.

Stein, J. A., Fox, S. A., and Murata, P. J. "The Influence of Ethnicity, Socioeconomic Status, and Psychological Barriers on Use of Mammography." *Journal of Health and Social Behavior,* 1991, *32,* 101–113.

Stephen, E. H., Foote, K., Hendershot, G. E., and Schoenborn, C. A. *Health of the Foreign-Born Population: United States, 1989–90.* Hyattsville, Md.: National Center for Health Statistics, 1994.

Suarez, L. "Pap Smear and Mammogram Screening in Mexican American Women: The Effects of Acculturation." *American Journal of Public Health,* 1994, *84,* 742–746.

Suarez, L., Weiss, N., Rainbolt, T., and Pulley, L. "Effect of Social Networks on Cancer-Screening Behavior of Older Mexican-American Women." *Journal of the National Cancer Institute,* 1994, *86,* 775–779.

SUDAAN: Survey Data Analysis Software, Release 6.34. Research Triangle Park, N.C.: Research Triangle Institute, Sept. 1993. Software.

Tortolero-Luna, G., and others. "Screening Practices and Knowledge, Attitudes, and Beliefs About Cancer Among Hispanic and Non-Hispanic White Women 35 Years Old or Older in Nueces County, Texas." *Journal of the National Cancer Institute,* 1995, *18,* 49–56.

Trapido, E. J., and others. "Epidemiology of Cancer Among Hispanics in the United States." *Journal of the National Cancer Institute,* 1995, *18,* 17–28.

U.S. Department of Commerce, Bureau of the Census. *The Nation's Hispanic Population—1994.* Washington, D.C.: U.S. Government Printing Office, 1995.

Valdez, R. B., Delgado, D. J., Cervantes, R. C., and Bowler, S. *Cancer in US Latino Communities: An Exploratory Review.* Santa Monica, Calif.: Rand, 1993.

Vega, W. A., and Amaro, H. "Latino Outlook: Good Health, Uncertain Prognosis." *Annual Review of Public Health,* 1994, *15,* 39–67.

Vernez, G., and Abrahamse, A. *How Immigrants Fare in US Education.* Santa Monica, Calif.: Rand, 1996.

Vernon, S. W., and others. "Breast Cancer Screening Behaviors and Attitudes in Three Racial/Ethnic Groups." *Cancer,* 1992, *69,* 165–174.

Williams, D. R. "Socioeconomic Differentials in Health: A Review and Redirection." *Social Psychology Quarterly,* 1990, *53*(2), 81–99.

Wolfgang, P. E., Semeiks, P. A., and Burnett, W. S. "Cancer Incidence in New York City Hispanics, 1982 to 1985." *Ethnicity and Disease,* 1991, *3,* 263–272.

Zambrana, R. E., and Ellis, B. "Contemporary Research Issues in Hispanic/Latino Women's Health." In D. L. Adams (ed.), *Health Issues for Women of Color: A Cultural Diversity Health Perspective.* Thousand Oaks, Calif.: Sage, 1995.

Zapka, J., and Estabrook, B. "Breast and Cervical Cancers—Early Detection and Control: Interpersonal Strategies and Channels." *Wellness Perspect: Research, Theory, and Practice,* 1995, *11*(2), 40–78.

Risk Factors for Invasive Cervical Cancer in Latino Women

Anna Nápoles-Springer
Eliseo J. Pérez-Stable
Eugene Washington

The authors review the factors that place Latinas at increased risk for cervical cancer, ranked the third most common cancer among Latinas (compared to sixth for White women). Although the study is limited to California, the findings are nevertheless of significance. California is one of eleven states where the cancer registry collects cancer morbidity data by race and ethnicity, and it is the home state to almost 40 percent of the Latinos who reside in the United States. Although the authors do not disaggregate the data by Latina subgroup, they provide comparisons with African Americans and Whites and systematically identify the areas of inquiry that are needed to understand Latinas' disproportionate burden of cervical cancer.

D espite significant advances in the prevention, early detection, and clinical management of invasive cervical cancer, this cancer continues to cause significant morbidity and mortality for thousands of women each year. Latin American countries report the highest rates of cervical cancer in the world (Morris and others, 1989), and it is arguably the most common cancer among women in the developing world (Parkin and Muir, 1992; Koutsky and others 1992). In the United States, invasive cervical cancer is the ninth most common cancer in women, affecting an estimated 15,000 women (American Cancer Society, 1995). Among Latino women, cervical cancer is the third most common cancer, while it ranks sixth for non-Latino women (NLW) women (American Cancer Society, 1991). Cervical cancer deaths rank thirteenth among all cancer deaths, with an estimated 4,600 women dying in 1994. Further contributing to the morbidity burden are the estimated 55,000 cases of cervical

We thank Diane Emer for her technical and administrative support.

212

carcinoma in situ and the even greater number of cytological abnormalities requiring further evaluation (American Cancer Society, 1994a).

Substantial reductions in the incidence and mortality of cervical cancer have been achieved in the past forty years, due largely to the increasing availability and use of Papanicolaou (Pap) smear screening. The age-adjusted incidence of cervical cancer has steadily declined, dropping 35 percent between 1973 and 1990, from a rate of 14.2 to 8.8 per 100,000 women. Similarly, age-adjusted mortality rates for cervical cancer have declined 41 percent from 1973 to 1990 from 5.2 to 3.0 per 100,000 women (Kosary, Schiffman, and Trimble, 1993). Nonetheless, cervical cancer continues to be a significant public health issue because more invasive cervical cancer cases could be prevented with timely screening and treatment. Data on cervical cancer outcomes by ethnicity and race are needed to effectively guide development of further research, prevention, and early detection strategies.

According to the 1990 U.S. Census, the California population was estimated to be 57.2 percent NLW, 25.8 percent Latino, and 7.0 percent African American, with Latinos comprising the fastest growing group (U.S. Bureau of the Census, 1993). Given Latinos' stated projected population growth, it is becoming increasingly important to examine ethnic differences in disease burden to identify protective practices and factors that increase risk for cancer. Thus, this chapter reviews the literature to identify differences in cervical cancer incidence and mortality rates for Latino women in California (compared to NLW women and African American women) and to examine possible explanations for existing ethnic disparities in invasive cervical cancer indicators of morbidity and mortality. The following questions guide the literature review: (1) Does the prevalence of risk factors associated with invasive cervical cancer differ between Latino and NLW women? (2) If there are differences, do these explain the disproportionately higher incidence of invasive cervical cancer in Latinos compared to NLW women?

METHODS

Population-based data on invasive cervical cancer incidence and mortality are collected for 9.6 percent of the U.S. population by the Surveillance, Epidemiology, and End Results (SEER) Program (Miller and others, 1993). SEER reports of national cancer incidence and mortality are available by African American/ White race but are not published by Latino ethnicity. Since the California tumor registry publishes its reports of cancer morbidity and mortality by race and ethnicity, we used this source to make racial and ethnic comparisons of the incidence and mortality experiences of Latino women with NLW and African American women.

California registry data for 1988 through 1992 marked the first time period for which Latino cases and deaths were identified by surname, in addition to medical record or death certificate information (Perkins and others, 1995). A study conducted by the Northern California Cancer Center (Stewart, Glaser, Horn-Ross, and West, 1993) found that the use of Spanish surname as a supplement to information about ethnicity obtained from the medical record resulted in improved sensitivity and accuracy of Latino cancer rates. However, we were unable to examine trends by race and ethnicity since race-specific rates presented in earlier California Cancer Registry reports are not comparable to those reported in earlier reports where race is identified through a different methodology.

A review of the medical and psychological literature was conducted using MEDLINE and PsychINFO databases. Articles on sexual behavior risk factors, cigarette smoking, genetic and biological factors, socioeconomic status, survival, Pap smear screening utilization, and barriers to preventive health services were reviewed to explain Latinos' elevated cervical cancer incidence and mortality and to suggest areas for future research.

Conceptual Model

In order to organize the specific factors that influence the disease burden associated with cervical cancer in Latino women, we developed the conceptual model depicted in Figure 10.1. Through a scientific literature review, we grouped factors associated with higher cervical cancer incidence into three categories: (1) structural factors, such as socioeconomic status, education, income and access to care; (2) behavioral factors, such as Pap smear use, cigarette smoking and sexual practices; and (3) biological and genetic factors, such as human papillomavirus (HPV) infection, host genetics, immune responses, and parity. These categories are not mutually exclusive, as a specific variable can have more than one dimension. For example, HPV infection, which is sexually transmitted, is also a biological precursor to cervical cancer. It is also heuristically useful to distinguish between factors related to etiology of cervical cancer and those related to screening practices. Etiological factors potentially affect incidence of cancer while the effects of screening factors are reflected in staging of disease and mortality indicators.

Incidence, Mortality, and Survival

In California, cervical cancer is the second most common cancer for Latino women, while it ranks sixth for African American women and sixteenth for NLW women. Latino and African American women in California experience an annual age-adjusted cervical cancer incidence approximately twice as high as that of NLW women (17.1, 12.5, and 7.5 per 100,000, respectively). Age-specific incidence rates by ethnic group indicate that cervical cancer occurs at higher rates for Latino women, particularly for younger women between the ages of

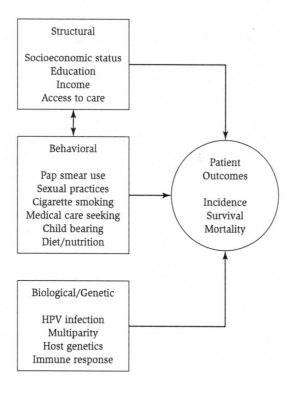

Figure 10.1. Conceptual Model of Patient Factors Relating to Cervical Cancer Mortality and Morbidity

30 to 45 years, and that rates increase for African American women after the age of 65 years (see Figure 10.2).

Latino and African American women also tend to die of this disease at twice the rate of NLW women (4.3, 5.0, and 2.2 per 100,000, respectively). For every 2.5 cases of cervical cancer, one African American woman dies, compared to one death for every 4 cases in Latino women and one in every 3.4 cases for NLW women (see Table 10.1; Perkins, and others, 1995). Age-specific mortality rates reveal increasing disparity in death rates over 30 years for all women, with dramatic increases for African American women older than 65 years (see Figure 10.3).

Follow-up data to assess survival following cervical cancer are not available statewide, but are collected for the five counties comprising the Region 8 registry. Table 10.2 shows differences in the survival rates of NLW, Latino, and African American women in the San Francisco Bay Area with invasive cervical cancer. The five-year relative survival rate for women diagnosed at a localized stage was 84 percent for African Americans and 84.8 percent for Latinos compared to 97.2 percent for NLWs for 1988 through 1992. Thus, NLW women

Table 10.1. Invasive Cervical Cancer Average Annual Age-Adjusted Incidence and Mortality Rates by Race/Ethnicity, California, 1988–1992

Race/Ethnicity	Incidence Rates		Mortality Rates	
	New Cases	Rate	Deaths	Rate
All races	8,337	9.9	2,292	2.8
Latino	2,502	17.1[a]	552	4.3[a]
African American	663	12.5[a]	253	5.0[a]
Non-Latino White	4,221	7.5[a]	1,264	2.2[a]

Note: Rates are per 100,000.

[a]Rate is significantly different for comparable rates for all races, 1988–1992 ($p < 0.05$).

Source: California Cancer Registry.

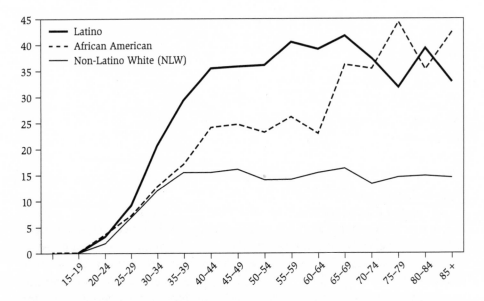

Figure 10.2. Invasive Cervical Cancer Average Annual Age-Specific Incidence by Race/Ethnicity California, 1988–1992

Source: California Cancer Registry.

with cervical cancer were more likely to survive when diagnosed at an early stage than the other two groups. Five-year survival rates for women diagnosed with regional cervical cancer indicate that African American women have the least likelihood of survival (20.9 percent), compared to Latinos (44 percent) or NLW women (50.7 percent). The greater rate disparities between African

Table 10.2. Invasive Cervical Cancer Five-Year Relative Survival Rates by Race/Ethnicity, San Francisco Bay Area, 1988–1992 (in percent)

Race/Ethnicity	Total Number	All Stages (SE)	Localized (SE)	Regional (SE)	Distant (SE)
Latino	139	49.5 (13.9)	84.8 (21.7)	44.0 (19.6)	0.0 (27.0)
African-American	122	51.9 (0.0)	84.0 (0.0)	20.9 (0.0)	0.0 (0.0)
Non-Latino White	233	72.3 (31)	97.2 (4.1)	50.7 (0.0)	0.0 (0.0)

Note: Region 8 includes Alameda, Contra Costa, Marin, San Francisco, and San Mateo counties. Rates are per 100,000.

Source: Northern California Cancer Center.

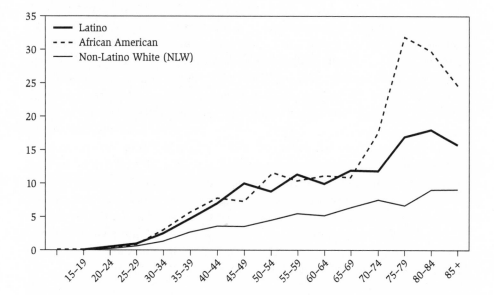

Figure 10.3. Invasive Cervical Cancer Average Annual Age-Specific Mortality by Race/Ethnicity, California, 1988–1992

Source: California Cancer Registry.

American and NLW women may be due to more advanced disease among African American women diagnosed at this stage. Although Latinos experience higher invasive cervical cancer rates and are screened less frequently in comparison to African American women, they tend to die less often from the disease and experience improved survival. These observations suggest protective cultural or biological factors operating, or alternatively, better access to follow-up care.

Table 10.3. Invasive Cervical Cancer Stage at Diagnosis by Race/Ethnicity,
California, 1988–1992 (in percent)

Race/Ethnicity	Local	Regional	Distant	Unstaged
Latino	48.9	34.6	8.3	8.2
African American	42.9	35.1	12.5	9.5
Non-Latino White	53.3	30.2	10.4	6.1

Note: Region 8 includes Alameda, Contra Costa, Marin, San Francisco, and San Mateo counties. Rates are per 100,000.

Source: Northern California Cancer Center.

One explanation for the poorer survival and higher mortality observed in African Americans and Latinos with cervical cancer compared to NLW women is that minority women tend to be diagnosed at later stages of disease. California African American and Latino women are diagnosed with localized cervical cancer less frequently than are NLW women (42.9 percent, 48.9 percent, and 53.5 percent, respectively; see Table 10.3). For example, crudeness of the cervical cancer rating system, which classifies disease extent as local, regional, or distant, underestimates racial variation in survival attributable to socioeconomic factors (Roach and Alexander, 1995). A study that evaluated the relative effects of age, race, and socioeconomic status on disease stage and survival for Connecticut women found African American women to be 50 to 60 percent more likely to be diagnosed with advanced disease. Stage of disease was an independent predictor of mortality adjusting for the effects of age at diagnosis, race, and socioeconomic status (as measured by census data for the percentage of high school graduates, percentage below poverty level, and median income) (Shelton, Paturzo, Flannery, and Gregorio, 1992). Unfortunately, such studies have not been published on Latino women with cervical cancer.

STRUCTURAL FACTORS

Socioeconomic Status and Ethnicity

In comparing ethnic differences across cancer sites, there are some types of cancer that are more highly correlated with socioeconomic status than others, which implies a stronger role for environmental factors than biological or genetic traits. Studies of invasive cervical cancer have found a strong association with lower socioeconomic levels. The challenge is to identify what these proxy measures represent in the real-life situations of Latino women faced with the risk of cervical cancer, that is, lifestyle practices, access to care, and delays in seeking care, among others.

Studies that have conducted multivariate analyses to examine racial or ethnic differences in the effects of socioeconomic factors on risk of cervical cancer have obtained mixed results. This issue has largely been studied in African American women using secondary data from national health surveys and SEER data with race-specific aggregate (census tract level) SES indicators (McWhorter, Schatzkin, Horm, and Brown, 1989). The various SES variables used in studies differed in the strength of their association with race depending on whether median family income, median education level, population density, or percentage below poverty level was used. Thus, differences may be due to lack of consistency in the SES indicators used. Nonetheless, most analyses have shown that adjusting for income, poverty, and education based on census tract level indicators appears to explain approximately half of the cervical cancer incidence differential between African Americans and NLWs (Baquet, Horm, Gibbs, and Greenwald, 1991; Devessa and Diamond, 1980; Samelson, Speers, Ferguson, and Bennett, 1994). Interestingly, in one study, stratification by a group-level poverty indicator revealed an interactive effect of race and social class on age-specific mortality rates, such that greater racial differences in mortality rates were observed for those groups in which poverty was less marked. Thus, available data indicate that racial and ethnic differences are confounded by poverty at lower income levels when comparing African American and NLW women (Samelson, Speers, Ferguson, and Bennett, 1994).

One study of Latino and NLW women in New Mexico, which controlled for HPV infection, other sexual risk factors, and cigarette smoking status, found that education independently predicted risk for high-grade cervical dysplasia (Becker and others, 1994b). Women having less than a high school education experienced a sixfold increase in risk compared to women with more than a high school education (Becker and others, 1994b). Another study found the single most important factor (controlling for the effects of sexual behavior factors) accounting for differences in incidence of cervical cancer between Latino and NLW women to be years of education in spite of matching of cases and controls on neighborhood (Peters, Bear, and Thomas, 1989). Thus, various socioeconomic factors may operate differently for distinct racial and ethnic groups.

Barriers to Preventive Health Services

Studies have shown that utilization factors such as having a place to obtain care, having a primary care provider, obtaining regular checkups, receiving care from an obstetrician-gynecologist, and use of preventive health services are significant predictors of regular screening for cervical cancer and thus affect staging of disease and mortality. One study evaluated the relative contribution of socioeconomic, utilization, attitudinal, and knowledge factors in 416 inner-city women from Baltimore at risk for cervical cancer (Mamon and others, 1990). Mamon and colleagues found that underscreened women were more likely to be 45 years of age or older, to have no medical insurance, to report never having been told by a clinician how often to get a Pap test, to feel that they did not see a physician as often as they thought they should, and, among older women, to lack knowledge about risk factors for cervical cancer (Mamon and others, 1990).

National and regional surveys have consistently shown that Latinos are significantly more likely to be uninsured than other ethnic groups (Treviño, Moyer, Valdez, and Stroup-Benham, 1991). According to the Centers for Disease Control and Prevention's Behavioral Risk Factor Surveillance System (BRFSS), which collects information in forty-eight states and the District of Columbia, 32.6 percent of Latino women reported lack of a health care plan versus 12.2 percent of NLW women during 1991–1992 (Centers for Disease Control and Prevention, 1994). These figures may actually underestimate the proportion of Latino women with limited access to health care since the survey is conducted by telephone and may exclude poorer segments of the population (Centers for Disease Control and Prevention, 1994). Unpublished analyses of California data from the 1989 National Health Interview Survey showed that 42 percent of Latinos younger than 65 years of age had no health insurance (personal communication, R. Wyn, Center for Health Care Policy, UCLA), which underscores the gravity of the access problem.

Misconceptions about cancer causes in general and fatalistic attitudes toward cancer diagnosis and treatment have been reported in both urban and rural Latino populations in comparison to NLWs (Pérez-Stable and others, 1992; Tortolero-Luna and others, 1995; Morgan, Park, and Cortes, 1995). However, studies in both a prepaid health plan and the community in general showed no significant differences in lifetime and interval Pap smear screening behavior among Latinos compared to NLWs, despite a perception that Latinos are less likely to get cancer (Pérez-Stable and others, 1994; Pérez-Stable, Sabogal, and Otero-Sabogal, 1995). Thus, the level of misconceptions about cervical cancer causes or fatalistic attitudes regarding cancer diagnosis does not appear to have a substantial impact on screening behavior.

Lack of physician referral is a primary reason for nonadherence with regular cervical cancer screening with Pap smears, especially for older women (Pérez-Stable and others, 1994; Pérez-Stable, Sabogal, and Otero-Sabogal, 1995). These women are underscreened despite being seen by a physician in some cases up to four times a year (Mamon and others 1990; Kleinman and Kopstein, 1981). A recent cross-sectional study of Colorado primary care clinicians found that nurses with more Latino patients more often perceived the Pap smear screening barriers to be associated with transportation, child care, and release time from work than were nurses with patient loads of fewer Latinos (Bakemeier and others, 1995). Several studies have found that factors such as embarrassment, fear of results, and concern about becoming a burden to family members if diagnosed with cancer are more frequently reported by Latinos, especially Spanish speakers, as reasons for not having regular screening examinations (Morris and others, 1989; Pérez-Stable, Sabogal, and Otero-Sabogal, 1995; Harlan, Bernstein, and Kessler, 1991; Peters, Bear, and Thomas, 1989). Another study found that Latinos were more likely to cite forgetfulness, lack of transportation, need for child care, and the long waits for not having had cancer screening examinations (Pérez-Stable and others, 1994; Pérez-Stable, Sabogal, and Otero-Sabogal, 1995).

A recent study of physician and patient beliefs about cervical cancer risk factors found greater discrepancies between Latino patients, particularly immigrants, and their clinicians, whereas NLW women's beliefs more likely resembled the physician biomedical model (Chavez and others, 1995). Interestingly enough, however, the differences manifested in underlying beliefs, rather than physician practices. For example, when Latino patients and their physicians agreed on a specific risk factor, such as multiple sex partners, the physicians viewed it as a sexually transmitted disease issue, whereas the Latinos saw it in moralistic terms (Chavez and others, 1995). In terms of physician practices, a study of New York City physician preventive practice patterns revealed no differences in Pap smear testing use between physicians mainly serving Latino or African American patients and those serving over 50 percent NLW patients (Gemson, Elinson, and Messeri, 1988). Further studies must address the interaction among clinicians' cultural competence, patients' beliefs and attitudes, preventive practice patterns, and system factors.

These studies underscore the importance of conducting interventions not only with women at risk, but also with clinicians and the clinics serving these populations. It is crucial to train physicians and other medical personnel on how to encourage cervical screening in a culturally competent manner. Provider and patient language discordance must also be further investigated as to their effects on the frequency of regular cervical screening.

Barriers to Diagnostic and Treatment Services

There is a paucity of information as to variations in practice patterns of diagnosis and treatment of cervical cancer by race and ethnicity. Differential delays in seeking treatment following an abnormal Pap smear might account for some of the excess mortality in minority women. Late-stage diagnosis can result from a number of factors, including infrequent screening or delays on the part of clinicians or patients in seeking diagnostic services. In a recent survey of 268 primary care physicians in Colorado whose practices included a median percentage of 15 percent Latino patients, only 54 percent of physicians recommended colposcopy as follow-up for minimally abnormal Pap smears (Bakemeier and others, 1995). A randomized study of over two thousand women with abnormal Pap smears in Los Angeles from twelve primary care health clinics that served low-income and ethnically diverse populations found significantly lower return rates for African American and Latino women than for NLW women (Marcus and Crane, 1992).

BEHAVIORAL FACTORS

Screening Rates

Another explanation for the poorer survival from cervical cancer of Latinos compared to NLW women is lack of timely Pap smear screening and early detection. National health surveys indicate that Pap smear screening rates are rising for ethnic minorities (American Cancer Society, 1994b). Nonetheless, Latino women consistently report lower rates of cervical cancer screening than NLW or African American women. An analysis of 1986 Access to Health Care Survey data found health insurance status, income, education, employment status, and race/ethnicity were independent predictors of having had a Pap test (Hayward, Shapiro, Freeman, and Corey, 1988). In this study, African American women were more likely than NLW and Latino women to have had a Pap smear within recommended time frames (odds ratio [OR] = 1.51, confidence interval [CI] 1.02–2.22). Similarly, an analysis of responses from 12,252 women who participated in the 1987 National Health Interview Survey (NHIS) found that Latino ethnicity, low income, never having been married, and age, especially in African American women, independently predicted underutilization of Pap tests. African American women overall were found more likely than NLW and Latino women to have had a Pap smear in the past year (42.4 percent versus 37.9 percent and 34.9 percent, respectively) (Calle, Flanders, Thun, and Martin, 1993). A recent analysis that compared trends for Pap smear testing based on 1987 and 1992 NHIS data found that Latinos continue to obtain Pap smears at lower rates than NLW women but that the differences have decreased substantially ("Getting a Handle on ASCUS," 1995).

In 1992–1993 among women in California with an intact uterus, 77 percent of Latinos reported having had a Pap test during the previous three years compared to 88 percent of NLWs and 92 percent of African American women (American Cancer Society, 1994b). These proportions reflect an increase of roughly 8 percent in NLW and Latino women and 9 percent in African American women over the preceding year. These data are not directly comparable since in the 1991–1992 survey, respondents were asked about Pap screening in the previous year, while in the second survey, the question concerned screening in the previous three years.

Increased intensity of Pap screening should initially result in increased rates of carcinoma in situ (CIS) followed by a decrease in invasive cervical cancer rates as diagnosis occurs at earlier stages of disease. According to estimates of the annual percentage change in rates in California between 1988 and 1992, CIS incidence rates have increased for all three ethnic groups, especially for African Americans. Incidence rates of invasive cervical cancer have decreased by 4.7 percent for African Americans and by 1.6 percent for NLWs, but have actually increased by 1.8 percent for Latinos. Mortality has decreased by 6.7 percent in African Americans and by 0.8 percent in NLWs, but it has increased by 3.9 percent in Latinos (Perkins and others, 1995). Another indicator of progress in early detection of cervical cancer is the rate ratios of CIS to invasive cancer, with higher ratios implying a more successful early detection program. The rate ratios for in situ versus invasive cervical cancer by ethnicity were 2.5 for African American, 2.2 for Latino, and 4.8 for NLW women in California for 1988 through 1992 (Perkins and others, 1995). These ratios indicate that programs for early detection of cervical cancer continue to lag for Latinos despite an increase in screening rates.

The need for Pap smear screening remains an important issue for the Latino community, and an assessment of whether women are receiving regular, ongoing screening may explain some of the variation in outcomes. It is likely that national and statewide screening rates among all ethnic groups based on telephone surveys are significantly overestimated when compared to medical records (Hiatt and others, 1995; Suarez, Goldman, and Weiss, 1995). However, in one study that compared Latino and NLW women, there was no significant difference in overreporting of screening tests by ethnicity (Hiatt and others 1995). Behavioral aspects of screening from the perspective of clinicians may also offer some explanation for the differences in screening rates. Differences in evaluation and treatment by race and ethnicity must also be assessed as possible explanatory factors for outcomes variations.

Sexual Behavior and HPV Infection

Epidemiological studies have demonstrated compelling evidence for an independent relationship between cervical cancers and genital human papillomavirus (HPV) infection (Koutsky and others, 1992; Muñoz and Bosch, 1992). Commercial dot hybridization assays have been replaced by more advanced HPV DNA detection methods using polymerase chain reaction techniques (PCR). Using more accurate and precise methods for the detection of HPV infection, recent studies provide evidence that the majority of cervical cancer cases are associated with some type of HPV infection (Bosch and others, 1994; Bosch and others, 1995; Schiffman and others, 1993). Further evidence has been found for geographic and ethnic variation of HPV types, which could indicate different relative risks for different geographic areas and populations (Bosch and others, 1995; Becker and others, 1991). In a recent international survey of invasive cervical cancer in twenty-two countries, the presence of HPV DNA was confirmed in 93 percent of one thousand cancer tumor specimens (Bosch and others, 1995). Although HPV 16 was dominant in all countries, HPV 39 and HPV 59 were almost entirely restricted to Central and South America.

In a study that evaluated risk factors for HPV and cervical intra epithelial neoplasia (CIN) in five hundred cases in Portland, Oregon, the associations of smoking and early age at first intercourse with increased risk for CIN were explained by number of sexual partners. Sexual behavior did not explain the elevated risk associated with education and income. Once HPV status was adjusted for, the increased risk of CIN associated with lifetime number of sexual partners and education and income was substantially diminished. Furthermore, adjustment for HPV infection disclosed a fairly strong association between parity and CIN (Schiffman and others, 1993). Another study conducted in four Latin American countries found a linear increased risk of cervical cancer associated with number of live births after controlling for sexual risk factors, HPV infection, interval since last Pap smear, age, and years of education (Brinton and others, 1989). The elevated risk associated with multiparity could be a result of physical trauma to the cervix during normal deliveries or possibly hormonal factors. Studies are beginning to emerge that show that persistence of HPV infection may play a critical role in determining whether women infected with HPV go on to develop advanced cervical cancer (Ho and others, 1995; Schiffman, 1995).

Two large case-control studies assessed risk factors for invasive cervical cancer in 759 women from four Latin American countries and 200 Latino women from Los Angeles, and both found that younger age at first intercourse and an increasing number of sexual partners were independently associated with increased risk for invasive cervical cancer (Peters, Bear, and Thomas, 1986; Herrero and others, 1990). After controlling for possible confounders, some researchers have found an independent contribution for both factors (Clarke, Hatcher, McKeown-Eyssen, and Lickrish, 1985; Swan and Brown, 1981), while others report a residual effect only for age at first intercourse (Lambert, Morisset, and Bielman, 1980; Singer, Reid, and Coppleson, 1976) or only for number of partners (Harris and others, 1980). Inconsistent results of earlier studies could be attributable to lack of advanced PCR techniques for detection and controlling for the confounding effects of HPV infection.

In the study of Latino women with cervical cancer in Los Angeles, the most important risk factors appeared to be Pap smear screening and barrier contraception, that is, preventive factors and not etiologic ones. This study found that if all women had received regular Pap smears and regularly used barrier contraceptives, an estimated 91 percent of the risk would have been avoided. In contrast, the two sexual behavior risk factors, interval between first menarche and first intercourse and number of sexual partners before age 20, together accounted for only 60 percent of the risk (Harris and others, 1986). Both of these sexual behavior risk factors are thought to be surrogates for exposure to the presumed etiologic agent of HPV infection.

A study of San Francisco Bay Area married Latino women and thirty-nine matched pairs of cervical cancer cases and controls found differences in the number of past sexual partners of husbands (Zunzunegui, King, Coria, and Charlet, 1986). Cases were 5.3 times more likely to be married to husbands who had twenty or more lifetime sexual partners. Cases and controls did not differ in their number of lifetime sexual partners, but women with cervical cancer were younger at first intercourse. The association of higher risk for cervical cancer with husbands' sexual history persisted after adjusting for women's sexual partners and age at first intercourse. Although the results did not reach statistical significance, this study indicates that increased risk for cervical cancer among Latino women may also be associated with their male partner's history of sexually transmitted diseases and cigarette smoking.

In another study of cancer incidence in Mexicans in Los Angeles, the risk for cervical cancer was found to be much higher for those who had grown up in Mexico than for those who emigrated to the United States as children. This observation suggests an environmental determinant that acts early in life and is consistent with either a venereal infection with a long latent period or early exposure to a potential carrier (Mack, Walker, Mack, and Bernstein, 1985).

Due to the disparities between Latino and NLW women in the incidence and mortality associated with cervical cancer in New Mexico, a series of studies was conducted comparing risk factors between these two populations (Becker and others, 1991, 1994a, 1994b; Becker, Wheeler, Key, and Samet, 1992; Apple, Becker, Wheeler, and Erlich, 1995). In a case-control study of 201 women with high-grade cervical dysplasia (64 percent of whom were Latino women), the largest ethnic differences were observed for the association of HPV 16 and HPV 18 and cervical cancer for Latinos (OR = 171, 95 percent CI, 22.8 to 1,280.5) compared to the association for NLW women (OR = 18, 95 percent CI, 6.4 to 50.5) (Becker and others, 1994b).

The studies above have important implications for Latinos. As Latino men and women become more acculturated, they tend to report a greater number of sexual partners (Sabogal, Faigeles, and Catania, 1993; Sabogal, Pérez-Stable, Otero-Sabogal, and Hiatt, 1995). An analysis of a national sample of 4,658 heterosexual Latinos for the 1990–1992 AIDS Behavioral Surveys showed that 17 percent of men and 4 percent of women reported multiple sexual partners in the previous year. Latino men were almost five times as likely as Latino women to report having multiple sexual partners (Sabogal, Faigeles, and Catania, 1993). Thus, research and prevention strategies for cervical cancer need to focus on Latino men as well as women, and be sensitive to differences in levels of acculturation.

Cigarette Smoking

Although many studies have demonstrated an association between cervical cancer and cigarette smoking after controlling for sexual behavior (Winkelstein, 1990), studies that examine racial and ethnic differences in smoking and cervical cancer are rare. Even when studies do look at racial and ethnic differences, they generally have insufficient power to detect significant differences due to small numbers of cases. Peters, Bear, and Thomas (1986) and Becker and others (1994a) in case-control studies of women with high-grade dysplasia found that current smoking was significantly associated with dysplasia after controlling for age, age at first intercourse, and lifetime number of sex partners in the case of NLW women but not for Latino women. They did not, however, control for the potentially confounding effects of HPV infection when they looked at ethnic differences.

Studies of the prevalence of cigarette smoking have consistently found lower rates in Latino compared to NLW women. According to the BRFSS for 1991–1992, the prevalence of smoking was 14.5 percent among Latino and 21.6 percent for NLW women (Centers for Disease Control and Prevention, 1994). Although there is evidence that as Latinos become more acculturated to the mainstream, their smoking rates tend to increase (Marin, Pérez-Stable, and Marin, 1989; Otero-Sabogal, Sabogal, Pérez-Stable, and Hiatt, 1995), overall, cigarette smoking does not appear to be a major contributor to the disproportionately higher incidence of cervical cancer in Latinos based on studies thus far and the relatively low prevalence of smoking for Latino women.

BIOLOGIC AND GENETIC FACTORS

In addition to investigations of possible geographic variation in the prevalence of different HPV types, studies have begun to evaluate genetic cofactors associated with HPV infection, which may explain ethnic differences in incidence of cervical dysplasia. Human leukocyte antigens (HLA) are molecules that regulate immune responses to foreign antigens. Certain classes of HLA types (class II haplotypes) have been found to be associated with an increased relative risk for cervical cancer in NLW (Wank and others, 1993) and African American women (Gregoire and others, 1994) independent of HPV type. These findings are consistent with the hypotheses that certain HPV associated cervical cancers may be mediated by some type of host response or defective cellular immunity. Race and ethnic differences in the immune responses to HPV antigens and their relation to the development of cervical cancer are unknown at this time. Thus, the relationship between host genetics and HPV variation requires further studies to determine if these factors explain a significant portion of racial and ethnic disparities in cervical cancer morbidity and mortality.

A study of 128 Latino women in New Mexico with dysplasia using PCR techniques recently found two HLA haplotypes associated with HPV-16-related severe dysplasia, but not among other HPV types. This study also found evidence of haplotypes that appear to confer a protective effect against HPV-16-related severe cervical dysplasia. This haplotype is common among American Indians and the investigators postulated is also present in their sample of Latino women due to population admixture (Apple, Becker, Wheeler, and Erlich, 1995). Clearly, more studies that compare biological factors and immune responses to HPV-type specific cervical cancers are needed.

If future studies show that certain ethnic groups are found to have a higher incidence of HPV types that are associated with a high risk of cervical cancer, this could have important implications for gynecological screening and public health. A new clinical trial that will attempt to identify which mild cervical lesions have a high risk of progressing to cancer along with available technology for detection of HPV types could significantly alter the standard for cervical screening ("Getting a Handle on ASCUS," 1995).

DISCUSSION

More studies are needed to better understand the relative impact of risk factors by language and ethnic subgroup. The relative roles of education, income, screening, early detection, sexual risk factors, HPV infection, immune responses, and parity in the development of cervical cancer must be examined across groups while simultaneously controlling for the effects of potential confounders. Future research should focus on ethnic differences in sexual risk factors, specifically, possible differences in HPV prevalence by type, multiparity, type of contraception, and prevalence of HPV in male partners. More information is also needed about the importance of age and persistence of infection, as well as the risks associated with parity, host response factors, and possibly nutrition.

Regarding our model of factors associated with Latino women's incidence and mortality of cervical cancer, these studies' contexts cannot be ignored. Inadequate regular Pap smear screening and barriers to access of diagnostic services continue to be widely experienced by Latino women in this country. Outreach programs that address structural and attitudinal impediments to and enablers of screening continue to be a public health priority. The results of such practices can be seen in the relatively poorer survival and later stage at diagnosis of Latino women compared to NLW women. Notable is an alarming gap in the information related to medical treatment services' quality and outcomes received by Latinos. As published literature becomes available, environmental factors should also be added to the model.

Most literature of U.S. Latinos and cervical cancer relates to Pap smear screening and incidence and mortality indicators. Other than one southwestern U.S. research team, biological differences in the epidemiology of cervical cancer in Latinos have largely been ignored. There have been several major case-control studies conducted in Latin American countries and more recently, international studies that shed light on issues such as geographical variation in HPV prevalence, which may explain ethnic variations in cervical cancer incidence and mortality along with differential access to screening, diagnostic and treatment services. Understanding Latinos' disproportionate burden of cervical cancer requires comprehensively assessing the full spectrum of structural, biological, behavioral, and environmental factors and their relative contributions for various populations.

References

American Cancer Society. *Cancer Facts and Figures for Minority Americans.* Atlanta, Ga.: American Cancer Society, 1991.

American Cancer Society. *Cancer Risk Report Prevention and Control—1994.* Atlanta, Ga.: American Cancer Society, 1994a.

American Cancer Society. *California Cancer Facts and Figures 1995.* Oakland, Calif.: American Cancer Society, 1994b.

American Cancer Society. *Cancer Facts and Figures—1995.* Atlanta, Ga.: American Cancer Society, 1995.

Anderson, L. M., and May, D. S. "Has the Use of Cervical, Breast, and Colorectal Cancer Screening Increased in the United States?" *American Journal of Public Health,* 1995, *85,* 840–842.

Apple, R. J., Becker, T. M., Wheeler, C. M., and Erlich, H. A. "Comparison of Human Leukocyte Antigen DR-DQ Disease Associations Found with Cervical Dysplasia and Invasive Cervical Carcinoma." *Journal of the National Cancer Institute,* 1995, *87,* 427–436.

Bakemeier, R. F., and others. "Attitudes of Colorado Health Professionals Toward Breast and Cervical Cancer Screening in Hispanic Women." *Journal of the National Cancer Institute Monograph,* 1995, *18,* 95–100.

Baquet, C. R., Horm, J. W., Gibbs, T., and Greenwald, P. "Socioeconomic Factors and Cancer Incidence Among Blacks and Whites." *Journal of the National Cancer Institute,* 1991, *83,* 551–557.

Becker, T. M., Wheeler, C. M., Key, C. R., and Samet, J. M. "Cervical Cancer Incidence and Mortality in New Mexico's Hispanics, American Indians, and Non-Hispanic Whites." *Western Journal of Medicine,* 1992, *156,* 376–379.

Becker, T. M., and others. "Cervical Papillomavirus Infection and Cervical Dysplasia in Hispanic, Native American, and Non-Hispanic White Women in New Mexico." *American Journal of Health,* 1991, *81,* 582–586.

Becker, T. M., and others. "Cigarette Smoking and Other Risk Factors for Cervical Dysplasia in Southwestern Hispanic and Non-Hispanic White Women." *Cancer Epidemiology, Biomarkers, and Prevention,* 1994a, *3,* 113–119.

Becker, T. M., and others. "Sexually Transmitted Diseases and Other Risk Factors for Cervical Dysplasia Among Southwestern Hispanic and Non-Hispanic White Women." *Journal of the American Medical Association,* 1994b, *271,* 1181–1188.

Bosch, F. X., and others. "Importance of Human Papillomavirus Endemicity in the Incidence of Cervical Cancer: An Extension of the Hypothesis on Sexual Behavior." *Cancer Epidemiology, Biomarkers, and Prevention,* 1994, *3,* 375–379.

Bosch, F. X., and others. "Prevalence of Human Papilloma Virus in Cervical Cancer: A Worldwide Perspective." *Journal of the National Cancer Institute,* 1995, *87,* 796–802.

Brinton, L. A., and others. "Parity as a Risk Factor for Cervical Cancer." *American Journal of Epidemiology,* 1989, *130,* 486–496.

Calle, E.E.C., Flanders, W. D., Thun, M. J., and Martin, L. M. "Demographic Predictors of Mammography and Pap Smear Screening in U.S. Women." *American Journal of Public Health,* 1993, *83,* 53–60.

Centers for Disease Control and Prevention. *Chronic Disease in Minority Populations.* Atlanta, Ga.: Centers for Disease Control and Prevention, 1994.

Chavez, L. R., and others. "Structure and Meaning in Models of Breast and Cervical Cancer Risk Factors: A Comparison of Perceptions Among Latinas, Anglo Women, and Physicians." *Medical Anthropology Quarterly,* 1995, *9,* 40–74.

Clarke, E., Hatcher, J., McKeown-Eyssen, G., and Lickrish, G. M. "Cervical Dysplasia: Association with Sexual Behavior, Smoking and Oral Contraceptive Use?" *American Journal of Obstetrics and Gynecology,* 1985, *151,* 612–616.

Devessa, S. S., and Diamond, E. L. "Association of Breast Cancer and Cervical Cancer Incidences with Income and Education Among Whites and Blacks." *Journal of the National Cancer Institute,* 1980, *65,* 515–528.

Gemson, D. H., Elinson, J., and Messeri, P. "Differences in Physician Prevention Practice Patterns for White and Minority Patients." *Journal of Community Health,* 1988, *13,* 53–64.

"Getting a Handle on ASCUS: A New Clinical Trial Could Show How." *Journal of the National Cancer Institute,* 1995, *87,* 787–790.

Gregoire, L., and others. "Association Between HLA-DQB1 Alleles and Risk for Cervical Cancer in African American Women." *International Journal of Cancer,* 1994, *57,* 504–507.

Harlan, L. C., Bernstein, A. B., and Kessler, L. G. "Cervical Cancer Screening: Who Is Not Screened and Why?" *American Journal of Public Health,* 1991, *81,* 885–890.

Harris, R., and others. "Characteristics of Women with Dysplasia or Carcinoma in Situ of the Cervix Uteri." *British Journal of Cancer,* 1980, *42,* 359–369.

Harris, R., and others. "Risk Factors for Invasive Cervical Cancer Among Latinas and Non-Latinas in Los Angeles County." *Journal of the National Cancer Institute,* 1986, *77,* 1063–1077.

Hayward, R. A., Shapiro, M. F., Freeman, H. E., and Corey, M. A. "Who Gets Screened for Cervical and Breast Cancer?" *Archives of Internal Medicine,* 1988, *148,* 1177–1181.

Herrero, R., and others. "Sexual Behavior, Venereal Diseases, Hygiene Practices, and Invasive Cervical Cancer in a High-Risk Population." *Cancer,* 1990, *65,* 380–386.

Hiatt, R. A., and others. "Agreement Between Self-Reported Early Cancer Detection Practices and Medical Audits Among Hispanic and Non-Hispanic White Health Plan Members in Northern California." *Preventive Medicine,* 1995, *24,* 278–285.

Ho, G.Y.F., and others. "Persistent Genital Human Papillomavirus Infection as a Risk Factor for Persistent Cervical Dysplasia." *Journal of the National Cancer Institute,* 1995, *87,* 1365–1371.

Kleinman, J. C., and Kopstein, A. "Who Is Being Screened for Cervical Cancer?" *American Journal of Public Health,* 1981, *71,* 73–76.

Kosary, C. L., Schiffman, M. H., and Trimble, M. D. "Section V Cervix Uteri." In B. A. Miller and others (eds.), *SEER Cancer Statistics Review: 1973–1990.* Bethesda, Md.: National Cancer Institute, 1993.

Koutsky, L. A., and others. "A Cohort Study of the Risk of Cervical Intra Epithelial Neoplasia Grade 2 or 3 in Relation to Papillomavirus Infection." *New England Journal of Medicine,* 1992, *327,* 1272–1278.

Lambert, B., Morisset, R., and Bielman, P. "An Etiologic Survey of Clinical Factors in Cervical Intra Epithelial Neoplasia: A Transverse Retrospective Study." *Journal of Reproductive Medicine,* 1980, *24,* 26–31.

Mack, T., Walker, A., Mack, W., and Bernstein, L. "Cancer in Hispanics in Los Angeles County." *National Cancer Institute Monograph,* 1985, *69,* 99–104.

Mamon, J. A., and others. "Inner-City Women at Risk for Cervical Cancer: Behavioral and Utilization Factors Related to Inadequate Screening." *Preventive Medicine,* 1990, *19,* 363–376.

Marcus, A. C., and Crane, L. A. "Improving Adherence to Screening Follow-Up Among Women with Abnormal Pap Smears: Results from a Large Clinic-Based Trial of Three Intervention Strategies." *Medical Care,* 1992, *30,* 216–229.

Marin, G., Pérez-Stable, E. J., and Marin, B. V. "Cigarette Smoking Among San Francisco Hispanics: The Role of Acculturation and Gender." *American Journal of Public Health,* 1989, *79,* 196–198.

McWhorter, W. P., Schatzkin, A. G., Horm, J. W., and Brown, C. C. "Contribution of Socioeconomic Status to Black/White Differences in Cancer Incidence." *Cancer,* 1989, *63,* 982–987.

Miller, B. A., and others. *SEER Cancer Statistics Review: 1973–1990.* Bethesda, Md.: National Cancer Institute, 1993.

Morgan, C., Park, E., and Cortes, D. E. "Beliefs, Knowledge, and Behavior About Cancer Among Urban Hispanic Women." *Journal of the National Cancer Institute Monograph,* 1995, *18,* 57–63.

Morris, D., and others. "Cervical Cancer, a Major Killer of Hispanic Women: Implications." *Health Education,* 1989, *20,* 23–28.

Muñoz, N., and Bosch, F. X. "HPV and Cervical Cancer: Review of Case-Control and Cohort Studies." In N. Muñoz, F. X. Bosch, K. V. Shah, and A. Meheus (eds.), *The Epidemiology of Human Papillomavirus and Cervical Cancer* (119th ed.). Lyon: IARC Scientific Publications, 1992.

Otero-Sabogal, R., Sabogal, F., Pérez-Stable, E. J., and Hiatt, R. A. "Dietary Practices, Alcohol Consumption, and Smoking Behavior: Ethnic, Sex, and Acculturation Differences." *Journal of the National Cancer Institute Monograph,* 1995, *18,* 73–82.

Parkin, D. M., and Muir, C. S. "Cancer Incidence in Five Continents. Comparability and Quality of Data." *Int. Agency Res. Cancer (WHO) Sci. Pub.,* 1992, *120,* 45–173.

Pérez-Stable, E. J., Sabogal, F., and Otero-Sabogal, R. "Use of Cancer-Screening Tests in the San Francisco Bay Area: Comparison of Latinos and Anglos." *Journal of the National Cancer Institute Monograph,* 1995, *18,* 147–153.

Pérez-Stable, E. J., and others. "Misconceptions About Cancer Among Latinos and Anglos." *Journal of the American Medical Association,* 1992, *268,* 3219–3223.

Pérez-Stable, E. J., and others. "Self-Reported Use of Cancer Screening Tests Among Latinos and Anglos in a Prepaid Health Plan." *Archives of Internal Medicine,* 1994, *154,* 1073–1081.

Perkins, C. I., and others. *Cancer Incidence and Mortality in California by Detailed Race/Ethnicity, 1988–1992.* Sacramento: California Department of Health Services, Cancer Surveillance Section, 1995.

Peters, R., Bear, M., and Thomas, D. "Barriers to Screening for Cancer of the Cervix." *Preventive Medicine,* 1989, *18,* 133–146.

Roach, M., III, and Alexander, M. "The Prognostic Significance of Race and Survival from Breast Cancer: A Model for Assessing the Reliability of Reported Survival Differences." *Journal of the National Medical Association,* 1995, *87,* 214–219.

Sabogal, F., Faigeles, B., and Catania, J. A. II. "Multiple Sexual Partners Among Hispanics in High-Risk Cities." *Family Planning Perspectives,* 1993, *25,* 257–262.

Sabogal, F., Pérez-Stable, E., Otero-Sabogal, R., and Hiatt, R. A. "Gender, Ethnic, and Acculturation Differences in Sexual Behaviors: Hispanic and Non-Hispanic White Adults." *Hispanic Journal of Behavioral Sciences,* 1995, *17,* 139–159.

Samelson, E. J., Speers, M. A., Ferguson, M. S., and Bennett, C. "Racial Differences in Cervical Cancer Mortality in Chicago." *American Journal of Public Health,* 1994, *84,* 1007–1009.

Schiffman, M. H. "New Epidemiology of Human Papillomavirus Infection and Cervical Neoplasia." *Journal of the National Cancer Institute,* 1995, *87,* 1345–1347.

Schiffman, M. H., and others. "Epidemiologic Evidence Showing That Human Papillomavirus Infection Causes Most Cervical Intraepithelial Neoplasia." *Journal of the National Cancer Institute,* 1993, *85,* 958–964.

Shelton, D., Paturzo, D., Flannery, J., and Gregorio, D. "Race, Stage of Disease, and Survival with Cervical Cancer." *Ethnicity and Disease,* 1992, *2,* 47–54.

Singer, A., Reid, B., and Coppleson, M. A. "Hypothesis: The Role of a High-Risk Male in the Etiology of Cervical Carcinoma." *American Journal of Obstetrics and Gynecology,* 1976, *126,* 110–115.

Stewart, S. L., Glaser, S. L., Horn-Ross, P. L., and West, D. W. *SEER Study of Methods to Classify Hispanic Cancer Patients (Final Report: Contract N01-CN-05224).* Union City, Calif.: Northern California Cancer Center, 1993.

Suarez, L., Goldman, D. A., and Weiss, N. S. "Validity of Pap Smear and Mammogram Self-Reports in a Low-Income Hispanic Population." *American Journal of Preventive Medicine,* 1995, *11,* 94–98.

Swan, S., and Brown, W. "Oral Contraceptive Use, Sexual Activity, and Cervical Carcinoma." *American Journal of Obstetrics and Gynecology,* 1981, *139,* 52–57.

Tortolero-Luna, G., and others. "Screening Practices and Knowledge, Attitudes, and Beliefs About Cancer Among Hispanic and Non-Hispanic White Women 35 Years Old or Older in Nueces County, Texas." *Journal of the National Cancer Institute Monograph,* 1995, *18,* 49–56.

Treviño, F. M., Moyer, M. E., Valdez, R. B., and Stroup-Benham, C. A. "Health Insurance Coverage and Utilization of Health Services by Mexican-Americans, Mainland Puerto Ricans, and Cuban Americans." *Journal of the American Medical Association,* 1991, *265,* 233–237.

U.S. Bureau of the Census. *1990 Census of Population and Housing: Population by Race and Hispanic Status.* Washington, D.C.: Economics and Statistics Administration, Bureau of the Census, 1993.

Wank, R., and others. "Cervical Intra-Epithelial Neoplasia, Cervical Carcinoma, and Risk for Patients with HLA-DQB1*0602, *0301, *0303 Alleles." *Lancet,* 1993, *341,* 1215–1219.

Winkelstein, W. "Smoking and Cervical Cancer—Current Status: A Review." *American Journal of Epidemiology,* 1990, *131,* 945–957.

Zunzunegui, M. V., King, M. C., Coria, C. F., and Charlet, J. "Male Influences on Cervical Cancer Risk." *American Journal of Epidemiology,* 1986, *123,* 302–307.

Perspectives of Pregnant and Postpartum Latino Women on Diabetes, Physical Activity, and Health

Edith C. Kieffer
Sharla K. Willis
Natalia Arellano
Ricardo Guzman

If there were a needle in the haystack concerning research and literature on diabetes among Latinas, then this chapter is it. Of all of the disease categories where little research has been conducted or reported on Latinas, it is diabetes, in spite of the fact that the Latino population has one of the highest rates in the United States. The findings reported in this chapter are based on focus groups that total twenty-two women and shed insight on several important issues: Latinas' perceptions about the cause and treatment of diabetes, the role of physical activity in reducing the risk of diabetes, and the structural and institutional factors that influence Latinas' health-seeking behaviors. This study represents a pilot that can serve as a point of departure for further inquiry.

Recent surveys document a sharply rising increase in obesity and Type 2 diabetes in the United States and throughout the world (Mokdad and others, 2000, 2001; Amos, McCarty, and Zimmet, 1997). Changes in the physical and social environment accompanying immigration and urbanization may exacerbate risks for these conditions by affecting diet, physical activity,

This study was conducted in collaboration with Community Health and Social Services (CHASS) with support from the University of Michigan's Center for Research on Women and Gender and School of Public Health, the W. K. Kellogg Foundation Community Health Scholars Program, and the Maternal and Child Health Bureau, Grant No. MC00115. The authors wish to thank the CHASS staff and focus group participants, and Anne Sebert, Rosalind Garcia, Marilyn Lugo, and Sudakshina Ceglarek for their assistance, time, and commitment to the project.

233

and other health behaviors (Amos, McCarty, and Zimmet, 1997). Obesity, impaired glucose tolerance (IGT), gestational diabetes mellitus (GDM), and Type 2 diabetes are prevalent among Latino women of child-bearing age, particularly in low-income and acculturating communities (Hazuda, Haffner, Stern, and Eifler, 1988; Pawson, Martorell, and Mendoza, 1991; Berkowitz, Lapinski, Wein, and Lee, 1992; Khan, Sobal, and Martorell, 1997; Harris and others, 1998; Kieffer and others, 1999). Among Latino women with GDM, more than half may develop Type 2 diabetes within five years postpartum (Kjos and others, 1995). This risk is greatest for obese women and those with the greatest prenatal to postpartum weight gain (Kjos and others, 1995; Buchanan and others, 1998).

Increased physical activity during and after pregnancy may contribute to weight control and improved metabolic status among women with, or at risk for, diabetes (Jovanovic-Peterson and Peterson, 1996; Gregory, Kjos, and Peters, 1993; Horton, 1991; Helmrich, Ragland, Leung, and Paffenbarger, 1991; Bourn and others, 1994). Repeated contact with health care providers during prenatal and postpartum care provides unique and underestimated opportunities for interventions designed to increase physical activity for Latino women (Kieffer, Martin, and Herman, 1999; Kieffer, 2000; Moran, Holt, and Martin, 1997; American Diabetes Association, 2001). However, physical activities recommended by care providers may not be perceived as appropriate or feasible by low-income, inner-city Latino women and their families or communities.

A few studies have assessed levels and correlates of physical activity among women self-identifying as Mexican American or Latino (Crespo, Keteyian, Heath, and Sempos, 1996; Kriska and Rexroad, 1998; Jones and others, 1998; Brownson and others, 2000). The proportion of women reported to engage in no leisure physical activity is higher among Mexican American than non-Hispanic White women (Kriska and Rexroad, 1998). In addition, fewer Latino than non-Hispanic White women participate in moderate levels of leisure physical activity (Jones and others, 1998). Studies conducted primarily with nonpregnant, middle-aged, and older-aged Latino women have identified examples of common physical activities and terminology used to describe them, barriers and incentives to increasing physical activity level, and potential intervention recruitment and retention strategies (Brownson and others, 2000; Eyler and others, 1998, 1999; Tortolero and others, 1999; Whitehorse, Manzano, Baezconde-Garbanati, and Hahn, 1999; Soto Mas and others, 2000).

Latino women's participation in physical activity during and after pregnancy is likely to be influenced by personal, family, and community beliefs and attitudes about physical activity itself and its relationship to health and disease (Strecher and Rosenstock, 1997). Beliefs about causes of diseases such as diabetes, personal susceptibility, and modifiability of risk, including cognitive links between physical activity and disease, may all influence women's motivation to undertake new activities. Pregnancy and new parenthood present additional issues and challenges to women who might participate in physical activity interventions (Devine, Bove, and Olson, 2000). Understanding beliefs about appropriate roles and activities for women during and after pregnancy, and the impact of specific physical activities on the health of mother, fetus, and baby, is critical to intervention planning (Devine, Bove, and Olson, 2000; Zhang and Savitz, 1996; Hatch and others, 1993). However, the published literature includes little information about physical activity–related beliefs and practices or specific issues associated with poverty, immigration, or the urban environment as they affect Latinas during and after pregnancy. Information about these beliefs and practices from the perspective of potential program participants should provide an essential foundation for the work of health educators and others responsible for health and social program and policy development.

This study was undertaken as part of a community-based participatory process to develop realistic and appropriate strategies for improving the metabolic and general health status of pregnant and postpartum Latino women, with a particular focus on physical activity. The purpose of this phase of the process was to engage pregnant and postpartum Latino women in discussion of (1) their perceptions of diabetes risk and impact; (2) their physical activity–related beliefs, attitudes, and practices; and (3) factors influencing their participation in regular physical activity during and after pregnancy.

METHOD

Design

A participatory research design, with an emphasis on shared ownership and analysis of the data, was employed (Kemmis and Mctaggart, 2000). This approach was based on the philosophy that women's own ideas about diabetes and physical activity, the kinds of explanations that they give for these beliefs, and the words they use to explain them are essential for intervention planning. The same women participated in a series of three focus groups, one during pregnancy and two following the birth of their baby. The series format facilitated open discussion and interaction among participants, in-depth exploration of topics, and inclusion of changes in perception with time and life events such as childbirth and parenting. This process moved beyond data collection for the purpose of informing intervention development by investigators as has most often been employed in chronic-disease research (Gettleman and Winkleby, 2000; Blanchard and others, 1999; Roubideaux and others, 2000; Moreno and others, 1997). Women were actively involved in both data analysis and intervention development while still maintaining the focused data collection function inherent to focus groups (Morgan, 1998).

Study Setting, Participants, and Recruitment

The project was conducted at the Community Health and Social Services Center (CHASS), a federally qualified comprehensive health center that serves the predominantly Latino community of southwest Detroit. This generally economically depressed area formerly housed much of Detroit's automobile industry and includes a mixture of open and vacant warehouses, factories, and small businesses, and old, frequently dilapidated detached homes. The community is experiencing a rapid increase in immigration, primarily from Mexico (Center for Urban Studies, 2001). Most Latino prenatal clients at CHASS are of Mexican ancestry (more than 90 percent), born outside of the United States (more than 80 percent), low income (mean family income less than $10,000), and uninsured (more than 60 percent). Approximately 60 percent report that they are married.

Focus group participants were recruited from Maternal Health and Pregnancy Outcomes Among Hispanics, a three-year, prospective longitudinal cohort study that included approximately 97 percent of all Latino mothers entering prenatal care at CHASS. Criteria for focus group participation included women who were Spanish speaking, at least age 18, and in the latter part of the third trimester of pregnancy but not less than four weeks from their estimated date of delivery at focus group session 1. Thirteen participants met these criteria. An additional nine postpartum women joined the second postpartum focus groups for the purpose of confirming and extending the findings of the earlier groups. They were similar to the rest of participants with regard to sociodemographic characteristics. The final study population included twenty-two women.

Except for two women who were born in Guatemala and one who was born in Detroit, the rest of the participants were born in Mexico. All but three women completed their education outside the United States, and most participants had less than twelve years of education, including 38 percent with less than nine years, 38 percent with nine to eleven years, and 24 percent with twelve or more years of education. Spanish was the primary language of all participants except one who was bilingual. The largest proportion of women were 30 years of age or older (41 percent), followed by 18 to 20 years (27 percent), 25 to 29 years (18 percent), and 21 to 24 years (14 percent). Just more than one-quarter of participants had GDM, IGT, or an abnormal screen result, which is similar to the proportion in the prenatal population at CHASS. Six women were primiparous at the time of the first focus group. The remaining women had between one and three children, including four women who had just had their first child at the time of the postpartum focus group. All participants were mailed a flier that described the study and invited them to participate. A bilingual research assistant telephoned women to discuss questions or concerns, scheduling, child care, and transportation arrangements. Participation was confirmed during this, and a follow-up, telephone call.

Focus Group Procedures and Content

A series of three focus groups were conducted: Session 1 when women were approximately thirty to thirty-six weeks pregnant, followed by Session 2 at four to twelve weeks postpartum, and Session 3 at ten to eighteen weeks postpartum. The content of each focus group session built on themes identified from earlier sessions. For example, following the discussion of barriers to physical activity during Session 1, the following common themes were identified: isolation, family responsibility, partners/spouses, community safety, lack of facilities, and health of self and baby. During Session 2, women discussed why these might be barriers, how commonly they acted as barriers, and generally how these barriers might be addressed for women in their community. During Session 3, participants reviewed ideas from Sessions 1 and 2 and then identified and discussed specific aspects of a program that could help them to exercise more regularly and meet other needs of women like themselves. Table 11.1 summarizes the content of each focus group session.

Transportation, child care, healthy snacks, and a $25 gift certificate to a local grocery store were provided at each meeting. Focus groups were facilitated by one of the investigators (S.W.) with extensive experience in qualitative research with Latino women. All groups were conducted in Spanish, the primary language of the participants and the great majority of CHASS prenatal patients. A bilingual

Table 11.1. Focus Group Topics

First session (third trimester of pregnancy)
  Women's beliefs about diabetes, including personal susceptibility
  Perceptions of inevitability or possibility of diabetes risk reduction
  Cognitive links between diabetes risk factors
  Physical activity beliefs, attitudes, practices
  Perceived barriers and facilitators to regular physical activity during and
  after pregnancy

Second session (at six weeks postpartum)
  Results of prenatal group session reviewed
  Perceived risk modifiability and barriers to physical activity discussed in depth
  Changes in participant perceptions following childbirth
  Ideas for addressing barriers

Third session (at twelve weeks postpartum)
  Potential prenatal and postpartum intervention strategies
  Interest in and perceived feasibility of specific program activities
  Program settings, staffing, and participants
  Ideas regarding recruitment and retention of participants

238 LATINA HEALTH IN THE UNITED STATES

research assistant took field notes that included the order of speakers and non-verbal cues. Focus groups lasted sixty to ninety minutes and were audiotaped.

Data Management and Analysis

Verbatim Spanish transcripts were developed and then translated to English. Both languages were included in the final transcript, along with field notes and speaker order. The research assistant responsible for taking field notes at each focus group session reviewed the session transcript for accuracy. Analysis took place at multiple levels to incorporate the community-based analysis vital to participatory research while ensuring scientific rigor, a lack of which is often criticized when evaluating participatory research (Hazuda, Haffner, Stern, and Eifler, 1988). The investigators conducted preliminary analysis during regular research team meetings and presented these findings within the second and third focus group sessions, during which women reviewed, confirmed, and expanded on ideas generated in earlier focus group sessions.

Further in-depth analysis was carried out as research team members carefully read the transcripts and developed codes that represented broad themes seen in the data, such as perceived risk of diabetes, reasons for risk, diet, physical activity, barriers, facilitators, and intervention strategies. Coding qualitative data is a way to group sections of data into categories, allowing for identification of themes and patterns across the data (Tesch, 1990; Miles and Huberman, 1994). A codebook was developed that, for each code, provided its definition, inclusion and exclusion criteria, and examples of text fitting the definition (Crabtree and Miller, 1999; Miles, 1994). ATLAS/ti qualitative data analysis software was used to code data and retrieve text for analysis. Codes were applied to the interviews by research assistants under close supervision of the investigators. Intercoder reliability between the research assistants responsible for coding was determined to test the codebook. Any codes with less than 80 percent agreement were defined more clearly and recoded (Carey, Morgan, and Oxtoby, 1996). The investigators analyzed coded data to identify patterns within the themes and in relation to other themes. Data are presented textually using direct quotations from the women to illustrate findings.

RESULTS

Diabetes Causes or Risk Factors

Women with GDM or IGT were similar to those with normal glucose tolerance during this pregnancy with respect to ideas about diabetes risk factors, whether diabetes risk could be reduced, and the seriousness of the disease. Many women, regardless of current glucose status, either had relatives with diabetes whose behavior and treatment regimens may have influenced their beliefs or had experienced diabetes themselves during this or an earlier pregnancy. Several women had lost family members to the disease: ("After she [mother] passed away, two brothers of hers also passed away from the same thing, and now there are only two brothers left from her side.").

Most women linked their probability of developing diabetes, or "sugar" as many referred to it, with the presence or absence of several factors, most frequently diet, *herencia* or family history, and temperament or the experience of intense emotions (see Table 11.2). Most women believed that family history of diabetes and dietary practices were major contributors to diabetes risk. Diet was

Table 11.2. Selected Quotations Regarding Diabetes Causes or Risk Factors and the Role of Physical Activity

Concept	Quotation
Heredity	"I only have probabilities because of heredity . . . because my mother died from sugar, of diabetes . . . all family of my mom, and they are sick from diabetes."
Diet	"Diabetes comes from sweets . . . when one eats a lot of sweets."
Intense emotion	"One of my aunts, it [diabetes] developed because they scared her: they assaulted her in the street and from there she developed diabetes."
Multifaceted	"They say we have diabetes because of pregnancy . . . only that if one has a diabetic family, well, yes, it does not go away from pregnancy."
	"Like in the culture . . . my mother is fat and so am I. We're fat. Many say it's because of the family, but it's not because of the family; it's due to laziness, not exercising."
Physical activity	"I think diabetes has only to do with food, and I don't think any kind of physical act that you do could have anything to do with that."
	"Exercise is important; but for the 'sugar'—more the diet, the food. That's what I've seen."
Physical activity as treatment	"I ended up having 'sugar' [in a previous pregnancy], and then since I was doing a diet, it quickly went away. I try to walk and eat the same thing that I did with my son to avoid that [with this pregnancy]."
	"Because my mother is diabetic, the nutritionist said, 'You help. When it is summer, go outside to walk; take your mother and you walk too,' because that is the risk that she has and I have. Exercise helps a lot."

mentioned slightly more frequently because specific dietary practices were seen as increasing diabetes risk even in people without a family history of the disease. However, many women described these factors as intertwined, with dietary practices either increasing or decreasing risk for those from "diabetic families." Many women were aware of dietary recommendations for people with diabetes, based on observations of family members or their own experiences.

Specific dietary practices mentioned as increasing diabetes risk were the frequent intake of sweet foods and drinks, and fat, whether obtained from cooking with oil or lard or within foods themselves. These dietary characteristics were seen as an integral part of a Latino cultural lifestyle pattern, although variations in individual behavior were noted, specifically with regard to frequent consumption of sweets and snacks. Weight, age, pregnancy, and temperament were less often discussed as single causes of diabetes, but rather believed to interact with family history and diet to precipitate its onset. Women were aware that diabetes could be present only during pregnancy but saw the disease as most likely to develop during, and less likely to go away after, pregnancy if one had family members with diabetes and if one ate sweets frequently.

Some women reported that the experience of intense emotion was a cause or precipitant of diabetes. Feelings associated with *susto* (fear or fright) and *coraje* (anger) were the most commonly reported, but worry or preoccupation and excitement were also mentioned. Women gave examples that related to sudden events, as well as to a general temperament, for example, easily angered, always worried. Several women explained that these emotions cause the body to "give out more sugar" or to "put forth more insulin." A remedy in the case of anger or fear that was suggested by several participants was to drink water with sugar or eat bread or tortilla to absorb the extra insulin.

Diabetes and Physical Activity

There was considerable disagreement about the role of physical activity in causing diabetes. Many women did not believe there was a relationship between physical activity and the risk of diabetes because dietary factors were seen as the primary cause. Other women saw lack of exercise as part of a general cultural lifestyle pattern that increased diabetes risk and indicated their belief that Latinas were more likely to sit and eat, whereas Anglos were perceived as more likely to exercise. Although physical activity was less often seen as a cause or preventive strategy, several participants identified it as part of diabetes treatment, based on their own experiences and observations of family members and friends with diabetes.

Physical Activity Beliefs and Practices

Focus group participants used both of the terms *physical activity* and *exercise*. Physical activity encompassed movement that resulted from employment, family and household responsibilities, or recreation. Work-related physical activity was seen as both necessary and often exhausting. Women described non-work-related exercise as having greater health benefits, particularly if it released them from the stress of daily work and social isolation. ("It [exercise] helps to keep the mind busy, to run, not to think that I am sick. It helps with circulation, to eliminate fat, calories, which is also for the sugar.") Physical activity was often seen as a diversion, with mood-improving outcomes. ("If one distracts oneself, you get out the sadness that one has.") However, few of these women engaged in purely recreational activity other than walking. Walking was seen as a socially acceptable way to obtain the beneficial aspects of exercise while fulfilling maternal responsibilities such as shopping or accompanying children to school. Walking while socializing with a companion was seen as having the greatest benefit.

Physical Activity Before and During Pregnancy

There were differences in the types of activities that women saw as appropriate and those that they enjoyed doing before pregnancy (most often dancing, walking, and bicycle riding) versus during pregnancy (most often walking). Some of these differences were attributed to pregnancy itself, whereas others were linked to other aspects of life before pregnancy, such as residence in Mexico ("We lived in the ranch . . . and we would grab the bikes and we would just go like that, pregnant") or being unmarried ("before marriage is when you have more activity"). Women also mentioned that physical activity is a part of the work of their daily lives. These activities included house cleaning, washing clothes, shopping, and child care. Women frequently walked their children to and from school and made frequent trips up and down several flights of stairs. ("I go to the children's schools, like a half an hour to go and return. I go four times. With that I think it's more than sufficient . . . every day that is my same routine.") Others mentioned employment that involved physical activity such as working in a laundry and waiting tables. ("I walk about a mile and a half a day: that's exercise!")

Walking was generally seen as safe and beneficial for pregnant women and their infants. Women had heard that exercise made labor easier, quicker, and less painful. Exercise was also mentioned as relaxing for the baby. Walking as a way to get out of the house and distract oneself from daily worries and work was frequently mentioned as a benefit of exercise during pregnancy. Women were concerned about possible negative effects of some kinds of exercise during pregnancy. They suggested that picking up heavy things or activity that resulted in becoming overtired was unwise during pregnancy.

Barriers to Physical Activity During and After Pregnancy

Women reported numerous barriers to physical activity (see Table 11.3). These included physical complaints or concerns such as tiredness, pain, and embarrassment about their appearance; lack of knowledge about how to exercise

Table 11.3. Selected Quotations Regarding Barriers to Physical Activity During and After Pregnancy

Concept	Quotation
Physical complaints and embarrassment	"You look like a cow standing up."
Lack of knowledge	"When they say exercise, one thinks that they will make you jump . . . one does not know much about exercises while pregnant."
Cuarentena	"One should take care for forty days. . . . Women should take care of themselves . . . sweeping and cleaning you cannot do."
Social isolation	"I really don't have friendships or female friends. All the time I am only there in the house. I don't have family. I don't have much communication with other people that I know. Here in the clinic we talk, but I will not see you again."
Family responsibilities	"One is only taking care of babies, keeping up the house, taking care of the husband. . . . The time that we have, we sit and rest. We can take advantage of it, exercising, but we get tired of going from here to there, and instead of exercising one sits down."
Partner and family attitudes and beliefs	"They [male partners] say, 'How are you going to go around like that; you are already a married woman and you have children.' . . . Machismo. Oh! . . . running around like a girl or riding a bike. . . . Many think, 'Sure, you want to be skinny so that others can see you, so they can talk to you.'"
	"He says, 'What are you going for? Take the kids . . . and you come back soon because you have to give me my dinner.' Well, then, I won't go."
	"Our mothers have told us . . . that to do much physical activity maybe would affect the baby . . . and now I realize that instead of affecting, it will be very much in your favor."
Lack of safety	"There are times when we can't go out because gunshots have been heard. . . . One has to cross to the store . . . and I am afraid."

safely while pregnant; environmental barriers, such as very hot, cold, or icy weather; lack of, or distance from, exercise facilities; unsafe streets and parks; and social barriers. Social barriers included the *cuarentena,* a traditional period of forty days postpartum during which aspects of lifestyle such as diet, bathing, housework, and other physical activity are prescribed or proscribed for the protection of mother and baby, and specific support is provided by family members. Women saw the *cuarentena* as part of the culture that helped them care for themselves and that must be respected. It was seen as limiting, but not precluding, physical activity.

Social isolation, expressed as being *encerrado* or being closed in the house, was perceived as a major barrier to physical activity. Social isolation was explained as the outcome of personal and family concerns about safety and appropriate maternal behavior, child and partner care responsibilities, severe weather, and the absence of close family or friends, English-speaking ability, or driving skills. Many women expressed their feelings of being trapped. ("Here, [there is] so much enclosure, one even feels like suffocating when one does not go out.") After women spent the day caring for children, preparing meals, washing clothes, and cleaning the house, little time or energy was perceived as available for exercise. If a choice was to be made between these responsibilities and taking the time for recreation, family responsibilities clearly came first. ("The family counts for more than to say to ourselves, 'I'm going to distract myself over there outside the house' . . . it's all right but one does not do it.")

The attitudes, whether disapproving or approving, and practices of husbands, partners, and family members were very important influences on the attitudes and practices of focus group participants. Disapproval appeared to be a potent barrier to physical activity. Several women reported that their male partners viewed physical activity outside the home as inappropriate for married women and mothers with household responsibilities. Women's mothers also sometimes cautioned women to avoid strenuous activity during pregnancy. Concerns about safety in the urban environment of Detroit were also very important. Activities that women had done in Mexico such as bicycling or walking were not seen as possible in Detroit because of a physical environment that was dilapidated and ridden with heavy traffic, groups of drunken or dangerous men, and prostitutes. Women said that a woman walking might be misperceived by others as a prostitute. ("[There are] a lot of men drinking or women waiting there so that someone could take them . . . what if they think that I'm also there looking for a 'ride.'") The few neighborhood parks were viewed as too dangerous for a woman or her children to use for physical activity.

Facilitators of Physical Activity During and After Pregnancy

Focus group participants also identified situations that did make, or could have made, it easier for them to engage in physical activity (see Table 11.4). Social support from husbands or partners, family, and friends was especially important. Some women's husbands gave general encouragement, whereas others accompanied women to walk or exercise in gymnasiums or parks. Several focus group participants identified family members and friends as companions for exercise, whereas others expressed their wishes for similar support. Community

Table 11.4. Selected Quotations Regarding Facilitators of Physical Activity During and After Pregnancy

Concept	Quotation
Partner/family support	"My husband tells me to do exercise and walk so that you can forget everything. . . . He is also very active. . . . He likes it a lot that me and the children do a lot of those things. . . . He gives me support."
Companions	"If one would combine the exercise, the companionship . . . to go out for at least an hour with another person to exercise . . . it would be a lot better."
Community safety	"Maybe they will give the parks a cleanup so that families can go walk . . . instead of . . . easy women and drunks, so the families can feel like going."
Transportation	"There is a great need for us to become independent. . . . I mean that we can also take our car and go because we also have many possibilities."
A center-based program	"There could be a center where they [women] could come together . . . where there are activities for women . . . like in Mexico." "We could do exercises too and like the rest say also have manual activities . . . to help one relieve the stress of being there in the house."

safety clearly played an important role in making regular exercise possible. Several women described neighborhoods where women felt free to walk, even at night, and where there were places for children to play. Learning to drive and to speak English were seen as skills that would make it easier to seek opportunities, including recreation, in safer places outside their neighborhood. Women also said that the availability of guidance or education about how to safely exercise during pregnancy and child care at recreational facilities would make it easier for them to be physically active.

Women's Primary Recommendation: A Group Activity Program

Focus group participants recommended the development of a center-based group activity program. Physical activities were seen as something that could be offered within the broader context of a program that provided a variety of activities. Women recommended that the program provide opportunities for developing knowledge and learning new skills. Suggestions included selecting and preparing healthy meals, learning and practicing safe and enjoyable exercises (dance lessons were suggested), creating handicrafts, and developing English and driving skills. Such a program was seen as providing opportunities for women to expand their social networks and make friends while relieving stress and boredom. Center-based group activities were seen as providing the necessary motivation and social support for physical activity while addressing safety and other environmental concerns. Ideas for involving both women and children in activities were explored because participants viewed the program as a means for both women and their children to become healthier. Women suggested several creative strategies for overcoming many barriers and promoting participation. They were excited about the ways their intervention ideas could enhance their lives.

DISCUSSION

The value of active involvement of potential participants in planning, designing, implementing, and evaluating interventions is strongly supported by a growing body of literature (Kriska and Rexroad, 1998; Whitehorse, Manzano, Baezconde-Garbanati, and Hahn, 1999; Lewis and others, 1993; Israel, Checkoway, Schulz, and Zimmerman, 1994; Marin and others, 1995; Baker and others, 1997; Schulz, Israel, Selig, and Bayer, 1998). Intervention strategies designed through community-based participatory research are more likely to reflect the cultural values, behavioral preferences, expectations, and environmental context of potential participants (Israel, Schulz, Parker, and Becker, 1998). This study, which is one of the first to address factors associated with diabetes, physical activity, and health among pregnant and postpartum Latino women, strengthens the basis for interventions by contributing new information regarding the dynamic context of pregnancy and the period surrounding childbirth for women in this stage of life.

This study found that pregnant and postpartum Latino women in Detroit believed that diabetes risk was primarily mediated by heredity and several aspects of Latino culture, the most prominent being dietary practice such as consumption of high levels of sugar and fat. Similar perceptions of diabetes causation among nonpregnant Latinas have been reported recently (Weller and others, 1999; Alcozer, 2000). Although physical activity was seen as helpful for improving both physical and emotional health, few women initially believed it played a role in reducing the risk of developing diabetes. As the focus group series proceeded, women with prior experience with diabetes (in themselves or family members) introduced ideas about the role of physical activity as a diabetes treatment and, less commonly, as a preventive strategy during pregnancy.

Regardless of the perceived potential benefits of physical activity, women discussed numerous social, cultural, and environmental barriers present in the context of their daily lives. Many barriers were similar to those found in studies conducted with nonpregnant minority women, including household responsibilities that left them with little time or energy, lack of knowledge about how to exercise safely, social isolation, weather, and lack of access to safe facilities (Eyler and others, 1998). Participants in the current study discussed several additional barriers that arose specifically from their ideas about Latino culture and their status as pregnant and postpartum women. Although many of our participants had enjoyed bicycling and dancing before arriving in Detroit, these activities were not seen as appropriate or safe during pregnancy. Restrictions on physical activity in public were seen as rooted both in the dangers of the urban environment to which they were even more vulnerable during pregnancy and in the demands by many husbands for behavior seen as appropriate for the roles of wife and mother. Fear of appearing to be sexually available was a reason given for not engaging in recreational activity, particularly alone outside of the home. The *cuarentena,* or forty-day period of postpartum recuperation, was seen primarily as a cultural strength that protected them from overexertion but did not necessarily preclude all activity.

Positive attitudes toward women's physical activity in the community and social support from partners, other family members, and friends are important influences on health-related behavior, including physical activity (Kriska and Rexroad, 1998; Eyler and others, 1998, 1999; Hovell and others, 1991; Wing and Jeffery, 1999; Schaffer and Lia-Hoagberg, 1997). The role of partners and extended family may be particularly salient in pregnancy and postpartum, given the importance of family unity and traditions such as the *cuarentena* in this culture (Cousins and others, 1992; Tamez and Vacalis, 1989; Vega, 1995). During pregnancy, the baby's father is often an important source of social support among Latino women (Norbeck and Anderson, 1989). Because the needs of the family were viewed as taking precedence over the individual needs of the women, it is not surprising that women whose partners emphasized the benefits of exercise for themselves and for women were the most likely to feel able to engage in recreational exercise. Partners supported women's exercise activities by encouraging them to participate and by accompanying them on walks to parks or gyms. Focus group participants also reported that friends and family members were, or could be, important sources of motivation, companionship, information, and instrumental support for exercise. However, several participants in this largely immigrant group of women noted that they did not have friends or family members living in the area. The social benefits of group physical activity may provide a powerful motivator for participation (Eyler and others, 1998, 1999).

LIMITATIONS

Because focus group recruitment was conducted by telephone, women with no telephone service were unable to participate. It is also probable that we were less likely to reach and recruit women who move frequently or are more socially isolated. However, several women said that they participated as a means to meet, and talk with, other women. Several of the strategies proposed by participants were suggested specifically for the purpose of reaching more isolated women. Some women who initially agreed to participate were unable to continue the process due to competing family responsibilities. Nine additional postpartum women joined the group. These women confirmed the themes introduced by the earlier participants, including issues associated with the postpartum *cuarentena* and the identification of needs of, and strategies for, women with families.

Focus group participants were slightly older than CHASS prenatal clients. Otherwise, participants were similar in characteristics to both CHASS prenatal clients and the previously described CHASS cohort study from which they were recruited. Because the focus group participants reported almost identical perceptions of diabetes susceptibility and risk factors as the first 600 women interviewed as part of the cohort study, it is likely that at least some of their views are representative of CHASS prenatal clients as a whole. The focus groups were composed almost entirely of women who recently immigrated from Mexico, so findings may not be representative of women with roots in other Latin American countries or those who have resided within U.S. borders for generations. Although CHASS serves the majority of pregnant Latino women in Detroit, further research will be needed to confirm if the perceptions expressed by focus group participant women are representative of other Latina women of childbearing age in this community. Nonetheless, the focus group participants clearly expressed perspectives that are likely to represent the needs of recent immigrants from Mexico, whose numbers have increased greatly in urban areas throughout the United States (Guzman, 2001).

IMPLICATIONS FOR RESEARCH AND PRACTICE

Interventions in this population should focus on promoting a supportive atmosphere for physical activity in both the family and the broader social environment because this support appears to help initiate engagement in physical activity (Eyler and others, 1999). Low-income pregnant women may greatly benefit from specific interventions designed to enhance social support because of limited resources (St. John and Winston, 1989). Interventions clearly must be able to fit into the framework of experiences in women's daily lives. For example, because walking was an important routine for many focus group participants and was considered to be pleasurable and safe, interventions designed to demonstrate methods for integrating brisk walking and other similar physical activities into daily routines could be recommended (Tortolero and others, 1999). Because concerns about safety and social acceptability affect the circumstances under which walking and other activities can take place, women suggested that organized group activities in a familiar and respected location would be the most likely to succeed. As has been found in other studies, focus group participants said that safe, clean, accessible, and convenient places to exercise that allowed the participation of children or provided child care and provided instruction in exercising safely would also facilitate engaging in physical activity during and after pregnancy (Kriska and Rexroad, 1998; Eyler and others, 1999; Miles, 1994).

Focus groups have recently been used in several studies to identify nonpregnant women's physical activity perceptions and practices as well as modifiable factors that influence these patterns (Eyler and others, 1998; Whitehorse, Manzano, Baezconde-Garbanati, and Hahn, 1999; Soto Mas, and others, 2000; Carter-Nolan, Adams-Campbell, and Williams, 1996). Latino participants in other studies have found focused discussion groups to be a useful strategy for health education interventions (Moreno and others, 1997). Women may perceive themselves as sharing a common problem and develop a sense of ownership of the solutions they suggest (Whitehorse, Manzano, Baezconde-Garbanati, and Hahn, 1999; Carter-Nolan, Adams-Campbell, and Williams, 1996). In this study, the three session series appeared to have such an effect, as information was shared and social bonds among women were developed. These bonds could form a solid foundation for the group activity intervention proposed by the women. This methodology may prove useful for health educators and others developing community-based interventions among Latino women.

Health care planners and providers must become aware of women's perceptions of the multiple barriers they face to engaging in regular physical activity for the purpose of improving health. Given the realities of daily life, these largely social and environmental barriers might seem insurmountable. However, the women became actively engaged in developing strategies that, if implemented, could improve their likelihood of becoming more physically active while addressing their primary interest in increased social support. The focus group itself served as a model for participants of the value of group activity. The challenge will be to identify resources needed to make such interventions a reality. The rising roll for individuals, families, and communities of obesity, diabetes, and their complications make such action imperative.

References

Alcozer, F. "Secondary Analysis of Perceptions and Meaning of Type 2 Diabetes Among Mexican American Women." *Diabetes Education,* 2000, *26,* 768–794.

American Diabetes Association. "Position Statement: Gestational Diabetes Mellitus." *Diabetes Care,* 2001, *24*(Suppl. 1), S77–S79.

Amos, A. F., McCarty, D. J., and Zimmet, P. "The Rising Global Burden of Diabetes and Its Complications: Estimates and Projections to the Year 2010." *Diabetic Medicine,* 1997, *14,* S7–S85.

Baker, E. A., and others. "The Latino Health Advocacy Program: A Collaborative Lay Health Advisor Approach." *Health Education and Behavior,* 1997, *24,* 495–509.

Berkowitz, G. S., Lapinski, R. H., Wein, R., and Lee, D. "Race/Ethnicity and Other Risk Factors for Gestational Diabetes." *American Journal of Epidemiology,* 1992, *135,* 965–973.

Blanchard, M. A., and others. "Using a Focus Group to Design a Diabetes Education Program for an African American Population." *Diabetes Education,* 1999, *25,* 917–924.

Bourn, D. M., and others. "Impaired Glucose Tolerance and NIDDM: Does a Lifestyle Intervention Program Have an Effect?" *Diabetes Care,* 1994, *17,* 1311–1319.

Brownson, R. C., and others. "Patterns and Correlates of Physical Activity Among US Women 40 Years and Older." *American Journal of Public Health,* 2000, *90,* 264–270.

Buchanan, T.A.M., and others. "Utility of Fetal Measurements in the Management of Gestational Diabetes Mellitus." *Diabetes Care,* 1998, *21,* B99–B106.

Carey, J., Morgan, M., and Oxtoby, M. "Intercoder Agreement in Analysis of Responses to Open-Ended Interview Questions: Examples from Tuberculosis Research." *Cultural Anthropology Methods,* 1996, *8,* 1–5.

Carter-Nolan, P. L., Adams-Campbell, L. L., and Williams, J. "Recruitment Strategies for Black Women at Risk for Noninsulin-Dependent Diabetes Mellitus into Exercise Protocols: A Qualitative Assessment." *Journal of the National Medical Association,* 1996, *88*(9), 558–562.

Center for Urban Studies. *1990 and 2000 Population by Census Tract—Southwest Detroit.* Detroit, Mich.: Wayne State University, 2001.

Cousins, J. H., and others. "Family Versus Individually Oriented Intervention for Weight Loss in Mexican American Women." *Public Health Report,* 1992, *107*(5), 549–555.

Crabtree, B. F., and Miller, W. L. "Using Code Manuals: A Template Organizing Style of Interpretation." In B. F. Crabtree and W. L. Miller (eds.), *Doing Qualitative Research.* Thousand Oaks, Calif.: Sage, 1999.

Crespo, C. J., Keteyian, S. J., Heath, G. W., and Sempos, C. T. "Leisure-Time Physical Activity Among US Adults. Results from the Third National Health and Nutrition Examination Survey." *Archives of Internal Medicine,* 1996, *156,* 93–98.

Devine, C. M., Bove, C. F., and Olson, C. M. "Continuity and Change in Women's Weight Orientations and Lifestyle Practices Through Pregnancy and the Postpartum Period: The Influence of Life Course Trajectories and Transitional Events." *Social Science and Medicine,* 2000, *50,* 567–582.

Eyler, A. A., and others. "Physical Activity and Minority Women: A Qualitative Study." *Health Education and Behavior,* 1998, *25*(5), 640–652.

Eyler, A. A., and others. "Physical Activity, Social Support and Middle- and Older-Aged Minority Women: Results from a US Survey." *Social Science and Medicine,* 1999, *49*(6), 781–789.

Gettleman, L., and Winkleby, M. A. "Using Focus Groups to Develop a Heart Disease Prevention Program for Ethnically Diverse, Low-Income Women." *Journal of Community Health,* 2000, *25,* 439–453.

Gregory, K. D., Kjos, S. L., and Peters, R. K. "Cost of Non-Insulin-Dependent Diabetes in Women with a History of Gestational Diabetes: Implications for Prevention." *Obstetrics and Gynecology,* 1993, *81,* 782–786.

Guzman, B. *The Hispanic Population: Census 2000 Brief.* Washington, D.C.: U.S. Department of Commerce, Economics and Statistics Administration, U.S. Census Bureau, 2001.

Harris, M. I., and others. "Prevalence of Diabetes, Impaired Fasting Glucose, and Impaired Glucose Tolerance in U.S. Adults. The Third National Health and Nutrition Examination Survey, 1988–1994." *Diabetes Care,* 1998, *21,* 518–524.

Hatch, M. C., and others. "Maternal Exercise During Pregnancy, Physical Fitness, and Fetal Growth." *American Journal of Epidemiology,* 1993, *137,* 1105–1114.

Hazuda, H. P., Haffner, S. M., Stern, M. P., and Eifler, C. W. "Effects of Acculturation and Socioeconomic Status on Obesity and Diabetes in Mexican Americans. The San Antonio Heart Study." *American Journal of Epidemiology,* 1988, *128,* 1289–1301.

Helmrich, S. P., Ragland, D. R., Leung, R. W., and Paffenbarger, R. S. "Physical Activity and Reduced Occurrence of Non-Insulin-Dependent Diabetes Mellitus." *New England Journal of Medicine,* 1991, *325,* 147–152.

Horton, E. S. "Exercise in the Treatment of NIDDM. Applications for GDM?" *Diabetes,* 1991, *40*(Suppl. 2).

Hovell, M., and others. "Identification of Correlates of Physical Activity Among Latino Adults." *Journal of Community Health,* 1991, *16,* 23–36.

Israel, B. A., Checkoway, B., Schulz, A., and Zimmerman, M. "Health Education and Community Empowerment: Conceptualizing and Measuring Perceptions of Individual, Organizational, and Community Control." *Health Education Quarterly,* 1994, *21,* 149–170.

Israel, B. A., Schulz, A. J., Parker, E. A., and Becker, A. B. "Review of Community-Based Research: Assessing Partnership Approaches to Improve Public Health." *Annual Review of Public Health,* 1998, *19,* 173–202.

Jones, D. A., and others. "Moderate Leisure-Time Physical Activity: Who Is Meeting the Public Health Recommendations? A National Cross-Sectional Study. *Archives of Family Medicine,* 1998, *7,* 285–289.

Jovanovic-Peterson, L., and Peterson, C. M. "Review of Gestational Diabetes Mellitus and Low-Calorie Diet and Physical Exercise as Therapy." *Diabetes/Metabolism Review,* 1996, *12,* 287–308.

Kemmis, S., and Mctaggart, R. "Participatory Action Research." In N. K. Denzin and Y. S. Lincoln (eds.), *Handbook of Qualitative Research.* Thousand Oaks, Calif.: Sage, 2000.

Khan, L. K., Sobal, J., and Martorell, R. "Acculturation, Socioeconomic Status, and Obesity in Mexican Americans, Cuban Americans, and Puerto Ricans." *International Journal of Obesity and Related Metabolic Disorders*, 1997, *21*(2), 91–96.

Kieffer, E. C. "Maternal Obesity and Glucose Intolerance During Pregnancy Among Mexican-Americans." *Paediatric and Perinatal Epidemiology*, 2000, *14*, 14–19.

Kieffer, E. C., Martin, J. A., and Herman, W. H. "Impact of Maternal Nativity on the Prevalence of Diabetes During Pregnancy Among U.S. Ethnic Groups." *Diabetes Care*, 1999, *22*, 729–735.

Kieffer, E. C., and others. "Glucose Tolerance During Pregnancy and Birth Weight in a Hispanic Population." *Obstetrics and Gynecology*, 1999, *94*, 741–746.

Kjos, S. L., and others. "Predicting Future Diabetes in Latino Women with Gestational Diabetes: Utility of Early Postpartum Glucose Tolerance Testing." *Diabetes*, 1995, *44*, 586–591.

Kriska, A. M., and Rexroad, A. R. "The Role of Physical Activity in Minority Populations." *Women's Health Issues*, 1998, *8*(2), 98–103.

Lewis, C. E., and others. "Promoting Physical Activity in Low-Income African-American Communities: The PARR Project." *Ethnicity and Disease*, 1993, *3*(2), 106–118.

Marin, G., and others. "A Research Agenda for Health Education Among Underserved Populations." *Health Education Quarterly*, 1995, *22*, 346–363.

Miles, M. B. *Qualitative Data Analysis: An Expanded Sourcebook.* (2nd ed.) Thousand Oaks, Calif.: Sage, 1994.

Miles, M. B., and Huberman, A. M. *Qualitative Data Analysis.* (2nd ed.) Thousand Oaks, Calif.: Sage, 1994.

Mokdad, A. H., and others. "Diabetes Trends in the U.S.: 1990–1998." *Diabetes Care*, 2000, *23*, 1278–1283.

Mokdad, A. H., and others. "The Continued Increase of Diabetes in the U.S." *Diabetes Care*, 2001, *24*, 412.

Moran, C. F., Holt, V. L., and Martin, D. P. "What Do Women Want to Know After Childbirth?" *Birth*, 1997, *24*, 27–34.

Moreno, C., and others. "Heart Disease Education and Prevention Program Targeting Immigrant Latinos: Using Focus Group Responses to Develop Effective Interventions." *Journal of Community Health*, 1997, *22*, 435–450.

Morgan, D. L. "The Focus Group Guidebook." In D. L. Morgan and R. A. Krueger (eds.), *The Focus Group Kit* (Vol. 1). Thousand Oaks, Calif.: Sage, 1998.

Norbeck, J. S., and Anderson, N. J. "Psychosocial Predictors of Pregnancy Outcomes in Low-Income Black, Hispanic, and White Women." *Nursing Research*, 1989, *38*, 204–209.

Pawson, I. G., Martorell, R., and Mendoza, F. E. "Prevalence of Overweight and Obesity in US Hispanic Populations." *American Journal of Clinical Nutrition*, 1991, *53*(Suppl. 6), 1522S–1528S.

Roubideaux, Y. D., and others. "Diabetes Education Materials: Recommendations of Tribal Leaders, Indian Health Professionals, and American Indian Community Members." *Diabetes Education,* 2000, *26,* 290–294.

Schaffer, M. A., and Lia-Hoagberg, B. "Effects of Social Support on Prenatal Care and Health Behaviors of Low-Income Women." *Journal of Obstetric, Gynecologic, and Neonatal Nursing,* 1997, *26,* 433–440.

Schulz, A., Israel, B., Selig, S., and Bayer, I. "Development and Implementation of Principles for Community-Based Research in Public Health." In R. MacNair (ed.), *Research Strategies for Community Practice.* New York: Haworth, 1998.

Soto Mas, F., and others. *"Camine con Nosotros:* Connecting Theory and Practice for Promoting Physical Activity Among Hispanic Women." *Health Promotion Practice,* 2000, *1,* 178–187.

St. John, C., and Winston, T. J. "The Effect of Social Support on Prenatal Care." *Journal of Applied Behavioral Science,* 1989, *25,* 79–98.

Strecher, V. J., and Rosenstock, I. M. "The Health Belief Model." In K. Glanz, F. M. Lewis, and B. K. Rimer (eds.), *Health Behavior and Health Education: Theory, Research and Practice.* (2nd ed.) San Francisco: Jossey-Bass, 1997.

Tamez, E. G., and Vacalis, T. D. "Health Beliefs, the Significant Other and Compliance with Therapeutic Regimens Among Adult Mexican American Diabetics." *Health Education,* 1989, *20,* 24–31.

Tesch, R. *Qualitative Research: Analysis Tapes and Software Tools.* New York: Falmar, 1990.

Tortolero, S. R., and others. "Assessing Physical Activity Among Minority Women: Focus Group Results." *Women's Health Issues,* 1999, *9,* 135–142.

Vega, W. A. "The Study of Latino Families—Familism and Continuity of Family Values." In R. Zembrana (ed.), *Understanding Latino Families: Scholarship, Policy, and Practice.* Thousand Oaks, Calif.: Sage, 1995.

Weller, S. C., and others. "Latino Beliefs About Diabetes." *Diabetes Care,* 1999, *22,* 722–728.

Whitehorse, L. E., Manzano, R., Baezconde-Garbanati, L. A., and Hahn, G. "Culturally Tailoring a Physical Activity Program for Hispanic Women: Recruitment Successes of La Vida Buena's Salsa Aerobics." *Journal of Health Education,* 1999, *30,* S18–S24.

Wing, R. R., and Jeffery, R. W. "Benefits of Recruiting Participants with Friends and Increasing Social Support for Weight Loss and Maintenance." *Journal of Consulting and Clinical Psychology,* 1999, *67*(1), 132–138.

Zhang, J., and Savitz, D. A. "Exercise During Pregnancy Among US Women." *Annals of Epidemiology,* 1996, *6,* 53–59.

PART FIVE

ALCOHOL, TOBACCO, AND OTHER DRUGS

CHAPTER TWELVE

Alcohol Use and Misuse Among Hispanic Women

Selected Factors, Processes, and Studies

Glorisa Canino

The research questions and issues that this chapter raises remain as relevant today as they did in 1994, when this chapter was originally published. These issues continue to require inquiry and study so as to inform and guide prevention and treatment programs and policies.

R ates of alcohol use and misuse and problems associated with drinking among Hispanic women have rarely been assessed using probability samples of the populations studied. Epidemiologic studies are important in providing information regarding who is at "risk" or more vulnerable and what are some of the factors or processes that protect individuals from excessive drinking or alcoholism. For example, epidemiologic studies provide information on whether socioeconomic factors, gender, marital status, and other factors are related to the distribution of alcohol use and misuse in a population (Helzer, Burnam, and McEvoy, 1991). The main advantage of epidemiological studies is the identification of factors that may be related to a higher probability of individuals' misusing alcohol. This information can then be used for prevention purposes and for generating an etiological hypothesis, which can then be tested with experimental designs. A disadvantage of this method of inquiry is that since large samples are needed to make inferences to the total population, in-depth analyses of the etiological mechanisms involved in the development of the condition are not possible. Cross-cultural epidemiology has the advantage of providing information regarding how groups differ from each other in the prevalence of alcoholism risk factors, as well as the meaning that drinking has in each culture.

Epidemiologic studies of alcoholism and patterns of alcohol use in general populations have been difficult to interpret because of variations in case definitions, diagnostic procedures, and methodology. These difficulties are greater in studies among Hispanics because of the use of instruments that have not been standardized or validated for those populations. In addition, as noted in Caetano's review of the literature (1983), with few exceptions, the published surveys conducted in the United States to study the prevalence of alcohol patterns and problems have not been developed to study Hispanics. Hispanics constitute a minority in the United States, and its assessment requires translation and adaptation of the instruments used. The numbers of respondents identified in these surveys as Hispanic have constituted small proportions of the samples, making it impossible to estimate prevalence by sex in that ethnic group with reasonable confidence. Furthermore, the Hispanic groups characteristically have not been disaggregated into component national groups (Caetano, 1983). This poses difficulties in the interpretation of the data since research has demonstrated that Hispanic groups differ in terms of their drinking patterns and prevalence of alcohol problems (Gordon, 1981; Gilbert and Cervantes, 1987; Page, Rio, Sweeney, and McKay, 1985). Societies differ in how they view alcohol consumption, in their accessibility to the substance, and even in their physiological tolerance of alcohol, factors that have all been associated with the prevalence of alcohol consumption and alcoholism (Babor, 1986). Thus, one would expect to find differences in alcohol use and misuse across cultures and within the same ethnic group. Gender differences are also expected inasmuch as societal mores prescribe different roles for each sex (Helzer and Canino, 1992). In spite of the paucity of research regarding alcoholism or alcohol use and misuse among Hispanics, some national studies of U.S. Hispanics, island Puerto Ricans, and Latin Americans have been carried out. The focus of these studies has not been the study of Hispanic women but mostly a description of alcohol use patterns or prevalence rates of alcoholism in the population. However, data are also presented that pertain to alcohol use or alcoholism among Hispanic women. Most of the studies describe alcohol use patterns that may range from very mild to more severe alcohol consumption patterns. Other studies, mostly those carried out in Latin America and Puerto Rico, focus on the extreme forms of drinking (misuse and dependence) associated with alcoholism. These last studies use operational definitions of alcoholism based on a medical model of disease such as the nosological system of the *Diagnostic and Statistical Manual* (DSM III, Third Revision) of the American Psychiatric Association (1983). Thus, it is important to note that in this chapter, alcohol use should not be equated with alcohol misuse or dependence or with alcoholism. Alcohol misuse or dependence involves extreme forms of drinking, which are usually associated with impairment in social or occupational roles or withdrawal or tolerance of the substance. Alcohol use, even when referring to heavy drinking, does not necessarily entail impairment in functioning. What follows is a critical review of the research on alcohol use and alcoholism, focusing on the results pertinent to Hispanic women. Recommendations for future research in this area are also given.

ALCOHOL USE IN LATIN AMERICAN WOMEN

The diversity of cultural experiences of Latin American nations is reflected in a wide variation in alcohol use. Latin American countries can be characterized not only by their political systems or level of economic development but also by national drinking patterns, beverage preference, attitudes toward alcohol consumption, and attention given to alcohol problems. There are wine-producing and wine-drinking countries such as Argentina and Chile; there are countries such as Puerto Rico where distilled spirits are preferred; and there are beer-drinking countries like Mexico (Canino, Burnam, and Caetano, 1992). Some of these differences in alcohol use arise from demographic factors, such as the presence of a large indigenous population, which may have contributed since colonial times to the development and survival of certain patterns of drinking in the non-European population. A possible example of this is the pattern of infrequent drinking with high consumption per occasion observed in Mexico, which may have emerged from ritual drinking among the natives in precolonial times (Heath, 1982; Taylor, 1979).

But if there is a wide variation in alcohol use among the different nations of Latin America from which U.S. Hispanics come, there is also some uniformity. Drinking and drunkenness by men and the young are more accepted than by women and the elderly (Caetano, 1984). Following these normative prescriptions, drinking in Latin America is predominantly a male activity, something that men do when they get together after work, during sports activities, or when socializing. Excessive drinking is also exhibited mostly by men, the great majority of women being either abstainers or very "light" drinkers. Thus, most of the people in treatment for alcohol problems are men (Caetano, 1984). Data on drinking patterns, attitudes, and norms toward alcohol consumption and alcohol problems among Hispanics in the United States and island Puerto Ricans reflect these patterns found in Latin American countries (Alcocer, 1982; Caetano, 1984; Gilbert and Cervantes, 1986; García, 1976).

ALCOHOL USE AMONG U.S. HISPANIC WOMEN

Most of the epidemiological work done on alcohol consumption among Hispanics has centered on Mexican American populations basically from just two states, Texas and California (Gilbert and Cervantes, 1987). Research on drinking patterns of mainland Puerto Ricans is limited to two studies, one reported in 1976 and a more recent investigation performed by researchers at the Hispanic Research Center of New York (García, 1976; Johnson and Gurin, 1994). Research on Cuban Americans and other Hispanic groups in the United States is practically nonexistent.

Few national studies of Hispanic populations have been done, and in most of these, the majority of the Hispanics sampled were Mexican Americans (Caetano, 1987). Most of these studies show that alcohol use and excessive drinking is a predominantly male activity. However, abstention rates, as well as patterns of drinking, vary among Hispanic women according to region, socioeconomic level, acculturation, and employment status.

To our knowledge, the only study that permits comparisons among the major groups of Hispanics in the United States is a 1984 survey reported by Caetano (1986). In this study, a national probability sample of Hispanics from forty-eight states was obtained ($n = 1,453$). The results pertaining to women showed that although the majority of Hispanic women in the United States have higher abstention rates than U.S. women, Mexican American women report more heavy drinking and alcohol-related problems than Cubans or Puerto Ricans (Caetano, 1986). Abstention rates were highest among Mexican American women (46 percent) and lowest for Puerto Rican women (33 percent). This lifetime abstention rate of mainland Puerto Rican women is almost identical to that reported by Canino, Burnam, and Caetano (1992) for island Puerto Ricans (32 percent) and that reported by P. Johnson (personal communication; 31 percent) for a probability sample of New York Puerto Rican women. The abstention rate of Cuban women as reported by Caetano's national survey (1986) was higher (42 percent) than that of Puerto Ricans. In addition, Cuban women exhibited the most moderate drinking patterns among the three groups.

Gilbert and Cervantes (1987), in their review of the literature of Mexican American alcohol use, provide evidence which indicates that Mexican American women from Texas as compared to those from California have a lower prevalence of alcohol use and higher abstention rates. The review of studies of low-income or blue-collar Hispanic populations indicates higher abstention rates and low frequency of use as well as lighter drinking patterns as opposed to white-collar women or women from more heterogeneous socioeconomic groups. Lower socioeconomic and educational status is usually associated with more traditional values, which strongly proscribe drinking among Hispanic women, thus accentuating differences when comparisons are made with Anglo women or Hispanic women of higher educational levels. For example, Gilbert and Cervantes (1987) quote a study of a low-income population in Houston in which the lifetime abstention rate among Mexican American women was 84 percent, in contrast with 38 percent of the Anglo population of females. Prevalence data from a more representative statewide Texas sample showed less difference in the abstention rate among Mexican American women (45 percent) as opposed to Anglo women (36 percent). Possibly this was due to the larger number of urban women from different generations in this statewide sample, as well as to the larger heterogeneity of the sample in terms of socioeconomic and educational levels. In fact, Gilbert and Cervantes quote the work of Holck, Warren, Smith, and Rochat (1984), which corroborates the link between education and greater consumption among Mexican American women. These researchers found that when educational level was held constant, the differences in consumption patterns between the Mexican American and Anglo women they studied disappeared.

The role of educational level in drinking behavior is also reported by Burnam's Epidemiological Catchment Area (ECA) study (1989) in Los Angeles. In this study, the prevalence of alcohol misuse and dependence among Mexican American women increased with higher educational levels. In contrast, the findings from the five ECA U.S. communities revealed the opposite trend. In these U.S. communities, alcohol misuse and dependence was significantly more common among individuals with lower educational levels, for example, less than high school diploma (Helzer, Burnam, and McEvoy, 1991). It is possible that the differences between the studies are explained by the fact that increasing educational levels among Mexican American women are accompanied by increasing levels of acculturation. As will be discussed later, acculturation among Hispanic women is strongly associated with an increase in alcohol consumption and alcohol problems.

Other studies of Hispanic women have found that lower alcohol consumption and lower alcohol problems are associated with marriage, being a housewife, and with blue-collar status (Caetano, 1984; Holck, Warren, Smith, and Rochat, 1984; Gilbert and Cervantes, 1987). These lower alcohol consumption patterns of blue-collar married housewives may also be related to acculturation status. Hispanic housewives are less exposed to the cultural values of American society, so that one would expect them to be less acculturated than those who are employed. In addition, adherence to more traditional values, which strongly disapprove of women drinking, is usually associated with lower educational levels (Gilbert and Cervantes, 1987).

The comparison of alcohol patterns of Anglo women in the United States with Hispanic women living in their culture of origin is informative since it provides baseline data for Hispanic women in the United States and can disentangle the effects of culture from other factors (such as prejudice, low socioeconomic status, and select migration) that may affect the consumption of alcohol among Hispanic women. Most important, Gilbert and Cervantes (1987) provide a review of a study by Roizen (1983) that compared probability samples from Mexico and San Francisco of rural and urban populations similar in demographic composition. In this study, abstention rates were significantly higher among Mexican women. San Francisco Anglo women drank at higher frequencies and in lower quantities than those few Mexican women who drank. Mexican women who drank did so only a few times a year. Thus, the data comparing U.S. women with women from Mexico consistently show different consumption patterns in both groups, which suggests differences in cultural attitudes toward drinking among women in both cultures. Drinking among Mexican women is certainly more strongly proscribed than in the U.S. culture.

ALCOHOL USE AND MISUSE IN ISLAND AND MAINLAND PUERTO RICAN WOMEN: A CROSS-CULTURAL COMPARISON

As previously stated, only two alcohol studies of mainland Puerto Ricans were identified in the literature. The first study, reported by Haberman and Sheinberg (1967), investigated the drinking patterns of a large sample of New York Puerto Ricans and found that all problem drinkers were male and that Puerto Ricans had the highest female/male ratio of reported nondrinking of all ethnic groups studied.

In the second epidemiologic study, 1,084 Puerto Rican adults who resided in the New York metropolitan area were surveyed (Johnson and Gurin, 1994). The study employed multistage probability sampling methods to survey the population aged 18 and older regarding alcohol drinking patterns and related problems. In addition, respondents completed the Center for Epidemiologic Studies Depression Scale (CES-D). Preliminary results of this study showed that Puerto Rican men reported more recent drinking problems (4.2 percent) than did women (1.2 percent), while Puerto Rican women reported more depressive symptoms than men (14.9 versus 6.8 percent). In addition, as previously stated, the lifetime abstention rate for Puerto Rican women (31 percent) was considerably higher than for men but similar to that reported for island Puerto Ricans (32 percent) (Canino, Burnam, and Caetano, 1992) and other U.S. women (36 percent) (Caetano, 1986). Comparison of the New York Puerto Rican women with Irish American women from the same region showed very different drinking practices (Johnson and Gurin, 1994). The lifetime abstention rate for Irish women was 4 versus 31 percent for Puerto Rican women, and while 73 percent of Puerto Rican women had never been intoxicated, 54 percent of Irish women reported no intoxication.

Different results among ethnic groups are obtained when comparing data obtained from an island Puerto Rican epidemiologic study of alcoholism with an analogous one done in five U.S. communities as part of the Epidemiologic Catchment Area Study (ECA) (Helzer and Canino, 1992). Similar diagnostic and sampling methods were used in these two studies. Alcohol misuse or dependence was ascertained in both studies with the Diagnostic Interview Schedule

(DIS; Robins, Helzer, Croughan, and Ratcliff, 1981), and both used probability sampling methods to survey the population. Thus, differences in results between the studies could not be due to variations in diagnostic definition or method of ascertainment. The results of the comparisons of these two studies showed higher lifetime abstention rates among island Puerto Rican females (31.7 percent) compared to those of Anglo females from Los Angeles (11.95 percent) or those of Mexican American origin (29.5 percent) (Canino, Burnam, and Caetano, 1992). Nevertheless, Mexican American women born in Mexico had higher abstention rates (44.2 percent) compared to Puerto Ricans. Furthermore, when comparing abstention rates by sex, it was found that while four times as many women abstain from drinking as compared to men in Puerto Rico, among Mexican American immigrants, the difference was fifteen times greater. These differences could be due to differences in socioeconomic status, since immigrant women are considerably poorer and less educated than a representative sample of island Puerto Rican women, where a more diverse group of socioeconomic status is found. In addition, Caetano (1985) has provided evidence that immigrant Mexican women are more abstemious (71 percent) than women in Mexico. It is possible that Mexican women who migrate become entrenched in their cultural values and norms when faced with the threat of losing their values to different mores from the host country. In fact, most studies consistently show that immigrant Mexican American women do not alter their drinking patterns during their lifetime (Gilbert and Cervantes, 1986). An exaggeration of cultural norms and values may be a defensive response against the threat of losing these values.

The pattern is once more repeated when comparing prevalence rates of alcohol misuse or dependence between Mexican Americans from Los Angeles and island Puerto Ricans. The results of the studies described above indicate that the male/female ratio is much higher among immigrant Mexican Americans (25:0) compared to Mexican Americans born in the United States (4:1) and island Puerto Ricans (12:1) (Canino, Burnam, and Caetano, 1992). Comparisons among the different ethnic groups of women again showed the same pattern. While *no* cases of alcohol misuse or dependence were identified among the immigrant group of women, lifetime prevalence rates for U.S.-born Mexican American women were 5 and 2.0 percent for Puerto Ricans. Thus, island Puerto Ricans have lower prevalence rates of alcoholism than U.S.-born Mexican American women but higher than immigrants, falling at the middle point between the two groups. The same pattern is thus observed for abstention rates and male/female ratios.

Comparison of alcohol misuse and dependence rates of island Puerto Ricans with five U.S. communities, Mexican American immigrants from Los Angeles, and three other regions of the world (Munich, Edmonton, Christchurch) have been made by Helzer and Canino (1992). These investigators compare several

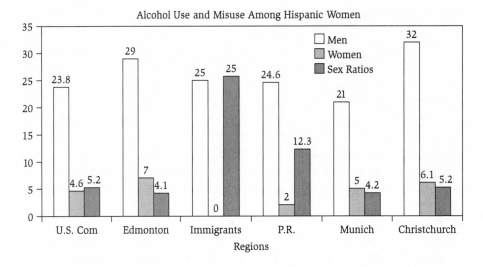

Figure 12.1. Lifetime Prevalence Rates by Sex for DIS/DSM-III Alcohol Misuse/ Dependence in Six Regions

studies that used similar methods and instruments of ascertainment, for example, probability samples and the Diagnostic Interview Schedule (DIS). The DIS is based on the DSM classificatory system of mental disorders of the American Psychiatric Association (1983). Alcohol misuse and dependence is the classification used for what is known as "alcoholism" in other classificatory or nosological systems. The results of these comparisons show that the male/ female ratio of alcohol misuse or dependence is considerably higher in the two Hispanic communities (Puerto Rico and Mexican Americans) compared to the other ethnic groups (see Figure 12.1, also reported in Helzer and Canino, 1992). Prevalence rates of alcohol misuse or dependence among the Hispanic women were considerably lower than in the other groups. Possible explanations for these observed differences include differential genetic risk, lower tolerance for alcohol among women, and greater social stigma attached to their drinking. In addition, the fact that the male/female ratio is considerably larger in the two Hispanic groups compared to the other ethnic groups also suggests an important societal effect that may be related to cultural values, differences among the ethnic groups and regions regarding industrialization and modernization, or both.

In order to test this possible societal effect empirically, Helzer and Canino (1992) disaggregated sex as a risk factor for heavy drinking and for alcoholism among heavy drinkers in these different ethnic groups and regions of the world (Figure 12.2). Considerable variation was observed in the male/female ratio for heavy drinking, ranging from a low of 1.7 among American Indians to 6.3 in Puerto Rico. The high sex ratio of heavy drinking in Puerto Rico may be explained

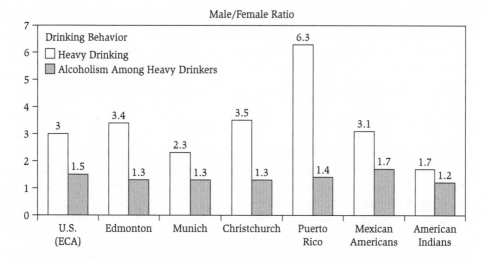

Figure 12.2. Sex Ratios for Heavy Drinkers and for Alcoholism Among Heavy Drinkers from Seven Regions

by societal values in which excessive drinking in women is strongly disapproved (Avilés-Roig, 1973). In this comparison, Mexican American immigrants were not disaggregated from the totality of Mexican Americans in Los Angeles. The data also showed that once the exposure variable was equalized by considering only those who drink "heavily," alcoholism rates by sex were more similar and more cross-culturally consistent, as evidenced by the lower and more constant sex ratios. The sex ratio in Puerto Rico, for example, was in the same range as at other sites. We interpret this set of findings to mean that cross-cultural differences in social disapproval of drinking by women have a major impact on alcoholism rates. Once the social stigma regarding "heavy" drinking has been overcome, the differences between men and women are more similar cross-culturally. However, these results need to be interpreted with caution. Even though uniformity of interview administration was achieved across the different cultures studied, this does not necessarily ensure that the same behaviors or symptoms are being measured, since the meaning ascribed to the items by respondents may systematically vary among cultures, as may willingness to reply candidly.

Differences across cultures are also observed regarding the severity of alcoholism in women versus men. Table 12.1 compares the mean number of symptoms by sex in three different cultures. As can be seen once more, while the mean number of symptoms in males is always higher than in females in all sites, in Puerto Rico, the gender difference is more dramatic, with women having a significantly lower number of alcohol symptoms compared to men. Multivariate regression analyses of the Puerto Rican alcoholic population, with

Table 12.1. Mean Number of Lifetime Alcohol Symptoms in Alcoholics, by Sex

Sex	St. Louis	Edmonton	Puerto Rico
Male	5.1	5.7	5.9
Female	4.6	5.1	4.2
Male/female ratio	1.1	1.1	1.4

the total number of symptoms as the dependent variable and age, sex, and education as independent variables, showed that alcoholic men tend to have more symptoms than alcoholic women. Thus, female alcoholism in Puerto Rico, as compared to other Western countries with an Anglo-Saxon tradition, appears to be significantly less common as well as less severe.

These cross-cultural data suggest that at least in two Latin American countries (Puerto Rico and Mexico), cultural mores prescribe strong social disapproval of alcohol use and misuse by women, which in turn may expose them less to the consequences of heavy drinking and to the risk of alcohol misuse or dependence. Various researchers have stressed the importance of interactions between gender and social roles in the etiology of psychological disorders. In this instance, we may speculate that an interaction between gender and social roles affects the vulnerability to excessive alcohol use and alcoholism. Thus, women and men have a different vulnerability or risk toward becoming alcoholics because of the way they are socialized. Men are expected to be at much higher risk of becoming alcoholic than women because the cultural mores are more permissive toward their use or misuse of alcohol. Women are at less risk or less vulnerable since cultural mores are more restrictive and condemn their misuse of alcohol. Cultural regulations of drinking prescribe not only how much may be drunk but also who may drink and under what circumstances. Ethnographic research has shown that in the traditional Hispanic culture, permissive norms for drinking in men and restrictive ones for women are predominant. Because of this, several investigators have hypothesized that Hispanic cultural norms protect women from the adverse consequences of excessive drinking (García, 1976; Caetano, 1983; Schaefer, 1982; White, 1982; Alcocer, 1982; Gomberg, 1982). It is hypothesized that the more traditional the Hispanic culture, the more this process of "cultural protection" will work. In both Mexico and Puerto Rico, traditional Hispanic family structures with their concomitant marked sex role differentiation still prevail (Bird and Canino, 1982). As a consequence, it is possible that the low prevalence of alcoholism and heavy drinking, as well as the low prevalence of negative consequences of excessive alcohol consumption, may be related to these cultural mores. This hypothesis nevertheless needs to be tested empirically.

Inasmuch as societal mores deviate from these traditional Hispanic values, one would expect an increase in alcohol consumption as well as in alcoholism rates among women. In Puerto Rico, for example, important changes in the traditional family structure and mores toward more liberal roles in the male–female relationship have been recently observed (Bird and Canino, 1982). We hypothesize that these changes in traditional roles will affect the "risk" for alcoholism in the near future for young generations of Puerto Rican women. In fact, data from the Puerto Rico epidemiologic study point toward this direction (Canino and others, 1987a). In this study, a trend was observed for sex differences to dissipate regarding alcohol misuse or dependence among women born in more recent decades. In addition, a trend was observed for diminished gender differences regarding the age of onset of first alcoholic symptom. These analyses should nevertheless be considered with caution since the number of alcoholic women in the Puerto Rico sample was small (lifetime prevalence rate of 2.0 percent).

Gilbert and Cervantes (1987), in their review of the literature of Mexican American adolescent drinking patterns, found no evidence that these girls were following in the abstinent footsteps of their mothers. In fact, Mexican American adolescents consistently appeared to have similar patterns of drug use compared to adolescents in the general U.S. population. Certainly there is a need for further research that examines the role that changes in cultural attitudes in younger generations may have in rates of alcohol consumption and alcoholism among Hispanic women.

ACCULTURATION AND THE RISK FOR ALCOHOLISM AMONG HISPANIC WOMEN

Data from a number of studies that examined the role of acculturation in drinking patterns among Hispanic women demonstrate the important role that cultural values have in diminishing or increasing the "risk" for alcoholism. Most of the studies consistently show that acculturation by Hispanic women to the U.S. culture is significantly related to an increase of alcohol consumption and to a greater risk for alcoholism. In the same 1984 national study of Hispanic Americans previously quoted, Caetano (1986) found that women who were 40 years of age and older, who were married, who had a job, who were born in the United States of U.S.-born parents, and who were highly acculturated had a particularly high rate of drinking once a week or more often, and drinking five or more drinks at a sitting at least once a week. When the relationship between "heavy" drinking and sociodemographic characteristics was examined with multivariate analysis (logistic regression), women who were highly acculturated were nine times more likely to be "heavy" drinkers than women in the low-acculturation group (Caetano, 1986). Acculturation was measured in this study with twelve items covering the respondents' ability to speak, read, and write English and Spanish, preference for media in English or Spanish, ethnicity of people with whom the respondent interacted the most, and a series of questions about values thought to be characteristic of the Hispanic culture.

Acculturation was also associated with attitudes toward drinking in various social settings. Hispanics who were high in acculturation were more liberal regarding drinking, especially drinking by women and by older people. Attitudes toward what is appropriate drinking across gender and age groups were more liberal among acculturated than nonacculturated Hispanics (Caetano, 1986).

In another study comparing Mexican Americans with Mexicans living in Mexico City, Caetano and Medina-Mora (1988) found that the rate of abstention among women born in Mexico was 61 percent and did not decline with number of years of life in the United States; very few of these women were highly acculturated to the United States. Acculturation was defined in the same way as in Caetano's previously stated study (Caetano, 1986). Almost all of those born in the United States were in the high-acculturation group, and the abstention rate was comparatively low (32 versus 61 percent).

As part of the Epidemiologic Catchment Area Study (ECA) of four U.S. communities, Burnam (1989) reported the prevalence rates of alcoholism and consumption patterns of Mexican Americans from Los Angeles. In this study, Burnam (1989) compared Mexican Americans born in the United States with those born in Mexico and found significant differences between both groups for rates of alcoholism and alcohol consumption by sex. Lifetime abstention rates by sex showed that immigrant Mexican American women abstained from drinking fifteen times more often than men. The pattern of abstention by sex for the native Mexican American was very different. In this group, women abstained from drinking only six times more frequently than men. Similarly, prevalence rates of alcoholism as measured by the DIS showed considerably higher rates of alcohol misuse or dependence for males than for females. The male/female ratio was significantly higher among immigrant Mexican Americans (25:0) compared to native Mexican Americans (4:1).

In an in-depth study of sixteen married Mexican American couples, Gilbert (1985) contrasted the drinking behavior in the traditional Mexican marriages, which emphasize sex-segregated activities, with those in the more acculturated marriages, where there were more liberal and sharing role functions. She found heavy drinking among men and little or no drinking among the women in the traditional marriages. In the acculturated marriages, the woman's assertiveness led to an increase in alcohol consumption by themselves as well as to a control of the spouse's excessive drinking. Interestingly, Corbett, Mora, and Ames (1991) found that drinking patterns among Mexican American women were similar to those of their spouses; if the husbands were drinkers, the wives were also drinkers.

Gilbert and Cervantes (1987) also compared the drinking patterns of Mexican American women of different generations. The results of this study indicated that although succeeding generations showed a movement out of the lowest frequency of drinking, Mexican American women from a third generation still did not equal those of U.S. women. Nevertheless, by the third generation, the drinking patterns of Mexican American women more closely resembled those of other U.S. women compared to those of women in Mexico (Gilbert, 1991).

The process of acculturation involves a change toward the host country's cultural values, habits, costume, and lifestyle, and this includes values toward drinking as well. U.S. family values tend to be more egalitarian and less restrictive regarding drinking behavior among women, and stress less sex role differentiation compared to Hispanic values. Thus, it is not surprising that whatever imputed protection Hispanic women have from developing an alcohol disorder seems to diminish with increased exposure to the Anglo American culture. Acculturation of Hispanic women to the U.S. culture appears to have a direct effect on their drinking behavior. It is nevertheless ironic that the traditional values of Hispanic society, which restrict women's individuation, their role in the labor force, and increase their risk for depressive disorders (Canino and others, 1987b), also protect them from alcohol disorders.

DIRECTIONS FOR FUTURE RESEARCH

This review of the literature has consistently pointed out that traditional Hispanic values seem to be related to high abstention rates and "light" drinking, as well as to low prevalence rates of alcoholism among different groups of Hispanic women. The findings seem to replicate whether they involve Hispanic women living in Mexico or Puerto Rico, or whether they are immigrants to the United States. However, although traditional Hispanic values seem to be protective against alcoholism in women, in general, the mechanisms involved in this "protective process" are generally unknown.

As Gilbert and Cervantes (1987) have pointed out, there is a need to operationalize and measure the alleged role attributes of the Hispanic culture and to systematically assess how these attributes are integrated to alcohol behavior in the different life cycles. There is a need to understand why such norms are still in effect among many Hispanic groups and why some women violate them while others do not.

Research also needs to address directly how changes in these role attributes, either through the process of acculturation in U.S. society or through the modernization or liberalization of sex roles in the Hispanic countries, are transformed to changes in drinking behavior among Hispanic women. What are the changes in the female/male roles that occur as a result of increased education, income, and exposure to U.S. culture that are related to increased levels of drinking and alcoholism among Hispanic women? Why is it that immigrant Mexican Americans and migrant Puerto Rican women exhibit drinking behavior patterns more traditional than the ones upheld by the women in their culture of origin? Is this exaggeration of cultural norms a result of a mechanism to protect their own cultural values in the face of the threat of losing them?

Until we are able to answer some of these questions, treatment and prevention of alcoholism among Hispanic women could be misguided. This type of in-depth research on the relationship of sociocultural values to drinking behavior can offer clues for the development of prevention strategies for younger Hispanic women, who seem to be at increased "risk" for higher levels of alcohol-related problems compared to their mothers. A simplistic approach to prevention would be to promote traditional values among young Hispanic women. However, the same traditional values that are protective against alcoholism also promote depression, inequality, and dependency in women. The in-depth analysis of these issues could probably provide clues for the promotion of healthy drinking attitudes, which are not necessarily accompanied by the negative consequences of the more traditional Hispanic values. There is no question that Hispanic values are related to the low prevalence of alcoholism and alcohol consumption among women. However, these extremely low prevalence rates could also be affected by the social stigma associated against women drinking, possibly producing a bias toward underreporting the behavior by women. All of the studies quoted in the literature rely on self-reports and thus are subject to this possible report bias. There is therefore a need to do studies that use other methods of ascertaining excessive alcohol use, such as laboratory tests and the use of other key informants.

Research is also needed to address the relationship between educational and income level and culture systematically. Since so many Hispanic women in the United States or in their countries of origin are impoverished, it is difficult to disentangle the effect of education and culture from their drinking behavior patterns (Canino, Burnam, and Caetano, 1992). We have observed that for immigrant Mexican American women from Los Angeles, an increase in education is associated with an increase in the prevalence rates of alcoholism. There is a need to test empirically whether this is the result of an interaction between education and acculturation. Most research among island Puerto Ricans and U.S. populations shows the opposite trend; that is, the risk for alcoholism is increased with lower educational levels (Canino and others, 1987a; Helzer, Burnam, and McEvoy, 1991). Caetano (1990) has warned researchers against simplistic models that rely on one major factor, such as acculturation stress or machismo, to explain drinking practices in the Hispanic culture. There is certainly a need to investigate how acculturation interacts with sex, age, and birthplace and to disentangle the complex ways in which this process affects drinking practices in Hispanic women. A systematic comparison of different Hispanic groups of different ages by acculturation levels and with women from their culture of origin could be informative in answering many of the unanswered questions that the research has left us.

References

Alcocer, A. M. "Alcohol Use And Abuse Among the Hispanic American Population." In *Alcohol and Health Monograph 4: Special Population Issues.* Rockville, Md.: Department of Health and Human Services, 1982.

American Psychiatric Association. *Diagnostic and Statistical Manual of Mental Disorders.* (3rd ed.) Washington, D.C.: American Psychiatric Association, 1983.

Avilés-Roig, C. A. "Aspectos socioculturales del alcoholismo en Puerto Rico." In E. Tongue, R. T. Lambo, and B. Blair (eds.), *Proceedings of the International Conference on Alcoholism and Drug Abuse.* San Juan, P.R.: ICAA Publication, 1973.

Babor, T. F. *Alcohol and Culture: Comparative Perspectives from Europe and America.* New York: New York Academy of Sciences, 1986.

Bird, H., and Canino, G. "The Puerto Rican Family: Cultural Factors and Family Intervention Strategies." *Journal of the American Academy of Psychoanalysis,* 1982, *10,* 257–268.

Burnam, A. "Prevalence of Alcohol Abuse and Dependence Among Mexican Americans and Non-Hispanic Whites in the Community." In D. L. Spigler, D. A. Tate, S. S. Aitken, and C. M. Christian (eds.), *Alcohol Use Among U.S. Ethnic Minorities.* Washington, D.C.: U.S. Government Printing Office, 1989.

Caetano, R. "Drinking Patterns and Alcohol Problems Among Hispanics in Northern California." *Dissertation Abstracts International* 44:08, 2389-B, 1983. (University Microfilms DA 8328811).

Caetano, R. "Self-Reported Intoxication Among Hispanics in Northern California." *Journal of Studies on Alcohol,* 1984, *45,* 349–354.

Caetano, R. "Drinking Patterns and Alcohol Problems in a National Sample of U.S. Hispanics." Paper presented at the National Institute on Alcohol Abuse and Alcoholism Conference, Epidemiology of Alcohol Use and Abuse Among U.S. Ethnic Minorities, Bethesda, Md., 1985.

Caetano, R. "Patterns and Problems of Drinking Among U.S. Hispanics." In *Report of the Secretary's Task Force on Black and Minority Health, Vol. VII: Chemical Dependency and Diabetes.* Washington, D.C.: U.S. Department of Health and Human Services, 1986.

Caetano, R. "Acculturation and Drinking Patterns Among U.S. Hispanics." *British Journal of Addiction,* 1987, *82,* 789–799.

Caetano, R. "Hispanic Drinking in the U.S.: Thinking in New Directions." *British Journal of Addiction,* 1990, *85,* 1231–1236.

Caetano, R., and Medina-Mora, M. E. "Acculturation and Drinking Among People of Mexican Descent in Mexico and the United States." *Journal of Studies on Alcohol,* 1988, *49*(5), 462–471.

Canino, G., Burnam, A., and Caetano, R. "The Prevalence of Alcohol Abuse and/or Dependence in Two Hispanic Communities." In J. Helzer and G. Canino (eds.), *Alcoholism in North America, Europe and Asia.* New York: Oxford University Press, 1992.

Canino, G., and others. "The Prevalence of Alcohol Abuse and/or Dependence in Puerto Rico." In M. Garrison and J. Arana (eds.), *Health and Behavior: Research Agenda for Hispanics.* Urbana: University of Illinois Press, 1987a.

Canino, G., and others. "Sex Differences and Depression in Puerto Rico." *Psychology of Women Quarterly,* 1987b, *2,* 443–459.

Corbett, K., Mora, J., and Ames, G. "Drinking Patterns and Drinking-Related Problems of Mexican American Husbands and Wives." *Journal of Studies on Alcohol,* 1991, *52*(3), 215–223.

García, C. S. *Magnitud del problema de alcoholismo en Puerto Rico.* Rio Piedras, P.R.: Universidad de Puerto Rico, 1976.

Gilbert, M. J. "Mexican Americans in California Cultural Variations in Attitudes and Behavior Related to Alcohol." In L. Bennet and L. Ames (eds.), *The American Experience with Alcohol: Contrasting Cultural Perspectives.* New York: Plenum Press, 1985.

Gilbert, M. J. "Acculturation and Changes in Drinking Patterns Among Mexican American Women: Implications for Prevention." *Alcohol Health & Research,* 1991, *15*(3), 234–238.

Gilbert, M. J., and Cervantes, R. C. "Patterns and Practices of Alcohol Use Among Mexican Americans: A Comprehensive Review." *Hispanic Journal of Behavioral Sciences,* 1986, *8,* 1–60.

Gilbert, M. J., and Cervantes, R. C. *Mexican Americans and Alcohol.* Los Angeles: University of California, 1987.

Gomberg, E.S.L. "Special Populations." In E. L. Gomberg, H. R. White, and J. A. Carpenter (eds.), *Alcohol, Science and Society Revisited.* Ann Arbor: University of Michigan Press, 1982.

Gordon, A. "The Cultural Context of Drinking and Indigenous Therapy for Alcohol Problems in Three Migrant Hispanic Cultures: An Ethnographic Report." *Journal of Studies on Alcohol,* 1981, *9,* 217–240.

Haberman, P. W., and Sheinberg, J. "Implicative Drinking Reported in a Household Survey." *Quarterly Journal of Studies on Alcohol,* 1967, *28,* 538–543.

Heath, D. "Historical and Cultural Factors Affecting Alcohol Availability and Consumption on Latin America." In *Legislative Approaches to Prevention of Alcohol-Related Problems: An Inter-American Workshop.* Washington, D.C., 1982.

Helzer, J., Burnam, A., and McEvoy, L. "Alcohol Abuse and Dependence." In L. Robins and D. Regier (eds.), *Psychiatric Disorders in America: The Epidemiologic Catchment Area Study.* New York: Free Press, 1991.

Helzer, J. E., and Canino, G. "Comparative Analysis of Alcoholism in Ten Cultural Regions." In J. Helzer and G. Canino (eds.), *Alcoholism in North America, Europe and Asia.* New York: Oxford University Press, 1992.

Helzer, J. E., and others. "Alcoholism: A Cross-National Comparison of Population Surveys with the Diagnostic Interview Schedule." In R. Rose and J. Barret (eds.), *Alcoholism: Origins and Outcome.* New York: Raven Press, 1988.

Holck, S. E., Warren, C., Smith, J., and Rochat, R. "Alcohol Consumption Among Mexican American and Anglo Women: Results of a Survey Along the U.S. Mexico Border." *Journal of Studies on Alcohol,* 1984, *45,* 149–153.

Johnson, P., and Gurin, G. "Negative Affect, Alcohol Expectancies and Alcohol Related Problems." *Addiction,* 1994, *89*(5), 581–586.

Page, J. B., Rio, L., Sweeney, L., and McKay, C. "Alcohol and Adaptation to Exile in Miami's Cuban Population." In L. Bennet and G. Ames (eds.), *The American Experience with Alcohol: Contrasting Cultural Perspectives.* New York: Plenum Press, 1985.

Robins, L. N., Helzer, J. E., Croughan, J., and Ratcliff, K. S. "The NIMH Diagnostic Interview Schedule: Its History, Characteristics, and Validity." *Archives of General Psychiatry,* 1981, *38,* 381–389.

Roizen, R. *Alcohol Dependence Symptoms in Cross-Cultural Perspectives: A Report of Findings from the World Health Organization Study of Community Response to Alcoholism.* Berkeley, Calif.: Alcohol Research Group, 1983.

Schaefer, J. M. "Ethnic and Racial Variations in Alcohol Use and Abuse." In *Alcohol and Health Monograph 4: Special Population Issues.* Rockville, Md.: Department of Health and Human Services, 1982.

Taylor, W. B. *Drinking, Homicide and Rebellion in Colonial Mexican Villages.* Stanford, Calif.: Stanford University Press, 1979.

White, H. R. "Sociological Theories of the Etiology of Alcoholism." In E. L. Gomberg, H. R. White, and J. A. Carpenter (eds.), *Alcohol, Science, and Society Revisited.* Ann Arbor: University of Michigan Press, 1982.

CHAPTER THIRTEEN

The Treatment of Alcohol Dependency Among Latinas

A Feminist, Cultural, and Community Perspective

Juana Mora

This chapter provides a comprehensive and informative overview of the subject of treating Latinas with alcohol problems and dependency. Although the literature cited is not current, the issues discussed remain pertinent and relevant. The cultural framework presented provides a culturally and linguistically responsive model for treatment and is worthy of consideration by those addressing the need.

Although a decade of research on Latino drinking patterns has revealed consistent evidence of increased alcohol use and abuse among some segments of the Chicana/Latina population (Caetano, 1985; Gilbert, 1987, 1991; Canino, 1994), there is a serious lack of research and information on effective treatment approaches and modalities for Latinas (Gilbert and Cervantes, 1988). The current state of knowledge on substance abuse treatment for Latinas is based on reports from treatment professionals and reviews of local and state treatment statistics (Gilbert and Cervantes, 1988; Woll, forthcoming; Mora and Gilbert, 1991). There are few empirical studies detailing the efficacy of various treatment approaches or modalities with this population. It is not known, for example, which forms of alcohol treatment are most effective or desirable for Latinas in general and for specific groups of Latinas, including Latina adolescents, Latina lesbians, and other Latinas who may be at risk for developing alcohol dependency problems.

There is currently not enough information available on the extent to which Latinas are at risk for developing alcohol dependency problems, which Latinas are most "at risk," or even the characteristics of Latinas in treatment. In fact, about the only information available is that Latinas are less represented in treatment programs than men (Gilbert and Cervantes, 1988) and face many barriers in securing adequate treatment (Beckman and Amaro, 1986). Latinas, for example, face a host of complicating factors and barriers to treatment, including stigma, fear of losing custody of children, lack of child care while in treatment, and language and financial barriers (U.S. Department of Health and Human Services, 1995).

The lack of systematic and empirical studies of treatment effectiveness with Latinas is partially due to the failure of traditional treatment programs to reach this population. Studies on substance abuse, like mental health research, have found that Latinas are less likely than other persons to seek treatment and less likely to complete treatment (Finn, 1994). Research on women has also found that women with a drinking problem may not initiate or continue treatment in a program that misunderstands or ignores important aspects of her life (McCrady and Raytek, 1993).

This chapter will explore the meaning of "culturally competent" and "gender-specific" programming for Latinas, address the impact of culture and gender on alcohol problems, and argue for the development of a theoretical framework for the treatment of alcohol abuse and dependency among Latinas based on feminist, cultural, and community perspectives.

CONCEPTS AND DEFINITIONS

Research on the treatment of alcohol and other drug abuse among women indicates that programs that incorporate and address the unique experiences and needs of women have best results and outcomes (McCrady and Raytek, 1993; U.S. Department of Health and Human Services, 1995). Because of this link between the understanding of the lives of women and positive treatment outcomes, it is important for treatment providers who serve Latina women to move beyond a basic cultural awareness and sensitivity and make serious efforts to become "competent" in the culture of the women in treatment. The concept of cultural sensitivity refers to an awareness and appreciation of one's own and other cultures (Orlandi, 1992). However, one can be "sensitive" but lack knowledge about the history, values, art, and music of another culture, and this lack of knowledge can be a barrier between the provider and the client. The concept of cultural competence refers to a set of cognitive, interpersonal skills, and deliberate actions that allow individuals to increase their understanding and appreciation of cultural differences (Orlandi, 1992; Gilbert, 1993). In this chapter, I argue that when working with Latina women, an important aspect of the "competence" providers must acquire to effectively work with this population is an understanding of the role of the Latina woman within traditional Latino culture and in contemporary U.S. society.

Traditionally, Latinas hold special but difficult roles in their families and communities. In Latino cultures, women are given special roles and are highly respected as the central figures in the extended family networks (Falicov, 1982). While this special cultural place gives women much prestige and cultural power, it is also a role that requires them to sacrifice their needs for the needs of others. In recent years, the traditional role of Latinas has gone through major modifications as a result of the large number of Latinas in the labor force and the influence of the women's movement (Padilla and Salgado de Snyder, 1995). Part of the change in the lives of Latina women is an apparent increase in alcohol use among some Latinas.

Because traditional treatment programs have not served Latinas well and this population is young and expected to grow, it is important to define and develop gender-specific and culturally competent alcohol treatment services and programs for Latinas (Beckman and Amaro, 1986; Hill, 1994; Woll, forthcoming; U.S. Department of Health and Human Services, 1995). Latinas, for example, represent 52 percent of the estimated 27 million Latinos living in the United States, and it is anticipated that by the year 2010, Latinas will represent nearly 11 percent of the total U.S. female population. It is also important to address the potential for alcohol problems in this populations because Latinos are young, with nearly half (48 percent) of the population being under the age of 24 (Herrell, 1993; U.S. Bureau of the Census, 1994).

Effective treatment programs for Latinas must include an understanding of the traditional role of women in Latino culture, the changing lives of Latina women in the United States, and the factors that contribute to the changes in their lives and how these play a role in the development of alcohol problems. An understanding of the dynamics of change, gender, and culture in the lives of Latina women will help counselors and others reduce the risk of alcohol dependency and support Latinas in their recovery.

This chapter will not address the efficacy of various treatment modalities, that is, residential versus outpatient. Instead, the focus will be on examining underlying and common themes related to the sociocultural context of alcohol use and abuse among Latinas and how these can be utilized to design culturally sensitive and competent programming.

Due to a lack of empirical data on effective alcohol treatment approaches for Latinas, the ideas expressed in this chapter are taken from and based on a variety of sources, including: (1) the Latino alcohol literature, (2) Chicana feminist literature, (3) women's alcohol literature, and (4) my experience as a consultant on a 1990–1993 national cross-site evaluation of Pregnant and Postpartum Women and Their Infants (PPWI) Demonstrations program funded by the Center for Substance Abuse Prevention.

CHICANA/LATINA HETEROGENEITY

It is difficult to articulate what "culturally competent" programming means for Latinas because there is great heterogeneity both across Latina groups and within specific groups. Among Mexican American women there are differences in values, language, and behaviors due to age, class, education, and generational status. Some Mexican American women have very recently immigrated to the United States; others are members of families who have lived in the United States for many generations. Generally, recently immigrated Latinas are less educated, work in lower-paying jobs, and are primarily Spanish speaking. Later-generation or U.S.-born Latinas are more likely to be English speaking or bilingual and have various levels of education (Buriel, 1993).

The major Latino groups in the United States are Mexican Americans, Puerto Ricans, Cubans, and Central Americans. Each group has a unique history and special relationship with the larger society. Each group has a sense of its own identity but shares common linguistic, religious, and family characteristics recognized across groups as Latino.

Mexican Americans are the largest of the Latino groups in the United States, representing more than half of all Latinos. The majority of Mexican Americans live in the South and midwestern parts of the United States. The next largest group are Puerto Ricans, who live primarily in or near the New York area, followed by Cubans, who live primarily in the city of Miami, Florida.

In some regions, there is a growing number of Central American immigrants and other Latin American immigrants. In New York City, Dominican and Colombian immigrants are prominent, and in Los Angeles there are large communities of Guatemalan, Salvadoran, and Nicaraguan immigrants.

DIVERSITY AMONG LATINAS: IMPLICATIONS FOR TREATMENT

The diversity in language, values, and backgrounds encountered across and within Latina groups is sometimes perceived as an obstacle to developing culturally competent and effective treatment programs for Latinas. However, if the diversity in cultures and backgrounds is respected and validated and if common themes, values, and experiences are identified and utilized in treatment, this approach can be a powerful method for helping Latinas address their common problems with alcohol. Validating cultural background can be a powerful tool in recovery. Mental health and cross-cultural counseling literature identifies cultural heritage and pride as positive tools for building self-esteem in culturally different clients (Sue, 1981). As program staff develop an understanding of the uniqueness in the cultural groups encountered in their service area, they can utilize this knowledge to build self-esteem and empower Latinas in treatment.

Two important common experiences across Latina groups that can be exploited for developing self-esteem and empowerment among Latina women in treatment is their similar gender socialization and acculturation experiences. Culturally, most Latinas grow up in patriarchal and authoritarian family environments that are reinforced and influenced by the Catholic church. In these settings, women are expected to nurture and care for others and to aspire to marriage and motherhood (Falicov, 1982; Williams, 1990). The significance for treatment is that although acculturated Latinas may reject these cultural expectations, the messages received in early childhood about the "proper" role of a "señorita" may remain very much a part of their cultural and personal identity. Stress and conflict associated with the integration of traditional cultural expectations with new cultural values, roles, and expectations may form part of the basis for alcohol abuse and should be explored in the treatment and recovery process.

Another common experience is that Latinas living in the United States must adapt and adjust to new cultural surroundings as they strive to retain their ethnic identity (Blea, 1992). This process can be very difficult and stressful for some Latinas, particularly younger women. There is some evidence that cultural conflict contributes to substance abuse among Latina adolescents (Szapocznik and Kurtines, 1989; Vega, 1995). It is possible that at least among some Latinas, conflicts and questions regarding cultural identity, acculturation pressures, and perceived or real discrimination form part of the context for alcohol abuse and should also be incorporated into the treatment and recovery process.

Program staff should strive to understand the commonalities across Latina groups for building trust and support but should also acknowledge important differences. There are, for example, differences across all groups associated with generational status. Newly arrived or recent immigrant Latinas have unique language, employment, educational, and psychological needs. These women are more likely to experience grief and loss associated with immigration and stress related to the lack of language and employment skills (Vargas-Willis and Cervantes, 1987; Vega, 1995). Later-generation or U.S.-born Latinas have different language, education, employment, and psychological needs. These women are more likely to be bilingual or English dominant and thus may experience less strain associated with lack of language skills, but they may be more likely to experience other types of stressors associated with the process of adaptation to new cultural values and behaviors (Buriel, 1993). These differences contribute to a different set of vulnerabilities and problems associated with the onset of alcohol problems for these women.

ALCOHOL USE AMONG LATINAS: WOMEN AT RISK

Several researchers have suggested, based on survey research studies, that some Latinas may be at risk for developing alcohol dependency and related problems (Gilbert, 1991; Roth, 1991; Ames and Mora, 1988; Canino, 1994). Epidemiological studies among Latinos have found differences in drinking patterns across Latino groups and by gender. For example, a 1984 national survey of drinking patterns among Latinos in the United States found that there is a higher proportion of Mexican American men who drink "heavily," defined as drinking five or more drinks at a sitting at least once a week or more often, followed by Puerto Rican and other Latino and Cuban men (Caetano, 1985). The same survey found that although the majority of Latina women in the United States have higher abstention rates than U.S. women (47 percent versus 36 percent), Mexican American women report more "heavy" drinking (14 percent) than Cuban (7 percent) or Puerto Rican (5 percent) women (Caetano, 1985).

Abstention rates were highest among Mexican American women (46 percent) and lowest for Puerto Rican women (33 percent). The abstention rate for Cuban women was higher than Puerto Rican women (42 percent) and similar to Mexican American women. In addition, Cuban women exhibited the most moderate drinking patterns among the three groups.

It seems paradoxical that Mexican American women have the highest rates of "heavy" drinking and also have high rates of abstention from drinking. This apparent paradox most likely reflects the large proportion of Mexican immigrant women in the population who are primarily abstainers compared to a smaller proportion of Mexican American women who are "heavy" drinkers.

High abstention rates among Latinas reflect the strict cultural sanctions against female drinking that are common in most Latin American cultures (Bacon, 1976). Drinking is viewed as primarily a male activity to be shared with other men. In the United States, this pattern is maintained, particularly in immigrant families, where drinking is viewed as an activity to be shared by the men after work or on weekends. Traditionally, Chicanas and other Latinas report less and less frequent drinking compared to men (Caetano, 1985) and are more likely to prefer mixed drinks than beer or wine (Trotter, 1985; Munch and others, 1981). Latinas, particularly immigrant women, tend to drink lightly, infrequently and primarily at family gatherings and holidays (Gilbert, 1987; Canino, 1994).

Research indicates that a larger proportion of Latina women abstain from drinking alcohol compared to other women in the U.S. population. This means that Latina women, as they immigrate to the United States, generally maintain their cultural norms and values regarding the proper role of women as occasional or nondrinkers. However, research also indicates that a small proportion of subsequent generations of Latina women, particularly Mexican American and Puerto Rican women, are beginning to drink alcohol in heavier quantities compared to immigrant women in their communities (Gilbert, 1987).

The important questions for treatment are: (1) To what extent are some of these women who are increasing their alcohol intake at risk for developing alcohol dependency? (2) Who are the Latina women who are most at risk and most likely to require treatment? (3) What are the factors that contribute to the increased risk, and how can treatment programs help the women at greatest risk? The following sections will explore some of these questions in more detail.

ACCULTURATION AND ALCOHOL USE

Most studies of alcohol use among Chicanas and Latinas indicate that acculturation to U.S. culture is related to an increase in the quantity and frequency of alcohol use. In the first national survey of alcohol use among Latinos in the United States, Caetano (1985) found that U.S.-born and more highly acculturated women, particularly Mexican American women, had higher rates of "heavy" drinking (14 percent).

Acculturation into U.S. culture and society, more than any other factor, appears to have a direct effect on changes in drinking behaviors on Latinas. Acculturation theory, as it relates to modifications in alcohol use, proposes that over time, the drinking patterns, norms, and behaviors of an immigrant population will look more like the patterns of the new culture than the culture of origin (Markides, Krause, and Mendes de Leon, 1988; Keefe and Padilla, 1987).

The degree to which Latinas acculturate to U.S. norms is usually influenced by the age of immigration to the United States, degree of exposure to the new culture, individual willingness to explore new environments, and self-confidence (Negy and Woods, 1992; Keefe and Padilla, 1987). Thus, degree and level of acculturation is highly variable and differs by individual experience.

For Latinas, a major acculturating force that has had an impact on gender roles, family dynamics, and alcohol use is the large number of Latinas employed outside the home (Zavella, 1987; Williams, 1990; Gilbert, 1991). Latina scholars argue that it is within the context of the workplace where traditional Latinas gain access to new sources of knowledge, information, and personal and economic power (Williams, 1990; Zavella, 1987). Working outside the home can thus form a major and important transformational experience for traditional Latina women. These changes associated with employment and being born or raised in the United States seem particularly important in lowering abstention and increasing rates of heavier drinking among Latina women. Holck, Warren, Smith, and Rochat (1984), for example, found a link between education and greater alcohol consumption among Mexican American women in Texas. Burnam (1989) also reported higher levels of alcohol abuse and dependency among more highly educated Mexican American women in Los Angeles. However, higher levels of consumption are also found among younger, acculturated inner-city Latinas (Gilbert, 1989; Beauvais and others, 1996).

Although increased alcohol use seems to be linked to education, acculturation is probably a stronger indicator of increased use among both highly educated and employed Latinas and younger, inner-city Latinas. In fact, there is increasing evidence that younger generations of Mexican American female adolescents are drinking more like their male counterparts or women in the general population than like their immigrant mothers (Gilbert, 1991). This has also been found among younger generations of Puerto Rican women, who have rates of alcohol consumption similar to their male counterparts and show few differences between themselves and young men in terms of the onset of the first alcoholic symptom (Canino and others, 1987).

If in fact employment and acculturation play key roles in the increased use of alcohol among some Latinas, what are the changes in the lives of Latinas that occur as a result of employment and acculturation that are related to increased alcohol use? And what are the implications for treatment?

LATINAS: CONTEMPORARY LIFESTYLES AND CHANGES IN GENDER ROLE

Several researchers have proposed that employment outside the home and changes in traditional gender roles increase the risk of alcohol dependency among Latinas (Canino, 1994; Gilbert, 1987; Corbett, Mora, and Ames, 1991). Several important questions for treatment are: (1) What are the changes in traditional female roles that influence changes in drinking behaviors, (2) how do employment and education opportunities affect drinking behavior, and (3) how can treatment providers make sense of these changes in order to reduce the risk and support women in the process of change and recovery?

Employment for Latinas, as for all other women in American society, creates some conflict and role transformation. For the Latina who is socialized within a traditional family structure that requires strict sex role differentiation, there are numerous stressors related to sex role changes and accommodations that are part of working outside the home (Vargas-Willis and Cervantes, 1987; Blea, 1992; Williams, 1990). Increasing employment among Latinas who would otherwise be involved in child rearing and other family obligations has significant personal and social implications. Working women have higher levels of social support, in part because they have income and are more likely to drive, but they may also experience rejection and resistance from spouses, children, or other family members (Williams, 1990; Blea, 1992; Zavella, 1987). Kelly and Garcia (1989), for example, compared employed Mexican immigrant women in Los Angeles and Cuban immigrant women in Miami and found that working was a difficult experience that challenged them to continually negotiate and justify their actions to other members of the family.

The prevailing view about employment and women's drinking through the 1970s was that employment outside the home has negative effects on women's mental health and drinking behavior, particularly when combined with marital or family roles. Explanations for the increased drinking associated with employment or with multiple roles include stress-related interpretations of role conflict as well as environmental explanations involving increased opportunities and more permissive drinking norms outside the home (McCrady and Raytek, 1993).

For Latinas, both stress and environmental explanations for alcohol abuse are possible. For example, acculturation stress and conflicts about new roles and expectations and the inability to meet these may form part of the onset and development of alcohol abuse among some Latinas. Other research has found that increased use of alcohol among some Latinas is due to environmental forces, including new opportunities to drink, greater exposure to public environments for drinking, and increased income (Gilbert, 1991; Mora, forthcoming). However, changes in drinking behavior among Latinas cannot be attributed entirely to employment trends or changes in gender roles. These demographic and social changes are very complex and are part of larger social, economic, and cultural forces impacting Latinas.

The current research literature does not provide sufficient information about how Chicana and Latina women balance two cultures, enter new careers, break old traditions, and refashion new identities and how these changes affect drinking behavior. We do know that the status and role of Latinas in the United States has been undergoing a process of change for several decades. Latinas are now not only more likely to work outside the home, but they are having fewer children, pursuing higher education, and working in the arts, business, medicine, and politics (Blea, 1992; Williams, 1990). These changes are not necessarily negative, and for many Latinas, these experiences constitute positive new experiences in their lives. In addition, we cannot disregard the fact that alcohol dependency in women is also related to individual risk factors, including family background, childhood sexual abuse, low self-esteem, and depression (McCrady and Raytek, 1993).

In a discussion of gender role conflict and drinking behavior, Hunter (1990) concluded that the intricate relationship between the women's movement and changes in women's roles to drinking behavior among women are complex, and although it may be more acceptable for women to drink in public, drinking excessively is still less acceptable for women than for men. In fact, there is some indication that rates of drinking and heavier drinking among employed women vary considerably by the type of employment (professional/managerial versus blue collar), suggesting that there is not a single, simple effect of employment per se. For example, Gilbert (1991) and Mora (forthcoming), in a study of nearly three hundred Latinas in Los Angeles, found that increased alcohol consumption was encountered among professional Latinas and not among blue-collar women.

It is too simplistic and problematic to suggest that the loss of traditional female roles leads to the development of drinking problems among women and consequently that the treatment and solution would be to help women accept traditional female gender roles. Feminist scholars suggest that it is in fact the lack of access to power within traditional families, including the power of choice and economic decision making, that causes feelings of powerlessness and a desire to relieve the strain by using or abusing alcohol (Bepko and Krestan, 1985). Beckman and Amaro (1984), for example, reported that alcoholic women are more likely to report drinking or feeling like drinking than are men when they feel powerless and inadequate.

If we frame alcohol problems among Latinas in a feminist and cultural perspective, the treatment of alcohol problems should not necessarily reinforce traditional and possibly oppressive cultural patterns for Latinas. Instead, treatment services and programs should be structured to support and empower Latinas to pursue new roles and make new choices, free of alcohol, guilt, and stigma.

DIVERSITY AND CHANGE: TREATMENT IMPLICATIONS

The treatment implications of diversity and change in the Latina population are that in order for services to be fully competent and effective, they must move beyond simple notions of cultural sensitivity. Effective and competent programs must incorporate a realistic understanding of the contemporary cultural life of Latina women and the complex interaction between traditional culture, change, and alcohol problems among Latina women.

Regardless of the modality utilized (inpatient versus outpatient, for example), the philosophical framework of a culturally competent program should be based on a complete understanding of the unique cultural and historical legacies of each Latina population served, of the traditional cultural expectations and changing lifestyles and roles of Latina women, and how all of these interact with individual and family factors in the development of alcohol problems for each woman in treatment. Programs can avoid "ineffective" approaches and strategies by hiring bilingual and bicultural and recovering female staff who understand the traditional and ideal expectations of Latinas, the realities of contemporary Latina lifestyles, and alcoholism.

The environment of culturally competent programs should be supportive, nonjudgmental, and empowering places where Latinas can find relief from stigma and guilt, support for their choices from other women like themselves, and understanding and insight into their own behaviors, education and job training, child care and parenting education, and family involvement in their treatment and recovery.

The role of culturally competent alcohol treatment programs for Latinas should be to lessen the risk of alcohol problems associated with changes in gender roles and lifestyles, reduce cultural and community stigma associated with female alcoholism, and empower Latinas to live better lives.

References

Aguirre-Molina, M. "Issues for Latinas: Puerto Rican Women." In P. Roth (ed.), *Alcohol and Drugs Are Women's Issues.* Metuchen, N.J.: Scarecrow Press, 1991.

Ames, G., and Mora, J. "Alcohol Problem Prevention in Mexican American Populations." In M. J. Gilbert (ed.), *Alcohol Consumption Among Mexicans and Mexican Americans: A Binational Perspective.* Los Angeles: Spanish Speaking Mental Health Research Center, University of California, 1988.

Bacon, M. K. "Cross Cultural Studies of Drinking: Integrated Drinking and Sex Differences in the Use of Alcoholic Beverages." In M. W. Everett, J. O. Waddell, and D. B. Heath (eds.), *Cross-Cultural Approaches to the Study of Alcohol.* The Hague: Mouton, 1976.

Beauvais, F., and others. "Drug Use, Violence and Victimization Among White American, Mexican American, and American Indian Drop-Outs: Students with Academic Problems and Students in Good Standing." *Journal of Counseling Psychology,* 1996, *43*(3), 292–299.

Beckman, L. J., and Amaro, H. "Patterns of Women's Use of Alcohol Treatment Agencies." In S. Wilsnack and L. Beckman (eds.), *Alcohol Problems in Women.* New York: Guilford Press, 1984.

Beckman, L. J., and Amaro, H. "Personal and Social Difficulties Faced by Women and Men Entering Alcoholism Treatment." *Journal of Studies on Alcohol,* 1986, *47*(2), 135–145.

Bepko, C., and Krestan, J. *The Responsibility Trap: A Blueprint for Treating the Alcoholic Family.* New York: The Free Press, 1985.

Blea, I. *La Chicana and the Intersection of Race, Class, and Gender.* Westport, Conn.: Praeger, 1992.

Buriel, R. "Childrearing Orientations in Mexican American Families: The Influence of Generation and Sociocultural Factors." *Journal of Marriage and the Family,* 1993, *55,* 987–1000.

Burnam, A. "Prevalence of Alcohol Abuse and Dependence Among Mexican Americans and Non-Hispanic Whites in the Community." In D. L. Spigler, S. S. Tate, S. Aitken, and C. Christian (eds.), *Alcohol Use Among U.S. Ethnic Minorities.* Washington, D.C.: U.S. Government Printing Office, 1989.

Caetano, R. "Drinking Patterns and Alcohol Problems in a National Sample of U.S. Hispanics." In D. L. Spigler, S. S. Tate, S. Aitken, and C. Christian (eds.), *Alcohol Use Among U.S. Ethnic Minorities.* Washington, D.C.: U.S. Government Printing House, 1985.

Canino, G. "Alcohol Use and Misuse Among Hispanic Women: Selected Factors, Processes and Studies." *International Journal of the Addictions,* 1994, *29*(9), 1083–1099.

Canino, G., and others. "The Prevalence of Alcohol Abuse and/or Dependence in Puerto Rico." In M. Garrison and J. Arana (eds.), *Health and Behavior: Research Agenda for Hispanics.* Urbana: University of Illinois Press, 1987.

Corbett, K., Mora, J., and Ames, G. "Drinking Patterns and Drinking Related Problems of Mexican American Husbands and Wives." *Journal of Studies on Alcohol,* 1991, *52*(3), 215–233.

Falicov, C. J. "Mexican Families." In M. McGoldrick, J. K. Pearce, and J. Girodano (eds.), *Ethnicity and Family Therapy.* New York: Guilford Press, 1982.

Fernandez-Kelly, M. P., and Garcia, A. "Informalization at the Core: Hispanic Women, Homework, and the Advanced Capitalist State." In A. Portes, M. Castells, and L. Benton (eds.), *The Informal Economy* (pp. 247–263). Baltimore: Johns Hopkins University Press, 1989.

Finn, P. "Addressing the Needs of Cultural Minorities in Drug Treatment." *Journal of Substance Abuse Treatment,* 1994, *11,* 4.

Gilbert, M. J. "Alcohol Consumption Patterns in Immigrant and Later Generation Mexican American Women." *Hispanic Journal of the Behavioral Sciences,* 1987, *9*(3), 299–313.

Gilbert, M. J. "Current Information on Drinking Behavior Among Hispanic Youth." In R. Wright Jr. and T. D. Watts (eds.), *Alcohol Problems of Minority Youth in America.* New York: Edwin Mellon Press, 1989.

Gilbert, M. J. "Acculturation and Changes in Drinking Patterns Among Mexican American Women: Implications for Prevention." *Alcohol Health and Research World,* 1991, *15*(3), 234–238.

Gilbert, M. J. "Anthropology in a Multidisciplinary Field: Substance Abuse." *Social Science and Medicine,* 1993, *37,* 1–3.

Gilbert, M. J., and Cervantes, R. "Alcohol Treatment for Mexican Americans: A Review of Utilization Patterns and Therapeutic Approaches." In M. J. Gilbert (ed.), *Alcohol Consumption Among Mexicans and Mexican Americans: A Binational Perspective.* Los Angeles: Spanish Speaking Mental Health Research Center, University of California, 1988.

Herrell, I. C. *Health Care Issues Affecting Hispanic Women, Infants, and Children.* Washington, D.C.: U.S. Department of Health and Human Services, Health Resources and Services Administration, 1993.

Hill, S. Y. *Mental and Physical Health Consequences of Alcohol Use in Women.* Pittsburgh, Pa.: Department of Psychiatry, University of Pittsburgh School of Medicine, 1994.

Holck, S. E., Warren, C. W., Smith, J. C., and Rochat, R. W. "Alcohol Consumption Among Mexican American and Anglo Women: Results of a Survey Along the U.S. Mexico Border." *Journal of Studies on Alcohol,* 1984, *45*(2), 149–154.

Hunter, J. (1990) "Violence Against Lesbian and Gay Male Youths." *Journal of Interpersonal Violence,* 1990, *5*(3), 295–300.

Keefe, F. E., and Padilla, A. M. *Chicano Ethnicity.* Albuquerque: University of New Mexico Press, 1987.

Markides, K., Krause, N., and Mendes de Leon, C. "Acculturation and Alcohol Consumption Among Mexican Americans: A Three-Generational Study." *American Journal of Public Health,* 1988, *9,* 1178–1181.

McCrady, B., and Raytek, H. "Women and Substance Abuse: Treatment Modalities and Outcomes." In E. S. Lisansky-Gomberg and T. D. Nirenberg (eds.), *Women and Substance Abuse.* Norwood, N.J.: Ablex, 1993.

Mora, J. *Learning to Drink: Early Drinking Experiences of Chicana and Mexicana Women.* University of California, Davis, forthcoming.

Mora, J., and Gilbert, M. J. "Issues for Latinas: Mexican American Women." In P. Roth (ed.), *Alcohol and Drugs Are Women's Issues.* Metuchen, N.J.: Scarecrow Press, 1991.

Munch, N., and others. "How Americans Say They Drink: Preliminary Data from Two Recent National Surveys." *Current Studies in Alcoholism*, 1981, *8*, 233–251.

Negy, C., and Woods, D. J. "The Importance of Acculturation in Understanding Research with Hispanic-Americans." *Hispanic Journal of Behavioral Sciences*, 1992, *14*(2), 224–247.

Orlandi, M. A. *Cultural Competence for Evaluators: A Guide for Alcohol and Other Drug Abuse Prevention Practitioners Working with Ethnic/Racial Communities.* Washington, D.C.: U.S. Department of Health and Human Services, Organization for Safety and Asepsis Procedures, 1992.

Padilla, A. M., and Salgado de Snyder, N. V. "Hispanics: What the Culturally Informed Evaluator Needs to Know." In M. A. Orlandi, R. Weston, and L. G. Epstein (eds.), *Cultural Competency for Evaluators: A Guide for Alcohol and Other Drug Abuse Prevention Practitioners Working with Ethnic/Racial Communities.* Rockville, Md.: Office of Substance Abuse Prevention, 1995.

Roth, P. "Introduction." In P. Roth (ed.), *Alcohol and Drugs Are Women's Issues.* Metuchen, N.J.: Scarecrow Press, 1991.

Sue, D. *Counseling the Culturally Different: Theory and Practice.* New York: Wiley, 1981.

Szapocznik, J., and Kurtines, W. M. *Breakthroughs in Family Therapy with Drug Abusing and Problem Youth.* New York: Springer, 1989.

Trotter, R. "Mexican Americans in South Texas: Differing Lifestyles and Alcohol." In L. Bennett and G. Ames (eds.), *The American Experience with Alcohol: Contrasting Cultural Perspectives.* New York: Plenum Press, 1985.

U.S. Bureau of the Census. *The Nation's Hispanic Population-1994, Statistical Brief.* Washington, D.C.: U.S. Department of Commerce, 1994.

U.S. Department of Health and Human Services. *White Paper: Effectiveness of Substance Abuse Treatment.* Washington, D.C.: U.S. Department of Health and Human Services, 1995.

Vargas-Willis, G., and Cervantes, R. "Consideration of Psychosocial Stress in the Treatment of the Latina Immigrant." *Hispanic Journal of Behavioral Sciences*, 1987, *9*(3), 315–329.

Vega, W. A. "The Study of Latino Families: A Point of Departure." In R. E. Zambrana (ed.), *Understanding Latino Families: Scholarship, Policy, and Practice.* Thousand Oaks, Calif.: Sage, 1995.

Williams, N. *The Mexican American Family: Tradition and Change.* Dix Hills, N.Y.: General Hall Press, 1990.

Woll, C. "What Difference Does Culture Make? Providing Treatment to Women Different from You." In B. Underhill (ed.), *Chemical Dependency: Women at Risk.* New York: Haworth Press, forthcoming.

Zavella, P. *Women's Work and Chicano Families: Cannery Workers of the Santa Clara Valley.* Ithaca, N.Y.: Cornell University Press, 1987.

CHAPTER FOURTEEN

Tobacco Use Among Multiethnic Latino Populations

Jon F. Kerner
Nancy Breen
Mariella C. Tefft
Joscelyn Silsby

*Because the focus of this chapter is on New York City Latinos, it provides one
of the few and better assessments of tobacco use among subgroups of Latinas
that are rarely studied: Colombian, Dominican, Ecuadorian, and Puerto
Rican. The authors offer important insights into the role of acculturation
on tobacco use and demonstrate subgroup variation and the critical
importance of disaggregating data.*

Effective health promotion programs, particularly those aimed at smoking cessation and prevention, require careful investigation into possible cultural and societal factors influencing predictors and barriers to preventive health behavior (Edwards and MacMillan, 1990). These data are largely absent with respect to many of the immigrant populations currently living in the United States and whose populations have grown significantly from 1980 through the 1990s (U.S. Bureau of the Census, 1991). The health beliefs, values, and practices of these groups may differ not only from the majority white, middle-class populations, but also within ethnic groups.

Tobacco use is the single most preventable cause of death and disease in the United States, with cigarette smoking accounting for approximately 434,000 deaths annually ("CDC Smoking-Attributable Mortality," 1991). Although it is

From the Cancer Prevention and Control Program, Vincent T. Lombardi Cancer Center,
Georgetown University, Washington, D.C. (J.F.K., M.C.T., J.S.); and the Applied Research
Branch, Division of Cancer Prevention and Control, National Cancer Institute. This research
was supported by grant R01 CA 53083 from the National Cancer Institute. The authors wish to
acknowledge the expert programming assistance of Todd Gibson, IMS, and Alex Cheng from the
NCI; and the constructive critiques of the manuscript offered by Kathryn Taylor, Ph.D., and Ann
O'Malley, M.D., M.P.H., from Georgetown University Medical Center.

widely known that smoking initiation, prevalence, and consumption vary according to ethnicity ("CDC Cigarette Smoking," 1992; Gritz and others, 1989; DeMoor and others, 1989; Martin, Cummings, and Coates, 1990; Rogers and Crank, 1998), occupation (Marcus, Shopland, Crane, and Lynn, 1989), education (Escobedo and others, 1990; Wagenknecth and others, 1990), age (Escobedo and others, 1990; Markides, Coreil, and Ray, 1987), and gender (Fiore and others, 1989; Marin, Pérez-Stable, and Marin, 1989), studies characterizing cigarette smoking behavior among nationally defined racial/ethnic groups (for example, black, Hispanic) have rarely examined the extent or importance of cultural variation within and among ethnic groups ("CDC Cigarette Smoking," 1992). For example, while a number of studies have shown that Hispanics have lower cigarette smoking prevalence rates than whites or African Americans (Rogers and Crank, 1998; Marcus, Shopland, Crane, and Lynn, 1989; Humble, Samet, Pathak, and Skipper, 1985), few studies have delineated the cultural predictors of smoking behavior in this population, and even fewer have examined differences among the many distinct groups that comprise the broadly defined category of "Hispanic."

A number of studies have suggested that acculturation to U.S. mainstream culture may influence cigarette smoking and initiation. However, acculturation's total effect remains somewhat unclear, as studies have revealed variable findings due in part to the different populations being studied, the different measures of acculturation used, and different methods of interviewing Spanish-speaking respondents. Studies in the Southwest, using data from the 1982–1984 Hispanic HANES, showed there were more female smokers identified in the highly acculturated versus less acculturated group, but found no consistent relationship among men (Haynes, Cohen, Harvey, and McMillen, 1990). Marin, Pérez-Stable, and Marin (1989) found that cigarette smoking prevalence rates were higher among less acculturated males (37.5 percent versus 26.7 percent) and among more acculturated females (22.6 percent versus 13.6 percent), and that regardless of gender, more acculturated individuals smoked a greater number of cigarettes per day (Marin, Pérez-Stable, and Marin, 1989). In contrast, a study among older Mexican Americans and their relatives showed that acculturation was not at all related to smoking prevalence (Markides, Coreil, and Ray, 1987). This suggests that smoking behavior among Hispanics may vary by country of origin.

In national surveys examining prevalence and predictors of cigarette smoking behavior, including the National Health Interview Survey (NHIS) and the Current Population Survey (CPS), the Latino populations sampled usually focus on the Mexican American populations in the southwestern United States (Rogers and Crank, 1998; Markides, Coreil, and Ray, 1987; Lee and Markides, 1991; National Center for Health Statistics, 1985), Puerto Ricans in the Northeast

(National Center for Health Statistics, 1985), and Cubans in Florida (National Center for Health Statistics, 1985). While these are the largest Latino populations nationally, many smaller Central and South American Latino populations are aggregated and cannot be analyzed separately because of sample size constraints, although in some parts of the United States, these are among the fastest-growing groups of Latinos (U.S. Bureau of the Census, 1996). Moreover, these national survey data are also limited methodologically. For example, the NHIS and the CPS do not exclusively use bilingual interviewers for all their Hispanic interviews and thus do not routinely offer Hispanic respondents the opportunity to choose to complete the interview in Spanish or English. Instead, untrained intermediaries from the family or neighborhood of the respondent often are used to "help" Spanish-speaking respondents interviewed by non-Spanish speakers (personal communication, U.S. Census staff, May 1995).

Special surveys of Hispanics have been conducted in San Francisco, Texas, and New Mexico (Marin, Pérez-Stable, and Marin, 1989; Humble, Samet, Pathak, and Skipper, 1985; Lee and Markides, 1991). Few of these studies, however, have examined the health status of Caribbean or Central or South American Latinos living in the eastern half of the United States. In a review of epidemiological information on Latinos in New York City, Thiel de Bocanegra, Gany, and Fruchter (1993) found that most of the available data are from Puerto Ricans, although New York's Latino population is becoming increasingly diverse to include Hispanics from the Dominican Republic, Colombia, Ecuador, Honduras, El Salvador, and Peru.

According to the 1990 census, over half of New York City's Latinos are not Puerto Rican, and some groups will soon outnumber Puerto Ricans if demographic trends continue. The increasing ethnic diversity among Hispanics in New York City (and other urban areas) creates challenges for health care providers and health promotion program planners who do not have access to population-specific data. While the Centers for Disease Control and Prevention (CDC) survey many health behaviors through state health departments on an annual basis, in many states the samples of Hispanics and other minority groups who are interviewed are so small that analyses within groups are impossible.

Thus, national and state survey data need to be complemented with local data, which may not be adequately sampled on a nationwide or statewide basis. This could be accomplished, for example, by regularly oversampling specific ethnic/racial groups in different years in national and state surveys (for example, NHIS, CPS, BRFSS). In this fashion, ethnic group diversity could be periodically captured (for example, every five years) within the major ethnic/racial groupings without the expense of oversampling all groups within the same year.

In this study, we examine self-reported cigarette smoking behavior from a 1992 telephone survey of New York City Puerto Rican, Dominican, Colombian, and Ecuadorian Hispanics and compare them to a sample of New York City Hispanics from the Tobacco Use Supplement to the 1992–1993 Current Population Survey. Descriptive statistics of population characteristics and cigarette smoking behavior are presented, as well as the results of logistic regression models for predicting cigarette smoking in both survey samples. These data assess the magnitude and significance of ethnic group differences in smoking behaviors in relation to acculturation, age, sex, and socioeconomic status (SES), and suggest different strategies for developing and evaluating interventions designed to reduce smoking prevalence among adult Hispanics. The purposes of comparing the findings from the two different survey samples are to (1) examine how different survey methodologies may contribute to convergent and divergent results and (2) explore the implications of divergent results with respect to the interpretation and external validity of Latin American health behavior survey findings.

METHODS

The New York City data were collected from May to October 1992 as part of a National Cancer Institute–funded survey of cancer control needs in three black and four Hispanic multiethnic populations (O'Malley and others, 1997; Taylor, Kerner, Gold, and Mandelblatt, 1997). The data on New York State Hispanics were collected in September 1992, January 1993, and May 1993 as part of the Tobacco Use Supplement to the 1992–1993 CPS. Where appropriate weights are used, the Tobacco Supplement yields population estimates for New York City Puerto Ricans and "Other Hispanics" as a group.

New York City Quota Survey

This survey used computer-assisted telephone interviews (CATI) conducted by the Response Analysis Corporation (RAC). The sample was selected from the telephone exchanges from all five boroughs of New York City. Potential respondents were New York City residents, between the ages of 18 and 74, who belonged to one of the following six ethnic/racial groups: Puerto Rican, Dominican, Colombian, Ecuadorian, U.S.-born black, and Caribbean-born, English-speaking black. Subsequent to the funding of the study, and at the request of the project's Community Advisory Board, an additional quota sample of Haitian-born black New York City residents was integrated into the sampling design. Eligibility for all groups was determined by screening questions pertaining to self-reported ethnicity, age, and gender.

Data were collected from subjects within eight age and gender categories. The categories were defined by four age groups (18–44, 45–54, 55–64, and 65–74) and by gender. The initial study design was to sample and complete fifty interviews in each age and gender category for the original six ethnic/racial groups. Only twenty-five Haitian interviews could be added to the sampling frame, in each of the eight age/gender categories, because no additional research funds were available and the addition of these two hundred interviews had to be integrated into the existing project survey budget. Thus, the overall goal of this quota sample was to complete twenty-six hundred interviews. For analytic comparisons between ethnic groups and subgroups, the survey with twenty-six hundred would have provided power of .80 at the .05 (two-sided) level of significance to detect differences of: (1) 8 percent or greater between any two ethnic groups ($n = 400$); (2) 12 percent or greater between any two ethnic-specific gender groups and Haitians both gender groups combined ($n = 200$); and (3) 18 percent or greater between any two ethnic-specific age groups ($n = 100$) (Cohen, 1988). The factorial model for analysis of variance (ANOVA) was used for these estimates.

Based on the advice of the project's Community Advisory Board, survey advertisements were placed on local radio stations, signs in subway stations, and bulletins in churches and social clubs. The campaign to promote survey participation was entitled "Health 92" and involved (1) pictures of representative participants talking on the telephone; (2) a listing of the community organizations on the advisory board supporting the project; (3) an announcement about a lottery for survey participants that entitled them to be entered into a drawing with two $1,000 first prizes, four $500 second prizes, and ten $100 third prizes; and (4) a slogan developed for the campaign that stated: "If you get called for the Health 92 survey, speak up, don't hang up."

Both list and random-digit dial (RDD) sampling techniques were used in combination to ensure coverage of those households with unlisted telephone numbers and to locate those households most likely to include members of the seven ethnic/racial groups. The targeting procedure for low-count ethnic groups began by defining, in terms of ZIP codes, the geographic areas in which the majority of each group resides. Next a "ZIP/exchange analysis" mapped the defined ZIP codes into their corresponding telephone exchanges. To increase the hit rate for Hispanic ethnic groups, the surnames associated with listed telephone households with the selected telephone exchanges were compared to a U.S. Census database of Hispanic surnames. The list sample, selected by surname and ZIP code targeting, was then analyzed to ascertain the most common telephone exchanges or those that appeared to include the most potential respondents. Random-digit dial telephone numbers were generated using these telephone exchanges, making it possible to include in the sample those members of ethnic groups with unlisted telephone numbers.

Calling took place from 8:00 A.M. to 9:00 P.M. on weekdays, from 9:00 A.M. to 9:00 P.M. on Saturdays, and from 11:00 A.M. to 6:00 P.M. on Sundays, unless a respondent requested an appointment during a time outside these hours. An original call and up to seven call-backs were placed in attempt to contract a respondent. The 800 number for Response Analysis Corporation (RAC) was given to those respondents who wanted to contact RAC at a more convenient time. It should also be noted that those respondents who objected to the lottery drawing on religious or moral grounds had the option of either donating their winnings to a charity or not entering their telephone number into the drawing. The overall response rate of 62.3 percent for the survey included calls made to identify homes of persons belonging to the ethnic, gender, and age groups of interest and was calculated using the formula:

Response rate = Actual completed interviews/estimated eligibles
Total estimated eligibles = eligibles + (eligibility rate × eligibility unknown)
Response rate = 2,462/[2,514 + (.194 × 7415.8)] = 62.3 percent

For Hispanics, the targeted sampling quotas consisted of equal portions of males and females within each of the four age groups across all four Hispanic ethnic groups, with an overall goal of sixteen hundred completed interviews. A total of 1,529 Hispanics completed the telephone interview. Ethnic group–specific response rates were unable to be calculated because, in the absence of ethnic group information from the eligibility screener, only an overall estimate of the number of eligible respondents could be calculated. It should be noted that Dominicans, ages 18 through 44, were inadvertently oversampled at the beginning of the survey.

Members of New York City Hispanic ethnic groups are typically much younger than are average New York City residents because many are recent immigrants, who tend to be young when they arrive. Because of their extremely low counts in the census, locating eligible older residents proved to be very difficult, even when screening was prolonged. In particular, difficulties were experienced locating older male Ecuadorians, Colombians, and Dominicans and older female Ecuadorians. In the end, it became necessary to revise the quotas for the oldest cells to take into account the limited number of these elderly respondents in the population as measured by the census. This resulted in unequal age cells in the quota sample, with fewer older Hispanics interviewed than was originally planned.

The questionnaire was designed to collect data on age, sex, socioeconomic status, ethnicity, acculturation, and selected knowledge, attitudes, and beliefs concerning cigarette smoking, food preparation and purchase practices, alcohol use, cancer screening utilization, and use of and access to general health services. The acculturation index included a five-point scale measuring English-Spanish language use with nine different types of people or situations. The reliability of the acculturation scale was assessed using Cronbach's alpha and revealed internal consistency among all nine items (alpha = .91). A Spanish translation (with back translation to English) of the survey instrument was completed and pilot tested. Even though some of the respondents were bilingual, all respondents were given a choice of which language they preferred to use during the interview. Other indicators of acculturation were also present in the data set (for example, proportion of life spent on the mainland United States, age of immigration to the United States).

With respect to the cigarette smoking section of the interview, respondents were asked whether they currently smoked, when they started smoking, how many cigarettes they smoked per day, and whether they had ever tried to quit smoking. Nonsmokers were asked whether they had ever smoked in the past and, if so, when they had stopped. These data were categorized two different ways: categorical (current, former, and nonsmokers) and dichotomous (ever versus never smoked) dependent variables.

Current Population Survey

A Tobacco Use Supplement was added to the basic Current Population Survey (CPS) instrument administered by the Census Bureau to about sixty thousand households in each interview wave during September 1992, January 1993, and May 1993. The CPS sample was selected from the 1980 Decennial Census files, with coverage in all states and the District of Columbia. The Tobacco Use Supplement was designed to evaluate the National Cancer Institute's American Stop Smoking Intervention Study (ASSIST) program. No household was interviewed more than once (except for approximately 3.4 percent who were reinterviewed to ensure data quality).

The CPS, with its large sample size and stratified sample design, provides population estimates of tobacco use behavior by state and for very large cities, such as New York City. All strata are defined within state boundaries. This enabled us to compare the 1992–1993 CPS data from New York City with the 1992 New York City Multi-Ethnic Survey data. The CPS sample was about 1 in every 1,600 New York households; 14,702 individuals aged 18 and older were interviewed, including 1,441 Hispanics (9.8 percent).

The CPS is designed to provide racial/ethnic-specific estimates for each state. Estimates can be made for a few large cities as well. Most Hispanics in New York State are concentrated in New York City. Prior to comparing results derived from the CPS randomized sample for New York City with the quota sample, we compared CPS estimates for Hispanics for both the state and the city. Since most Hispanics in the state reside in New York City, the means and standard errors for Hispanics in the state and the city are similar. Thus, we decided to present estimates for the New York City Hispanic population from the CPS and the quota sample here. The CPS sampled 1,264 Hispanics from New York City (1,441 Hispanics for the entire state) from September 1992 to May 1993. Data were weighted, using replicate weights (discussed below) to derive Hispanic population estimates. CPS results shown are population estimates and percentages based on them.

Approximately one week before the start of interviewing, each new or returning sample household received an advance letter that explained the voluntary nature of the survey and cited the legal authority for conducting it. Field representatives informed the returning respondents that supplements might be administered.

Since self-respondent data have been found to be more reliable than proxy data for most tobacco use, special efforts were made to maximize self-response interviews for the Tobacco Use Supplement. The supplement questionnaire was printed on a form separate from the labor force questions, and interviewing for the supplement was extended for a second week (there is a one-week limit for labor statistics collection). These procedures were expected to increase self-response from 70 to 83 percent; the actual rate exceeded 80 percent. After two call-backs, proxy interviews for the supplement, conducted with a knowledgeable household respondent, aged 15 years or older, were accepted.

The survey instrument was translated into Spanish and verified by an independent reviewer. As with the English version of the questionnaire, the Spanish translation underwent a cognitive testing process with approximately ten Spanish-speaking respondents to ensure its accuracy. The CPS origin variable included the following precoded options for Hispanics: Mexican American, Chicano, Mexican (Mexicano), Puerto Rican, Cuban, Central or South American. Unlike the New York quota sample, which distinguished among Dominicans, Colombians, and Ecuadorians, the CPS grouped all these nationalities under "Central or South American."

A single data collection instrument was used, though field representatives were provided with a Spanish translation of the Tobacco Use Supplement to use as needed. Generally, in fielding the CPS with a Spanish-speaking respondent who does not understand English, a Spanish-speaking interviewer from the regional office is sought, or, if one is not available, a Spanish-speaking person from a nearby university or a household member is sought. This was also the procedure with the Tobacco Use Supplement; however, the Spanish-speaking person also had the Spanish Tobacco Use Supplement available to use during the interview. Field representatives indicated on the instrument whether interviews were administered in English, Spanish, or some other language. This indicator is the basis for the CPS variable "language of interview."

STATISTICAL METHODS

Descriptive data for cigarette smoking, demographic, and language use predictors of smoking are presented for the NYC and CPS data sets. Chi square analyses were performed to compare the frequency distributions of cigarette smoking and sociodemographic characteristics among the different Hispanic groups in the quota and CPS data sets.

Because of the relatively small percentage of the non–Puerto Rican population who reported to be current smokers (particularly among females) in the quota sample, the three-level categorical smoking status variable (current, former, and never smokers) could not be used reasonably as the dependent variable. Thus, the ever-smoked versus never-smoked dichotomous measure was chosen as the dependent variable for all univariate and multivariate analyses. The relative odds and confidence intervals for univariate and multivariate analyses of individual predictors of having ever smoked are presented, and case scenarios exploring tobacco control intervention and implications are discussed.

Categorical variables including gender, ethnicity, religious preference, and employment status were compared with smoking status using contingency table analyses. Continuous variables, such as age and education, were examined by means of univariate logistic regression analyses. All variables whose univariate tests had p-values ≤ 0.30 were candidates for the multiple logistic regression analyses (Hosmer and Lemeshow, 1989). Both backward and forward stepwise approaches were used to develop the most parsimonious model (Hosmer and Lemeshow, 1989). Variable selection was performed manually, based on change in log-likelihood, effect, on other parameters in the model, and validity considerations. Once we arrived at a main effects model that contained the essential variables, we checked the assumption of linearity in the logit for the continuous variables of age and education. The Box-Tidwell test (Hosmer and Lemeshow, 1989) was applied, but only age gave evidence for nonlinearity in the logit. Therefore, a quadratic term for age was added to the chosen main effects model. Each possible interaction term was examined with the chosen main effects model. The only interactions that provided a significant improvement over the chosen main effects model were between interview language and gender and between interview language and education.

Because the CPS is a complex sample, special weights must be computed to generate correct variance estimates. Replicate weights[a] were computed by the Census Bureau for estimating variances for the nation and the most populous states, including New York. Appropriate use of these replicate weights with the WESTVAR statistical package (Flyer, Rust, and Morganstein, 1989) will generate approximately correct variance estimates for parameters of interest (Judkins, 1990). Proxy responses were deleted from the CPS sample prior to analysis to improve the accuracy of the estimates.

---

[a]Replicate weights are computed by generalized replication, a variance estimation method developed by Dr. Robert Fay of the Census Bureau, and used for several U.S. government surveys. Replicate weights are used to estimate variances and covariances of any statistics computed from the CPS data.

RESULTS

Six tables present smoking rates and sociodemographic characteristics, and the univariate and multivariate relationship between them for the multiethnic quota and CPS surveys. The frequency distribution of smoking status and socio-demographic characteristics among the ethnic groups under study are shown for the quota (Table 14.1) and CPS (Table 14.2) samples. Relative odds of having

Table 14.1. Percentage Distribution of Smoking Behavior and Sociodemographic Characteristics Among Latino Groups: NYC Quota Sample

	Ethnic Group				
Characteristic	Colombian	Dominican	Ecuadorian	Puerto Rican	Total
Smoking status*	(n = 324)	(n = 489)	(n = 253)	(n = 444)	(n = 1,510)
Current	14.5	13.9	13.0	22.1	16.3
Former	16.0	8.2	11.9	17.6	13.2
Nonsmoker	69.4	77.9	75.1	60.4	70.5
Gender	(n = 329)	(n = 492)	(n = 258)	(n = 450)	(n = 1,529)
Male	38.6	37.4	41.5	45.1	40.6
Female	61.4	62.6	58.5	54.9	59.4
Age*	(n = 329)	(n = 492)	(n = 258)	(n = 450)	(n = 1,529)
18–44	35.0	45.5	40.7	33.1	38.8
45–54	29.2	20.5	33.3	22.2	25.0
55–64	23.7	20.7	17.8	22.7	21.5
65 and over	12.2	13.2	8.1	22.0	14.7
Mean age	47.7	45.6	45.0	50.1	47.3
(±SD)	(13.9)	(15.6)	(14.2)	(15.8)	(15.3)
Marital status	(n = 329)	(n = 492)	(n = 255)	(n = 448)	(n = 1,524)
Married/living as married	54.1	54.7	55.7	49.8	53.3
Single/divorced/ widowed	45.9	45.3	44.3	50.2	46.7
Language[a]*	(n = 328)	(n = 492)	(n = 258)	(n = 448)	(n = 1,526)
Only-mostly English	4.0	3.0	5.8	19.9	8.7
English and Spanish equally	24.4	20.7	19.4	42.0	27.5
Only-mostly Spanish	71.6	76.2	74.8	38.2	63.8

Table 14.1. (Continued)

Characteristic	Ethnic Group				
	Colombian	Dominican	Ecuadorian	Puerto Rican	Total
Interview language*	(n = 329)	(n = 492)	(n = 258)	(n = 450)	(n = 1,529)
English	11.6	14.0	14.0	41.8	21.6
Spanish	88.4	86.0	86.0	58.2	78.4
Birthplace*	(n = 329)	(n = 492)	(n = 258)	(n = 450)	(n = 1,529)
In mainland United States	4.3	7.1	3.9	23.8	10.9
Outside United States	95.7	92.9	96.1	76.2	89.1
Years of education*	(n = 325)	(n = 478)	(n = 253)	(n = 446)	(n = 1,502)
1–8	23.4	36.2	26.1	28.3	29.4
9–11	11.1	11.9	19.0	17.3	14.5
12	31.1	22.2	26.5	24.4	25.5
13–15	19.1	18.2	19.4	16.6	18.1
16 and over	15.4	11.5	9.1	13.5	12.5
Mean years of education	11.2	10.4	10.7	10.6	10.7
(±SD)	(3.9)	(4.1)	(3.6)	(4.1)	(4.0)
Employment*	(n = 327)	(n = 489)	(n = 256)	(n = 448)	(n = 1,520)
Currently employed	54.7	43.1	59.8	50.7	50.7
Unemployed less than three years	13.5	14.3	14.5	6.9	12.0
Out of labor force[a]	31.8	42.5	25.8	42.4	37.4
Income*	(n = 329)	(n = 492)	(n = 258)	(n = 450)	(n = 1,529)
Less than $20,000	38.0	45.3	39.1	32.2	38.8
$20,000 or more	36.8	27.4	30.6	43.6	34.7
Missing[b]	25.2	27.2	30.2	24.2	26.4
Health insurance*	(n = 321)	(n = 482)	(n = 251)	(n = 439)	(n = 1,493)
Medicaid/care only	16.8	35.1	20.3	35.3	28.7
Other insurance	45.8	33.6	38.2	53.1	42.7
No insurance	37.4	31.3	41.4	11.6	28.5
Religion*	(n = 329)	(n = 489)	(n = 255)	(n = 443)	(n = 1,516)
Catholic	88.4	78.5	86.7	75.8	81.3
Protestant/other	9.1	13.1	12.2	17.6	13.4
None	2.4	8.4	1.2	6.5	5.3

[a]Includes students, homemakers, and retired/disabled people.

[b]Only missing data frequencies of 10 percent or more are recorded.

*$p \leq 0.0001$.

ever smoked are shown by these characteristics in Tables 14.3 and 14.4. Table 14.5 presents the relative odds from multivariate logistic regression models of the two samples; Table 14.6 presents the best-fitting model using the NYC quota sample only, for which national origin groups and religion were measured (unlike the CPS, which did not collect detailed data on Hispanic national origin groups or religion).

Table 14.1 describes the ethnic group differences among New York City Hispanics in terms of the smoking status variable and other independent variables that have been shown to predict smoking status in the past. Puerto Ricans were significantly more likely to be current smokers and ever smokers than the other three Latino groups. While no significant gender differences were observed among Latino groups, Puerto Ricans had a significantly higher percentage of respondents 65 years of age or older. This was primarily due to the difficulty in finding potential respondents 65 and older among the other three Latino groups.

As noted in the methods section, the quota survey provides information on more Hispanic countries of origin than does the CPS. However, it is possible to single out Puerto Ricans in both surveys and compare them with the other ethnic groups in the quota sample and with "other Hispanics" in the CPS. In this way, it is possible to compare the quota sample data, which are not based on a random sample of the Hispanic population, with those data from the CPS. It is important to keep in mind that the quota was stratified not only by ethnic group but also by age, so that ethnic groups under study in the quota survey appear older (mean ages range from 45 to 50 years) than they do in the CPS (mean ages range from 38 to 42 years). However, there is consistency to the extent that Puerto Ricans are older than the other ethnic groups of Hispanics.

With respect to other sociodemographic characteristics, significant differences among Latino groups were observed with respect to education, employment, health insurance, religion, and income (Table 14.1). Finally, in terms of potential indexes of acculturation, Puerto Ricans were significantly different from the other three Latino groups. They were more likely to have been born in the U.S. mainland, more likely to have completed the interview in English, and more likely to speak English and Spanish equally or to use English with friends, family, and in social and work situations.

Table 14.2 compares CPS data for Puerto Rican and "other" Hispanics. With respect to smoking and sociodemographic characteristics, Puerto Ricans are more likely than other Hispanics to be current or former smokers. Consistent with the data in Table 14.1, women were more likely to be survey respondents, Puerto Ricans were less likely to be married than other Hispanics, and more likely to complete the interview in English. Reported years of educational attainment vary between the two surveys. The quota survey suggests all groups of Hispanics have more college than reported in the CPS. The CPS, in addition to having a sample

Table 14.2. Percentage Distribution of Smoking Behavior and Sociodemographic Characteristics Among Latino Groups: CPS Sample of New York City Data—September 1992, January 1993, May 1993 (unweighted counts and percentages)

	Ethnic Group		
Characteristic	Puerto Rican (n = 624)	Other Hispanics (n = 640)	Total (n = 1,264)
Smoking status*			
Current	24.7	15.9	20.3
Former	13.5	8.4	10.9
Nonsmoker	61.9	75.6	68.8
Gender			
Male	35.7	41.1	38.5
Female	64.3	58.9	61.6
Age*			
18–44	60.4	71.3	65.9
45–54	18.1	14.7	16.4
55–64	10.1	7.8	8.9
65 and over	11.4	6.3	8.8
Mean age	42	38	40
(±SD)	(15.8)	(14.7)	(15.2)
Marital status*			
Married[a]	39.6	50	44.9
Single/divorced/widowed	60.4	50	55.1
Interview language*			
English	74.2	64.8	69.5
Spanish	24.7	33.6	29.2
Years of education			
0–8	19.1	25.5	22.3
9–11	28.7	19.5	24.1
12	27.4	28.3	27.9
13–15	18.9	18.3	18.6
16 or more	5.9	8.4	7.2
Employment*			
Currently employed	40.7	51.3	46.0
Unemployed	7.9	9.8	8.9
Out of labor force	51.4	38.9	45.1
Income			
Less than $20,000	56.7	56.7	56.7
$20,000 or more	38.5	37.8	38.1
Missing	4.8	5.5	5.1

[a]No precoded "living as married" option on CPS.

*$p < 0.001$.

reporting less educational attainment than that observed in the quota survey, also has a higher percentage of respondents reporting being out of the labor force than was observed in the quota survey. Both samples reflected Puerto Ricans as older than the other Hispanics. The CPS showed similar and relatively low incomes for both groups of Hispanics, while the quota survey showed more variation; however, about a quarter of income responses were missing in the quota survey. Health insurance status and religion were not asked by the CPS. Some of the differences between the CPS and quota study findings may have been related to the noteworthy and far higher percentage of respondents who took the interview in Spanish in the quota survey compared with the CPS.

While sociodemographic characteristics are similar but not identical, in the two NYC surveys under study, the relative odds of ever smoking, shown for the quota survey (Table 14.3) and the CPS Survey (Table 14.4), are in the same direction and of similar magnitudes. Without adjusting for other factors, Hispanic men are more than twice as likely as Hispanic women to have ever smoked. Older age, being Puerto Rican, taking the interview in English, current employment, and more education (though the relationship between ever smoking and education is not linear as shown in Table 14.4) also put Hispanics at greater risk of having ever smoked. Table 14.3, which presents additional predictors measured in the quota sample, further confirms that higher levels of acculturation (being born in the United States, greater English proficiency), and reporting being a Catholic are predictors of increased smoking risk.

In Table 14.5, a multivariate logistic regression model was constructed to compare smoking status among Hispanics in the two NYC surveys. The independent

Table 14.3. Relative Odds of Ever Smoking Across Sociodemographic Indicators: NYC Quota Sample

| Characteristic | Smoking Status | | | |
	Ever Smoked	Never Smoked	Relative Odds	95% CI
Gender	(n = 446)	(n = 1,064)		
Male	238	373	2.12	1.69–2.65
Female	208	691	1.00	—
Age[b]				
45			1.46	1.11–1.92
25[a]			1.00	—
Ethnicity	(n = 446)	(n = 1,064)		
Colombians	99	225	0.67	0.49–0.91
Dominicans	108	381	0.43	0.32–0.57
Ecuadorians	63	190	0.50	0.36–0.71
Puerto Ricans[a]	176	268	1.00	—

Table 14.3. (Continued)

Characteristic	Ever Smoked	Never Smoked	Relative Odds	95% CI
		Smoking Status		
Marital status	(n = 445)	(n = 1,061)		
Married/living as married	237	563	1.01	0.81–1.26
Single/divorced/ widowed[a]	208	498	1.00	—
Birthplace	(n = 446)	(n = 1,064)		
In United States	68	96	1.81	1.30–2.53
Outside United States[a]	378	968	1.00	—
Language	(n = 445)	(n = 1,062)		
Only–mostly English	52	80	1.96	1.35–2.87
English and Spanish equally	154	260	1.79	1.40–2.29
Mostly–only Spanish[a]	239	722	1.00	—
Interview language	(n = 446)	(n = 1,064)		
English	138	191	2.05	1.59–2.64
Spanish[a]	308	873	1.00	—
Years of education[c]				
16			1.52	1.21–1.91
8[a]			1.00	—
Employment	(n = 446)	(n = 1,055)		
Currently employed	244	514	1.62	1.26–2.08
Unemployed less than three years	75	107	2.40	1.68–3.42
Out of labor force[d]	127	434	1.00	—
Health insurance	(n = 433)	(n = 1,042)		
Medicaid/care only	107	318	0.81	0.60–1.09
Other insurance	202	427	1.13	0.87–1.48
No insurance	124	297	1.00	—
Religion	(n = 440)	(n = 1,058)		
Catholic	371	845	1.36	1.01–1.83
All others[e]	69	213	1.00	—

[a]Fixed reference category.

[b]Age is a continuous variable; highlighted is a comparison between 45 and 25 years of age. The effect of age is obtained by $\exp[\beta_1(Age_2 - Age_1) + \beta_2(Age_2^2 - Age_1^2)]$.

[c]Education is a continuous variable; highlighted is a comparison between 16 and 8 years of education.

[d]Includes students, homemakers, and retired/disabled people.

[e]Includes Protestants, Muslims, and people with no religion.

Table 14.4. Relative Odds of Ever Having Smoked by Sociodemographic Indicators: CPS Study Sample, New York City (September 1992, January 1993, May 1993)

Characteristic	Ever Smoked (N = 394)	Never Smoked (N = 870)	Relative Odds[a]	95% CI
Gender				
Male	205	281	2.30	1.78–2.96
Female[b]	189	589	1.00	—
Age				
45			1.85	0.65–5.28
25[b]			1.00	—
Ethnicity				
Other Hispanics	156	484	.54	0.43–0.68
Puerto Ricans[b]	238	386	1.00	—
Marital status				
Married[c]	174	393	0.99	0.71–1.38
Single/divorced/widowed[b]	220	477	1.00	—
Interview language[d]				
English	282	596	1.18	0.87–1.59
Spanish[b]	107	262	1.00	—
Years of education				
1–8[b]	65	217	1.00	—
9–11	124	180	2.35	1.45–3.82
12	101	251	1.40	0.95–2.06
13–15	77	158	1.62	1.03–2.56
16 or more	27	64	1.46	0.90–2.38
Employment				
Currently employed	209	373	1.57	1.24–2.00
Unemployed	33	79	1.17	0.84–1.63
Out of labor force[b]	152	418	1.00	—

[a]Relative odds are based on population estimates; actual counts of ever and never smokers are not weighted.

[b]Fixed reference category.

[c]No precoded "living as married" option on CPS.

[d]Five "ever smoked" respondents and twelve "never smoked" respondents were deleted from this analysis because their language status was missing from the CPS data set.

Table 14.5. Relative Odds with 95 Percent CI from Multivariate Logistic Regression Models of NYC Quota and CPS Sample Data

	New York City (Quota)		New York City (CPS)	
Covariate	Adjusted Relative Odds	95% CI	Adjusted Relative Odds	95% CI
Age[a]				
45	1.84	1.36–2.50	1.94	1.60–2.35
25[b]	1.00	—	1.00	—
Ethnicity				
Other Hispanics	0.57	0.44–0.75	0.53	0.40–0.70
Puerto Ricans[b]	1.00	—	1.00	—
Interview language and gender interaction				
English interview				
Males	1.28	0.81–2.02	6.29	4.61–8.57
Females[b]	1.00	—	1.00	—
Spanish interview				
Males	2.38	1.81–3.12	3.70	2.36–5.81
Females[b]	1.00	—	1.00	—
Interview language and education interaction				
English interview/years of education				
1–8[b]	1.00	—	1.00	—
13–15	0.89	0.28–2.79	0.89	0.54–1.48
12	0.83	0.30–2.32	0.85	0.55–1.31
13–15	0.85	0.31–2.36	0.03	0.02–0.05
16 or more	0.48	0.17–1.38	0.22	0.12–0.41
Spanish interview/years of education				
1–8[b]	1.00	—	1.00	—
9–11	1.24	0.81–1.88	1.55	0.76–3.18
12	1.21	0.83–1.76	1.10	0.53–2.26
13–15	1.61	1.05–2.47	0.29	0.07–1.18
16 or more	1.33	0.81–2.17	0.64	0.13–3.20

[a]Age is a continuous variable; highlighted is a comparison between 45 and 25 years of age. The effect of age is obtained by $\exp[\beta_1(\text{Age}_2 - \text{Age}_1) + \beta_2(\text{Age}_2^2 - \text{Age}_1^2)]$.

[b]Fixed reference category.

variables used in the model were restricted to those included in the CPS Smoking Supplement. The model for each data set included age, Puerto Rican versus other Hispanic ethnicity, interview language as it interacts with gender, and interview language as it interacts with education. These interaction variables were chosen after considerable variable testing as described in the methods section. Outcomes were similar in the two surveys, although not identical. Adjusting for the factors listed above, older age and Puerto Rican ethnicity remained significant positive predictors of having ever smoked. Men who completed the interview in Spanish were significantly more likely to smoke compared with women who completed the interview in Spanish, according to both surveys. This pattern can also be seen for men and women who took the interview in English, although it is significant only in the CPS estimates. Finally, smoking rates may fall with more years of education for those who took the interview in English; however, this result is merely suggestive because it is not confirmed by consistently significant results. For those completing the quota survey in Spanish, there was an inconsistently significant finding suggesting that more highly educated Spanish-speaking respondents were more likely to have ever smoked, although this finding was not confirmed in the CPS survey data.

The best multivariate logistic regression model for the quota sample data, which provides considerably more information than the CPS does, is shown in Table 14.6. Older age, Puerto Rican ethnicity (versus other Hispanic groups), being Catholic, being male when taking the interview in Spanish, and more education (as a continuous variable) when taking the interview in Spanish were all significant predictors of having ever smoked in the New York City quota sample data.

DISCUSSION

The comparison of the quota sample data and the CPS data suggests that the New York City quota sample was comparable to the weighted probability sample of New York City Hispanics on several demographic parameters unrelated to the quota sampling framework (such as age) and the language of the interview. These included gender, years of education, and employment status. Moreover, these data sets reflect similar findings concerning smoking behavior among New York City Hispanics. First, Puerto Ricans reported the highest prevalence rates of current smoking of all Hispanic groups surveyed, and this rate (22 to 25 percent) is comparable to the national rate for U.S. white male and female population combined in 1993 (approximately 25 percent) (Shopland, Burs, Thompson, and Lynn, 1995). Among other Hispanics in general, and among Dominicans, Colombians, and Ecuadorians in particular, current smoking

Table 14.6. Relative Odds with 95 Percent CI from Multivariate Logistic Regression: NYC Quota Sample

Covariate	Adjusted Relative Odds	95% CI
Age[a]		
45	1.77	1.31–2.41
25[b]	1.00	—
Ethnicity		
Colombians	0.68	0.48–0.96
Dominicans	0.48	0.35–0.67
Ecuadorians	0.49	0.33–0.72
Puerto Ricans[b]	1.00	—
Religion		
Catholic	1.77	1.28–2.44
All others[b]	1.00	—
Interview language and gender interaction		
English interview		
Males	1.27	0.80–2.02
Females[b]	1.00	—
Spanish interview		
Males	2.56	1.94–3.38
Females[b]	1.00	—
Interview language and education interaction[c]		
English interview/years of education		
16	0.64	0.33–1.27
8[b]	1.00	—
For each additional year of education	0.95	0.87–1.03
Spanish interview/years of education		
16	1.37	1.02–1.83
8[b]	1.00	—
For each additional year of education	1.04	1.002–1.079

[a]Age is a continuous variable; highlighted is a comparison between 45 and 25 years of age. The effect of age is obtained by $\exp[\beta_1(Age_2 - Age_1) + \beta_2(Age_2^2 - Age_1^2)]$.

[b]Fixed reference category.

[c]Education is a continuous variable; highlighted is a comparison between sixteen years and eight years of education.

rates in 1992 were at or below the National Cancer Institute goal of 15 percent adult smoking prevalence by the year 2000 (Greenwald and Sondik, 1986).

Because of the low current smoking prevalence rates among all Hispanics except Puerto Ricans, we analyzed predictors of having ever smoked. With respect to predictors of having ever smoked, apart from the Puerto Rican versus other Hispanic comparison, both data sets indicated that men were significantly more likely to have ever smoked than women, currently employed respondents were more likely to have ever smoked than those out of the labor force, and, contrary to what has been observed in other U.S. resident populations, Hispanics with more years of education completed were more likely to have ever smoked.

The two completely consistent findings from the quota and CPS samples, reflected in Table 14.5, suggest that smoking cessation programs may need to be culturally tailored and targeted to older Puerto Rican populations, while adult-focused smoking prevention programs may need to be developed to prevent Hispanics of Central and South American origin from taking up the tobacco habit after they arrive in the United States. While tobacco use rates may differ between recent immigrants and those who choose to remain in their countries of origin, multinational tobacco industries continue to move production facilities overseas and aggressively promote their tobacco products in the developing world. If the impact on smoking prevalence rates of multinational tobacco industry production and promotion in Latin America is similar to that observed in Asia and Africa, then we may observe an upsurge in tobacco use in Latin America. Thus, it is important for the U.S. and international public health communities to compare smoking prevalence rates among recent immigrants and comparable populations in their countries of origin and to identify the cultural and socioeconomic forces that have contributed to keeping smoking prevalence low in these more recent immigrant populations.

A review of the interaction between acculturation and other predictors of smoking behavior indicates that Hispanic males were more likely to have ever smoked than Hispanic females, though this was only consistently significant between the quota and CPS sample data when the male respondent completed the interview in Spanish. This is consistent with findings previously reported from San Francisco (Marin, Pérez-Stable, and Marin, 1989). When the interview was completed in English, the male/female smoking difference was greatly reduced and became nonsignificant in the quota sample, while the male/female smoking difference was inflated in the CPS sample. This may have been a consequence of the different methodological pathways by which respondents could complete the interview in Spanish in the quota or CPS surveys.

In the New York City quota sample, any respondent wishing to take the interview in Spanish was free to do so, because all interviewers were fully bilingual and all Spanish-language questions were programmed into the CATI system. Latinos who took the interview in English took it by choice rather than by necessity. In contrast, Spanish-speaking respondents in the CPS had a good chance of being assigned to an interviewer who did not speak Spanish. For these individuals, an interpreter may have been found; the interview may have been completed in English despite the respondent's preference; or the individual may have refused to participate. There are no estimates of the exact impact of this process on who was interviewed in the CPS and how their responses to questions may have been affected. If language use is a reasonable indicator of acculturation, as is suggested by the high correlations between language use variables and other indexes of acculturation (Marin, Sabogal, and Marin, 1987), and if acculturation is linked to health risk behaviors such as smoking, then our understanding of the relationship between acculturation and smoking behavior is likely to be heavily impacted by these methodological dilemmas.

Consistent with the Marin, Pérez-Stable, and Marin (1989) findings, Hispanic women in the quota sample who chose to complete the interview in English were eight times more likely to have said they ever smoked compared with Hispanic women who chose to complete the interview in Spanish (data not shown). This had the effect of greatly reducing the male/female smoking differences when respondents completed the interview in English. Interestingly, Hispanic males who chose to complete the interview in English were four times more likely to report having ever smoked compared with males who completed the interview in Spanish. Given the larger effect of acculturation (as measured by the interview language choice) among Hispanic females, the net effect on male/female smoking differences was most clearly seen among Spanish-language respondents. The relationship between acculturation and smoking behavior appears to be complex and sensitive to methodological issues of sampling and interview language.

The finding that more highly educated Hispanics were more likely to have ever smoked contradicts most research for the past two decades with respect to the relationship between tobacco use and education. However, upon examining the interaction between interview language and education (as a continuous variable) with respect to having ever smoked, the data from the quota survey in Table 14.6 reflect a nonsignificant trend suggesting that among the relatively small percentage of Hispanic respondents who chose to complete the interview in English, those with more education were less likely to have ever smoked. Among the large majority of Latino respondents who chose to complete the interview in Spanish, those with more education were significantly more likely to have ever smoked than their less educated counterparts. Thus, the relationship between education and smoking may also be mediated by acculturation. If we are to make tobacco control programs culturally and educationally appropriate for an increasingly diverse U.S. population, more research exploring these complex relationships needs to be conducted. It may be important to examine this interaction effect with other measures of acculturation as well as examining where immigrant populations completed their education.

Several limitations to this research need to be considered. First, the New York City quota sample was designed and funded as a cross-section survey of a sample not specifically drawn to be representative of New York City Hispanics. Rather, quota sampling was used to ensure adequate representation of Hispanics from the four major countries of origin in New York City, males and females, and older as well as younger Hispanics. Differences observed among Hispanics from different countries of origin, different ages, and males and females appear to justify this approach. Nevertheless, only by comparing these findings with findings from area-probability sample data, such as in the CPS, are we able to increase our confidence about the universal nature of these results obtained by the quota sample design. A limitation caused by these comparative analyses is that only common data elements (such as interview language as a common measure of acculturation) can be examined across surveys, narrowing the number of variables that can be analyzed.

Ideally, these phenomena should be studied longitudinally. Particularly with respect to the influence of acculturation, samples of Hispanic smokers, former smokers, and nonsmokers need to be identified and followed to better understand how the processes of acculturation and perhaps assimilation may influence health risk behaviors such as tobacco use. However, such an endeavor would be costly and difficult to replicate across the varied and rapidly growing groups of Latin Americans immigrating to and residing in the United States. A less costly alternative is to routinely conduct rolling oversamples among different Latin American groups, so that national and regional time trends can be monitored for any group within a span of three to five years.

As the number and diversity of the Hispanic population in the United States continue to grow, it will be necessary to refine methods to regularly and reliably measure health behaviors, like smoking, so as to ensure that Hispanics at all levels of acculturation, speaking Spanish or English, can fully participate in health behavior surveys. The data from these two surveys strongly suggest that the relationship between smoking behavior and acculturation (as measured by language usage) is complex and sensitive to methodological issues of sampling and interview language. Further research to elucidate these complexities should be a high priority in the U.S. public health community.

References

"CDC Cigarette Smoking Among Chinese, Vietnamese, and Hispanics—California, 1989–1991." *MMWR*, 1992, *41*, 362–367.

"CDC Smoking-Attributable Mortality and Years of Potential Life Lost. United States, 1988." *MMWR*, 1991, *40*, 62–63, 69–71.

Cohen, J. *Statistical Power Analysis for the Behavioral Sciences.* (2nd ed.) Mahwah, N.J.: Erlbaum, 1988.

DeMoor, C., and others. "Generic Tobacco Use Among Four Ethnic Groups in a School Age Population." *Journal of Drug Education,* 1989, *19,* 257–270.

Edwards, N. C., and MacMillan, K. "Tobacco Use and Ethnicity: The Existing Data Gap." *Canadian Journal of Public Health,* 1990, *81,* 31–35.

Escobedo, L. G., and others. "Sociodemographic Characteristics of Cigarette Smoking Initiation in the United States." *JAMA,* 1990, *264,* 1550–1555.

Fiore, M. C., and others. "Trends in Cigarette Smoking in the United States: The Changing Influence of Gender and Race." *JAMA,* 1989, *261,* 49–55.

Flyer, P., Rust, K., and Morganstein, D. "Complex Survey Variance Estimation and Contingency Table Analysis Using Replication." *ASA Proceedings of Survey Research Methods Section,* 1989, 110–119.

Greenwald, P., and Sondik, E. (eds.). *Cancer Control Objectives for the Nation: 1985–2000. NCI Monographs,* 1986, *2,* 1–105.

Gritz, E. R., and others. "Ethnic Variations in the Prevalence of Smoking Among Registered Nurses." *Cancer Nursing,* 1989, *12,* 16–20.

Haynes, S. G., Cohen, B., Harvey, C., and McMillen, M. "Cigarette Smoking Among Mexican Americans: HHANES, Southwest United States, 1983–1984." *American Journal of Public Health,* 1990, *80*(Suppl.), 47–53.

Hosmer, D. W., and Lemeshow, S. *Applied Logistic Regression.* New York: Wiley, 1989.

Humble, C. G., Samet, J. M., Pathak, D. R., and Skipper, B. J. "Cigarette Smoking and Lung Cancer in 'Hispanic' Whites and Other Whites in New Mexico." *American Journal of Public Health,* 1985, *75,* 145–148.

Judkins, D. R. "Fay's Method for Variance Estimation." *Journal of Official Statistics,* 1990, *6,* 223–239.

Lee, D. J., and Markides, K. S. "Health Behaviors Risk Factors, and Health Indicators Associated with Cigarette Use in Mexican Americans: Results from the HHANES." *American Journal of Public Health,* 1991, *81,* 859–864.

Marcus, A. C., Shopland, D. R., Crane, L. A., and Lynn, W. R. "Prevalence of Cigarette Smoking in the United States: Estimates from the 1985 Current Population Survey." *National Cancer Institute,* 1989, *81,* 409–414.

Marin, G., Pérez-Stable, E. J., and Marin, B. V. "Cigarette Smoking Among San Francisco Hispanics: The Role of Acculturation and Gender." *American Journal of Public Health,* 1989, *79,* 196–198.

Marin, G., Sabogal, F., and Marin, B. V. "Development of a Short Acculturation Scale for Hispanics." *Hispanic Journal of Behavioral Science,* 1987, *9,* 183–205.

Markides, K. S., Coreil, J., and Ray, L. A. "Smoking Among Mexican Americans: A Three Generational Study." *American Journal of Public Health,* 1987, *77,* 708–711.

Martin, R. V., Cummings, S. R., and Coates, T. J. "Ethnicity and Smoking: Differences in White, Black, Hispanic, and Asian Medical Patients Who Smoke." *American Journal of Preventive Medicine,* 1990, *6,* 194–199.

National Center for Health Statistics. *Plan and Operation of the Hispanic Health and Nutrition Examination Survey, 1982–1984.* Washington, D.C.: Government Printing Office, Sept. 1985.

O'Malley, A. S., and others. "Continuity of Care and the Use of Breast and Cervical Cancer Screening Services in a Multiethnic Community." *Archives of Internal Medicine,* 1997, *157,* 1462–1470.

Rogers, R. G., and Crank, J. "Ethnic Differences in Smoking Patterns: Findings from NHIS." *Public Health Report,* 1998, *103,* 387–393.

Shopland, D. R., Burs, D. M., Thompson, B., and Lynn, W. R. "Smoking Control and the COMMIT Experience—Summary and Overview." In *Community-Based Interventions for Smokers. The COMMIT Field Experience.* Bethesda, Md.: National Cancer Institute, Aug. 1995.

Taylor, K. L., Kerner, J. F., Gold, K. F., and Mandelblatt, J. S. "Ever vs. Never Smoking Among an Urban Multiethnic Sample of Haitian, Caribbean and U.S.-Born Blacks." *Preventive Medicine,* 1997, *26,* 855–865.

Thiel de Bocanegra, H., Gany, F., and Fruchter, R. "Available Epidemiological Data on New York's Latino Population: A Critical Review of the Literature." *Ethnicity and Disease,* 1993, *3*(4), 413–426.

U.S. Bureau of the Census. *Statistical Abstract of the United States: 1990.* (100th ed.) Washington, D.C.: U.S. Government Printing Office, 1991.

U.S. Bureau of the Census. Public Use File of the March 1996 Supplement of the Current Population Survey.

Wagenknecth, L. E., and others. "Cigarette Smoking Behavior Is Strongly Related to Educational Status: The CARDIA Study." *Preventive Medicine,* 1990, *19,* 158–169.

CHAPTER FIFTEEN

Illicit Drug Use Among Mexicans and Mexican Americans in California

The Effects of Gender and Acculturation

William A. Vega
Ethel Alderete
Bohdan Kolody
Sergio Aguilar-Gaxiola

This chapter reports the findings of a study of illicit drug use among Mexican Americans in Fresno County, California, an agricultural community with only one metropolitan area. The findings, derived from a sample of 3,012 subjects between the ages of 18 and 59, demonstrate the important influence of acculturation on Latinas' behaviors. Once again this study, like so many others in this book, identifies Latinos' increased vulnerability for illicit drug use with increased acculturation. This situation exists for both men and women but is stronger among women.

Mexicans and Mexican Americans are the second largest ethnic minority group in the United States, and the most rapidly increasing. The epidemiology of illicit drug use among adults of Mexican origin residing in the United States has received insufficient attention in the literature despite the very rapid growth of this population and their apparent high-risk status. The lack of information is due in part to the combining of Mexican origin with diverse Hispanic nationalities in studies on drug use, thereby lowering the precision of estimates (U.S. Department of Health and Human Services, 1993;

This research was supported by a grant from the National Institute of Mental Health, MH 51192, William A. Vega, Principal Investigator.

Warner and others, 1995). Thus, the possibilities of identification and comparison of specific ethnic group patterns and trends are limited.

Only two field studies, each more than a decade old, have been the main sources presenting detailed epidemiological profiles on Mexican American adult drug use. The Los Angeles Epidemiologic Catchment Area Project (LAECA, Karno and others, 1987) and the Hispanic Health and Nutrition Examination Survey (HHANES; Amaro, Whitaker, Coffman, and Heeren, 1990) provided important historical data for assessing drug use patterns. In the LAECA, only urban rates of drug abuse/dependence were assessed. The LAECA reported lifetime DIS/DSM-III drug abuse/dependence rates over four times higher for white non-Hispanics compared with Mexican Americans (13.2 versus 3.7). Mexican American rates were lowest among women, men over 40 (Karno and others, 1987), and immigrant males (Burnam and others, 1987). Drug use however, was prevalent among younger Mexican American men. Lifetime rates of drug abuse/dependence among Mexican American men were 9.0 among those 18 to 39 years of age and 0.5 among those 40 years or older. Among Mexican American women, the rate for those between 18 and 39 years of age was only about three times higher than for those 40 years or older (3.7 versus 1.1).

Data from the 1985 HHANES were used to produce two important reports on the use of illicit drugs among the three major Hispanic groups: Mexican Americans, Cubans, and Puerto Ricans (National Institute on Drug Abuse, 1987). Mexican Americans differed not only in rates of drug use from other Hispanic subgroups, but also in their preferences for certain types of drugs. Mexican American men had age-adjusted rates of lifetime marijuana use (48.8) similar to Puerto Ricans (49.5) and higher rates than Cubans (30.7). However, their lifetime cocaine use rate (19.6) was about half the rate for Puerto Ricans (40.6), and similar to the rate for Cubans (20.3). The age adjusted lifetime marijuana use rate for Mexican American females (19.4) was lower than for Puerto Ricans (30.8) and higher than for Cubans (11.5). The Mexican American female lifetime cocaine use rate (6.4), however, was only one-third the rate for Puerto Rican women (21.2) and slightly lower than the rate for Cuban women (7.2) (Amaro, Whitaker, Coffman, and Heeren, 1990). Mexican Americans were more likely to have used inhalants than Puerto Ricans. The use of cocaine and marijuana was highest among Mexican Americans 18 to 24 years of age. Furthermore, Mexican American single males between the ages of 18 and 24, whose primary language was English, had the highest prevalence of illegal drug use (National Institute on Drug Abuse, 1987). Also, Mexican Americans with incomes above the poverty level were more likely to utilize marijuana and cocaine than those who lived in poverty (De la Rosa, Khalasa, and Rouse, 1990).

Vega and others (Vega, 1993a; Vega, Kolody, Noble, and Porter, 1997) used anonymous urine toxicology screening methodology to estimate the prevalence of prenatal substance exposure in the birthing population in California

($n = 30,000$). The subsample of Latinas born in the United States, mostly of Mexican origin, was eight times more likely to have used illicit drugs than were immigrant women. Higher odds ratios among those born in the United States were associated with no prenatal care, no insurance, and the age range of 25 to 34 years. Zambrana and Scrimshaw (1997) conducted a prospective study of patterns of substance use before and during pregnancy among low-income pregnant women in twenty-two prenatal clinics in Los Angeles. The study included 255 black women, 525 Mexican Americans, and 764 Mexican immigrant women. In this study, however, data on drug use were collected in face-to-face interviews. Mexican-origin women were less likely than African American women to report use of substances before and during pregnancy.

ACCULTURATION

Acculturation and the psychosocial changes that occur upon immigration into the United States and exposure to the American culture have been hypothesized to increase the risk of drug use. Burnam and others (1987) examined the effect of acculturation on drug abuse or dependence among Mexican Americans using LAECA data. The multidimensional acculturation measure included language preference, ethnic background and identification, and ethnic activities. Prevalence rates increased with level of acculturation. Respondents with low acculturation levels had lifetime prevalence of drug abuse or dependence of 0.4. The prevalence rate increased to 4.3 and 8.3 for those with medium and high levels of acculturation, respectively. Drug abuse or dependence was also higher among U.S.-born Mexican Americans (8.1) than among immigrants (1.6). When controlling for nativity, acculturation was not related to drug abuse or dependence among U.S.-born Mexican Americans.

Analyses based on the 1982–1984 HHANES showed that acculturation measured as language preference was significantly associated with marijuana and cocaine use in the previous year (Amaro, Whitaker, Coffman, and Heeren, 1990). The odds of using marijuana were eight times greater, and those of using cocaine were twenty-five times greater, for Mexican Americans who were English speaking than among Spanish-speakers. These results also suggested that the relation of acculturation to drug use differs across education levels. Acculturation had the strongest relation to drug use among those who were least educated. Mexican Americans who were highly acculturated but had low education levels were most likely to report marijuana and cocaine use. The relation between acculturation and drug use also varied by sex. Once socioeconomic factors were considered, the gender gap in marijuana use was relatively small among Spanish-speaking Mexican Americans. This contrasts with the rates of drug use among those who were predominantly English speaking, for whom the rates were much higher among men than among women. Yet the relative difference in drug use between Spanish and English speakers was larger among women than among men. These results indicate that acculturation is more strongly associated with drug use among Mexican American women than among Mexican American men. The effect of nativity on drug use was not significant. However, English speaking was more strongly associated with cocaine use among those who were born in the United States compared to those born in Mexico.

An assessment of the association between acculturation and use of crack cocaine among Hispanic Americans living in the United States was conducted using epidemiological data from three national surveys conducted in 1988, 1990, and 1991. Results showed that Mexican Americans interviewed in Spanish, as opposed to English, were less likely to have used the drug. This was true even after controlling for environmental and demographic characteristics. Hispanic women were less likely than men, and older Hispanics less likely than younger cohorts, to have used crack. Although Spanish-speaking Mexican Americans had lower odds ratios of crack smoking than English-speaking Mexican Americans, this association was not found for other Hispanics in the study population (Wagner-Etchegaray, Schutz, Chilcoat, and Anthony, 1994).

These limited risk factor profiles exhaust what is known from epidemiological survey data about illicit drug use among adult Mexican Americans. Recent studies with Latina adolescents, including Mexican American girls, suggest that patterns of illicit drug use are changing, with increased acculturation creating parity of lifetime rates across ethnic groups and genders (Chavez, Beauvais, and Oetting, 1986; Koury and others, 1996). Patterns of drug use are fluid and responsive to multiple personal, cultural, and environmental factors and influences. Therefore, the state of current knowledge on this topic must be considered fragmentary and awaiting replication and extension.

This study uses a gender-specific approach to address the current status of illicit drugs or inhalants used among adult Mexican Americans in California. The aim is to assess similarities and differences by sex in prevalence rates and to test for associations of illicit drug use with acculturation and nativity variables. Data are current and stem from a large epidemiological survey of Mexican-origin adults that collected information on health, mental health, and drug use using structured household interviews.

METHODS

Research Site

The research site, Fresno County, is approximately 6,000 square miles. It includes the city of Fresno and adjacent Clovis, but it is primarily a low-density agricultural region with scattered small towns and rural hamlets. The county population is approximately 764,800, with 463,600 people located in the Fresno–Clovis metropolitan area (United Way of Fresno, 1996). Hispanics, almost all of whom are of Mexican origin, constitute 38.3 percent of the total county population. Fresno County is representative of the illicit drug use levels in California, as indicated by epidemiological surveillance (U.S. Department of Health and Human Services, 1993; SAMSA Drug Abuse Warning Network, 1996).

Sampling

The design was based on a survey of individuals of Mexican origin between the ages of 18 and 59 years in Fresno County. The 3,012 subjects were selected under a fully probabilistic stratified, multistage cluster-sampling design. The sample was stratified by gender and place of residence in Fresno county, with total sub-sample sizes as follows: urban $n = 1,006$, town $n = 1,006$, and rural $n = 1,000$. Urban respondents were selected from the Fresno–Clovis urbanized area that ranged from 2,500 to 25,000 people, and the rural sample was drawn from the remainder unincorporated areas and isolated residences in the county. The 200 primary sampling units (PSUs) in each stratum (urban, town, rural) were census blocks or block aggregates selected with a probability proportionate to the size of their Hispanic population. In the second sampling stage, a quota of five households was selected randomly in each PSU. In the final stage, one person per household was selected randomly. Because within-PSU quotas were, in some instances, either not met or slightly exceeded due to differential interview refusal rates, a system of PSU weights to adjust for the design requirement of equal PSU sample sizes was developed. Data collection was completed in October 1996. Response rates were 87.8 percent for the urban strata, 90.6 percent for small towns, and 92.3 percent for the rural strata among eligible households. They were calculated as refusals $\times$ 100/refusals + completed interviews.

Instrument

The survey instrument is a modified version of the World Health Organization's Composite International Diagnostic Interview (CIDI), designed to be administered by law interviewers (Robins and others, 1988). The CIDI is a structured clinical interview that was developed jointly by the World Health Organization (WHO) and the former U.S. Alcohol, Drug Abuse and Mental Health Administration (ADAMHA) as the research instrument of choice for large-scale, international psychiatric epidemiological research. The CIDI incorporated the core diagnostic questions of the Diagnostic Interview Schedule (Robins, Helzer, Croughan, and Ratcliff, 1981) and was designed to be used cross-culturally on populations with diverse levels of education and literacy (Wittchen and others, 1991). The survey instrument is available in English and Spanish and was specifically adapted and tailored for use with respondents of Mexican origin. Translation into Spanish was accomplished by the translation and back-translation method. Besides the psychiatric diagnostic and utilization core, demographic information includes acculturation patterns, migration, employment, family, and social dynamics questions. A computer-assisted personal interview (CAPI) system was developed for instrument administration. The CAPI version of the instrument is designed to have an average face-to-face administration time of approximately seventy minutes for those respondents without extensive psychiatric histories.

Definition of Variables

Lifetime Illicit Drug or Inhalant Use. Information on drug use was obtained from questions on type of drugs, frequency of use, and time frame. Respondents were considered illicit drug users if they had ever used marijuana, cocaine, inhalants, hallucinogens, or heroin.

Acculturation. The acculturation process poses many conceptual and measurement challenges to researchers because its content is expansive and multifactorial. However, in our opinion, the use of multifactorial acculturation scales in descriptive studies has not been adequately justified. Therefore, in this study, a language preference scale was used to assess acculturation. The seven-item acculturation measure was based on the Cuellar, Harris, Jasso scale (Cuellar, Harris, and Jasso, 1980; Vega and Gil, 1998). The scale measures preference for using Spanish versus English language in different social contexts (for example, work, home, with friends). It is structured in a Likert format, and each item has a range of five responses. A grand mean score of 1 indicates low acculturation and 5 indicates high acculturation (Cronbach's alpha = 0.95).

In validity studies leading to the development of the seven-item measure used in this survey, acculturation factors other than the social/behavioral language factor had inconsistent or insignificant statistical associations with drug and alcohol use in a multiethnic sample of Hispanics (Vega and Gil, 1998). Similarly, Burnam and others (1987) used a multidimensional acculturation scale in the LAECA and reported it was not predictive of drug abuse or dependence in a multivariate model. Cobas and others (1996) recently reported from another large survey that language use, rather than ethnic identity, had a superior predictive value for drug use among Mexican Americans. We conclude that the language use factor has been shown to be an efficient, albeit imperfect, proxy for acculturation in describing the distribution of drug use and assessing correlates (Vega and others, 1993b).

Other Covariates. Respondents were classified into two nativity groups according to country of birth (United States versus other country). Urban, town, and rural place of residence were ascertained according to the sampling stratification scheme. Demographic information was obtained using standard measures of education, annual family income, age at last birthday, marital status, and number of children.

Data Analysis

For data analysis, SUDAAN, version 6.40, was used. Prevalence estimates of lifetime illicit drug use were calculated by gender and by place of residence, using appropriate weights and sample design adjustments. Prevalence rates were age adjusted to the sex-specific Mexican American age distribution of Fresno County. The age adjustment incorporated five-year intervals employed by the U.S. Census. In addition, weights to adjust for household size (the number of eligibles) were calculated, as well as weights to conform the sample to the census age–sex distribution. The combined weights were designed to yield weighted sample sizes equal to the raw data. Given our multistage sampling design, all standard error estimates reported here are based on the first-order Taylor series approximation employed by the SUDAAN statistical software. Chi-square tests were used to examine the associations of lifetime illicit drug use with acculturation and demographic variables. Logistic regression was used to generate multivariate models of lifetime and past-year use of illicit drugs or inhalants, as well as separate models for the two most prevalent drugs: marijuana and cocaine. More than 50 percent of respondents used two or more drugs. Therefore, our last and most comprehensive multivariate models were constructed with any illicit drug or inhalants use composite outcome variable. Models included the following categorical covariates: sex, age, education, marital status, children, nativity, and place of residence. Income and acculturation produced no evidence of nonlinearity with lifetime drug use. Therefore, the standardized scores of these covariates were included in the logistic regression models. We tested two-way interactions between sex and all covariates, and acculturation and place of residence, acculturation and nativity, and place of residence and nativity. Covariates with significant two-way interactions were tested for three-way interactions. Interaction terms were tested one at a time. The final model included all significant interaction terms.

RESULTS

Table 15.1 presents sociodemographic variables by gender. The majority of the sample (60.1 percent) was born in Mexico and earned an annual family income of less than $18,000 (70.1 percent). Women had significantly lower annual family income than men, were less likely to be employed, were more likely to be born in the United States, and were less likely to prefer the use of English language.

Prevalence Rates of Lifetime Illicit Drug Use

Table 15.2 presents lifetime prevalence rates and standard errors of estimates for marijuana, cocaine, hallucinogens, inhalants, and heroin. Also presented are

Table 15.1. Sociodemographic Characteristics by Gender, Mexican-Origin Population, Fresno County, California ($n = 3,012$)

	Female (%)	Male (%)
Age (years)		
18–25	27.1	24.7
26–39	45.8	45.4
40–60	27.0	29.0
Marital status**		
Not married	19.9	31.5
Married	65.4	59.7
Divorced/widowed	14.7	8.8
Children**		
No	12.7	28.9
Yes	87.3	71.1
Education (years)		
0–6	33.0	36.0
7–12	51.7	48.6
12 or more	15.3	15.5
Family income*		
Less than $18,000	75.6	69.8
$18,000 or more	24.4	30.2
Currently employed**		
No	32.3	67.9
Yes	67.7	32.1
Acculturation*		
Low	33.6	28.0
Medium	34.6	41.0
High	31.8	31.1
Nativity*		
Foreign	57.9	63.8
U.S. born	42.1	36.1
Place of residence		
Urban	33.6	28.0
Town	34.6	41.0
Rural	31.8	31.1

Chi-square test: $p \leq 0.05$. *$p \leq 0.01$. **$p \leq 0.001$.

Table 15.2. Lifetime Illegal Drug Use Prevalence Rates by Residence and Gender, Mexican-Origin Population, Fresno County, California

	Rural			Town			Urban			Total		
	Female n = 499 % (SE)	Male n = 501 % (SE)	Total n = % (SE)	Female n = 512 % (SE)	Male n = 493 % (SE)	Total n = % (SE)	Female n = 504 % (SE)	Male n = 500 % (SE)	Total n = % (SE)	Female n = 1516 % (SE)	Male n = 1497 % (SE)	Total n = % (SE)
Marijuana	16.4 (2.3)	34.4 (3.0)	26.1 (1.9)	19.5 (2.3)	41.5 (2.9)	30.4 (1.8)	31.2 (2.6)	52.0 (2.8)	40.4 (2.0)	23.7 (1.7)	45.7 (1.9)	35.4 (1.3)
Cocaine	5.8 (1.5)	16.2 (2.1)	11.1 (1.3)	5.5 (1.2)	22.6 (2.5)	14.1 (1.3)	12.6 (1.8)	31.9 (2.9)	21.7 (1.7)	9.0 (1.1)	25.9 (1.8)	18.1 (1.1)
Hallucinogens	3.0 (1.2)	8.0 (1.5)	5.5 (0.9)	4.7 (1.3)	10.4 (1.6)	7.6 (1.0)	8.7 (1.5)	14.6 (1.7)	11.4 (1.2)	5.9 (0.9)	12.5 (1.2)	9.4 (0.8)
Inhalants	2.4 (1.2)	5.1 (1.2)	3.5 (0.8)	1.7 (0.6)	6.7 (1.3)	3.4 (0.7)	5.1 (1.2)	11.0 (1.8)	8.1 (0.7)	3.5 (0.7)	8.8 (1.1)	6.4 (0.7)
Heroin	0.4 (0.4)	1.5 (0.5)	1.1 (0.3)	0.2 (0.1)	3.6 (1.0)	2.0 (0.6)	1.4 (0.6)	5.3 (1.2)	3.2 (0.6)	0.8 (0.3)	4.0 (0.7)	2.5 (0.4)
Any illicit drug	16.6 (2.3)	36.8 (3.0)	27.2 (1.9)	20.3 (2.3)	45.1 (3.0)	32.3 (1.9)	32.8 (2.67)	57.0 (2.9)	43.5 (2.1)	23.2 (1.4)	46.3 (1.7)	37.9 (1.4)
Use of more than one drug	38.2 (7.4)	39.0 (6.3)	42.5 (4.0)	44.9 (4.8)	44.1 (4.9)	49.7 (3.5)	53.6 (4.6)	57.7 (4.0)	53.4 (3.1)	43.2 (3.9)	54.5 (2.9)	51.0 (2.4)

prevalence rates and standard errors for polydrug use. All gender and strata comparisons were statistically significant at $p \leq 0.05$. Lifetime prevalence of any illicit drug use was 46.3 percent for men and 23.2 percent for women. Urban rates were higher than rural for all drugs, for both women (32.8 percent versus 16.6 percent) and men (57.0 percent versus 36.8 percent). For the total sample, 46.7 percent of males had used marijuana compared to 23.7 percent of women. The prevalence of past-year marijuana use (not shown) was 13.7 percent for men and 4.7 percent for women. Lifetime cocaine prevalence rates were 25.9 percent for men and 9.0 percent for women. Previous-year rates for cocaine use were 6.4 percent for men and 1.4 percent for women. Multiple drug use was common, with 54.5 percent of men and 43.2 percent of women users reported using more than one drug. In addition, 89.7 percent of cocaine users reported using marijuana, and 45.0 percent of marijuana users also used cocaine (not shown).

Multivariate Analysis

Table 15.3 shows the adjusted odds ratios for marijuana, cocaine, and any illicit drug or inhalant use over the lifetime. Results are similar for the three drug use measures. Males had over four times greater likelihood of lifetime use of marijuana, cocaine, and illicit drugs or inhalants compared with women. Respondents 26 to 39 years of age had highest risk of cocaine use, compared with those 18 to 25 years of age. Respondents with children had increased risk of lifetime use of illicit drugs or inhalants compared with those who had no children. Being born in the United States, urban place of residence, and acculturation significantly increased the likelihood of illicit drug or inhalants, cocaine and marijuana use.

Similar results were obtained with three logistic regression models using as dependent variables past-year use of illicit drugs or inhalants, use of marijuana, and use of cocaine (not shown). Compared with females, males were about four times more likely to have used any illicit drugs or inhalants in the previous year (adjusted odds ratio [OR] = 4.67; 95 percent confidence intervals [CI] = 3.05–7.16) or marijuana (adjusted OR = 4.08; 95 percent CI = 2.61–6.38). Men were also over nine times more likely than women to have used cocaine in the previous year (adjusted OR = 9.79; 95 percent CI = 4.84–19.80).

Table 15.4 displays the most comprehensive model of lifetime use of illicit drugs or inhalants, including two-way interaction effects. Significant interaction effects were found between sex and nativity (chi square = 47, $df = 1$, $p < 0.001$), sex and acculturation (chi square = 8.5, $df = 1$, $p < 0.02$), and place of residence and acculturation (chi square = 10.3, $df = 2$, $p < 0.001$). Three-way interaction effects among sex, nativity, and acculturation were not significant.

The Effect of Nativity by Gender. The effect of nativity on the likelihood of lifetime use of illicit drugs or inhalants was greater among women than among

Table 15.3. Multiple Logistic Regression for Lifetime Use of Illicit Drugs or Inhalants, Cocaine, and Marijuana, According to Sociodemographic and Acculturation Characteristics, Mexican-Origin Population, Fresno County, California

	Any Illicit Drug: Adjusted OR (95% CI)	Cocaine: Adjusted OR (95% CI)	Marijuana: Adjusted OR (95% CI)
Sex			
Female	1	1	1
Male	4.75 (3.61–6.26)	5.28 (3.77–7.40)	4.29 (3.28–5.62)
Age (years)			
18–25	1	1	1
26–39	1.45 (0.99–2.12)	1.70 (1.15–2.49)	1.43 (0.97–2.13)
40–60	0.64 (0.41–0.99)	0.61 (0.37–1.03)	0.68 (0.44–1.07)
Marital status			
Not married	1	1	1
Married	0.76 (0.49–1.19)	0.75 (0.43–1.31)	0.98 (0.63–1.53)
Divorced/widowed	1.16 (0.66–2.04)	1.20 (0.57–2.52)	1.24 (0.70–2.20)
Children			
No	1	1	1
Yes	1.68 (1.04–2.73)	1.56 (0.88–2.75)	1.46 (0.89–2.38)
Income			
Mean	1	1	1
+1 SD	1.05 (0.93–1.18)	1.00 (0.87–1.16)	1.06 (0.94–1.9)
Education (years)			
12 or more	1	1	1
7–12	0.95 (0.69–1.32)	0.80 (0.54–1.18)	1.05 (0.76–1.45)
0–6	1.12 (0.77–1.65)	0.94 (0.61–1.44)	1.11 (0.76–1.62)
Acculturation			
Mean	1	1	1
+1 SD	1.75 (1.43–2.13)	1.65 (1.30–2.11)	1.76 (1.43–2.15)
Nativity			
Foreign	1	1	1
U.S. born	3.51 (2.49–4.95)	2.36 (1.44–3.14)	3.80 (2.70–5.34)
Place of residence			
Rural	1	1	1
Town	1.17 (0.82–1.66)	1.09 (0.73–1.61)	1.13 (0.80–1.60)
Urban	1.74 (1.28–2.38)	1.82 (1.25–2.67)	1.57 (1.15–2.16)

Table 15.4. Adjusted Odds Ratios and 95 Percent Confidence Intervals for Lifetime Use
of Illicit Drugs or Inhalants, According to Sex, Nativity Acculturation, and Place
of Residence, Mexican-Origin Population, Fresno County, California

	Lifetime Use of Illicit Drugs or Inhalants[a]	
	Adjusted OR	*(95% CI)*
Female		
Foreign born		
Acculturation (mean)/rural	1.00	
Acculturation (mean)/town	1.22	(0.86–1.74)
Acculturation (mean)/urban	1.62	(1.15–2.28)
Acculturation (+1 SD)/rural	2.21	(1.49–3.27)
Acculturation (+1 SD)/town	2.34	(1.47–3.71)
Acculturation (+1 SD)/urban	4.66	(2.89–7.50)
U.S. born		
Acculturation (mean)/rural	6.27	(3.36–11.73)
Acculturation (mean)/town	7.66	(3.79–15.49)
Acculturation (mean)/urban	10.19	(5.15–20.13)
Acculturation (+1 SD)/rural	13.84	(8.25–23.22)
Acculturation (+1 SD)/town	14.67	(8.28–26.00)
Acculturation (+1 SD)/urban	29.26	(16.53–51.80)
Male		
Foreign born		
Acculturation (mean)/rural	1.00	
Acculturation (mean)/town	1.22	(0.86–1.74)
Acculturation (mean)/urban	1.62	(1.15–2.28)
Acculturation (+1SD)/rural	1.45	(1.04–2.04)
Acculturation (+1SD)/town	1.54	(1.02–2.33)
Acculturation (+1SD)/urban	3.07	(2.05–4.61)
U.S. born		
Acculturation (mean)/rural	2.40	(1.57–3.66)
Acculturation (mean)/town	2.93	(1.68–5.11)
Acculturation (mean)/urban	3.89	(2.27–6.67)
Acculturation (+1SD)/rural	3.49	(2.31–5.26)
Acculturation (+1SD)/town	3.70	(2.27–6.02)
Acculturation (+1SD)/urban	7.38	(4.56–11.93)

[a]Multiple regression model also includes the following variables: age, marital status, children, income, employment, and education.

men. Being born in the United States increased women's odds of lifetime illicit drugs or inhalants use by more than six times (adjusted OR, 6.27) compared with foreign-born women. However, the risk for U.S.-born men was only 2.4 times greater (adjusted OR = 2.40) than for foreign-born men.

The Effect of Acculturation by Gender. The effect of acculturation on lifetime use of illicit drugs or inhalants was stronger for women than for men. U.S.- and foreign-born women with acculturation 1 SD above the mean had more than four times the risk of women with mean acculturation (adjusted OR = 4.66). Among men, acculturation increased the risk of illicit drug use by three times (adjusted OR = 3.07).

The Effect of Urban Residence by Acculturation. The main effect of urban residence was not significant. However, acculturation had a more acute effect on urban than on rural residents, men and women alike. Acculturated (+1 SD) urban respondents had significantly higher risk of having ever used illicit drugs or inhalants than acculturated rural respondents (adjusted OR = 2.11; 95 percent CI = 1.45–3.07; not shown).

The combined effect of nativity and acculturation was stronger for women than for men. The likelihood of lifetime use of illicit drugs or inhalants was almost thirty times greater (adjusted OR = 29.26) for acculturated U.S.-born urban women compared with rural foreign-born women, with mean acculturation levels. Among urban men, the combined effect of acculturation and nativity resulted in about eight times greater risk (adjusted OR = 7.4), compared with rural foreign-born men with mean acculturation levels.

Nevertheless, compared with women, men had far greater lifetime use of illicit drugs or inhalants. Table 15.5 shows adjusted odds ratios and 95 percent confidence intervals for lifetime use of illicit drugs or inhalants for foreign-born and U.S.-born respondents by sex, acculturation, and place of residence. Among men, the combined effect of nativity, acculturation, and place of residence resulted in odds ratios over seventy times greater than for women who did not have any of these risk factors (adjusted OR = 75.45; 95 percent CI = 40.08–138.57).

DISCUSSION AND CONCLUSIONS

These findings suggest that Mexican American men and women have relatively high lifetime use ratios for illicit drugs and inhalants. Our results replicate the essential findings of the HHANES and LAECA (Karno and others, 1987; Amaro, Whitaker, Coffman, and Heeren, 1990) surveys, but also suggest that lifetime illicit drug use rates among men and women of Mexican origin have not

Table 15.5. Adjusted Odds Ratios and 95 Percent Confidence Intervals for Lifetime Use of Illicit Drugs or Inhalants, According to Nativity, Sex, Acculturation, and Place of Residence, Mexican-Origin Population, Fresno County, California (n = 2,828)

	Lifetime Use of Illicit Drugs or Inhalants[a]	
	Adjusted OR	(95% CI)
Foreign born		
Female		
Acculturation (mean)/rural	1.00	
Acculturation (mean)/town	1.23	(0.87–1.74)
Acculturation (mean)/urban	1.63	(1.16–2.30)
Acculturation (+1SD)/rural	2.21	(1.49–3.27)
Acculturation (+1SD)/town	2.34	(1.47–3.71)
Acculturation (+1SD)/urban	4.66	(2.90–7.51)
Male		
Acculturation (mean)/rural	10.23	(6.26–16.71)
Acculturation (mean)/town	12.49	(7.09–22.02)
Acculturation (mean)/urban	16.60	(9.34–29.49)
Acculturation (+1 SD)/rural	14.88	(8.22–26.94)
Acculturation (+1 SD)/town	15.77	(8.38–29.66)
Acculturation (+1 SD)/urban	31.45	(16.53–59.86)
U.S. born		
Female		
Acculturation (mean)/rural	6.28	(3.36–11.72)
Acculturation (mean)/town	7.66	(3.79–15.48)
Acculturation (mean)/urban	10.19	(5.15–20.13)
Acculturation (+1 SD)/rural	13.84	(8.25–23.23)
Acculturation (+1 SD)/town	14.67	(8.28–25.99)
Acculturation (+1 SD)/urban	29.26	(16.3–51.80)
Male		
Acculturation (mean)/rural	24.54	(13.10–42.72)
Acculturation (mean)/town	29.96	(15.95–56.28)
Acculturation (mean)/urban	39.82	(21.30–74.46)
Acculturation (+1 SD)/rural	35.69	(20.70–61.53)
Acculturation (+1 SD)/town	37.82	(20.84–68.62)
Acculturation (+1 SD)/urban	75.45	(41.08–138.57)

[a]Multiple regression model also includes the following variables: age, marital status, children, income, employment, and education.

decreased in the past decade. Using the HHANES data, Amaro, Whitaker, Coffman, and Heeren (1990) had previously reported lifetime rates of marijuana use of 48.8 percent for men and 19.4 percent for women (Fresno men 45.7 percent, women 23.7 percent). Lifetime cocaine prevalence rates in this study were higher than those reported in the HHANES for Mexican Americans (HHANES men, 19.6 percent versus Fresno men 25.9 percent; HHANES women, 6.4 percent versus Fresno women 9.0 percent). However, current use levels may be lower. For example, a comparison with the HHANES past-year prevalence for marijuana showed lower rates for both women and men (HHANES women 6.6 percent versus Fresno, 4.7 percent; HHANES men 22.0 percent versus Fresno, 13.7 percent (Amaro, Whitaker, Coffman, and Heeren, 1990). Previous-year rates for cocaine use in Fresno were also lower than those from the HHANES (HHANES women 2.1 percent versus Fresno, 1.3 percent; HHANES, men 10.8 percent versus Fresno, 6.4 percent). Lifetime rates in the cohort between 26 and 39 years of age may have actually increased, especially for marijuana and cocaine. There appears to be a cohort effect attributable to the fact that individuals in this age group were adolescents in the peak drug use period of the 1970s.

Accelerated risk for illicit drug use is a consequence of the "Americanization" process on healthy development of adolescents and early adulthood among Mexican Americans (Vega, Hough, and Romero, 1983). Nativity, acculturation, and urban residence each contribute to increases in illicit drug use, with nativity having the strongest risk and protective effects. The finding of a more pronounced effect of acculturation among women than men is similar to results reported by Amaro, Whitaker, Coffman, and Heeren (1990). Low acculturation is protective even in urban settings for the foreign and U.S. born.

Apparently, socialization in the United States has deep, erosive effects on protective family and environmental socialization against drug use, particularly on the disreputable definition given to illicit drug use in Mexican culture. This effect is compounded by U.S. nativity, especially among women. These results are fundamentally similar to the effects of acculturation and nativity on alcohol use (Gilbert, 1991; Zapata and Katims, 1994; Lavato and others, 1994; Welte and Barnes, 1995). Alcohol and drug use rates are far lower in Mexico (Caetano and Medina-Mora, 1989; Medina-Mora and others, 1989). Public drinking for Mexican women is considered a negative reflection on moral character, but this influence weakens among the U.S. born, especially if they are highly acculturated (Markides, Krause, and Menendez de Leon, 1988). Mexican men, by contrast, drink less frequently than their U.S.-born counterparts but are known for "fiesta drinking," or consuming large quantities on special occasions. This is similar to the pattern we report: Mexican men are more likely to be lifetime users of illicit drugs than Mexican women but also have lower lifetime rates than those who are U.S. born. Acculturation effects on illicit drug use over multiple generations of Mexican Americans remain unknown. Paradoxically, the rapid increase in the foreign-born component of the Mexican-origin population will have the effect of lowering past-year prevalence for the total Mexican American population, especially in California, where Mexican immigrants constitute 50 percent of the total. However, this impact may be less obvious in lifetime rates because of the progressive increments in lifetime illicit drug use among immigrants over time.

Future comparative studies may explore how acculturation is related to predisposing socialization and risk behaviors among Mexican Americans, with a special focus on child and adolescent development. Since immigrants have far lower illicit drug use levels than the American population, it would be useful to identify the reasons for these differences by examining key aspects of early socialization (Gil and Vega, 1996). Recommended areas for research include perceptions of personal achievement as well as economic and educational attainment; sibling and peer attitudes about drug use; gender roles and relationships among family members, spouses, girlfriends, and boyfriends; family process and social support; shared identity, cultural pride, and collective orientation; and experiences of discrimination and racism (Mayers, Kail, and Watts, 1993; Moore, 1994; Felix-Ortiz and Newcomb, 1995). While it is impossible to prevent acculturation into American society, it may be feasible to design interventions that decrease exposure to risk factors for illicit drug use or reinforce culturally based protective factors.

References

Amaro, H., Whitaker, R., Coffman, G., and Heeren, T. "Acculturation and Marijuana and Cocaine Use: Findings from HHANES 1982–84." *American Journal of Public Health,* 1990, *80*(Suppl.), 54–60.

Burnam, M. A., and others. "Acculturation and Lifetime Prevalence of Psychiatric Disorders Among Mexican Americans in Los Angeles." *Journal of Health and Social Behavior,* 1987, *28*, 89–102.

Caetano, R., and Medina-Mora, M. E. "Acculturation and Drinking Among People of Mexican Descent in Mexico and the United States." *Journal of Studies in Alcohol,* 1989, *49*, 462–470.

Chavez, E. L., Beauvais, F., and Oetting, E. R. "Drug Use by Small Town Mexican American Youth: A Pilot Study." *Hispanic Journal of Behavioral Sciences,* 1986, *8*, 243–258.

Cobas, J. A., and others. "Acculturation and Low-Birthweight Infants Among Latino Women: A Reanalysis of HHANES data with Structural Equation Models." *American Journal of Public Health,* 1996, *86*, 394–396.

Cuellar, I., Harris, L. C., and Jasso, R. "An Acculturation Scale for Mexican Normal and Clinical Populations." *Hispanic Journal of Behavioral Sciences,* 1980, *2*, 199–217.

De la Rosa, M. R., Khalasa, J. H., and Rouse, B. A. "Hispanics and Illicit Drug Use: A Review of Recent Findings." *International Journal of the Addictions,* 1990, *25,* 665–691.

Felix-Ortiz, M., and Newcomb, M. D. "Cultural Identity and Drug Use Among Latino and Latina Adolescents." In G. J. Botvin, S. Schinke, and M. A. Orlandi (eds.), *Drug Abuse Prevention with Multiethnic Youth.* Thousand Oaks, Calif.: Sage, 1995.

Gil, A. G., and Vega, W. A. "Two Different Worlds: Acculturation Stress and Adaptation Among Cuban and Nicaraguan Families." *Journal of Social Personal Relationships,* 1996, *13,* 437–458.

Gilbert, M. J. "Acculturation and Changes in Drinking Patterns Among Mexican-American Women." *Alcohol Health & Research World,* 1991, *15*(3), 234–238.

Kail, B. L., and Watts, T. D. "Patterns and Predictors of Drug Abuse Within the Chicano Community." In R. S. Mayars, B. L. Kail, and T. D. Watts (eds.), *Hispanic Substance Abuse.* Springfield, Ill.: Charles C. Thomas, 1993.

Karno, M., and others. "Lifetime Prevalence of Specific Psychiatric Disorders Among Mexican Americans and Non-Hispanic Whites in Los Angeles." *Archives of General Psychiatry,* 1987, *44,* 695–701.

Koury, E. L., and others. "Gender and Ethnic Differences in the Prevalence of Alcohol, Cigarette, and Illicit Drug Use over Time in a Cohort of Young Hispanic Adolescents in South Florida." *Women and Health,* 1996, *24,* 21–40.

Lavato, C. Y., and others. "Cigarette and Alcohol Use Among Migrant Hispanic Adolescents." *Family and Community Health,* 1994, *24,* 21–40.

Markides, K., Krause, N., and Menendez de Leon, C. "Acculturation and Alcohol Consumption Among Mexican-Americans: A Three Generation Study." *American Journal of Public Health,* 1988, *78,* 1178–1181.

Mayers, R. S., Kail, B. L., and Watts, T. D. (eds.). *Hispanic Substance Abuse.* Springfield, Ill.: Charles C. Thomas, 1993.

Medina-Mora, M. E., and others. "Extension del consumo de drogas en Mexico: Escuela Nacional de Adicciones. Resultados nacionales [A study of the scope of the consumption of drugs in Mexico]." *Salud Mental,* 1989, *12,* 7–12.

Moore, J. "The *Chola* Life Course: Chicana Heroin Users and the Barrio Gang." *International Journal of the Addictions,* 1994, *29,* 1115–1125.

National Center on Addiction and Substance Abuse. *Substance Abuse and the American Woman.* New York: Columbia University, 1996.

National Institute on Drug Abuse. *Hispanic Health and Nutrition Examination Survey: Use of Selected Drugs Among Hispanics.* Rockville, Md.: U.S. Government Printing Office, 1987.

Robins, L. N., Helzer, J. E., Croughan, J. L., and Ratcliff, K. S. "National Institute of Mental Health Diagnostic Interview Schedule: Its History, Characteristics and Validity." *Archives of General Psychiatry,* 1981, *38,* 381–389.

Robins, L. N., and others. "The Composite International Diagnostic Interview: An Epidemiologic Instrument Suitable for Use in Conjunction with Different Diagnostic Systems and in Different Cultures." *Psychiatry,* 1988, *45,* 1069–1077.

SAMSA Drug Abuse Warning Network. *Preliminary Estimates of Drug Related Emergency Department Episodes, Jan–June 1995.* Rockville, Md.: Office of Applied Studies, Department of Health and Human Services, 1996.

U.S. Department of Health and Human Services, Substance Abuse and Mental Health Services. *National Household Survey on Drug Abuse: Main Findings.* Rockville, Md.: Department of Health and Human Services, Substance Abuse and Mental Health Services, 1993.

United Way of Fresno. *Vision 20/20: Snapshot of Fresno County.* Fresno, Calif.: United Way of Fresno, 1996.

Vega, W. A., and Gil, A. G. *Drug Use and Ethnicity in Early Adolescence.* New York: Plenum Press, 1998.

Vega, W. A., Hough, R. L., and Romero, A. "Family Life Patterns Among Mexican Americans." In G. Powell and others (eds.), *The Psychosocial Development of Minority Group Children.* New York: Brunner/Mazel, 1983.

Vega, W. A., Kolody, B., Noble, A., and Porter, P. "Perinatal Drug Abuse Among Immigrant and Native Born Latinas." *Substance Use and Misuse,* 1997, *32,* 43–60.

Vega, W. A., and others. *Profile of Alcohol and Drug Use During Pregnancy in California, 1992.* Sacramento: State of California, Health and Welfare Agency, Department of Alcohol and Drug Programs, 1993a.

Vega, W. A., and others. "Acculturation Strain Theory: Its Application in Explaining Drug Use Behavior Among Cuban and Other Hispanic Youth." In M. De la Rosa and J. L. Recio (eds.), *Drug Abuse Among Minority Youth.* Rockville, Md.: National Institute of Drug Abuse, 1993b.

Wagner-Etchegaray, F. A., Schutz, C. G., Chilcoat, H. D., and Anthony, J. C. "Degree of Acculturation and the Risk of Crack Cocaine Smoking Among Hispanic Americans." *American Journal of Public Health,* 1994, *84,* 1825–1827.

Warner, L. A., and others. "Prevalence and Correlates of Drug Use and Dependence in the United States." *Archives of General Psychiatry,* 1995, *52,* 219–229.

Welte, J. W., and Barnes, G. M. "Alcohol and Other Drug Use Among Hispanics in New York State." *Alcoholism: Clinical and Experimental Research,* 1995, *19,* 1061–1066.

Wittchen, H. U., and others. "Cross-Cultural Feasibility, Reliability and Sources of Variance of the Composite International Diagnostic Interview (CIDI)." *British Journal of Psychiatry,* 1991, *159,* 645–653.

Zambrana, R. E., and Scrimshaw, S. C. "Maternal Psychosocial Factors Associated with Substance Use in Mexican-Origin and African-American Low-Income Pregnant Women." *Pediatric Nursing,* 1997, *23,* 253–259.

Zapata, J., and Katims, D. S. Antecedents of Substance Use Among Mexican-American School-Age Children." *Journal of Drug Education,* 1994, *24,* 233–251.

CHAPTER SIXTEEN

Substance Abuse Treatment

Critical Issues and Challenges in the Treatment of Latina Women

Hortensia Amaro
Rita Nieves
Sergut Wolde Johannes
Nirzka M. Labault Cabeza

The findings in this study, based on a small sample of Latinas in a residential substance abuse treatment program, confirm previous observations regarding the importance of gender-appropriate treatment approaches for women, but with their own focus on Latinas. The findings also demonstrate the importance of a comprehensive assessment to identify comorbidity among Latinas with substance abuse. Recommendations for treating Latinas and areas in need of additional research provide important contributions to work on substance abuse and treatment issues confronting Latinas.

Among both Latinos and non-Latinos in the United States, addiction has long been considered a "male disease," and much of the research in this field has been based on male samples or has included women but has not investigated gender differences in the nature and course of addiction (Blumenthal, 1998; Kandall, 1998a, 1998b). Yet it is estimated that more than 4.4 million women in the United States need treatment for drug use (National Institute on Drug Abuse, 1994). Although Latinos represent the second-fastest-growing population in the United States, few studies of drug addiction among Latinas appear in the literature (Anglin, Hser, and Booth, 1987; Anglin, Hser, and McGlothlin, 1987; Moore and Dewitt, 1989; Moore and Mata, 1981).

Most research on Latino substance use has focused on alcohol use rather than on illicit drug use. This body of work indicates that heavy drinking among Latinas is significantly lower than that of Latino men (Caetano, 1990). Yet data on illicit drug use suggest a different picture. Data from the National Institute on Drug Abuse (1989) indicate that although Latinas report lower rates of alcohol use than non-Hispanic Whites, they report similar rates of cocaine use and higher rates of crack use than non-Hispanic White women. Data from the Hispanic Health and Nutrition Examination Study (Amaro, Whitaker, Coffman, and Heeren, 1990) indicate important differences between Hispanic groups in illicit drug use, wherein Puerto Ricans living in the U.S. mainland have the highest rates in comparison to other Hispanic groups. Furthermore, a number of studies indicate that increased acculturation is associated with higher rates of illicit drug use among Hispanics (Amaro, Whitaker, Coffman, and Heeren, 1990; Booth, Castro, and Anglin, 1990). The latest data from Monitoring the Future Study indicate that Hispanic youth have rates of drug use that are similar to that of non-Hispanic Whites (National Institute on Drug Abuse, 1998). In lower grades, Hispanic youth have higher use of cocaine, crack, and marijuana than other groups (National Institute on Drug Abuse, 1998). Even among high school seniors who are a select group that does not include dropouts, Hispanics have the highest prevalence of cocaine and crack use (National Institute on Drug Abuse, 1998). Initiation of substance use is important because it is a major predictor of substance abuse disorders in adulthood (Kandel, Warner, and Kessler, 1998).

Biological, psychological, and social consequences of alcohol and drug addiction are also known to vary for women and men (National Institute on Drug Abuse, 1998). Compared to men, women suffer disproportionately from the consequences of addiction. For example, female alcoholics have death rates that are 50 to 100 percent higher than those of male alcoholics (National Institute on Alcohol Abuse and Alcoholism, 1990). Women also have different treatment needs compared to men. For example, studies have indicated that compared to men, women enter treatment with fewer educational and job-related skills (Beckman and Amaro, 1984, 1986; Wallen, 1998). Women—even women who are addicted to alcohol or drugs—continue to be the primary caretaker of children; thus, child treatment and parenting training have also been noted as critical elements of women's treatment (Beckman and Amaro, 1984, 1986; National Institute on Drug Abuse, 1998).

Another clinically significant gender difference is the prevalence of comorbidity of drug dependence with other psychiatric disorders. Compared to men, women are much more likely to have comorbid psychiatric conditions of anxiety disorders and affective disorders (Brady and Sonne, 1995; Hesselbrock, Meyer, and Keener, 1985; Kandel, Warner, and Kessler, 1998). Depression and anxiety disorders, which are known to be more prevalent in women (Culbertson, 1997; Nolen-Hoeksema, 1987; Silverman, 1968), have also been found to increase the risk of abuse of alcohol and nonprescription drugs (Christie and others, 1988). The higher rate of psychiatric comorbidity among women has significance for substance abuse treatment because it is a major predictor of treatment outcome. Individuals with comorbidity have higher levels of impairment (Stoffelmayr and others, 1989) and have poorer treatment outcomes (Safer, 1987).

Posttraumatic stress disorder, often resulting from sexual or physical abuse, has also been found to be more prevalent in women compared to men (Helzer, Robins, and McEvoy, 1987). A review of data on victimization, posttraumatic stress disorder, and substance use and abuse by Kilpatrick and colleagues (Kilpatrick, Resnick, Saunders, and Best, 1998, p. 285) noted, "Substance use disorders are more prevalent in individuals with a history of criminal victimization." Recent data in the literature indicate that compared to men, women substance users report higher rates of sexual abuse (Brady, Grice, Dustan, and Randall, 1993; National Institute on Drug Abuse, 1994; Rohsenow, Corbett, and Devine, 1988; Wallen, 1992) and that sexual abuse increases the risk of psychiatric and substance use disorders (Kilpatrick, Resnick, Saunders, and Best, 1998; Winfield, George, Swartz, and Blazer, 1990). In addition, the study by Kilpatrick, Resnick, Saunders, and Best (1998) revealed that the risk of new assaults is increased by substance abuse. These studies clearly establish the high prevalence of history of victimization among women with substance abuse dependence and the importance of this factor in women's substance abuse treatment.

The aims of this study are to describe the history of childhood abuse (emotional, physical, and sexual), mental health problems, and medical problems in a sample of Latinas in residential treatment for substance abuse dependence and to discuss the implications of these issues for the treatment of Latina women.

METHODS

Participants

The study population includes all clients ($n = 66$) admitted to a residential substance abuse treatment program for Latina mothers and their children in Boston between May 1986 and December 1989. After being informed of the study by a Latina researcher, all clients agreed to participate. A certificate of confidentiality was obtained to protect clients' interviews from being subpoenaed. The internal review board of the agency where the study took place approved the research.

The Treatment Context

All participants were residents of a twelve-month gender- and culturally specific residential substance abuse treatment program for Latina mothers and their children. Clients are referred to the program through detoxification programs, social service agencies, courts, and correctional facilities and enter of their own free will and are free to leave the program at any time. The program provides comprehensive services including (1) individual counseling; (2) case management; (3) psychoeducational and group counseling on substance abuse, relapse prevention, family relationships, parenting, life skills, health education, family dynamics, trauma, self-esteem, and relationships; (4) linkage to medical, psychiatric, mental health, social, educational, and vocational services; (5) family reunification services; and (6) children's services including therapeutic child care; case management; individual and group play therapy; and linkage to medical, psychiatric, mental health, and specialized developmental interventions. Treatment is organized into four phases, which are based on client progress through specific recovery and behavioral goals. Phase 1 is crisis stabilization, orientation to the residential treatment community, and assessment; Phase 2 is carrying out a specific plan of activities to change cognitive and behavioral patterns of addiction to those who are supportive of recovery; Phase 3 is continued focus on relapse prevention, increased responsibilities within and outside the residential setting, and engagement in educational, vocational, and community service activities; and Phase 4 is preparation for transition to community living and assuming a leadership role within the residential community. Services in the program are provided by an interdisciplinary team of bilingual and bicultural professional and para-professional staff.

Procedure

A trained Latina researcher conducted interviews in a private office in the treatment program, which lasted approximately one hour. The interview was composed of closed-ended questions on demographic characteristics, history of drug use, drug treatment, childhood or adolescent abuse, medical and mental health problems, and criminal justice involvement.

Instruments

The intake assessment interview was developed for a national cross-site study of treatment outcomes for programs funded by the Substance Abuse, Mental Health Services Administration (National Evaluation Data and Technical Assistance Center, 1999). The program in which the clients received services is part of an ongoing national study. The variables used in this analysis are described below.

The interview gathered self-reported information on the following demographic variables: age (continuous), Latino group (Puerto Rican, Dominican, Cuban, Mexican, Central American, South American, and other), preferred language (English, Spanish), education (less than eighth grade, ninth through twelfth grade, high school graduate, some college, college graduate), employment status prior to entry into the program (employed, not employed), and number of children (continuous). In addition, the interview obtained self-reported information on the history of (1) abuse in childhood and/or adolescence (yes/no); (2) relationship to abuser (parent, family member, nonfamily member, other); (3) primary drug of choice (cocaine/crack, heroin, alcohol, other); (4) age at first use (continuous); (5) major health problems in the year prior (presence of health problems related to respiratory system, tuberculosis, hepatitis, nervous system, sexually transmitted diseases, HIV/AIDS, and other were collapsed into yes/no categories); (6) history of major mental health problems in the year prior (antisocial personality, anxiety disorder, bipolar disorder, depression, eating disorder, and psychological trauma were collapsed into yes/no categories); (7) history of involvement with the criminal justice system (yes/no); (8) substance abuse treatment in the year prior (yes/no); and (9) type of treatment received (detoxification program, inpatient hospital program, in jail, residential program, and outpatient). Program phase completed by participants was also measured (coded into three phases). These phases were reflective of achieved treatment goals and treatment progress. The interview protocol was translated into Spanish by a trained Latina researcher and reviewed by individuals familiar with the various Latino groups represented in the sample. The instrument was finalized after field testing.

Data Analysis

Descriptive statistics are presented to profile the sample. Comparisons of clients with and without a history of childhood abuse were conducted using chi-square analysis (categorical variables) and t-tests (continuous variables).

RESULTS

Table 16.1 presents the demographic profile of the sample. The majority of participants were Puerto Rican mothers between the ages of 18 and 30, who were not married, had not completed high school, and were not employed just prior to program entry. Almost half did not have stable housing (for example, homeless, shelter, institution, staying temporarily with friends or family members). All participants were mothers, and the majority had three or more children. The most common drug of choice was cocaine/crack, followed by heroin. Approximately three-fourths had been in treatment prior to this admission. Nearly half of the sample reported involvement with the criminal justice system, more than two-thirds reported a past year history of health problems, two thirds reported a past-year history of mental health problems, and more than two-thirds reported childhood history of abuse. In 87 percent of cases, participants reported a combination of two or more major risk characteristics.

Abuse in childhood or adolescence was reported by 80.3 percent of participants, wherein emotional, physical, and sexual abuse were equally common and usually co-occurring (see Table 16.1). Related to this was also the finding of multiple sources of abuse. The sources of sexual abuse were reported to be fathers (79 percent), relatives (85 percent), and nonrelatives (13 percent). The sources of emotional abuse were reported to be mothers (87 percent), fathers (81 percent), and relatives (23 percent). The sources of physical abuse were mothers (90 percent), fathers (85 percent), relatives (15 percent), and nonrelatives (2 percent). Thus,

Table 16.1. Sample Profile ($n = 66$)

Variable	Number	Percentage
Hispanic group		
Puerto Rican	52	78.79
Cuban	2	3.03
Dominican	7	10.60
Other	5	7.56
Primary language		
English	36	54.54
Spanish	30	45.45
Age		
18–19	2	3.03
20–24	15	22.73
25–29	17	25.76
30–34	16	24.24
35 and older	16	24.24
Marital status		
Married	8	12.12
Separated or divorced	18	27.27
Single	38	57.58
Missing	2	3.03
Level of education		
Less than sixth grade	5	7.57
Seventh to twelfth grade	44	66.67
High school graduate or GED	8	12.12
Vocational or college	6	9.09
Missing	3	4.55
Employment prior to treatment entry		
Employed	3	4.55
Not employed	63	95.45
Housing one year prior to admission		
Stable housing	34	51.51
Unstable housing	28	42.42
Missing	4	6.06
Number of children		
Fewer than two children	20	30.30
Three to four children	28	42.42
Five or more children	18	27.27

Table 16.1. (Continued)

Variable	Number	Percentage
Primary drug		
Cocaine/crack	32	48.48
Heroin	24	36.36
Alcohol	10	15.15
Substance abuse treatment in the prior year	49	75.38
Type of treatment received		
Detoxification	19	38.77
Inpatient	21	42.86
Outpatient	9	18.37
Criminal justice involvement	28	42.42
Mental health problems in prior year	50	75.76
Type of mental health diagnosis (multiple possible)		
Antisocial personality	1	2.00
Anxiety	13	26.00
Bipolar	8	16.00
Depression	35	70.00
Eating disorder	5	10.00
Psychological trauma	13	26.00
Medical problems in prior year	45	68.18
Type of medical problems (multiple possible)		
Respiratory system (asthma, bronchitis)	24	53.33
Tuberculosis	3	6.67
Hepatitis	4	8.89
Nervous system (seizures, blackouts)	6	13.33
Sexually transmitted diseases	5	11.11
HIV or AIDS	3	6.67
History of childhood abuse	53	80.30
Type of abuse		
Emotional	47	88.68
Physical	48	90.57
Sexual	48	90.57
Age at first experimentation with illegal drugs		
$n = 66$		
Range (low, high) = (9, 42)		
$M = 19.12$		
$SD = 6.21$		

the vast majority of participants who reported abuse experienced both multiple types of abuse (98.1 percent) as well as multiple sources of abuse (94.3 percent).

Table 16.2 shows results of comparisons between participants with a history of childhood and adolescent abuse history and those without such history.

Table 16.2. History of Abuse and Background, and Medical and Mental Health Problems (in percentages)

Variable	Abuse (n = 53)	No Abuse (n = 13)	p
Hispanic group			.85
Puerto Rican	79.25	76.92	
Other Hispanic	20.75	23.08	
Language			.01
Spanish	62.26	23.08	
English	37.74	76.92	
Age at program entry	30.26	27	11
Education			.56
Less than high school	76.92	69.23	
More than high school	23.08	30.76	
Number of children			.08
Fewer than four	67.92	92.31	
Four or more	32.08	7.69	
Drug of choice			.45
Cocaine/crack	46.15	53.85	
Heroin	40.38	23.08	
Alcohol	13.46	23.08	
No substance abuse treatment in prior year	73.58	83.33	.48
Type of treatment (n = 49)			.07
Detoxification	30.77	70.00	
Inpatient or residential	48.72	20.00	
Outpatient	20.51	10.00	
Criminal justice involvement	47.17	23.08	.12
Mental health problems	73.58	84.62	.41
Health problems	75.47	38.46	.01
Child removed from custody	57	15	.008
Age at first illicit drug use			.67
Range (low, high)	(9, 42)	(12, 29)	
M	18.98	19.90	
SD	6.45	5.08	

Results indicate that women with a history of abuse were more likely to be predominantly Spanish speakers ($p = .01$), report significantly higher levels of health problems ($p = .01$), and have children removed from their custody ($p = .008$). Other trends that did not reach statistical significance, perhaps due to the sample size, suggest that those with a history of abuse were more likely to have been in inpatient or outpatient treatment in the year prior to program entry, whereas those who were not abused were more likely to have only received detoxification treatment ($p = .07$). Another trend in the data suggests that those with a history of abuse were also were somewhat more likely to have more children ($p = .08$) and to be somewhat older than those who were not abused ($p = .11$).

A comparison of those with a history of abuse and those without such a history indicates a significant difference in the phase of the program completed ($p = .01$). Women who reported a history of abuse had higher rates of dropping out of treatment in the first place (75 percent). In contrast, those without a history of abuse had higher rates of completion of the last two phases of treatment (69 percent) compared to those with a history of abuse (11 percent).

DISCUSSION AND IMPLICATIONS FOR TREATMENT

To identify treatment issues of special concern, this study sought to describe the profile of a sample of sixty-six Latina women in a residential substance abuse treatment program. Because of the high prevalence of comorbidity of mental health and history of childhood and adolescent abuse in women (Brady and Sonne, 1995; Helzer, Robins, and McEvoy, 1987; Hesselbrock, Meyer, and Keener, 1985; Kandel, Warner, and Kessler, 1998) and the importance of these for treatment (Safer, 1987; Stoffelmayr and others, 1989), we were specifically interested in investigating whether these conditions were also highly prevalent among Latina women with substance abuse disorders.

The sample demographic profile demonstrates characteristics similar to those of Latina women entering substance abuse treatment programs statewide (Massachusetts Department of Public Health, 1998). The majority of participants were single heads of households, Puerto Rican mothers in their mid- to late twenties, with low educational attainment and had little employment experience. Nearly half had unstable housing situations. The most commonly reported drug of choice was cocaine/crack, and the majority had received prior substance abuse treatment.

A wide variety of studies have noted that women with substance abuse disorders, compared to similar men, have significantly lower levels of education and job-related skills and experience (Amaro, Beckman, and Mays, 1987; Beckman and Amaro, 1984, 1986; Robles and others, 1998; Wallen, 1998). These findings highlight the importance of including services in substance abuse treatment that connect Latina women to GED and other educational opportunities and to job training and job placement services. Latina women in our sample faced not only the challenge of recovery from addiction but also building English-language skills, completing their basic education, and gaining job-related skills and experiences that would enable them to build economic self-sufficiency once they exited the program. Recent reforms in welfare make it more critical than ever before that substance abuse treatment programs address these issues. Poor Latina mothers in recovery, even those with small children, face lessened government support and the pressing need to find employment.

Nearly half of the women in our sample were living in highly unstable conditions prior to program entry. Many were temporarily staying with family members or friends, whereas others came from jail, shelters, or other residential and transitional programs. Among those who had an apartment that they rented, many were living in public housing, which are often characterized by high rates of drug dealing and crime. Shortage of affordable and drug-free housing in many large urban areas makes it difficult for women in recovery to find stable housing after completion of residential treatment. In addition, discrimination by landlords based on history of drug dependence creates additional barriers to housing. Case management to assist women in finding appropriate housing is an essential part of substance abuse treatment. Typically, long waiting periods for housing and for government housing vouchers require that this process be started at program entry. Public policy changes are needed to facilitate the process of locating appropriate housing for mothers completing residential treatment.

Similar to other studies (Kessler and others, 1996), we found a high rate of mental health problem in this sample of Latina women. However, the prevalence of mental health problems was much higher in this sample (80.3 percent) compared to that reported (approximately 50 percent) in national samples of women with drug dependence (Kessler and others, 1996). The most common mental health disorder among Latinas in this sample was depression. This contrasts to results from the National Comorbidity Study (Warner and Kessler, as cited in Kandel, Warner, and Kessler, 1998), which indicates that anxiety disorders are highest among women. The high level of comorbidity of mental health problems among Latina participants in this study brings up a challenge for treatment. It is evident that programs must include appropriate assessment and referral to mental health practitioners. The shortage of bilingual and culturally competent mental health practitioners as well as those trained in the comorbidity of addiction and mental illness can be a barrier to identifying and obtaining services for Latina clients. We have found that identification of even a few providers in the community who can meet this need is critical to the successful treatment of clients. We have also found that staff training on comorbidity and psychiatric conditions, information that is often not part of substance abuse counselor education, is essential. Such training can change traditional norms against psychotropic drug use that may be held by staff who have a history of working in other treatment programs.

As in other studies of women in substance abuse treatment (Kilpatrick, Resnick, Saunders, and Best, 1998; National Institute on Drug Abuse, 1994; Nelson-Zlupko, Kauffman, and Dore, 1995; Wallen, 1992), we found that an overwhelming majority (80.3 percent) of Latinas in this sample had a history of abuse in childhood or adolescence. In this sample of Latina women in treatment, the rate of diagnosis of psychological trauma (26 percent), however, was significantly lower than the reported history of childhood abuse (80.3 percent). We also did not find a significant difference between those with a history of abuse and those without it in previous-year history of mental health problems. This suggests a possible underidentification and diagnosis of women with posttraumatic stress disorder as well as other mental health problems among women with a history of abuse. Alternatively, it is possible that some portion of women in our sample experienced abuse in childhood or adolescence but did not meet the criteria for posttraumatic stress disorder. For many women, history of abuse preceded onset of substance abuse–related problems and is clearly an underlying aspect of their addiction and should be addressed as part of their recovery process. As in the case of other psychiatric comorbidity, appropriate assessment and referral to specialists need to be part of substance abuse treatment. Here, again, we found specific challenges to identifying personnel trained in treatment of abuse who were also bilingual and knowledgeable of the Latino culture. Our approach to this dilemma has been to work with community providers trained in the treatment of trauma and also to train in-house staff on issues of trauma. An additional challenge in handling issues of abuse among Latina women is the particularly strong cultural norms against speaking about issues of family abuse (Gil and Vasquez, 1997). When the abuse is by a male partner, traditional culturally based gender norms can also make it especially difficult for women to even name their experience as abuse and to talk about it (Gil and Vasquez, 1997). We have found that psychoeducational group approaches that do not force women to speak of their experiences but that provide information and build understanding about emotional and physical boundaries, intimacy and mutuality, self-esteem, a sense of empowerment and choices in relationships, family myths and secrets, and forgiveness work best with Latina women in recovery (see Harris, 1998).

The majority of Latina women in our sample also experienced major health problems. Similar findings have been reported among other samples of women with substance abuse dependence (Curtis, Lenz, and Frei, 1993; Nyamathi, Stein, and Brecht, 1998; Wallen, 1998). Close working relationships with medical care providers is critical for the comprehensive care of women in recovery. In this program, an initial health examination is conducted as part of the assessment process, and case management for medical problems is conducted through the entire process of treatment. In addition, health education regarding all aspects of women's health, especially sexuality and reproductive health, is essential. Yet such education is often not included in women's treatment programs (Nelson-Zlupko, Dore, Kauffman, and Kaltenbach, 1996).

A central feature of the profile of Latinas in our sample was their role as mothers. Nearly three-fourths of our sample had three or more children. Although only 39 percent entered treatment with their children, for most women, entering treatment was motivated by the desire to improve their relationship with their children. Mothers who did not have custody of their children upon treatment entry typically prioritized regaining custody of their children as their primary immediate treatment goal. Although the opportunity for mothers to have their children with them during treatment is a major motivator for entering treatment among diverse groups of women (Colten, 1980), the centrality of the mother role in Latino cultures (Gil and Vasquez, 1997) may make this an especially relevant factor for Latina women. For this reason, it is especially critical for substance abuse treatment programs serving Latinas to provide services that support appropriate family reunification, facilities that allow children to live in the program with their mothers, child treatment services, child care, and parenting education and training. Although these same services are often found to be lacking in programs that serve women (Beckman and Amaro, 1984, 1986; Blume, 1988; Institute of Medicine, 1990; Wilsnack, 1991), evidence indicates that provision of these services improves outcomes for women and their children (Kumpfer, 1998). In our experience, provision of comprehensive services for children, not just live-in services for children, is essential as motivators for Latina mothers to enter treatment and for addressing the multiple and complex issues of adjustment and development that their children face. We have found that a family-focused model of treatment is well suited for Latinas. This has required training of counselors and other staff on child development, behavior management, child maltreatment, and parenting support. To accommodate the needs of children in a residential setting, the entire milieu, not just targeted children's services, needs to be child friendly and appropriate.

The profile of participants in this study indicates the need for a comprehensive approach to treatment of addiction among Latina women. Comprehensive treatment models, with many of the components described and suggested here, have been identified as the standard of care for women (Center for Substance Abuse Treatment, 1994; Goldberg, 1995; Institute of Medicine, 1990; Mactas, 1998). The most significant obstacle to comprehensive treatment for women, including Latina women, is the system of payment for these services. Common obstacles to the implementation of comprehensive models of care for women include (1) reimbursement rates that are insufficient to cover costs of care, (2) categorical funding that impedes blending of financial sources, (3) historical separation and somewhat antagonistic relationship of agencies responsible for funding and providing mental health and substance abuse services, and (4) an individualistic rather than family-focused approach to substance abuse treatment funding. Factors that disproportionately affect services for Latinas and their children also include (1) the lack of bilingual and culturally competent staff trained in the comorbidity of addiction, psychiatric disorders, and treatment of trauma and (2) lack of programs that specifically target Latina women and that can provide a culturally and linguistically sensitive approach to treatment.

This study provides data on a limited sample of Latina women in residential treatment, and its findings may not be generalizable to other populations or clients from other programs. The study sample size did not allow for multivariate analyses that would be useful in ascertaining the relative importance of multiple client characteristics in predicting treatment phase completion. This study also did not consider other factors, such as social support, that may be important in treatment retention.

Further research is needed on larger samples to more fully understand the problems of addiction among Latina women, their unique treatment issues, the characteristics that predict treatment outcomes, and the efficacy of varied approaches to substance abuse treatment in this population.

References

Amaro, H., Beckman, L. J., and Mays, V. M. "A Comparison of Black and White Women Entering Alcoholism Treatment." *Journal of Studies on Alcohol,* 1987, *48,* 220–227.

Amaro, H., Whitaker, R., Coffman, G., and Heeren, T. "Acculturation and Marijuana and Cocaine Use: Findings from the Hispanic HANES." *American Journal of Public Health,* 1990, *80,* 54–60.

Anglin, D., Hser, Y., and Booth, M. "Sex Differences in Addict Careers. 4. Treatment." *American Journal of Drug and Alcohol Abuse,* 1987, *13,* 253–280.

Anglin, D., Hser, Y., and McGlothlin, W. "Sex Differences in Addict Careers. 2. Becoming Addicted." *American Journal of Drug and Alcohol Abuse,* 1987, *13*(1/2), 59–71.

Beckman, L. J., and Amaro, H. "Patterns of Women's Use of Alcohol Treatment Agencies." In S. C. Wilsnack and L. J. Beckman (eds.), *Alcohol Problems in Women.* New York: Guilford, 1984.

Beckman, L. J., and Amaro, H. "Personal and Social Difficulties Faced by Males and Females Entering Alcoholism Treatment." *Journal of Studies on Alcohol,* 1986, *47,* 135–145.

Blume, S. B. *Alcohol/Drug Dependent Women: New Insights into Their Special Problems, Treatment, Recovery.* Minneapolis, Minn.: Johnson Institute, 1988.

Blumenthal, S. "Women and Substance Abuse: A New National Focus." In *National Institute on Drug Abuse, Drug Addiction Research and the Health of Women.*

Rockville, Md.: U.S. Department of Health and Human Services, National Institutes of Health, 1998.

Booth, M., Castro, F., and Anglin, D. *What Do We Know About Hispanic Substance Use? A Review of the Literature.* New Brunswick, N.J.: Rutgers University Press, 1990.

Brady, K. T., Grice, D. E., Dustan, L., and Randall, C. "Gender Differences in Substance Use Disorders." *American Journal of Psychiatry,* 1993, *150,* 1707–1711.

Brady, K. T., and Sonne, S. C. "The Relationship Between Substance Abuse and Bipolar Disorder." *Journal of Clinical Psychiatry,* 1995, *56*(Suppl. 3), 19–24.

Caetano, R. "Hispanic Drinking in the U.S.: Thinking in New Directions." *British Journal of Addiction,* 1990, *85,* 1231–1236.

Center for Substance Abuse Treatment. *Practical Approaches in the Treatment of Women Who Abuse Alcohol and Other Drugs.* Rockville, Md.: U.S. Department of Health and Human Services, SAMHSA, 1994.

Christie, K. A., and others. "Epidemiological Evidence for Early Onset of Mental Disorders and Higher Risk of Drug Abuse in Young Adults." *American Journal of Psychiatry,* 1988, *145,* 971–975.

Colten, M.E.A. "A Comparison of Heroin-Addicted and Non-Addicted Mothers: Their Attitudes, Beliefs and Parenting Experiences." In *Heroin-Addicted Parents and Their Children: Two Reports.* Rockville, Md.: National Institute on Drug Abuse, 1980.

Colten, M.E.A., and others. *Addicted Women, Family Dynamics, Self Perceptions, and Support Systems.* Rockville, Md.: National Institute on Drug Abuse, 1979.

Culbertson, F. M. "Depression and Gender." *American Psychologist,* 1997, *52,* 25–31.

Curtis, M. A., Lenz, K. M., and Frei, N. R. "Medical Evaluation of African American Women Entering Drug Treatment." *Journal of Addiction and Disease,* 1993, *12,* 29–44.

Gil, R. M., and Vasquez, C. I. *Maria Paradox: How Latinas Can Merge Old World Traditions with New World Self-Esteem.* Berkeley, Calif.: Berkeley Publishing, 1997.

Goldberg, M. E. "Substance-Using Women: False Stereotypes and Real Needs." *Social Work,* 1995, *40,* 789–798.

Harris, M. *Trauma Recovery and Empowerment.* New York: Free Press, 1998.

Helzer, J. E., Robins, L. N., and McEvoy, L. "Post-Traumatic Stress Disorder in the General Population." *New England Journal of Medicine,* 1987, *317,* 1630–1634.

Hesselbrock, M. N., Meyer, R. E., and Keener, J. J. "Psychopathology in Hospitalized Alcoholics." *Archives of General Psychiatry,* 1985, *42,* 1050–1055.

Institute of Medicine. *Treating Drug Problems.* Washington, D.C.: National Academy Press, 1990.

Kandall, S. R. "Women and Addiction in the United States—1850–1920." In *Drug Addiction Research and the Health of Women.* Rockville, Md.: U.S. Department of Health and Human Services, National Institutes of Health, 1998a.

Kandall, S. R. "Women and Addiction in the United States—1920-Present." In *National Institute on Drug Abuse, Drug Addiction Research and the Health of Women.*

Rockville, Md.: U.S. Department of Health and Human Services, National Institutes of Health, 1998b.

Kandel, D. B., Warner, L. A., and Kessler, R. C. "The Epidemiology of Substance Use and Dependence Among Women." In *National Institute on Drug Abuse, Drug Addiction Research and the Health of Women*. Rockville, Md.: U.S. Department of Health and Human Services, National Institutes of Health, 1998.

Kessler, R. C., and others. "The Epidemiology of Co-Occurring Mental Disorders and Substance Use Disorders in the National Comorbidity Survey: Implications for Prevention and Service Utilization." *American Journal of Orthopsychiatry,* 1996, *66,* 17–31.

Kilpatrick, D. G., Resnick, H. S., Saunders, B. E., and Best, C. L. "Victimization, Posttraumatic Stress Disorder, and Substance Use and Abuse Among Women." In *National Institute on Drug Abuse, Drug Addiction Research and the Health of Women*. Rockville, Md.: U.S. Department of Health and Human Services, National Institutes of Health, 1998.

Kumpfer, K. L. "Links Between Prevention and Treatment for Drug-Abusing Women and Their Children." In *National Institute on Drug Abuse, Drug Addiction Research and the Health of Women*. Rockville, Md.: U.S. Department of Health and Human Services, National Institutes of Health, 1998.

Mactas, D. "Treatment of Women with Substance Abuse Problems." In *National Institute on Drug Abuse, Drug Addiction Research and the Health of Women*. Rockville, Md.: U.S. Department of Health and Human Services, National Institutes of Health, 1998.

Massachusetts Department of Public Health, Bureau of Substance Abuse Services. *Overview 1998*. Boston: Massachusetts Department of Public Health, 1998.

Moore, J. W., and Dewitt, M. "Addicted Mexican-American Mothers." *Gender and Society,* 1989, *3,* 53–78.

Moore, J. W., and Mata, A. "Women and Heroin in Chicano Communities." Unpublished manuscript, Chicano Pinto Research Project, Los Angeles, 1981.

National Evaluation Data and Technical Assistance Center. "Minimum Evaluation Data Set: Cone Data Lists." Fairfax, Va., 1999.

National Institute on Alcohol Abuse and Alcoholism. "Alcohol and Women." *Alcohol Alert*. Bethesda, Md.: National Institute on Alcohol Abuse and Alcoholism, 1990.

National Institute on Drug Abuse. *National Household Survey on Drug Abuse: Population Estimates 1988*. Washington, D.C.: Government Printing Office, 1989.

National Institute on Drug Abuse. *Women and Drug Use*. Rockville, Md.: National Institutes of Health, 1994.

National Institute on Drug Abuse. *Drug Addiction Research and the Health of Women*. Rockville, Md.: U.S. Department of Health and Human Services, National Institutes of Health, 1998.

Nelson-Zlupko, L., Dore, M. M., Kauffman, E., and Kaltenbach, K. "Women in Recovery." *Journal of Substance Abuse Treatment,* 1996, *13,* 51–59.

Nelson-Zlupko, L., Kauffman, E., and Dore, M. M. "Gender Differences in Drug Abuse Treatment: Implications for Social Work Intervention with Substance-Abusing Women." *Social Work*, 1995, *40*, 45–64.

Nolen-Hoeksema, S. "Sex Differences in Unipolar Depression: Evidence and Theory." *Psychological Bulletin*, 1987, *101*, 259–282.

Nyamathi, A., Stein, J. A., and Brecht, M. L. "Psychosocial Predictors of AIDS Risk Behavior and Drug Use Behavior in Homeless and Drug-Addicted Women of Color." In *National Institute on Drug Abuse, Drug Addiction Research and the Health of Women*. Rockville, Md.: U.S. Department of Health and Human Services, National Institutes of Health, 1998.

Robles, R. R., and others. "Social and Behavioral Consequences of Chemical Dependency." In *National Institute on Drug Abuse, Drug Addiction Research and the Health of Women*. Rockville, Md.: U.S. Department of Health and Human Services, National Institutes of Health, 1998.

Rohsenow, D. J., Corbett, R., and Devine, D. "Molested as Children: A Hidden Contribution to Substance Abuse." *Journal of Substance Abuse Treatment*, 1988, *5*, 13–18.

Safer, D. J. "Substance Abuse by Young Adult Chronic Patients." *Hospital Community Psychiatry*, 1987, *38*, 511–514.

Silverman, C. *The Epidemiology of Depression*. Baltimore, Md.: Johns Hopkins University Press, 1968.

Stoffelmayr, B. E., and others. "Substance Abuse Prognosis with an Additional Psychiatric Diagnosis: Understanding the Relationship." *Journal of Psychoactive Drugs*, 1989, *21*(2), 145–152.

Wallen, J. "A Comparison of Male and Female Clients in Substance Abuse Treatment." *Journal of Substance Abuse Treatment*, 1992, *9*, 243–248.

Wallen, J. "Need for Services Research on Treatment for Drug Abuse in Women." In *National Institute on Drug Abuse, Drug Addiction Research and the Health of Women*. Rockville, Md.: U.S. Department of Health and Human Services, National Institutes of Health, 1998.

Wilsnack, S. C. "Barriers to Treatment for Alcoholic Women." *Addiction Recovery*, 1991, *11*, 10–12.

Winfield, I., George, L. K., Swartz, M., and Blazer, D. G. "Sexual Assault and Psychiatric Disorders Among a Community Sample of Women." *American Journal of Psychiatry*, 1990, *147*, 335–341.

PART SIX

MENTAL HEALTH

CHAPTER SEVENTEEN

Latinas

Melba J. T. Vasquez

This chapter presents a useful and relevant description and analysis of the mental health needs of Latinas, although the demographic data and referenced literature are not current. In addition to offering important background and cultural context, Vasquez describes a clinical counseling framework for treating Latinas. The author notes that the work examined here does not address Latina subgroups and makes specific recommendations for future work, including the importance of Latina and Latino subgroup mental health research. The data in this area remain inadequate due to research protocols that are not culturally or linguistically appropriate.

Understanding the conditions that make for Latinas' mental health requires both an awareness of factors specific to Hispanic culture and a sensitivity to individual variation. We must become adequately informed and respectful of the Latinas' relevant individual, sociocultural, and environmental influences if we are to provide her competent, ethical, and responsible services. Mental health practitioners who ignore cultural values, attitudes, behaviors, and experiences different from their own deprive themselves of crucial information. From that ignorance comes a tendency to impose their own worldviews and assumptions on clients in an erroneous and destructive manner. Yet clinicians must avoid making simplistic, unfounded assumptions on the basis of ethnicity and gender. Many clinicians, sometimes even well-meaning ones, apply ethnic stereotypes rather than carefully assessing a particular Latina woman's experience. Knowledge about cultural and socioeconomic contexts is best used as the basis for informed inquiry rather than as blanket group characteristics with which to stereotype the client.

This chapter will present a clinical/counseling framework (Casas and Vasquez, 1989) for the competent and ethical treatment of Latina women. The framework comprises three categories. The first category identifies personal and professional attitudes, beliefs, and knowledge of the therapist. The second identifies individual, sociocultural, and environmental experiences of Latina women that must be understood and addressed in psychotherapy. The third category

345

describes therapeutic approaches to counseling Latinas, including the importance of empowering clients through acknowledgment of the positive aspects of their culture. Critical issues in the delivery of both individual and group psychotherapy will be described. The terms *Latino* and *Latina* are growing in preference over the term *Hispanic* (Chapa and Valencia, 1993), and will thus be used throughout the chapter.

THE CLINICIAN

Language and cultural differences, as well as personal and professional biases, can serve as barriers to the delivery of mental health services to Latinas. Pope (Pope and Vasquez, 1991) interviewed several prominent therapists with expertise in identifying and responding to suicidal risk, among them Ricardo Munoz, Ph.D., a principal investigator in National Institute of Mental Health (NIMH) depression prevention research involving English-, Spanish-, and Chinese-speaking populations. Munoz presented a worst-possible scenario that could evolve from lack of language compatibility:

> Recently, a Spanish-speaking woman, suicidal, came to the emergency room talking of pills. The physician, who spoke limited Spanish, obtained what he thought was her promise not to attempt suicide and sent her back to her halfway house. It was later discovered that she'd been saying that she'd already taken a lethal dose of pills and was trying to get help [p. 167].

A study (Wampold, Casas, and Atkinson, 1981) investigating the attitudes of practicing psychotherapists toward African Americans, Chinese Americans, Japanese Americans, Jews, and Mexican Americans found that of all the responses provided by the therapists, 79.2 percent indicated the presence of subtle stereotypic attitudes, and 22.6 percent demonstrated blatant stereotypic attitudes. The stereotypes most frequently ascribed to Latinos tended to be negative (lazy, dumb, dirty, overemotional). Other research also supports the reality that therapists are personally and professionally biased. Furthermore, the risk of miscommunication in psychotherapy is thought to be highest when the client is an ethnic minority female and the therapist is an Anglo American male (Wilkinson, 1980).

Therapists face many challenges in identifying, understanding, and transcending differences between therapist and Latina client. Each of us must accept the reality that we are indeed influenced by our socialization, which includes assumptions, values, attitudes, biases, and stereotypes. We must remain constantly vigilant and engage in ongoing professional training to free us from our personal and professional biases.

Perhaps the therapist's biggest challenge is to work to prevent in the therapeutic relationship replication of various inequities of opportunity and other prejudices that the client encounters in society. To do so, therapists must recognize the personal and professional assumptions that determine and direct their interactions with clients. A healthy clinical relationship is difficult, perhaps impossible, if the counselor is unaware of his or her own perceptions and attitudes about particular differences, such as gender, race, ethnicity, skin color, socioeconomic status, nationality, and sexual orientation. Without awareness, the exploration that should occur regarding these issues cannot take place honestly and openly in the therapeutic relationship (Casas and Vasquez, 1989; Pinderhuges, 1989).

A fundamental set of cultural values forms the core of the therapeutic profession, regardless of therapeutic orientation. Those values reflect the majority culture: rugged individualism, autonomy, competition, action orientation, the Protestant work ethic, progress and future orientation, the scientific method of inquiry, the nuclear family structure, assertiveness, and rigid timetables. These are *not* universal values. A Latina woman who strongly identifies with traditional Latino culture may hold values in sharp contrast to some of them. She may emphasize family and group achievement over individual achievement; value extended family as well as nuclear family; lack the "proper" amount of assertiveness; or reveal a less rigid, present-focused time orientation. If so, she displays some traditional Latino values that may conflict with those of her counselor. Alternately, a highly acculturated Latina may espouse values, attitudes, and beliefs more similar to the White majority culture, varying only in manner and degree.

Yet some therapists ascribe blind and unquestioning importance to those cultural factors, perceiving them as universal (Casas and Vasquez, 1989). Imposing one's culture-specific values or assuming pathology in the absence of those values is prejudicial and destructive, however well-meaning one's intent. Often our treatment process intrudes our prejudicial attitudes in both the assessment and the treatment of culturally different individuals (Goodyear and Sinnett, 1984). Quite simply, without awareness of one's biases, a therapist is incapable of providing ethical and competent services for culturally different clients.

Several writers (Casas and Vasquez, 1989; Corvin and Wiggins, 1989; Katz and Ivey, 1977) have challenged psychotherapists to explore their own racism. They believe avoidance of this process allows mental health providers the luxury of denying responsibility for or connection with the racist system that oppresses others. In truth, too many mental health providers continue to view culturally different populations as inherently inferior and White American as superior to all existing cultures. We too often fail to realize that racism is not the result of cultural differences, but the consequence of White ethnocentrism

(Corvin and Wiggins, 1989) and that that ethnocentrism is a pervasive and problematic attitude for us all.

Despite the wide range of differences among people, diversity is not yet valued and celebrated. We do not yet fully respect those who differ from the majority. Indeed, racism is often an attempt to control diversity, for differences still make us feel uncomfortable, less secure, and, above all, threatened. Ironically, those therapists most prone to ethnocentrism seldom allow themselves to recognize that imposition of monoculturalism is identified by some theorists as a characteristic of the adolescent developmental stage, or that such a "herd instinct" cannot be easily reconciled with a quest for autonomy. The inability to accommodate ambiguity, the tendency to polarize, and the simplistic reasoning of duality are all characteristics of less-than-mature emotional and cognitive development. They are also central to the mind-set of racism.

Psychotherapists must be aware of the possibility of the insidious, pervasive, and inadvertent internalization of intolerance, which may take the form of disdain for deviations from their preferred standard, and must be particularly sensitive to their role in working with members of oppressed groups. Hare-Mustin, Marecek, Kaplan, and Liss-Levinson (1979) describe how members of these groups often enter therapy in a help-seeking posture, not a self-protective one; that the therapy situation is a novel one for most clients; and that some clients who have been denied power historically may not be prepared to assert their rights, especially if their complaints are typically unheeded. Therapists who must obtain informed consent for a particular technique or disclosure, for example, must be especially careful to ensure that genuine informed consent is in fact obtained.

Finally, therapists must be aware of how training and learning about human behavior take place in a sociocultural context. Our typical training does not emphasize the unique frame of reference and psychosocial history of culturally different clients. Moreover, our learning process entails development of a "cognitive map of the counseling process and a related 'psychology' of humanity" (Holiman and Lauver, 1987). The counselor's own cultural background and experiences serve as powerful filters to the acquisition of that cognitive map and view of humanity. This filtering process not only inhibits learning about cultural diversity, but also results in the tendency and desire to work with clients most culturally similar to oneself. It also discourages our appreciation of the importance of understanding behavior, attitudes, and feelings from the perspective of the culturally different individual. As a result, either we do not bond with our culturally different clients, or we risk errors in assessment, diagnosis, and treatment of those clients—sometimes both. Before we try to understand our clients, we must first be aware of our tendencies toward inappropriate inferences when we assess others' behaviors different from our own worldviews.

KNOWLEDGE OF THE CLIENT

Gender, ethnicity, and socioeconomic class are core components of an individual's identity. The Latina woman's culture, history, and experience with oppression cause variations in human behavior and development. Visible behavior may not mean the same to the client as it seems to the clinician, so that understanding these aspects of Latinas' cultural context is crucial for the psychotherapist. At the same time, we must remember that the descriptions that follow in this section are applicable to some Latinas, some of the time, for a period of time. Many differences exist within groups, and the groups that make up Latina women in the United States are dynamic and constantly in flux, as are values, behaviors, and attitudes. Conceptions of gender roles are changing for men and women as we enter the twenty-first century, both for White cultures and for the cultures of Latinos.

The following scenarios are created from years of clinical observation and experience, as well as from research conducted about Latina women. Some are fictional, others are composites of cases and have been modified to protect confidentiality. No case identifies any one person. There are no clear ways to conceptualize or intervene, but the cases are presented to stimulate discussion, and to encourage the reader to draw conclusions based on the information presented in this chapter. I also refer to these cases later in the chapter.

- *Scenario 1.* A 35-year-old Chicana woman enters therapy, reporting depressive symptoms. She reports that she has been distraught about and feels "stuck" in her grief for an aged aunt who died several months previously. As you explore, you discover that the aunt had served as the primary nurturer in this woman's life. Furthermore, you discover that this woman, who is a professional with advanced degrees, is suffering from incredible guilt because she "failed" to be at her aunt's deathbed, even though the aunt had asked for her. Your client had chosen to attend a professional meeting to do networking, basing her decision on the fact that her aunt had been sick on and off for several months. How do you proceed?
- *Scenario 2.* You colead a Latina women's support group that consists of Chicana, Puerto Rican, and Mexicana group members. You discover that all but one of the ten members of your group has either been sexually molested as a child or has experienced rape or other sexual assault. The question arises in your mind. Is there a higher incidence of sexual abuse among Latino groups?
- *Scenario 3.* A 32-year-old Chicana whose gentle, polite style has resulted in being "run over" and mistreated both at work and at home enters therapy as a result of a white woman's suggestion. She cannot afford your fee. After negotiating a sliding scale fee, she reports that she can only come once a month. Furthermore, she reports doubt about the "assertive style" that her friend uses

and is fearful that the therapist will also insist that the Chicana client use that style, as her friend has been insisting. How should you proceed?

• *Scenario 4.* A 23-year-old university female student enters therapy in crisis over a racist statement that a roommate made about Latinos. The client, half European American (father) and half Latina (mother), has never claimed her identity to herself, much less to peers such as roommates. She had been told by both parents to "pass" as White if she could. She has become very concerned about gender, race, and class issues, recently gave a talk about feminism, and is now confused about the ethnic aspect of her identity. She is beginning to be aware of the hurt and anger that is emerging toward her roommates and her parents. What direction should therapy take?

Demographics

The term *Latina* comprises a very diverse group of people. A publication from the U.S. Census Bureau (1991) reports that Latinos increased by 53 percent to 22.4 million since 1980, 9 percent of the U.S. population, compared to a 9 percent increase for the total population. Approximately half of this growth was due to foreign immigration and half was due to births to Latinos in the United States (Chapa and Valencia, 1993). Unfortunately, research surveys, census information, and other statistics rarely provide breakdowns of information within Latino groups. This is a problem since Latinos comprise an aggregation of several distinct national origin subgroups (Chapa and Valencia, 1993), and research has found differences among Puerto Rican, Mexican, and Cuban, Central, and South Americans (Amaro, Russo, and Johnson, 1987). Latinos living on the U.S. mainland have the following backgrounds: the Mexican-origin population constitutes 60 percent; South Americans, Central Americans, and other Latinos 22 percent; Puerto Ricans 12 percent; and Cubans 5 percent of the total Latino population.

The various Latino groups are concentrated in different regions of the country: Mexicans in the Southwest and Midwest, Puerto Ricans in the Northeast, Cubans in the Southeast. The other Latino populations are found in areas with concentrations of Mexican, Puerto Rican, or Cuban populations (Chapa and Valencia, 1993). Chapa and Valencia (1993) point out that Latinos are highly urbanized and that 67 percent of all U.S. Latinos reside in 16 metropolitan areas.

Various sociodemographic characteristics of Latinos are relevant to mental health, including education attainment, employment, generation and immigration status, family income, family size, and language status. Chapa and Valencia (1993) provide a thorough overview of those data for Latinos. It is important to note that a large percentage of Latinos are of the lower class, regardless of generational status in the United States (Padilla, Salgado de Snyder, Cervantes, and Baezconde-Garbanati, 1987). Any study involving Latinos should therefore control for social class, either experimentally or statistically. Unfortunately, many studies have been conducted comparing lower-class Latinos to middle-class Anglo Americans in which differences were attributed to culture rather than social class (Padilla, Salgado de Snyder, Cervantes, and Baezconde-Garbanati, 1987). More research is needed to determine the effects of poverty on Latinos, especially since Chapa and Valencia (1993) point out that many educational and economic measures show no indication that Latinos are achieving parity, and some measures indicate relative and absolute declines even among Latino families who have been in the United States for a number of generations. There is no doubt that poverty is clearly stressful, damaging to a sense of well-being, and results in numerous and complex disadvantages. Yet we must not automatically assume knowledge about the effects of poverty on each geographical cultural group. A report by Winkler (1990) in the *Chronicle of Higher Education* cited evidence of "cultural vitality," coined by David E. Hayes-Bautista, a professor of medicine at UCLA. Researchers examined some of California's poor Latina population, and their findings promoted debate over the traditional definitions of the "underclass." Some of Hayes-Bautista's research findings clearly invalidated characteristics typically associated with the "underclass" portrayed in other reports.

For example, poor Latinos were twice as likely to live in traditional family structures compared to either poor Blacks or Whites; Latinos had the highest rates of working males, higher life expectancy, with a 50 percent lower rate of violent deaths compared to Blacks, and 20 percent lower compared to Whites. Furthermore, immigrant Latinos exhibited healthier behavior than Latinos born in this country. These unexpected findings point to the importance of using well-conducted research as a foundation for our understanding of Latinos rather than speculative assumptions.

As the United States shifts to an economy based on technology and information, the American worker must become increasingly skilled, trained, and educated. Unfortunately, the educational rates of attainment for Latinos remain low. Educational demographics are important, since attainment of education is highly correlated to success and power in U.S. society, which in turn are related to well-being and mental health. In a study of 18- and 19-year-old Latinos, the National Council of La Raza found that in 1988, 31 percent had dropped out of high school, compared to 18 percent of African Americans, and 14 percent of European Americans at the same age. According to other figures, 40 to 50 percent of all Latino students leave school before the tenth grade. A report (1990) by the U.S. Census Bureau found that three out of ten Latino high school graduates aged 18 to 24 were enrolled in college in 1988, about the same percentage as in 1978; thus, over the past decade, there appears to have been little or no improvement in the Latino overall college attendance rates. A recent (1991) report from the American College Testing service indicated that Latinos had the lowest educational attainment rates compared to other groups.

There is some evidence that Latina women, particularly Mexican Americans, fare even worse. Mexican American women are reported in some studies to have the lowest educational attainment rates, the highest levels of unemployment, and the highest poverty levels of any group in the United States, including Mexican American men, African Americans of both sexes, and women of all groups (Chacon and others, 1985). The problem of educational attainment for Latinos is a complex one and cannot be adequately addressed here. Suffice it to say that the relatively low levels of educational attainment, low income, and lack of access to key resources in society contribute to many of the problems for Latina women.

Ethnic and Gender Identity

Identity is a very important factor affecting mental health. It involves the way one views oneself in regard to qualities, characteristics, and values. Social psychologists describe the development of one's identity as partly based on the messages one receives from significant others about oneself. In addition, identity is formed as a result of messages in society about one's primary reference group.

What are the messages in society about Latinas? The lack of positive images in the media, the lack of positive role models in positions of power, and the promotion of negative stereotypes and expectations of Latinas contribute to their second-class status. Some exceptions are emerging, such as the national newspaper *Vista*, which highlights positive contributions and achievements of Hispanic men and women. Nevertheless, Latinas are still generally affected by the triply oppressive experiences associated with being female, ethnic, and, often, poor. Latinas frequently come from families who themselves have had few opportunities and options in life, and do not have options in their repertoire to offer to their daughters.

Ramirez (1991) describes how minorities often experience "feeling different," including feelings of alienation and loneliness. He describes how the majority society imposes pressures on minority cultures to conform, to abandon their individuality, and to force themselves into the fictional ideal molds and patterns created by those who have power and influence. The members of these cultures are made to feel different and inferior, as if there were something wrong with them. The end result is often the rejection of oneself in order to fit in and to appear less different.

Teresa Bernardez, a professor of psychiatry in the College of Human Medicine at Michigan State University, in describing the various sources of depression for women at a Women and Self-Esteem conference (1990), noted that when a woman is not provided with people around her who are able to communicate appreciation for that woman's uniqueness and difference, damage to the self occurs. When caretakers, significant others, and society do not convey a caring attitude, with expectations that women will succeed, these women then fail to discover the abilities in themselves. Confidence does not develop or is eroded. When a Latina does not experience individuals who register with sensitivity and admiration the possibilities and visions for that woman, she then runs the risk of resigned despair, of finding herself on a "dead-end street."

Unfortunately, the restrictive gender and sex role stereotyping that characterizes early socialization fails to equip girls with skills and competence, undermines self-confidence, and lays a foundation for the development of mental health problems in adulthood (Gilligan, Rogers, and Tolman, 1991). Indeed, one of the most pervasive issues for women, including Latinas, is lack of confidence, tendency to blame self or lack of ability for failures, and failure to take credit for successes.

Encounters with racism, regardless of age, are traumatic. Early in life, those experiences result in a feeling of lack of safety and create dissonance and confusion. These experiences may result in a variety of responses and coping strategies. If one has been "inoculated" with a sense of self-pride and given strong messages of entitlement and appreciation of one's group, then an individual may not internalize the negative messages so much. However, most people have to develop a cognitive, emotional, and behavioral map of how to deal with the hurt, including denial, anger and rage, achievement, perfectionism, defensiveness, and strategizing.

Recurring racist events may lead to depression, anxiety, and posttraumatic stress disorder. Increased anxiety, nightmares, feelings of lack of safety, and irritability are some symptoms that Latinas may exhibit in response to such traumas. Each individual who experiences discriminatory behavior has to struggle to incorporate and deal with the painful experience. It takes extra effort not to feel badly about oneself; it takes extra effort to know what to do with hurt and anger. It is important in psychotherapy to talk openly about these aspects of a Latina woman's life and to discuss these issues as due more to institutional and systemic discrimination than to personal inadequacy. At the same time, skills (assertiveness, conflict management) and strategies (positive self-talk, seeking support strategies) in dealing with discrimination are part of the process of empowerment for a Latina. The negative expectations a college professor has of a Latina advisee and the glass ceiling she experiences at work because her boss assumes that her style would not be effective in advanced positions are examples of subtle but painful oppression. Helping a Latina client face these issues can contribute to a more positive sense of identity, which is a major aspect of mental health and well-being.

Cultural Characteristics

The importance and value of the family is perhaps one of the most salient and empirically supported characteristics of the Latino culture. Ramirez and Arce (1981) reviewed relevant empirical literature on the Chicano family, for example, in an attempt to explore the validity of various family issues that have been conceptually confusing and distorted in the social science literature. They present the following characteristics of Chicano families:

> a strong, persistent familistic orientation; a widespread existence of highly integrated extended kinship systems, even for Chicanos who are three or more generations removed from Mexico; and the consistent preference of Chicanos for relying on the extended family for support, as the primary means for coping with emotional stress [p. 15].

In an investigation of Latino familism and acculturation, Sabogal and others (1987) identified three separate dimensions of familism: family obligations (perceived obligation to provide material and emotional support to extended family members), perceived support from family (perception of family members as reliable providers of help), and family as referents (relatives as behavioral and attitudinal models of identity). They found that acculturation was a salient variable in predicting both the familial obligations and family as referent aspects of familism. Perceived support from the family seemed to be the most stable dimension of familism, as it did not decrease significantly with acculturation. Although two of the dimensions decreased with acculturation, even highly acculturated Latinos were more familistic than White non-Hispanics on all dimensions that were examined. Furthermore, the dimensions of family obligations, support from family, and family as referents were found to be core characteristics of Latino culture that did not vary among the subgroups that participated in the study—Mexican Americans, Cuban Americans, and Central Americans—despite levels of acculturation.

The implication of this research is that the individuation process, a salient therapeutic issue in most Western psychotherapies, may proceed differently for those from Latino cultures. Additionally, the importance of such values as independence, individuality, and competition may be different for Latinas than the traditional psychotherapist may expect.

Indeed, the client in Scenario 1, despite the fact that she was a third-generation, relatively acculturated Latina, still experienced the dilemma of pulls in the professional world to make professional responsibilities high priority, despite her family norm of honoring older members of the family by one's presence, particularly at times of illness and death. Helping her struggle through the guilt meant not diminishing the importance of either of her competing values and regrets about choices, but rather encouraging her to let go of the perfectionistic harshness with which she judged herself. She could do so when the therapist allowed her to have her regrets, grief, and wishes about different choices.

Gender Roles

Much has been written about the rigidity of gender roles in the traditional Latino culture. Many mental health workers automatically assume that derogatory portrayals of the socialization processes regarding gender roles in the Latino family are true. The most common stereotype is that of an authoritarian husband and submissive wife. In fact, very few studies have actually assessed the socialization processes of Latino families. A study by Zapata and Jaramillo (1981) used Adlerian-style interviews to examine the socialization of sex role stereotypes. They concluded that gender-related interactions within the Mexican American family were more complex than previously assumed. Parents did not perceive themselves as prescribing rigid sex roles to their children, but siblings reported perceptions that females acted in a more socially cooperative manner. Zapata and Jaramillo suggested that the socializing processes of Mexican American families may not be as different from majority culture as was earlier believed. They further concluded that a dynamic view of the Latino family may be more accurate than the static, rigid view that has been taken in past research. Indeed, the myth of male dominance in the Latino family, especially in regard to decision making, has been reviewed by others (Bernal, 1982; Comas-Díaz, 1989; Cromwell and Ruiz, 1979). Cromwell and Ruiz (1979), for example, concluded that the notion of male dominance in marital decision making was a myth. Their conclusion was based on an intensive analysis of four major studies on marital decision making within Mexican and Chicano families. While they did acknowledge that Latino males may behave differently from non-Latino males in their family and marital lives, they concluded that such behavior did not necessarily take the inappropriate forms suggested by the myth of the macho, with its strong connotations of social deviance.

In my experience, families that are relatively healthy and functional, where roles are traditionally assigned, exhibit a mutuality and respect for the ascribed roles. In those healthy families, the traditional roles (working father, homemaker mother) do not exclude equity in decision making and conflict resolution. However, in dysfunctional families, traditional roles are carried out in a more oppressive and pathological manner, with power battles, abusive behavior, poor conflict resolution, and low marital satisfaction. There is some evidence that Latinas internalize the expectation to nurture, care for, and maintain the family unity and connections. The Latina may therefore deny or ignore her needs in order to keep the family intact, even in the face of abuse, lack of happiness, or unsuccessful marriage. In addition, there is evidence that family support is positively associated with success in college for Chicanas (Gandara, 1982; Vasquez, 1982) and that Chicanas' strong emphasis on domestic responsibilities is related to poor progress in academic programs (Chacon, Cohen, and Strover, 1986).

The actual dynamic variation that exists among Latino families must be considered, and the tendency to pathologize Latino families simply because of traditional values must be avoided. Yet some elements of the assignment of traditional roles to men and women in any culture, while adaptive in agricultural and other societies, may become problematic in a dynamic technological society

(Vasquez, 1984). Especially for those women who are in traditional and dysfunctional relationships, symptoms of mental and physical illnesses, such as depression, anxiety, and psychosomatic symptoms, may be evident.

Mental Health Issues

Latina women are at high risk of experiencing mental health problems. However, the extent of this risk for Latinos in general, and to some degree for Latina women, is only beginning to be understood. Epidemiological studies on topics such as alcoholism among Latinos are relatively recent and often do not break down gender differences.

Depressive disorders and depressive symptomatology have been examined, as well as risk factors associated with depression. Most studies (Canino and others, 1987; Salgado de Snyder, 1987) are consistent with previous research on other groups, which shows that depression is significantly more prevalent in Latino (in these studies Puerto Rican and Mexican) women than in men. Gender differences are typically hypothesized to be due to social causation. That is, many of women's traditional roles are given low societal value; roles may be unrewarding; women's work outside the home may be associated with gender, ethnic, and class discrimination; in women, overt manifestation of anger is discouraged; and women feel (and often have) less control in their lives.

Some research is beginning to shed light on the specific manifestations of depression for Latinas. For example, Salgado de Snyder (1987) found that women immigrants who in the past three months experienced discrimination, sex role conflicts, and concern about starting a family in this country had significantly higher depression scores than did women who did not report experiencing those situations. Thus, Mexican women immigrants with those experiences may be at a higher risk for the development of psychological problems.

In a study examining family and work predictors of psychological well-being among Latina women professionals, Amaro, Russo, and Johnson (1987) found that income was the most consistently related demographic factor across all measures of psychological well-being.

This study of a very select population of highly educated, high-income Latina women in professional and managerial positions also showed that Latina women's psychological well-being is related to the experience of discrimination, reported by more than 82 percent of the sample. Furthermore, women in some Latino groups enjoyed better mental health than others. For example, Puerto Rican women were more likely than Mexican American women to report psychological distress symptoms, whereas Cubans reported less stress in balancing partner and professional roles than did Mexican Americans. These findings point to the critical need for research involving separate analyses for women of diverse Latino backgrounds; clinically, they imply that we must remain abreast of such research developments and carefully assess the situations of our individual clients. Never assume that a general finding for a particular Latino group applies to all Latino groups or to all individuals within the particular group.

A report by the American Psychological Association's National Task Force on Women and Depression (McGrath, Keita, Strickland, and Russo, 1990) more fully described the risk factors, research, and treatment issues in regard to women and depression, including Latinas. While no one theory or set of theories fully explains gender differences in depression, many helpful considerations for therapists are provided. For example, the rate of sexual and physical abuse of females is a major factor in women's depression. One-third to one-half of all women have had a significant experience of physical or sexual abuse before the age of 21. This points to the probability that depressive symptoms may be long-standing effects of posttraumatic stress syndrome for many women. Additionally, women in unhappy marriages are three times as likely to be depressed as married men and single women. Mothers of young children, especially several young children, are highly vulnerable to depression. Finally, the report summarizes that poverty is a "pathway to depression" (p. xii).

Violence against Latinas is an issue of concern to clinicians. Wife abuse is found in all social, economic, religious, ethnic, and educational levels. Mixed data are found in regard to variations of incidence among those groups. Studies report a range of 26 to 60 percent incidence for all couples (Torres, 1986). Although no studies have indicated a higher or lower incidence of spousal abuse among Latino groups, some research does indicate a higher incidence of wife abuse in lower socioeconomic classes. Other factors contributing to spousal abuse include violent behavior in previous generations, high levels of stress, social isolation, pregnancy, sex role stereotyping, and prevalence of alcohol and drugs (Walker, 1989).

As with wife abuse, rape is suspected to be underreported by Latina women, as it is in the general population. Nevertheless, perhaps because of the distrust of public agencies, women of color are less likely to report rape than nonminority women (Feldman-Summers and Ashworth, 1981). Violence against women is a major problem in society; for the Latina, it is an additional oppressive experience that can result in depression, poor self-esteem, and other physical and mental disorders.

Very little information is available in regard to sexual abuse among Latino families. In one study, however, the prevalence rates of child sexual victimization were reported to be lower for Latinos (3.0 percent) when compared to non-Latino Whites (8.7 percent) (Siegel and others, 1987). Thus, as clinicians, we must be aware that individual and group clients are a self-selected group of individuals, and a large proportion of sexually abused or assaulted clients means that these clients are suffering from long-term adjustment difficulties. Therapists must not generalize from situations such as that in Scenario 2, where nine out of ten group members had experienced some form of sexual violence.

Clinicians must remember that clients often self-select for treatment in appropriate ways—for example, to work through wounds from earlier emotional damage—but characteristics such as a high incidence of rape experiences among clients should not alone be considered evidence of high incidence in the Latina population quite generally. Wyatt (1990) maintains that there may be some aspects of ethnic minority children's lives that affect long-term adjustment to these traumatic experiences. Other forms of victimization (discrimination, poverty), may evoke posttraumatic stress disorder, for example.

Adolescent pregnancy has become a major social problem with the increase in pregnancy rates in the past decade. In 1978, over 19 percent of all teenage women in the United States had had unplanned pregnancies. Recent figures indicate that teen birthrates among Latinos are higher than those of non-Latino White women (Padilla, Salgado de Snyder, Cervantes, and Baezconde-Garbanati, 1987). Interestingly enough, Becerra and De Ana (1984, as cited in Padilla, Salgado de Snyder, Cervantes, and Baezconde-Garbanati, 1987), who conducted one of the few studies on Mexican American adolescent pregnancies, found that high level of acculturation was related to high levels of sexual activity and to low usage of contraceptive devices. That is, the more acculturated Mexican American adolescents are at higher risk for unwanted pregnancies than are those less acculturated. Padilla, Salgado de Snyder, Cervantes, and Baezconde-Garbanati (1987) point out that many factors other than acculturation have not been adequately studied in Latino adolescents, such as educational level of mothers, social support received from the mother, adolescents' self-esteem, use and nonuse of contraception, and information about human reproduction.

Suicide risk among Latinos has also been ignored among researchers. Padilla, Salgado de Snyder, Cervantes, and Baezconde-Garbanati (1987) summarized two studies, which reported lower rates of suicide among Latinos when compared to Whites. Important differences with respect to gender and age were found. The ratio of male to female suicides among Latinos was almost twice that of the male–female suicide ratio evidenced for non-Latinos. Additionally, 25 percent of Latina females and 33 percent of Latino males who committed suicide were found to be under 25 years of age. Unfortunately, the incidence of Latino homicide rates appears to be quite high: two and a half times the homicide rates found for Whites. Socioeconomic conditions and stressful urban living conditions are offered as possible reasons for the higher rates. These distressful realities either directly or indirectly affect the lives and well-being of the Latina women with whom we work.

AIDS as an issue for Hispanics and women was reported in the February 1991 issue of the *Monitor* (American Psychological Association). A study by Hortensia Amaro found misconceptions about AIDS and transmission of HIV that causes AIDS in large portions of four Latino subgroups studied, including women of childbearing age. The other groups were drug users, adolescents, and gay men. At the time of the study, Latinos accounted for more than 15 percent of the total AIDS cases diagnosed in the United Sates but made up only 7.8 percent of the U.S. population. The study reported that many programs have attempted to educate women about the need for condom use with their partners but have sometimes overlooked the critical role of educating men. This health crisis has numerous implications for mental health.

Employment issues are also of concern for Latina women. A person's employment and her attitude toward work are important characteristics affecting mental health. For most persons, work is a major life activity. A good job may represent a goal allowing escape from poverty for immigrants, or it can be an occupation that contributes to a positive sense of identity or well-being. It can also constitute a tedious, unavoidable task. We know that stress in the workplace is pervasive and has extensive costly consequences in dollars and physical health and psychological well-being. We also know that while high-stress jobs can have negative consequences, worker control (the fact or the perception that one has some degree of choice in work tasks, for example), or lack thereof, is the more meaningful predictor of physical problems such as cardiovascular response.

As of 1990, 75 percent of those entering the American workforce are minorities and women. Thus, women and ethnic minorities are predicted to dominate our labor pool in the near future. Patterns of prejudice, bias, and in-group preference will consequently have to be modified (Jones, 1990). Women and minorities face a glass ceiling that limits their advancement toward top management in organizations throughout U.S. society. The glass ceiling is a popular concept of the 1980s, describing a barrier so subtle that it is transparent, yet so strong that it prevents women and persons of color from moving up in the management hierarchy (Morrison and Von Glinow, 1990). Morrison and Von Glinow cite data that dispute that sex and race deficiencies account for the lack of representation in management ranks. Discrimination and other systemic barriers, including sexual harassment, are proposed as explanations. Discrimination was one of the factors described by Amaro, Russo, and Johnson (1987) as associated with Latina professional women's mental health distress symptoms and with their lower satisfaction in their personal lives.

The unique experience of the Latina must be assessed as an overlay to other more traditional sociohistorical life factors that differentiate all individuals (such as family size, birth order, childhood illnesses, family mobility, family deaths and divorces, and type of parenting received). Each Latina's experiences must be assessed to determine more accurately her particular reality and mental health needs. This section has articulated issues that, recognized and addressed, can contribute to the therapist's better understanding of Latinas.

THERAPEUTIC INTERVENTION

Individual Psychotherapy

Regardless of theoretical approach to treatment, effective therapy with Latina women incorporates elements of both feminist therapy and multicultural treatment. Both feminist and cross-cultural therapies are based on philosophies that hold as a basic tenet that external factors are examined as causative in the client's problems. Approaches are endorsed that result in empowerment of the client to engage in change if she so chooses rather than those that pathologize or blame her. Her strengths rather than her weaknesses are emphasized and validated. Care, respect, and conditions conducive to trust are promoted. Perhaps one of the most important functions of the therapist of a Latina is to communicate a caring attitude that discovers the abilities in the client, registers with sensitivity, respect, and admiration the possibilities and visions for the client, and is able to delight in what is unique, special, and novel in that client. Believing in a Latina client can do much to promote the confidence that has probably been eroded by the experience of life in this society.

For example, consider the group members in Scenario 2. Nine out of ten experienced sexual abuse and felt some degree of guilt and responsibility for that abuse. In addition to facilitating expressions of care, anger, and concern for each other about the experiences, the effective therapist would help group members understand how society condones such behavior toward women. The group would explore the differences between the socialization of the genders: that men are seen as entitled to having their needs met, without regard to women's feelings; that women are socialized to feel responsible for the well-being of others. This is an important intervention in decreasing the toxic guilt that women carry when they have been abused. Women in general tend to assume blame and responsibility for failure or for negative, painful experiences. The role of the therapist is to help the client have compassion and care for herself and to learn to expect it from significant others.

As therapists, we must guard against our tendency to apply psychotherapy in a manner that encourages our clients to adapt to unhealthy environments rather than empowering them to change those environments or leave them. Amaro and Russo (1987) call for the cultural sensitivity of services for Latina women, and they cite feminist criticism of psychotherapy as a form of social control. We cannot afford to ignore the truth that exists in that generalization. For example, "helping" a woman modulate her anger or express it in a "sensitive, tactful" manner to an abusive, sadistic husband or to an oppressive boss, rather than exploring other options such as to leave those environments, may collude with the oppression she is experiencing. Offering choices while examining potential consequences of those options is more freeing, empowering, and effective.

Often, well-meaning therapists discourage women's drive to maintain and need relationships by labeling women as dependent or codependent in the pathological sense, for wanting to care for others. The effective therapist validates the qualities and characteristics of care and nurturing of the Latina; in addition, the effective therapist teaches the Latina client to apply the same principles of care and nurturing to herself. Discouraging a Latina mother from caring "too much" for her children can be confusing. A more effective approach would be to validate her care and to also help her learn to listen to her inner voice in regard to the point at which "giving too much" violates her own needs and identity as a person. One client, for example, found herself constantly depressed in response to the life struggles of her three adult children. In therapy, we discussed the value of caring for her children, but also the notion of balancing her own care for herself. For a period of time, we practiced figuring out the ways in which she could indeed care, listen, and help within certain bounds, but not feel she had to come up with the resolution of every problem, and especially not take on the pain, depression, and angst of her children, which was conceptualized as a natural part of life's struggle.

Comas-Díaz (1987) challenges therapists to apply carefully the integration of feminist principles into practice with Latina women. She urges feminist therapists to appreciate the unique experiences of power and oppression, transculturation (process whereby a conflict in opposing cultural values results in emergence of a new culture, a very different process from acculturation), and other cultural experiences of Latinas. She also describes how assertiveness training can be effectively used with Puerto Rican women, when a cultural component incorporated into the training translates the concept to Puerto Rican women in an acceptable manner.

The Chicana in Scenario 3, who was fearful of having to be assertive like her white female friend, was much more willing to consider developing communication skills that articulated how she felt, what she preferred, and what was experienced as disrespectful to her. These assertive skills were incorporated into her style and conveyed in a manner with which she felt comfortable. She did leave her job for one with more responsibility (which she had been told by her previous boss that she could not handle) and has since received two promotions.

Traditional definitions or models of "power over" or "power for oneself" often leave Hispanic women feeling unable to act, since they perceive such behavior as incompatible with consideration of others, or they anticipate it may lead away from connection and bonding. Miller's (1988) proposed definition of *power* as the "capacity to move or to produce change" rather than "power over" is a preferred construct. Additionally, Surrey (1987) defines empowerment as the motivation, freedom, and capacity to act purposefully, with mobilization of the energy, resources, strengths, or power of each person through a mutual relational process. The therapist can better help many Latinas by exploring direct and healthy ways to be powerful and by empowering through awareness and expression of feelings, reactions, and needs in more effective ways.

Vasquez-Nuttal, Romero-Garcia, and De Leon (1987) describe how cultural sensitivity should incorporate recognition of the changes in Latina women's roles and circumstances rather than reinforcing disadvantaged social and economic status for such women. In particular, they review more recent psychosocial studies that question the traditional portrayal of male–female roles and allocation of power in Latino families. More research is needed to determine how Latinas are guiding their lives in ways that are compatible with cultural expectations, societal demands, and dynamic changes in gender roles.

Group Psychotherapy

Group psychotherapy has long been regarded as the treatment of choice for subgroup populations. Latina women's groups may be geared to those likely to benefit from validation of gender and ethnic identity. Group members help one another realize that they can nurture themselves as well as others, that they can give and receive support and nurturance from other women. Latinas often better learn to value themselves and other women as a result of group membership; consequently, group leaders should promote interaction that builds connection and enhances everyone's personal power.

Empowering group interactions increase zest, knowledge, self-worth, salience, and desire for more connection. The capacity for connection depends on the maintenance of fluid ego boundaries and responsiveness to the thoughts, perceptions, and feeling states of others (Surrey, 1987). In the tradition of feminist therapy, an effective group leader would model such behaviors, being careful to promote self-nurturance as well as nurturance of others. She would recognize and reinforce the positive aspects of Latinas' tendency to care for others and raise the possibility that some group members may not be applying the same concept of care to themselves.

The leader of a Latina women's group may need to rethink frequently asked questions. As these women deviate from the traditional models of power and action, they will encounter the widely recognized "fear of owning one's power," "identification with the victim," and "fear of success." Instead of asking, "Is she being too passive?" or, "Can she learn to be more active on her own behalf?" it may prove more growth enhancing and validating to ask, "Is she being responsibly interactive?" or, "Has she established a relational context where mutual power is encouraged and facilitated?" (Surrey, 1987). And as with individual therapy, it is important for group therapy leaders to individualize the members, knowing that they may be of different socioeconomic class, different acculturation levels, or different subgroup populations.

Groups provide members an opportunity to focus on issues that are uniquely or primarily the concerns of Latina women and explore them from the Latina's perspective. I (with Ay Ling Han) have developed a theme-oriented group for Latina women. The themes, around which various activities have been designed, include family relationships (mother, father, siblings); relationships with significant others (spouses, partners, friends); cultural conflicts, strengths, and identification; barriers to achievement; confidence enhancement; dealing with anger and other feelings; empowerment; skill building (communication, assertiveness, and risk taking); and sexuality. Typically, each of these themes take one to three ninety-minute weekly sessions, during which structured activities may be used to stimulate issues to be worked upon.

For example, the very first session is begun with an activity designed to elicit the Latina's identity issues, which are often related to relationship with mother. Members are asked to introduce themselves to group members the way their mothers would introduce themselves. After each member has done so, members express reactions, feelings, and concerns to one another, based on the nature of the introductions. While the group is structured with activities such as this one, lots of room is provided for in-depth exploration of feelings and issues.

Advocacy

Often, improving a Latina client's mental health may require direct advocacy activities, such as writing a letter (with appropriate releases) for a student to reenter school. Advocacy may also include engaging in efforts to effect policies, laws, and judicial decisions. Using one's expertise and knowledge of how the various forces effect the mental health of Latinas to educate others and effect situational change is a shared responsibility of all therapists of Latinas.

A CLINICAL CASE

The following is a summary of an illustrative case. Identifying data have been changed in order to protect confidentiality.

Angela was a 22-year-old Latina who was a junior when she came to the university counseling center. Her presenting concern was depression, which she reported experiencing for most of high school. She also reported high degrees of isolation and loneliness and the feeling that she belonged to no part of any group (social, cultural, professional, or otherwise). She came from a poor, working-class background and was the daughter of a single parent. She had two younger siblings. She and her mother and siblings had lived with several relatives over the years. Her father had been briefly married to her mother, but lived with them only infrequently despite ten years of marriage. Angela rarely saw her father, and he had provided virtually no child support on a regular basis. Angela still lived at home and complained of her mother's being overly involved, protective, and demanding. Yet she had few resources with which to consider moving into either a dorm or an apartment. She occasionally worked, but found it difficult and time-consuming to keep up with her studies. Her grade-point average was approximately 2.8 (on a 4.0 scale), and her mother wanted her to be an engineer.

The initial treatment plan consisted of developing a warm and trusting relationship, assessing sources of depression, and having a psychiatric evaluation, given the chronic and severe nature of the depression. While women tend to be overmedicated for treatment of depression, and while I am conservative in regard to referral for psychotropic intervention, this case clearly presented the possibility of chemical, biological depression.

In establishing the relationship, Angela's insecurities and ambivalence about her need for me in her life became clear. She quickly bonded, but often apologized for existing, called me "Dr. Vasquez" long after I offered the option of calling me by my first name, and often called me or telephone counseling with her fears and anxieties about a negative assumption she had made in "second-guessing" some aspect of our last session. I began to recognize in her behavior a terror of being abandoned and an incredible lack of confidence in general, but especially in her right to be a client. Given the time-limited nature of our agency's policies, I quickly decided that I would advocate for a lengthy extension for this client. It was important that I use my "chip" to see a long-term client in my organization with someone who did not have resources to get outside community help and who I judged could benefit especially from a Latina therapist. Given her identity confusion and loneliness, I felt that a Latina therapist would help her introject some positive elements of her cultural identity. As in many modern Latino families, some cultural traditions were maintained, and others were not. For example, her family had an important extended family network, with many advantages and disadvantages. My client often felt supported by extended family relatives, but the grandmother in particular frowned upon her living alone without being married. Other cultural characteristics were not present; my client did not speak Spanish, for example.

In addition to accessing extended therapy for Angela as an advocacy activity, the psychiatrist and I also provided key referral sources for Angela and her mother to seek methods to acquire regular child support from the father for the younger children. The state had new laws that allowed for garnishing of wages, and when the family had no money to pay for Angela's antidepressants, this intervention came to mind. This type of advocacy is one seldom used by most mental health professionals, with the exception of social workers. Yet it was a powerful way to enlist the support of the mother for Angela's continuance in therapy (which had been threatening to the mother). Naturally, appropriate and limited releases were acquired from Angela to engage in this process.

Angela's initial behavior during the first few weeks of therapy was typical of those clients often labeled "dependent." My approach consisted of validating her need to feel connected and assuring her that as long as it was within my power, she was not to be abandoned, due to her "mess-ups" in therapy. In addition, it was important that I be clear about my personal and professional limitations, as well as those of the agency, in meeting her needs in order for her not to interpret them as rejection of her. In other words, it was important during the first few weeks of therapy to be clear about our termination time (thus clearly identifying our time together), the times in which she could try to reach me, and about what issues (crisis, suicidal ideation, need for reassurance, and so forth). This boundary setting was done in as humanistic and interactive a manner possible, with some flexibility for negotiation, so that she could feel power in the relationship. In other words, I did not lay the rules out for her, but the boundaries emerged from two or three sessions (and occasionally later as needed) of negotiation of what her needs were and what would work for her, as well as for me and for the agency. At all times, I validated her needs as normal to her situation and did not convey that she was wrong or bad for wanting what she wanted.

In examining possible external sources of depression, we found several. While she had a generally positive nurturing experience from her mother, Angela and her family often lived with extended family members, some of whom were kind, but some of whom were physically, emotionally, and sexually abusive to Angela. Therapy consisted of helping Angela realize and work through the notion that some members of her extended family were dysfunctional and that despite the wonderful network and kinship of her Latino culture, it was tragic that some members of that family were abusive. It was also a tragedy that her mother had to work long hours, often evening hours. This resulted in Angela's inconsistent nurturing and experience of abandonment. She also came to understand the abandonment she experienced from her father, who was mostly a shadowy, distant figure to her, even during the brief times he was around. She also felt overly responsible and sad about the caretaking of her siblings. She was very devoted to them, but often made them a priority over her own needs, frequently canceling her own social plans if one of them wanted her attention.

The treatment itself involved several aspects: she did take antidepressants, which helped. Additionally, we explored the various forms of abuse, which were painful and resulted in the lack of confidence, low self-esteem, and lack of efficacy she felt. Not only did I insist over and over that she was not to blame for the abuse, but that she was a wondrous survivor, who had accomplished much, given the lack of support. The exploration of memories often evoked posttraumatic stress disorder symptoms, such as anxiety, nightmares, irritability, increased feelings of vulnerability, and suicidal ideation, which we had to attend to. We also explored her mixed feelings about the role of her mother. Facilitating anger for her mother's lack of protection is a traditional therapeutic intervention, but for many Latina women, especially in this case, where her mother was one of the few sources of support, that anger had to be balanced with an understanding that despite her historical (and current) parenting errors, her mother did the best she knew how to do and was herself a survivor of much abuse and distressful living. We worked on skills in communication and conflict management that would allow her to deal more effectively with her mother (in getting some degree of separation) and with other family members, professors, and peers. Her challenge of a professor who made a racist implication in class was a very powerful and important experience for her. Although she ended up dropping the class because of his hostile rebuke, she felt empowered, supported by a couple of students, and more assertive. She felt that she had spoken up for her integrity and identity.

Perhaps one of the most important elements of the therapeutic intervention was my attempt to be someone in her life who conveyed a consistent caring attitude that allowed her to discover her abilities. She was able to explore options other than engineering and discover that her grade-point average went up both when the anti-depressants worked and when she chose a major more to her liking and "fit." I was able to convey in all kinds of ways that her uniqueness, despite her lack of a beauty similar to that of White women or her lack of ability to speak Spanish, like that of other Latinos, was indeed special. She was beautiful; she was a "legitimate" full-blown Latina. Referring her to the Hispanic woman's group and encouraging her to join the professional Hispanic organization in her major were helpful strategies in that regard. My ability to convey genuine respect for her as a person and to listen without defensiveness when she was finally able to express anger and disappoint-ment in me were key elements in her empowerment in her relationship with me.

Therapy consisted of almost two years of regular weekly therapy. At termination, she declared that the most important thing I did for her was demonstrate that I "believed in her." My consistency and my ability to be honest and genuine about my care as well as negotiate my limits in a respectful way were important. Indeed, I was able to convey and mirror the admiration that she evoked and that she was then able to see in the eyes of others. The seeds of confidence, which were fortunately planted by her mother's positive aspects of parenting, grew and allowed her to take more risks in her life and to envision more options than a Latina woman in her experience had been allowed. This former client, who at one point was told by an engineering profes-sor that she'd "never make it" in graduate school (and which she heard as "you're not graduate school material at all," and which her grade-point average at the time con-firmed) has successfully completed a graduate program in another, better-suited field.

SUMMARY

Effective psychotherapy with Latinas requires knowledge of the clinician's per-sonal and professional attitudes, beliefs, and knowledge. Despite the challenges, we as clinicians must avoid negative and inappropriate stereotypes and prevent the replication of the experience of discrimination in the therapeutic experience. Knowledge and understanding of the individual and her sociocultural and envi-ronmental experiences as a Latina are important as tools to assess appropriate applications of the client's reality. We must also be aware of the aspects of our training that are irrelevant or even harmful to our clients. Labeling Latinas' need to nurture, care, and connect as "dependent" in a pathological manner can be inappropriate, as can be the failure to help a Latina learn to apply the same standard of care to herself.

Since Latinos make up almost 10 percent of the U.S. population and will by the year 2020 be the largest minority group, it behooves the therapist to learn to appreciate, value, and work effectively with differences. By then, one of every three Americans will be a person of color.

Feminist and multicultural approaches to both individual and group psychotherapy contribute a philosophy, more than technique, that encourages the examination of external factors as causative in the client's problems. The client's strengths rather than weaknesses are emphasized and validated, and approaches are endorsed that result in empowerment of the client to engage in change if she chooses. The Latina often enters therapy with a significant lack of confidence, resulting from the lack of societal validation of her worth, and a clear message that she is responsible for her problems. The role of the therapist is thus not only to impart skills and understanding, but to convey a caring attitude that discovers the abilities of the client, registers with sensitivity and admiration the possibilities and visions for that client, and delights in what is unique, different, and special about her (Bernardez, 1990).

Advocacy, undertaking activities that enhance the ultimate well-being of Latinas, is an unavoidable responsibility. Resources have much to do with one's sense of well-being, and often those with the least access to those resources (economic power, political power, decision making in organizational structures) are Latina women. Using our resources to provide access to resources directly for a client or to change policies, laws, and other institutions that affect Latinas is a social, moral, and professional responsibility.

Through ongoing training, supervision, consultation, and other mechanisms, therapists can greatly enhance their potential to provide competent and ethical psychotherapy to Latinas.

References

Amaro, H., and Russo, N. F. "Hispanic Women and Mental Health: An Overview of Contemporary Issues in Research and Practice." *Psychology of Women Quarterly,* 1987, *11,* 393–408.

Amaro, H., Russo, N. F., and Johnson, J. "Family and Work Predictors of Psychological Well-Being Among Hispanic Women Professionals." *Psychology of Women Quarterly,* 1987, *11,* 505–522.

American College Testing. *Reference Norms for Spring, 1990 ACT-Tested High School Graduates.* Iowa City: Research Services Department, American College Testing Service, 1991.

American Psychological Association. "Hispanics Lack Knowledge About AIDS." *American Psychological Association Monitor,* Feb. 1991, p. 31.

Bernal, G. "Cuban Families." In M. McGoldrick, J. K. Pearce, and J. Giordano (eds.), *Ethnicity and Family Therapy.* New York: Guilford Press, 1982.

Bernardez, T. *Older Women: Inventing Our Lives.* Topeka, Kans.: Menninger Foundation, 1990. Audiotape.

Canino, G. J., and others. "Sex Differences and Depression in Puerto Rico." *Psychology of Women Quarterly,* 1987, *11,* 443–460.

Casas, J. M., and Vasquez, M.J.T. "Counseling the Hispanic Client: A Theoretical and Applied Perspective." In P. B. Pedersen, J. G. Draguns, W. J. Lonner, and J. E. Trimble (eds.), *Counseling Across Cultures.* (3rd ed.) Honolulu: University of Hawaii Press, 1989.

Chacon, M., Cohen, E., and Strover, S. "Chicanas and Chicanos: Barriers to Progress in Higher Education." In M. A. Olivas (ed.), *Latino College Students.* New York: Teachers College, Columbia University Press, 1986.

Chacon, M., and others. *Chicanas in California Post-Secondary Education: A Comparative Study of Barriers to Program Progress.* Stanford, Calif.: Center for Chicano Research, 1985.

Chapa, J., and Valencia, R. R. "Latino Population Growth, Demographic Characteristics, and Educational Stagnation: An Examination of Recent Trends." *Hispanic Journal of Behavioral Sciences,* 1993, *15,* 165–187.

Comas-Díaz, L. "Feminist Therapy with Mainland Puerto Rican Women." *Psychology of Women Quarterly,* 1987, *11,* 461–474.

Comas-Díaz, L. "Culturally Relevant Issues and Treatment Implications for Hispanics." In D. R. Koslow and E. P. Salett (eds.), *Crossing Cultures in Mental Health.* Washington, D.C.: SIETAR International, 1989.

Corvin, S. A., and Wiggins, F. "An Antiracism Training Model for White Professionals." *Journal of Multicultural Counseling and Development,* 1989, *17,* 107–114.

Cromwell, R. E., and Ruiz, R. A. "The Myth of Macho Dominance in Decision Making Within Mexican and Chicano Families." *Hispanic Journal of Behavioral Sciences,* 1979, *1,* 355–373.

Feldman-Summers, S., and Ashworth, C. D. "Factors Related to Intentions to Report Rape." *Journal of Social Issues,* 1981, *4,* 53–70.

Gandara, P. "Passing Through the Eye of a Needle: High-Achieving Chicanas." *Hispanic Journal of Behavioral Sciences,* 1982, *4,* 167–179.

Gilligan, C., Rogers, A. G., and Tolman, D. L. (eds.). *Women, Girls and Psychotherapy: Reframing Resistance.* Binghamton, N.Y.: Harrington Park Press, 1991.

Goodyear, R. K., and Sinnett, E. R. "Current and Emerging Ethical Issues for Counseling Psychology." *Counseling Psychologist,* 1984, *12,* 87–98.

Hare-Mustin, R. T., Marecek, J., Kaplan, A. G., and Liss-Levinson, N. "Rights of Clients, Responsibilities of Therapists." *American Psychologist,* 1979, *34,* 3–16.

Holiman, M., and Lauver, P. J. "The Counselor Culture and Client-Centered Practice." *Counselor Education and Supervision,* 1987, *26,* 184–191.

Jones, J. M. "Psychology Goes to Work." *Advancing the Public Interest,* 1990, *11,* 3.

Katz, J. H., and Ivey, A. G. "White Awareness: The Frontier of Racism Awareness Training." *Personnel and Guidance Journal,* 1977, *55,* 485–489.

McGrath, E., Keita, G. P., Strickland, B. R., and Russo, N. F. *Women and Depression: Risk Factors and Treatment Issues.* Washington, D.C.: American Psychological Association, 1990.

Miller, J. B. *Connections, Disconnections and Violations*. Wellesley, Mass.: Stone Center, 1988.

Morrison, A. M., and Von Glinow, M. A. "Women and Minorities in Management." *American Psychologist*, 1990, *45*, 200–208.

National Council of La Raza. *Hispanic Education: A Statistical Portrait*. Washington, D.C.: National Council of La Raza, 1990.

Padilla, A. M., Salgado de Snyder, N., Cervantes, R. C., and Baezconde-Garbanati, L. "Self-Regulation and Risk-Taking Behavior: A Hispanic Perspective." In *Research Bulletin*. Los Angeles: Spanish Speaking Mental Health Research Center, Summer 1987.

Pinderhuges, E. *Understanding Race, Ethnicity and Power: The Key to Efficacy in Clinical Practice*. New York: Free Press, 1989.

Pope, K. S., and Vasquez, M.J.T. *Ethics in Psychotherapy and Counseling: A Practical Guide for Psychologists*. San Francisco: Jossey-Bass, 1991.

Ramirez, M. III. *Psychotherapy and Counseling with Minorities: A Cognitive Approach to Individual and Cultural Differences*. New York: Pergamon Press, 1991.

Ramirez, O., and Arce, C. "The Contemporary Chicano Family: An Empirically-Based Review." In A. Baron (ed.), *Explorations in Chicano Psychology*. New York: Praeger Press, 1981.

Sabogal, F., and others. "Hispanic Familism and Acculturation: What Changes and What Doesn't?" *Hispanic Journal of Behavioral Sciences*, 1987, *9*, 397–412.

Salgado de Snyder, N. V. "Factors Associated with Acculturative Stress and Depressive Symptomatology Among Married Mexican Immigrant Women." *Psychology of Women Quarterly*, 1987, *11*, 475–488.

Siegel, J. M., and others. "The Prevalence of Childhood Sexual Assault: The Los Angeles Epidemiology Catchment Area Project." *Journal of Epidemiology*, 1987, *126*, 1141–1153.

Surrey, J. I. *Relationship and Empowerment*. Wellesley, Mass.: Stone Center, 1987.

Torres, S. "A Comparative Analysis of Wife Abuse Among Anglo-American and Mexican-American Battered Women: Attitudes, Nature, Severity, Frequency, and Response to the Abuse." Unpublished doctoral dissertation, University of Texas at Austin, 1986.

U.S. Bureau of the Census. "School Enrollment—Social and Economic Characteristics of Students: October 1987 and 1988. In *Current Population Reports*. Washington, D.C.: U.S. Government Printing Office, 1990.

U.S. Bureau of the Census. *Resident Population Distribution for the United States, Region, and States by Race and Hispanic Origin: 1990*. Washington, D.C.: U.S. Government Printing Office, 1991.

Vasquez, M.J.T. "Confronting Barriers to Participation of Mexican American Women in Higher Education." *Hispanic Journal of Behavioral Sciences*, 1982, *4*, 147–165.

Vasquez, M.J.T. "Power and Status of the Chicana: A Social-Psychological Perspective." In J. L. Martinez and R. H. Mendoza (eds.), *Chicano Psychology.* (2nd ed.) Orlando, Fla.: Academic Press, 1984.

Vasquez-Nuttal, E., Romero-Garcia, I., and De Leon, B. "Sex Roles and Perceptions of Femininity and Masculinity of Hispanic Women: A Review of the Literature." *Psychology of Women Quarterly,* 1987, *11,* 409–426.

Walker, L.E.A. *Terrifying Love: Why Battered Women Kill and How Society Responds.* New York: HarperCollins, 1989.

Wampold, B. E., Casas, J. M., and Atkinson, D. R. "Ethnic Bias in Counseling: An Information Processing Approach." *Journal of Counseling Psychology,* 1981, *28,* 498–503.

Wilkinson, D. Y. "Minority Women: Sociocultural Issues." In A. Brodsky and R. Hare-Mustin (eds.), *Women and Psychotherapy.* New York: Guilford Press, 1980.

Winkler, K. J. "Evidence of 'Cultural Vitality.'" *Chronicle of Higher Education,* Oct. 10, 1990, pp. A5, A8.

Wyatt, G. E. "Sexual Abuse of Ethnic Minority Children: Identifying Dimensions of Victimization." *Professional Psychology: Research and Practice,* 1990, *21,* 338–343.

Zapata, J. T., and Jaramillo, P. T. "The Mexican American Family: An Adlerian Perspective." *Hispanic Journal of Behavioral Sciences,* 1981, *3,* 275–290.

PART SEVEN

THE NEXT GENERATION

Latina Adolescents

CHAPTER EIGHTEEN

The Protective Role of Social Capital and Cultural Norms in Latino Communities

A Study of Adolescent Births

Jill Denner
Douglas Kirby
Karin Coyle
Claire Brindis

This chapter examines the impact and importance of a community's social capital and its contribution to reducing teen pregnancy among poor and at-risk Latinas. The study examined here is based on a sample of Latina adolescents from California and therefore provides insight based on findings from the state with the largest Latino community in the United States. Although subgroup data are not reported, the authors nevertheless make a compelling case for the positive impact of social capital and identify the assets present in Latino communities.

Research on communities typically focuses on risk factors, especially poverty and the paucity of resources or opportunities available to youth in poor communities (W. J. Wilson, 1987). Poverty is associated with an urban underclass that cannot provide adequate resources, resulting in a range of negative youth outcomes including teen childbearing (Coulton and Pandey, 1992; Hogan and Kitagawa, 1985; Kirby, Coyle, Denner, and Gould, 2001; Massey, Gross, and Eggers, 1991; Murry, 1996). Less is known about the characteristics of

This research was supported by a grant from The California Wellness Foundation (TCWF). Created in 1992 as a private and independent foundation, TCWF's mission is to improve the health of the people of California through proactive support of health promotion and disease prevention programs. The authors gratefully acknowledge Marcy Lopez Golden, Jeff Gould, Tony Zepeda, Deborah Ivie, Tiffany Chinn, and the community informants who generously shared their wisdom with us.

communities that thrive despite economic hardship. A cultural-ecological model provides a framework for understanding how residents in poor communities use social organization and cultural values to cope with environmental demands (Ogbu, 1981). Studies that identify social and cultural resources in economically poor communities raise questions about the relevance of the underclass concept for immigrant Latino communities (Vélez-Ibáñez, 1993). This study investigates how four communities limit rates of teenage childbearing among Latinas, despite high rates of poverty. The findings show how high social capital and protective cultural norms can minimize the negative effects of poverty.

HOW COMMUNITIES CAN PROTECT ADOLESCENTS

Most studies of communities focus on risk factors associated with demographic characteristics and the physical environment and pay less attention to the social processes that protect youth (see Table 18.1). For example, studies of adolescents suggest that higher rates of childbearing or sexual behavior are found in urban communities with high crime rates, few positive role models, high rates of unmarried childbearing, and limited countywide economic opportunities (Billy, Brewster, and Grady, 1994; Brooks-Gunn, Duncan, Klebanov, and Sealand, 1993; Coulton and Pandey, 1992). Other risk factors associated with adolescent childbearing include isolation of families, civic disengagement, loss of socialization consistency, and the marginalization of youth (Benson, Leffert, Scales, and Blyth, 1998).

In contrast, a few recent studies have begun to look at resilient communities, ones that successfully respond to adversity (Sampson, Raudenbush, and Earls, 1997; Sonn and Fisher, 1998). Several theories suggest the ways that social processes in communities can protect adolescents from engaging in risky behavior. For example, social ecology models suggest that negative community effects can be mediated by relationships between adolescents and their family, peers, and others in their communities (Bronfenbrenner, 1989). Similarly, sociological models identify the mechanisms through which communities influence adolescents. For example, *collective socialization* models suggest social norms established by adult behavior are internalized by teens, *social comparison* models suggest that inequality in wealth leads to disillusionment and negativity for the future, and *cultural conflict or social competition* models suggest that perceptions of blocked opportunities result in resistance or competition for scarce resources (Jencks and Mayer, 1990).

Based on these models, communities that are high in social capital protect adolescents from the negative effects of poverty. A community that is high in social capital offers parental and kin support, relationship networks that provide collective supervision and resources for youth to pursue goals, positive

Table 18.1. Commonly Measured Community Characteristics

Characteristic	Key Indicator	Data Source
Demographics	Age	U.S. census
	Race/ethnicity	
	Birthplace	
	Employment	
	Educational attainment	
	Head of household	
	Household income	
	Residential mobility	
Physical environment	Crime	Observations
	Density	Local data
	Facilities	
	Graffiti	
	Housing	
	Organizations	
	Services	
Social processes	Social capital	Surveys
	Cultural norms	Interviews
		Local data

opportunities, safe places, and norms that emphasize education, social control, and rule enforcement (Aber, Gephart, Brooks-Gunn, and Connell, 1997; Benson, Leffert, Scales, and Blythe, 1998; Chaskin, 1995; Coleman, 1988; Cook, Shagle, and Degirmencioglu, 1997; Denner, Kirby, and Coyle, 2000; Furstenberg and others, 1999; Garmezy, 1991; Kretzmann and McKnight, 1993; Portes, 1998; Valenzuela and Dornbusch, 1994; T. D. Wilson, 1998). These factors result in a collective efficacy, a willingness of residents to organize and intervene on behalf of the neighborhood and its youth (Jessor, 1993; Sampson, Raudenbush, and Earls, 1997). Although perceived social capital has been linked with general measures of self-reported health in individuals (Kawachi, Kennedy, and Glass, 1999), it has not been linked directly to adolescent birthrates.

Social capital can intersect with cultural norms in immigrant communities to provide unique protection for youth. Some immigrants live in ethnic enclaves that are poor but maintain cultural norms about staying on the good or moral path, and parental authority (Cooper, Denner, and Lopez, 1999; Portes and Zhou, 1993). For example, many recent Central American immigrants in Los Angeles live in poverty but are oriented toward family and community and often have professional and community organizing skills that result in informal networks of support (Chinchilla, Hamilton, and Loucky, 1993; Dorrington, 1995; T. D. Wilson, 1998). Mexican immigrants also rely on well-developed informal networks to find jobs and other assistance (Hayes-Bautista, Schink, and Chapa, 1988; Menjivar, 1997), avoiding government systems that may jeopardize their chances of remaining in the United States. Strong cultural norms found in less acculturated Latinos include respect for the family, which may be a protective factor against early sexual behavior (Flores, Eyre, and Millstein, 1998; Ford and Norris, 1993; Rumbaut, 1999). However, being born outside the United States decreases the likelihood of condom use and increases the likelihood of early pregnancy (Aneshensel, Becerra, Fielder, and Schuler, 1990; Sabogal and Catania, 1996). These studies suggest that social capital and norms can be protective, but we need a better understanding of how they protect adolescents from engaging in risky behavior.

In summary, most research focuses on risk factors in communities. Furthermore, there is little understanding of the social and cultural processes that protect youth from the negative effects of poverty. This chapter aims to partially fill this gap, focusing on Latinas because as a group they have the highest national adolescent birthrates of any major ethnic group (Curtin and Martin, 2000; Ventura, Mathews, and Curtin, 1998) and are the largest ethnic group in California.

METHOD

Like earlier studies designed to enhance our understanding of how community factors influence adolescents (Korbin and Coulton, 1997), this study uses multiple methods. This was an exploratory study designed to generate, rather than test, particular hypotheses or theories. Thus, no formal predictions were specified at the outset. Instead, our goal was to allow potential explanations for known differences in community birthrates to surface from people in the communities. Our strategy included two tasks: (1) to identify Latino communities with adolescent birthrates that were either much lower or much higher than expected given their level of poverty, and (2) to interview adults and youth in the community to elicit possible explanations for the differing birthrates.

To identify Latino communities for inclusion in this study, we obtained data on birthrates for 15- to 17-year-old females in the years 1990 to 1994 for more than two thousand ZIP codes in California.[1] ZIP codes in which fewer than one thousand teens lived over a period of five years (two hundred per year) were dropped from further analysis because the low numbers reduced the stability of the birthrates and increased the likelihood of chance error. ZIP codes that had lower than predicted teen birthrates for Latinas ages 15 to 17 years were identified using multiple regression with teen birthrate as the dependent variable.

Four independent variables that previous research found to be predictive of teen birthrates were used: percentage in ZIP code below poverty, percentage of college graduates, percentage of females between the ages 15 and 25 years who have never been married, and percentage of females employed. A scatter plot was created with the standardized residual on the y-axis and the number of teens on the x-axis. Outliers were ZIP codes with birthrates that were more than two standard deviations below or above the predicted mean. The four ZIP codes with lower-than-predicted birthrates were compared with four ZIP codes with higher-than-predicted birthrates, matched on median household income and the number of Latina teens.

Once the data were identified, quantitative and qualitative data were collected to examine demographics and physical environment (see Table 18.1). The 1990 U.S. census was the source for data on head of household, professional jobs, housing, public assistance, poverty, birthplace, linguistic isolation, and high school graduation. Data on high school dropout, student and teacher demographics, and college enrollment were obtained from the California Education Data Partnership profiles of California public schools Web site (data1.cde.ca.gov/dataquest) and a Web site called theschoolreport.com. Other data from CACI Marketing Systems include median household income, population, median age, and race/ethnicity (CACI, 1997). Data on each of the ZIP codes were also compiled from city maps and visits to the communities.

To collect data on the possible explanations for the differing birthrates, we identified informants who worked with youth-serving agencies through Internet searches, phone books, and existing contacts. All known agencies that had contact with youth in the target ZIP codes were contacted. On the phone, we asked to speak with the person who knew about youth and youth programs in the community. We explained our study of teen birthrates in California, but did not tell the informant whether their site was high or low. Initial interviews conducted by phone were designed to gather information on youth programs and opportunities, community collaboration, social services, schools, parental monitoring, and community norms about teenage sex and pregnancy. We also asked for the names of other people who were familiar with the community. Informants included representatives from social service agencies, clinics, libraries, government institutions, churches, and schools. Although this sample is not representative of all residents in the ZIP code, we followed up all leads to reach people who were most involved with youth and knowledgeable about their community.

Field-based methods of data collection were used to supplement the telephone interviews. We visited each ZIP code to collect data on visible indicators of community characteristics and to conduct more in-depth interviews with professionals from youth-serving agencies who were identified as key resources during the phone interviews. These professionals introduced us to youth to interview at the programs. We also questioned a convenience sample of teens and adults on the street, in local restaurants and stores, and in local businesses. In either English or Spanish, we asked them about programs, attitudes toward youth, community norms, and adult involvement with youth. In urban areas, institutions outside the ZIP code that served many teens from the ZIP code of interest were also visited. For sites with low teen birthrates, 103 people were interviewed, averaging 25 per community. For sites with high teen birthrates, 64 people were interviewed, averaging 16 people per community. Only themes that were repeated in more than one interview are reported here.

RESULTS

Demographic Characteristics

Our analyses focused on California ZIP codes that had more than one thousand Latinas ages 15 to 17 years residing over a five-year period. The mean annual birthrate for these Latinas was 80 births per 1,000 for the years 1990 to 1994. In contrast, the four low-birthrate ZIP codes averaged 50 births per 1,000, which was especially low when compared with the rate predicted by economic factors in those communities (90 per 1,000). The high-birthrate ZIP codes averaged 131 births per 1,000 Latinas ages 15 to 17 years, compared with the 91 per 1,000 predicted by economic indicators. Of the four low-teen-birthrate sites, two were rural farming towns, one was urban, and one was suburban. Of the four high teen birthrate sites, two were urban and two were suburban. Table 18.2 contains data for each of the low- and high-teen-birthrate ZIP codes on key indicators. Some of the ZIP codes included an entire town (for example, Calexico), whereas other ZIP codes were one small part of a city (for example, Los Angeles). School-level data were not available for one low-birthrate ZIP code because we were not able to identify any high school attended by the majority of students.

Demographic differences across high- and low-teen-birthrate sites partially supported previous studies of which community characteristics are associated with high rates of teen births. As others have found, high birthrates were associated with a higher percentage of married females ages 15 to 25 years, a larger population, and fewer new housing or business improvements. Findings that are inconsistent with previous studies are that, compared with high-teen-birthrate sites, the low-birthrate sites had a lower median household income, higher male unemployment, fewer home owners, more dense population, and fewer high school graduates. Low-birthrate sites also had a higher percentage of Hispanics and a lower percentage of adults born in the United States.

Social Capital

In addition to the demographic differences just described, data collected from interviews and observations distinguished the low- and high-teen-birthrate ZIP

Table 18.2. Comparison of Communities Across Demographics, Physical Environments, and Social Processes

	Low Teen Birthrate by ZIP Code				High Teen Birthrate by ZIP Code					
	Calexico	San Ysidro	Los Angeles	Gonzales	Bakersfield	Redwood City	Stockton	Los Angeles	Mean (low rates)	Mean (high rates)
Hispanic 15 to 17 year old										
Birthrate, 1990–1994	43	45	73	39	136	137	106	146	50	131
Number female, 1990–1994	4,235	4,186	2,257	1,016	2,566	1,725	1,801	1,621	2,923	1,928
Demographics										
Median household income										
1990	20,050	19,768	15,760	28,861	20,475	30,969	27,909	18,724	21,109	24,519
1997	18,851	24,310	19,045	34,250	23,698	39,676	26,859	23,964	24,114	28,549
Population	22,452	30,253	19,003	12,930	33,961	28,627	31,397	35,606	21,159	32,397
Ages 15 to 25 never married (%)	75	70	59	75	68	63	65	49	70	61
Male employment (%)	53	40	71	18	61	70	51	71	45	63
Female employment (%)	33	37	46	40	38	60	35	49	39	45
Professional jobs (%)	14	14	9	7	16	13	11	16	11	14
Median age, 1990	26.3	26.0	25.7	28.7	26.7	28.5	28.8	28.8	26.7	28.2
Own housing (%)	21	32	9	43	46	38	55	8	26	36
Public assistance (%)	25	29	13	13	22	8	27	12	20	17

(Continued)

Table 18.2. Comparison of Communities Across Demographics, Physical Environments, and Social Processes (Continued)

	Low Teen Birthrate by ZIP Code				High Teen Birthrate by ZIP Code				Mean (low rates)	Mean (high rates)
	Calexico	San Ysidro	Los Angeles	Gonzales	Bakersfield	Redwood City	Stockton	Los Angeles		
Below poverty level (%)	31	29	42	26	30	15	27	29	32	25
Same house 1985 (%)	54	40	46	42	45	43	51	33	45	43
Hispanic (%)	95	77	87	57	53	56	41	56	79	51
Adult U.S. born (%)	34	44	10	65	79	50	75	21	38	56
Child U.S. born (%)	84	82	66	77	92	72	88	61	77	78
Foreign born who came to United States, 1987–1990 (%)	10	10	26	14	16	24	13	29	15	20
Linguistic isolation (%)	37	28	51	18	12	19	12	42	33	21
High school graduate (%)	36	35	26	52	55	60	47	51	37	53
Hispanic high school graduate (%)	34	35	17	26	35	37	35	22	28	32
High schools										
Hispanic students (%)	97	68	NA	82	67	37	53	88	82	61
Hispanic teachers (%)	45	24	NA	NA	19	11	17	21	34	17
Total dropout rate	3.1	4.2	NA	NA	5.2	1.3	3.2	11.9	3.6	5.4
Hispanic dropout rate	6.4	9.8	NA	NA	10.8	9.6	8.1	22.9	8.1	12.8
Enroll junior college (%)	70	45	NA	23	50	30	30	45	57	39
Enroll four-year college (%)	5	35	NA	24	32	51	15	25	20	31

Physical environment									
Population density/ square mile	9,316	9,781	14,641	1,765	11,602	9,693	11,619	24,360	8,875	14,318
Vacant housing (%)	2	4	6	9	7	4	4	8	5.10	5.75
County crime per 1,000	3,267	2,631	3,527	2,108	2,692	1,394	3,402	3,527	2,883	2,753
Number of parks	12	5	2	NA	2	4	5	3	6.1	3.2
New improvement	Yes	Yes	Yes	Yes	No	No	No	No	Yes	No
Clinics three-mile radius	2	1	3+	0	3+	3+	2	3+	1+	2+
Hospital in ZIP code	0	0	0	0	1	1	0	0	0	0.5
Community center	No	Yes	Yes	No	No	Yes	No	Yes	Yes/no	Yes/no
Teen center in ZIP code	No	No	No	No	No	Yes	No	No	No	No/yes
Colleges in ZIP code	Yes	Yes	Yes	No	Yes	No	No	Yes	Yes/no	Yes/no
Social processes										
Social networks	High	Medium	Medium	High	Low	Low	Low	Low	Medium/ high	Low
Institutional collaboratives	Yes	Yes	No	No	No	No	No	No	Yes/no	No
Staff from community	Yes	Yes	Yes	Yes	No	No	No	No	Yes/no	No
Cultural context	Mexican border	Mexican border	Urban/ immigrant	Rural/ farming	Urban Suburban	Suburban	Suburban	Urban	All	Suburban/ urban

Table 18.3. Factors That Mediate the Impact of Community Economic
Factors on Hispanic Teen Birthrates

Factor	Example
Social capital	Shared adult monitoring
	Connection to adults
	Information channels
	Locally run agencies
	Reciprocal obligations
	Shared norms about teen behavior
	Social networks
	Staff educated and from the community
	Youth know and look out for each other
	Youth are viewed positively by adults
Cultural norms	Commitment to family
	Connection to country of origin
	Intergenerational families
	Religious values
	Respect for adults

codes, suggesting that the low-teen-birthrate communities had a wealth of resources that could not be measured with traditional indicators alone. Two major themes emerged: social capital and cultural norms, which are summarized in Table 18.3.

There were several indications that the low-teen-birthrate ZIP codes had levels of social capital higher than expected given their poverty level. The low-birthrate towns had more social networks, institutional collaboratives, and staff from the community than the high sites. Although poverty was higher in the ZIP codes with lower-than-predicted teen birthrates, residents chose to live and work in these more homogeneous communities with stronger informal support systems and a shared culture because they viewed them as better places for their children. Despite the comparable levels of crime at the county level, several parents shared the following view: "Many people stay in [the community] because it is not as violent, it is a good place to raise kids." All of the low-teen-birthrate sites were undergoing changes that included new business, new housing, increased police presence, and efforts to reduce gangs and crime. In one community where several residents cited increased police presence and community improvements as possible explanations for low teen birthrates, an educator said there is a "sense of quietness in schools . . . more sense of hope, that things are moving in a forward direction." These informants suggested that collaboration within the community increased monitoring and residents' sense of safety.

Much of the social capital was informal, such as residents sharing child rearing and mutual support, due to long histories of relationships and extended family. For example, a school secretary lived next door to her mother, who took care of her children while she worked. Although the census data indicated small differences between low- and high-birthrate sites in the numbers who had been in the same house since 1985, interviews suggested that in the low-teen-birthrate sites, more people were related and knew each other due in part to immigration patterns and the multiple generations that lived there. Therefore, although people did move, many of those who moved in were already connected to the community and moved to be near friends or family.

The high- and low-teen birthrate communities also differed in the level of staff investment and connection to the community. Most of the low-birthrate communities had a nonprofit organization (health center, community center, or youth program) that had existed for twenty years or more, was run by a longstanding member of the community, and had a positive reputation for serving the Latino community. Many of the staff had grown up in the area, left to get an education, and returned because they wanted to give back to the community and be near family. As one youth worker told us, he went to the center as a child and was committed to "giving back." He devoted so much time to the center that "[my] wife says I give too much. . . . I can't be a father to everyone." In one school district, the principal reported that 60 percent of the teachers had graduated from the local high school. At another school, staff said, "Teachers are surrogate fathers . . . [they] show the kids tough love." Parents at this school said it was "staffed by people who really care about the neighborhood and the kids' futures." For the ZIP codes in which we could identify a high school, data from the California Department of Education show that low-teen-birthrate ZIP codes had a higher proportion of Hispanic teachers, suggesting a greater potential for role models. Agencies and schools in the high-teen-birthrate communities were also run by caring individuals, but fewer were Hispanic, from the community, or connected to other youth-serving agencies.

Cultural Norms

The data suggested differences in cultural norms between the two groups of ZIP codes. As shown in Table 18.2, compared with the ZIP codes with high teen birthrates, low ZIP codes had a higher percentage of Hispanic residents, fewer adults born in the United States, and more households that were linguistically isolated. Visits to the communities revealed that two of the low-teen-birthrate ZIP codes were located on the United States–Mexico border, and the other two had ethnic enclaves of families who had immigrated from Mexico or Central America. Residents suggested that the community was "seen as part of Mexico . . . the closest thing to it and still be in the U.S." Interviews with local residents and staff showed that these ties resulted in the maintenance of traditional values about commitment to family and community, respect for family and family reputation, close ties to religious institutions, and the control, close monitoring, and protection of girls. Proximity to the home country and the constant return or influx of immigrants helped maintain these values. One teacher said, "Many of the residents have close relatives in the middle-class in [Mexico] and I believe some of the family traditions and norms are influenced by those linkages." In contrast, nobody in the high-teen-birthrate sites described the community as strongly identified with Latino culture, consistent with the lower percentage of Hispanic residents. All of the low-teen-birthrate communities were described as closely knit. One social service agency director explained that "because all speak Spanish, [they] share a background. There are no high-income areas, ethnic areas, [or] language differences. It feels like a community wherever you go. You don't have to self-identify as Chicano, Mexicano, because all are the same. There is no contrast, no comparison to rich people." In a different town, another social service agency director said, "This community sticks together . . . small town feel amongst residents, culturally homogenous surrounded by White communities helps them stick together. Forty-four percent of the community is pedestrian-based, information is shared that way." Residents said that "[it] feels that family is very important and that family, school, and community agencies all work together to ensure their kids have a future." Most agreed that most residents in the community know each other.

In contrast, high-teen-birthrate communities were more ethnically diverse, and interviews with people who were not Latino revealed the perspective that Latinos had moved in and negatively changed the culture of the community. One Korean shop owner felt that Latinos had displaced what was once an Asian community: "They come here like everywhere in L.A. . . . everybody move away." The White director of a community center complained that Mexican-descent residents who are new to the neighborhood took advantage of the food program, saying that "they abuse the system." These comments reflect a lack of unity across ethnic groups in these communities.

Views on youth varied as well. In the small communities with low teen birthrates, adult feelings about teens were mostly positive. Agency staff said, "Adults think teens are good kids and want them to get a good education." School staff said they have "good kids, all know each other and watch each others' back . . . they have respect." In the high-teen-birthrate communities, attitudes toward youth were either neutral or negative. Many of the staff lived outside the community or were less familiar with youth needs. Negative attitudes toward youth were demonstrated by the words of one program director, who, when asked about gender differences during adolescence, stated that "the girls are just as mouthy as the boys."

The residents of the low-teen-birthrate communities had more clear opinions about adolescent pregnancy in their community. Even though these communities had lower birthrates than expected given their poverty level, most believed birthrates were still too high. As one very devoted high school principal stated, "Don't tell me we don't have a [teen pregnancy] problem!" Many residents in the low sites stated that teen pregnancy was not desirable and described a growing acceptance of reproductive health services to prevent pregnancy despite strong religious views. Residents lamented the lack of communication between parents and children about issues related to sex and birth control; they also reported an increase in acceptance of birth control and parent willingness to have schools teach sex education. Two mothers described parents who "put their daughter on the Pill but don't talk about it." Indeed, teens reported that most had some knowledge of where to get contraception. As reported by an 18-year-old female, "Most who get pregnant knew where to go [for contraception]."

In contrast, in the communities with high teen birthrates, there was no clearly stated consensus on whether teen pregnancy was a problem in the community or what attitude parents had toward contraception. Residents of these communities were less informed or involved in what teenagers were doing.

DISCUSSION

The findings suggest that economic indicators alone are not sufficient for understanding the protective role of communities (Coulton and Pandey, 1992). In this study, high social capital and strong, shared, cultural norms were associated with lower-than-predicted teen birthrates for 15- to 17-year-old Latinas. Specific protective characteristics included small size, low density, low proportion of adults born in the United States, and high percentage of Hispanic residents. Low-teen-birthrate communities had characteristics of *colonias,* which have a Latino majority and close ties to their home country (Rochín and Castillo, 1993). Residents chose to live or work in these communities to be close to family, have informal networks of support, and shared monitoring of children. When community residents share cultural norms, this strengthens family messages about sexual behavior, supporting the family connectedness and monitoring that lowers teen pregnancy (Resnick and others, 1997).

The findings support previous assertions that social capital protects Latino communities from some of the negative effects of poverty (Vélez-Ibáñez, 1993). This may be because many Latino communities are characterized by intergenerational networks of support, monitoring, and political organization that build on cultural traditions (Valenzuela and Dornbusch, 1994; Vélez-Ibáñez, 1993). In the more homogeneous communities, residents identified more strongly with each other and their home country, reducing social competition and comparison (Matute-Bianchi, 1991; W. J. Wilson, 1987). Informal economies that include day laboring, street vending, services performed in the home, and local businesses reinforce cultural and ethnic identity (Chinchilla, Hamilton, and Loucky, 1993) and build local networks by minimizing reliance on services or support from outside the community. In the more heterogeneous communities, recent changes in the population created divisions along ethnic lines and undermined social cohesion.

When this study began, interviews were focused on how programs and other services distinguished ZIP codes with low and high teen birthrates for Latinas ages 15 to 17 years. In fact, programs and agencies in low-teen-birthrate ZIP codes did have some of the characteristics considered to be part of successful programs: integrated services were available, they were run by local community members, staff were invested and trained, and teens were involved in running the program (Kirby, Denner, and Coyle, 2000). However, there were relatively few programs in any of the communities, and it was the social processes that seemed to be more important.

The findings have implications for strengthening communities. Despite the apparent benefits of living in a homogenous community, we do not recommend segregation because there may be negative effects on other aspects of adolescent functioning, such as opportunities for employment and higher education. Instead, interventions should focus on building social capital within diverse communities by building communication across youth-serving agencies and between youth-serving agencies and diverse community members, helping residents see that the success of their community rests in part on their investment in youth (Cooper, Denner, and Lopez, 1999).

There are four important limitations to this study. First, the sample of communities is small and may not be generalized to all communities with similar birthrates, although consistent themes were found within the four low- and four high-birthrate communities. Second, the community informants were selected based on a convenience and snowball sample so that their views cannot be generalized to each community as a whole. Fewer interviews were conducted in the high-teen-birthrate communities, which were larger and more challenging to understand, and there were minimal data collected on family strategies associated with resilience among children (Jarrett, 1995). A third limitation is that interviews were conducted in 1998 and 1999, while the teen birthrate data were from 1990 to 1994. After the analyses were completed, data from 1995 to 1996 became available and showed similar birthrate trends, but even these data were three years old at the time of the interviews and observations. Finally, ZIP codes were used to define a community and may not reflect how residents define their own community or current social conditions (Furstenberg, 1993).

In spite of these limits, this study adds to the small but growing body of research on the social organization of resilient communities. It is a pilot study intended to contribute to the development of a language that will help communities identify and build on existing resources (Benson, Leffert, Scales, and

Blyth, 1998; Kretzmann and McKnight, 1993). The findings point to several promising strategies, including training local staff for leadership positions, supporting parents to sustain cultural norms, and nurturing informal networks of support across families and generations. In contrast to current intervention strategies that focus on individuals, the current findings suggest there are strengths in the shared culture and social capital of communities that may minimize the negative effects of poverty on teen birthrates. Informal social organization is difficult to measure with quantitative indicators but appears to be an important mechanism that can modify links between poverty and teen birthrates. The current challenges are to develop (1) clearer definitions of social capital and methods of measuring both it and community norms, (2) more rigorous methods of measuring the impact of social capital on adolescent behavior, and (c) interventions to support communities to build and maintain informal networks and shared values while also increasing children's access to resources outside their community.

Note

1. The database was created by Jeffrey B. Gould, professor of maternal and child health, University of California, Berkeley, School of Public Health. It integrated the Improved Perinatal Outcome Data Management database, census data, and California birth certificate data files.

References

Aber, J. L., Gephart, M. A., Brooks-Gunn, J., and Connell, J. P. "Development in Context: Implications for Studying Neighborhood Effects." In J. Brooks-Gunn, G. J. Duncan, and J. L. Aber (eds.), *Neighborhood Poverty: Context and Consequences for Children.* New York: Russell Sage, 1997.

Aneshensel, C. S., Becerra, R. M., Fielder, E. P., and Schuler, R. H. "Onset of Fertility-Related Events During Adolescence: A Prospective Comparison of Mexican American and Non-Hispanic White Females." *American Journal of Public Health,* 1990, *80,* 959–963.

Benson, P. L., Leffert, N., Scales, P. C., and Blyth, D. A. "Beyond the 'Village' Rhetoric: Creating Healthy Communities for Children and Adolescents." *Applied Developmental Science,* 1998, *2,* 138–159.

Billy, J.O.G., Brewster, K. L., and Grady, W. R. "Contextual Effects on the Sexual Behavior of Adolescent Women." *Journal of Marriage and the Family,* 1994, *56,* 387–404.

Bronfenbrenner, U. "Ecological Systems Theory." *Annals of Child Development,* 1989, *6,* 185–249.

Brooks-Gunn, J., Duncan, G. J., Klebanov, P. K., and Sealand, N. "Do Neighborhoods Influence Child and Adolescent Development?" *American Journal of Sociology,* 1993, *99,* 353–395.

CACI. *The Sourcebook of ZIP Code Demographics: 12th Edition.* Chantilly, Va.: CACI, 1997.

Chaskin, R. J. *Defining Neighborhood: History, Theory, and Practice.* Chicago: Chapin Hall Center for Children, University of Chicago, 1995.

Chinchilla, N., Hamilton, N., and Loucky, J. "Central Americans in Los Angeles: An Immigrant Community in Transition." In J. Moore and R. Pinderhughes (eds.), *In the Barrios: Latinos and the Underclass Debate.* New York: Russell Sage, 1993.

Coleman, J. S. "Social Capital in the Creation of Human Capital." *American Journal of Sociology,* 1988, *94,* 95–121.

Cook, T. D., Shagle, S. C., and Degirmencioglu, S. M. "Capturing Social Process for Testing Mediational Models of Neighborhood Effects." In J. Brooks-Gunn, G. J. Duncan, and J. L. Aber (eds.), *Neighborhood Poverty: Context and Consequences for Children.* New York: Russell Sage, 1997.

Cooper, C. R., Denner, J., and Lopez, E. M. "Cultural Brokers: Helping Latino Children on Pathways Toward Success." *Future of Children,* 1999, *9,* 51–57.

Coulton, C. J., and Pandey, S. "Geographic Concentration of Poverty and Risk to Children in Urban Neighborhoods." *American Behavioral Scientist,* 1992, *35,* 238–257.

Curtin, S. C., and Martin, J. A. *Births: Preliminary Data for 1999.* Hyattsville, Md.: National Center for Health Statistics, 2000.

Denner, J., Kirby, D., and Coyle, K. "How Communities Can Promote Positive Youth Development: Responses from 49 Professionals." *Community Youth Development,* 2000, *1,* 31–35.

Dorrington, C. "Central American Refugees in Los Angeles." In R. E. Zambrana (ed.), *Understanding Latino Families: Scholarship, Policy, and Practice.* Thousand Oaks, Calif.: Sage, 1995.

Flores, E., Eyre, S. L., and Millstein, S. G. "Sociocultural Beliefs Related to Sex Among Mexican American Adolescents." *Hispanic Journal of Behavioral Sciences,* 1998, *20,* 60–82.

Ford, K., and Norris, A. E. "Urban Hispanic Adolescents and Young Adults: Relationship of Acculturation to Sexual Behavior." *Journal of Sex Research,* 1993, *30,* 316–323.

Furstenberg, F. F., Jr. "How Families Manage Risk and Opportunity in Dangerous Neighborhoods." In W. J. Wilson (ed.), *Sociology and the Public Agenda.* Thousand Oaks, Calif.: Sage, 1993.

Furstenberg, F. F., Jr., and others. *Managing to Make It: Urban Families and Adolescent Success.* Chicago: University of Chicago Press, 1999.

Garmezy, N. "Resiliency and Vulnerability to Adverse Developmental Outcomes Associated with Poverty." *American Behavioral Scientist,* 1991, *34,* 416–430.

Hayes-Bautista, D. E., Schink, W. O., and Chapa, J. *The Burden of Support: Young Latinos in an Aging Society.* Stanford, Calif.: Stanford University Press, 1988.

Hogan, D. P., and Kitagawa, E. M. "The Impact of Social Status, Family Structure, and Neighborhood on the Fertility of Black Adolescents." *American Journal of Sociology,* 1985, *90,* 825–855.

Jarrett, R. L. "Growing Up Poor: The Family Experiences of Socially Mobile Youth in Low-Income African-American Neighborhoods." *Journal of Adolescent Research,* 1995, *10,* 111–135.

Jencks, C., and Mayer, S. E. "The Social Consequences of Growing Up in a Poor Neighborhood." In L. E. Lynn Jr. and M.G.H. McGeary (eds.), *Inner-City Poverty in the United States.* Washington, D.C.: National Academy Press, 1990.

Jessor, R. "Successful Adolescent Development Among Youth in High-Risk Settings." *American Psychologist,* 1993, *48,* 117–126.

Kawachi, I., Kennedy, B. P., and Glass, R. "Social Capital and Self-Rated Health: A Contextual Analysis." *American Journal of Public Health,* 1999, *89,* 1187–1193.

Kirby, D., Coyle, K., Denner, J., and Gould, J. "Manifestations of Poverty and Birthrates Among Teenagers in California Zip Code Analysis." *Family Planning Perspectives,* 2001, *33*(2), 63–69.

Kirby, D., Denner, J., and Coyle, K. *Building the Ideal Community or Youth Program: An Expert Panel Rates the Key Characteristics for Reducing Teen Pregnancy.* Washington, D.C.: National Campaign to Prevent Teen Pregnancy, 2000.

Korbin, J. E., and Coulton, C. J. "Understanding the Neighborhood Context for Children and Families: Combining Epidemiological and Ethnographic Approaches." In J. Brooks-Gunn, G. J. Duncan, and J. L. Aber (eds.), *Neighborhood Poverty: Policy Implications in Studying Neighborhoods.* New York: Russell Sage, 1997.

Kretzmann, J. P., and McKnight, J. L. *Building Communities from the Inside Out: A Path Toward Mobilizing a Community's Assets.* Chicago: ACTA Publications, 1993.

Massey, D. S., Gross, A. B., and Eggers, M. L. "Segregation, the Concentration of Poverty, and the Life Chances of Individuals." *Social Science Research,* 1991, *20,* 397–420.

Matute-Bianchi, M. E. "Situational Ethnicity and Patterns of School Performance Among Immigrant and Non-Immigrant Mexican Descent Students." In M. Gibson and J. Ogbu (eds.), *Minority Status and Schooling: A Comparative Study of Immigrant and Involuntary Minorities.* New York: Garland, 1991.

Menjivar, C. "Immigrant Kinship Networks: Vietnamese, Salvadoreans, and Mexicans in Comparative Perspective." *Journal of Comparative Family Studies,* 1997, *28,* 1–24.

Murry, V. M. "Inner-City Girls of Color: Unmarried, Sexually Active Nonmothers." In B.J.R. Leadbeater and N. Way (eds.), *Urban Girls: Resisting Stereotypes, Creating Identities.* New York: NYU Press, 1996.

Ogbu, J. U. "Origins of Human Competence: A Cultural-Ecological Perspective." *Child Development,* 1981, *52,* 413–429.

Portes, A. "Social Capital: Its Origins and Applications in Modern Sociology." *Annual Review of Sociology,* 1998, *24,* 1–24.

Portes, A., and Zhou, M. "The New Second Generation: Segmented Assimilation and Its Variants Among Post-1965 Immigrant Youth." *Annals of the American Academy of Political Social Science,* 1993, *530,* 74–96.

Resnick, M. D., and others. "Protecting Adolescents from Harm: Findings from the National Longitudinal Study on Adolescent Health." *Journal of the American Medical Association,* 1997, *278,* 823–832.

Rochín, R. I., and Castillo, M. D. *Immigration, Colonia Formation, and Latino Poor in Rural California: Evolving "Immiseration."* Claremont, Calif.: Tomás Rivera Center, 1993.

Rumbaut, R. G. "Assimilation and Its Discontents." In C. Hirschman, J. De Wind, and P. Kasinitz (eds.), *The Handbook of International Migration: The American Experience.* New York: Russell Sage, 1999.

Sabogal, F., and Catania, J. A. "HIV Risk Factors, Condom Use, and HIV Antibody Testing Among Heterosexual Hispanics: The National AIDS Behavioral Surveys (NABS)." *Hispanic Journal of Behavioral Sciences,* 1996, *18,* 367–391.

Sampson, R. J., Raudenbush, S. W., and Earls, F. "Neighborhoods and Violent Crime: A Multilevel Study of Collective Efficacy." *Science,* 1997, *277,* 918–924.

Sonn, C. C., and Fisher, A. T. "Sense of Community: Community Resilient Responses to Oppression and Change." *Journal of Community Psychology,* 1998, *26,* 457–472.

Valenzuela, A., and Dornbusch, S. M. "Familism and Social Capital in the Academic Achievement of Mexican Origin and Anglo Adolescents." *Social Science Quarterly,* 1994, *75,* 18–36.

Vélez-Ibáñez, C. "U.S. Mexicans in the Borderlands: Being Poor Without the Underclass." In J. Moore and R. Pinderhughes (eds.), *In the Barrios: Latinos and the Underclass Debate.* New York: Russell Sage, 1993.

Ventura, S. J., Mathews, T. J., and Curtin, S. C. *Declines in Teenage Birth Rates, 1991–1997: National and State Patterns.* Hyattsville, Md.: National Center for Health Statistics, 1998.

Wilson, T. D. "Weak Ties, Strong Ties: Network Principles in Mexican Migration." *Human Organization,* 1998, *57,* 394–403.

Wilson, W. J. *The Truly Disadvantaged: The Inner City, the Underclass, and Public Policy.* Chicago: University of Chicago Press, 1987.

CHAPTER NINETEEN

Smoking Acquisition Among Adolescents and Young Latinas

The Role of Socioenvironmental and Personal Factors

Celia P. Kaplan
Anna Nápoles-Springer
Susan L. Stewart
Eliseo J. Pérez-Stable

The research findings reported in this chapter present a comprehensive examination of an array of predictor variables ranging from tobacco experimentation to regular use for Latina adolescents. The focus on young Latinas has special merit in that the findings contribute to the design and implementation of prevention programs designed for this population. The findings also highlight the importance of analyzing smoking at various stages of adoption among Latinas. Although the authors do not describe the Latino population in their cohort, the participants were selected from Planned Parenthood clinics in Los Angeles County. Given this information, it is safe to assume that the vast majority of the cohort was likely of Mexican descent. However, the findings are not immediately generalizable to the larger Latina population.

Cigarette smoking represents a significant public health problem and has been identified as the single most preventable cause of disease and premature death in the United States. Although adolescent smoking rates as a whole have increased in the United States in the past decade, data from California studies indicate that teen smoking remained fairly stable between 1990 and 1993. However, recent studies among California adolescents identify an increase in smoking-related behavior since 1993 (Pierce and others, 1994,

We would like to acknowledge funding support from the University of California, Tobacco-Related Disease Research Program (Grant 2KT004).

1998). Furthermore, these studies show a greater increase among girls than boys. Smoking in young women is of particular concern, not only because it poses long- and short-term hazards to the smoker's health, but also due to its potential immediate impact on reproductive function, health of children, and birth outcomes (Berman and Gritz, 1991; Gritz, 1984).

Latino populations have been identified as being at high risk for smoking (Glynn, Anderson, and Schwartz, 1991), particularly as they become increasingly targeted by the media (Ernster, 1985) and adopt the patterns of behavior of non-Latino populations. Current data indicate that Latino adolescents of both sexes are more likely to report current cigarette use than African American adolescents but less likely than non-Latino whites (Pierce and others, 1998). The 1989 Teenage Attitudes and Practices Surveys found that 49.5 percent of whites, ages 12 to 18 years, reported having ever smoked compared with 43.1 percent of Latinos and 36.4 percent of African Americans (U.S. Department of Health and Human Services, 1994). While young adolescent Latino males tend to smoke in similar proportion to their non-Latino white counterparts (Burns and Pierce, 1992), Latina adolescents report somewhat lower rates of smoking than non-Latino white adolescents (Burns and Pierce, 1992). The difference in smoking prevalence between Latino boys and girls reflects the gender-specific nature of smoking and suggests that there may be unique processes that lead to initiation and maintenance of smoking behaviors in each gender. For example, Latinas may be particularly susceptible to smoking as they become more acculturated (Escobedo and Remington, 1989; Marin and others, 1989; Sabogal, Otero-Sabogal, Pérez-Stable, and Marin, 1989) due to greater sensitivity to cigarette advertisements or use of smoking as a method to reduce acculturative stress (Epstein, Botvin, and Diaz, 1998), whereas young males may be more influenced by risk-taking behavior (Flay, Hu, and Richardson, 1998).

Previous research has certainly increased our understanding of the process of smoking initiation among all ethnic groups, including Latino adolescents (Landrine, Richardson, Klonoff, and Flay, 1994; Lovato and others, 1994; Moreno and others, 1994; Otero-Sabogal, Sabogal, and Pérez-Stable, 1995; Sallis and others, 1994; Vega and others, 1993). However, significant information has been occluded because data concerning onset, experimentation, and regular smoking processes have been combined in analyses or only one of these stages has been examined in isolation. Consequently, these studies have failed to identify the unique factors that may affect the transition from one stage of the smoking continuum to another and to clarify how these antecedents vary across the different stages of smoking intake. In addition, studies that examined separately the stages of smoking acquisition have not included relevant cultural elements essential to the explanation of Latino health behavior (Flay, Hu, and Richardson, 1998).

Smoking initiation primarily begins in adolescence when the consequences to morbidity and mortality seem irrelevant or distant. In fact, among adults who smoke daily, almost 90 percent began using cigarettes by age 18 (U.S. Department of Health and Human Services, 1994). The choice about whether to smoke can be conceptualized as the end point in a series of decisions that reflect the individual's environment and cultural background, as well as personal characteristics. The process comprises several distinct stages beginning with an individual's first attempts to smoke and then further experimentation that can lead to regular smoking. Several frameworks have been developed to describe the progression through the smoking continuum (Flay, Ockene, and Tager, 1992; Flay and others, 1983; Leventhal and Cleary, 1980). In general, these schema divide the period of smoking uptake into successive and progressive stages based on level of cigarette consumption and regularity of smoking (Flay and others, 1983; Pierce and others, 1998; Stern, Prochaska, Velicer, and Elder, 1987). We will evaluate socioenvironmental and personal characteristics as predictors of stages of smoking, as previously identified in the literature for two important stages of the smoking continuum: onset and regular smoking.

The goal of this chapter is to identify whether similar or different socioenvironmental and personal predictors are associated with each of the two stages of the smoking uptake continuum—onset and regular smoking—among a sample of Latinas recruited at two federally funded family planning clinics. Particular emphasis will be placed on the role of cultural factors in each of these stages. Identification of specific antecedents for each of these stages has important implications for the primary and secondary prevention of cigarette smoking among Latino youth. We expect that understanding the unique factors affecting each of the smoking stages will lead to the development of programs to promote specific smoking prevention and cessation interventions targeting adolescents and young Latinas.

ANALYTIC FRAMEWORK AND HYPOTHESES

Socioenvironmental Factors

While an adolescent's decision to experiment or to smoke regularly reflects an individual choice, it is shaped by the social environment, including his or her cultural milieu, the smoking-related behavior of family and peers, and social behavior related to smoking.

Cultural Indicators. Latinos enjoy a relative advantage with respect to several physical health indicators (Markides and Coreil, 1986; Scribner, 1996), despite their overall lower economic and educational status. Studies indicate that, particularly for women, this advantage may be partly attributable to important lifestyle preferences that may be culturally determined, such as low smoking prevalence, balanced diet, and relatively low drinking rates (Alaniz, 1994;

Guendelman and Abrams, 1995; Markides, Coreil, and Ray, 1987). However, this comparative advantage may be disappearing as Latinos adopt the behavioral patterns of the dominant society (Canino, 1994; Markides, Coreil, and Ray, 1987).

One strategy that attempts to identify cultural influences on smoking behavior is to explore the impact of acculturation. There has been extensive debate regarding the definition of acculturation (Barret, Joe, and Simpson, 1991; Burnam, Telles, Hough, and Escobar, 1987; Domino and Acosta, 1987; Garza and Gallegos, 1985). In general, it has been defined as a dynamic, multidimensional phenomenon encompassing "values, ideologies, beliefs . . . attitudes . . . language, cultural customs and practices" (Cuellar, Harris, and Jasso, 1980). As a result of immigration and increasing participation in American life, Latinas are influenced simultaneously by their own cultural heritage and by the social and economic realities of the majority society. Such acculturative or biculturative processes are usually accompanied by changes in attitudes, behaviors, norms, and values that may affect health-related behavior. In particular, among Latina women, acculturation has been linked with changes in attitudes toward smoking (Campbell and Kaplan, 1996; Marin and others, 1989) and an increase in cigarette or alcohol consumption (Canino, 1994; Epstein, Botvin, and Diaz, 1998).

According to Betancourt, the concept of acculturation has helped to measure cultural influences (Betancourt and Lopez, 1993). However, acculturation has also been criticized for its lack of specificity, particularly when the construct is limited to linguistic changes that serve as markers for multifaceted changes in cultural attitudes, norms, and behaviors. To measure acculturation more precisely, we expanded our examination to include other domains that are part of the process of adaptation to a different culture and that usually accompany linguistic changes. Therefore, in addition to linguistic acculturation, we considered beliefs about women's roles within the family and strength of family loyalty (familialism), two important aspects of Latino culture, as relevant dimensions of the acculturation process. A woman's beliefs about the role of women in the family may influence the role she envisions for herself, and her role expectations may, in turn, affect her health behaviors. Women who smoke are often portrayed in media advertisements as professional and independent. With increased acculturation, Latinas may begin to view themselves as less traditional, leading them to identify with these media images and initiate smoking. For instance, one study found increased smoking and decreased cessation efforts among more language-acculturated Latina women related to relaxed cultural norms about women who smoke (Wolff and Portis, 1996).

Another empirically substantiated characteristic of Latino culture is the importance of family loyalty or familialism (Moore, 1970; Sabogal and others, 1987). Familialism includes strong attachments to, emphasis on, and identification with family interests and welfare; a preference for living in geographical proximity to other family members; and an emphasis on family interdependence, reciprocity, and mutual support. The family network provides emotional support to its members, protecting them from external and psychological stresses (Keefe, 1980) while influencing patterns of health behavior. Therefore, women with strong family values may be less likely to initiate and adopt smoking than those with weaker family values, particularly if their reasons for smoking are to alleviate stress.

Smoking-Related Behavior of Parents and Peers. Parental factors have been hypothesized to affect the development of adolescent health behaviors through several mechanisms. One of the most evident mechanisms of influence is modeling (Best and others, 1988; Flay and others, 1983; Flay, Hu, and Richardson, 1998). Various studies have shown that parental smoking increases the risk that their children will smoke (Bauman, Foshee, Linzer, and Koch, 1990; Moreno and others, 1994). Peers also have been identified as exerting a strong influence on adolescent behavior (Landrine, Richardson, Klonoff, and Flay, 1994); however, the relative effect of peers varies by ethnic group (Landrine, Richardson, Klonoff, and Flay, 1994). Adolescence is considered a period of increasing influence of peers, leading to the initiation of high-risk behavior to gain recognition and acceptance. Generally, research on peer modeling indicates that adolescents who associate with peers engaging in specific high-risk behaviors (such as smoking) tend to display more of those behaviors themselves (Flay, Hu, and Richardson, 1998). In addition to the role modeling effect, exposure to other smokers, whether they be peers or family, provides the adolescent easy access to tobacco products.

Smoking-Related Norms. Family and peers also influence the adolescent's smoking behavior through a complex system of norms that sanction or discourage smoking. Through these norms, family and friends communicate explicitly or implicitly the acceptability or unacceptability of the behavior and the individual and social consequences of smoking (Chassin, Presson, Sherma, and Edwards, 1991).

Personal Factors

While the social environment shapes and may facilitate the decision to smoke, the adolescent's personal profile may enhance or reduce the chances of smoking. For example, the propensity for rebelliousness has been associated with smoking, as well as with other risk behaviors (Jessor and Jessor, 1977). Jessor and Jessor have argued that there is a propensity for high-risk behavior (behavior that departs from regulatory norms) to cluster.

Behavioral health research has also shown strong links between people's personal beliefs and their health behavior. The Theory of Reasoned Action (Ajzen and Fishbein, 1980) hypothesizes that behavior (smoking) can be predicted by the attitudes about that behavior and the individual's intention to act in a certain way. The theory further hypothesizes that attitudes toward a behavior can be predicted from specific beliefs about the likely consequences of the behavior and the personal evaluation of those consequences. According to this theory, an individual's evaluation of both the risks and benefits of smoking determines the likelihood of smoking initiation and continued use (Ajzen and Fishbein, 1980; Gerber, Newman, and Martin, 1988).

METHODS

The data were obtained in a study assessing the smoking practices, attitudes, and beliefs of young Latinas, ages 14 to 24 years, who were clients at two family planning clinics in Los Angeles County between May 1992 and March 1993. All adolescents (ages 14 to 19 years) receiving services at the participating clinics during the study period were eligible to participate. Family planning clinics offer a good setting to sample potentially high-risk adolescents who may not be attending school and may be at increased risk of smoking. Given the large number of women 20 to 24 years of age receiving services at these clinics, a 25 percent random sample of women in this age group was also invited to participate. The overall response rate was 80.1 percent, and the final sample contained 1,411 respondents. Comparison of respondents and nonrespondents indicates that nonrespondents were less educated than respondents (Kaplan and Tanjasiri, 1996).

Procedures

The original study was also designed to compare two interview modalities, face-to-face and telephone interviews, to ascertain smoking behaviors and attitudes. For the analyses, data resulting from both collection methods were combined since Kaplan and Tanjasiri (1996) found that the two methods yielded comparable results in assessing smoking behaviors and attitudes in this population.

Each eligible woman was approached by the interviewer and asked to participate in the survey. Subjects who agreed were randomly assigned to the two interview modalities. Subjects selected for the face-to-face modality were interviewed at the time they agreed to participate in the survey. Subjects assigned to the telephone interview modality completed a form indicating their telephone number and basic demographic information, such as age, level of education, and smoking behavior. Within two weeks of identification, three bicultural/bilingual interviewers conducted telephone interviews.

Survey Instrument

Development of the survey required several stages that included a review of existing surveys and implementation of focus groups and open-ended interviews. Because the majority of the population was Spanish speaking, all survey items were translated into Spanish by bilingual/bicultural staff and evaluated by a group of bilingual English and Spanish speakers. Finally, the Spanish version of the interview was back translated into English and compared to the original, and the principal investigator and the team of translators resolved inconsistencies. Pretesting of the instrument was conducted on sixty-one members of the target population. The final version included 105 items, and the average length of the survey was twenty-five minutes.

Measures

Outcome Measures. The principal outcome measures classified respondents into the three stages of the smoking continuum:

1. Never smokers: Respondents who have never tried cigarettes, not even a few puffs.

2. Experimenters: Respondents who indicated having tried or experimented with cigarette smoking, even a few puffs, but have smoked less than 100 cigarettes.

3. Regular smokers: Respondents who indicated smoking one hundred cigarettes or more in their lifetime regardless of current smoking status. This criterion for regular smokers is derived from Pierce and others (1998), who identified those addicted to cigarettes as having reported smoking one hundred cigarettes or more.

Predictor Variables

• Demographic indicators. Information about the respondent's age, marital status, highest grade of regular school completed, birthplace, and income was collected.

• Socioenvironmental factors. Socioenvironmental factors were measured by three cultural indicators, four items regarding the smoking-related behavior of family and peers, and three groups of questions pertaining to smoking-related norms.

Cultural indicators. Cultural indicators included linguistic acculturation, beliefs about women's roles within the family, and familialism.

Linguistic acculturation. The linguistic acculturation indicator used in this investigation was based on the acculturation scale developed by Cuellar, Harris, and Jasso (1980) and used in the Hispanic Health and Nutrition Survey (HHANES). Participants responded to eleven items regarding language preferences for speaking, writing, and reading. Response categories were Spanish only, mostly Spanish, both equally, mostly English, and English only. These items were collapsed into three constructs indicating the language the respondent preferred to speak, read, and write. The linguistic acculturation indicator (Cronbach's alpha = 0.90) was created by taking a rounded average of these three constructs, resulting in a five-point scale from 1 (*Spanish only*) to 5 (*English only*).

Beliefs about women's roles within the family. Women's beliefs about family roles were assessed using five items adapted from the National Longitudinal Survey of Youth. Respondents were asked whether they agreed, had no opinion, or disagreed with respect to five items assessing beliefs about women's roles within the family. (See the chapter appendix for a list of items.) All items were combined into a single scale ranging from 1 (traditional) to 3 (less traditional). An internal consistency estimate of 0.80 was obtained for this scale.

Familialism. Four items assessed respondents' perceived obligation to support family members. (See the appendix for a list of items.) These items were a subset of those developed by Sabogal and others (1987) and modified for this population. Respondents were asked whether they agreed (item score = 1), disagreed (item score = 3), or had no opinion (item score = 2). All the items were combined into a single scale that demonstrated modest reliability (Cronbach's alpha = 0.51). This scale ranged from 1 (*traditional*) to 3 (*less traditional*).

Parental and peer smoking-related behavior. Exposure to smoking among friends and family was assessed by reading a list of relatives and friends and asking respondents whether these individuals currently smoke cigarettes. Responses were grouped into two categories: smoking behavior of peers and smoking behavior of parents. Smoking behavior of peers was defined as a continuous variable assessing the total numbers of friends, brothers, sisters, and significant others who smoke. Responses ranged from 0 (no sibling, friend, or significant other smokes) to 4 (friend, sibling, and significant other smoke). Parents' smoking status was dichotomized into whether any parent smoked (coded as 1) or none smoked (coded as 0).

Smoking-related norms. Norms were classified into three groups: friends' norms, parental norms, and siblings' norms. Norms were ascertained by three questions addressing each of the referent groups: (1) How do you think your best friends would feel about you smoking one or more packs of cigarettes a day? (2) If you lit up a cigarette in front of your parents, how do you think they would react? and (3) If you lit up a cigarette in front of your brothers or sisters, how do you think they would react? For each question, response categories included: (1) tell you to stop; (2) disapprove but not tell you to stop; (3) not care if you smoke; and (4) approve of your smoking. Responses indicating "Tell you to stop" were coded as 1 while all other responses were coded as 0.

- Personal factors:

Risk-taking behaviors. Three measures were used to assess an individual's inclination to engage in high-risk behaviors. First, respondents were asked whether they agreed, disagreed, or had no opinion with the statement: "I get a kick out of doing things every now and then that are a little dangerous or risky." This item was derived from the California Tobacco Survey as one of the indicators of rebelliousness (Burns and Pierce, 1992). Respondents who agreed with the statement were classified as reporting risky attitudes (coded as 1); all others were considered as reporting low-risk attitudes (coded as 0). The second measure combined respondent's lifetime utilization of substances such as marijuana, cocaine, amphetamines, or barbiturates. Any use of these substances was sufficient for that individual to be classified as having used drugs (coded as 1). No reported use was classified as never having used drugs (coded as 0). The third measure assessed whether the respondent had ever consumed alcoholic beverages (ever consumed alcohol coded as 1; never consumed alcohol coded as 0).

Intention to smoke in the future. All respondents were asked whether they planned to smoke in a year. Any response other than "definitely not" was considered as an intention to smoke at some point in the future (coded as 1). The other options were "definitely yes," "probably yes," and "probably no."

Data Analysis Procedures

Reliability estimates (Cronbach's alpha) allowed us to examine the relationships between items in each of the linguistic acculturation, beliefs about women's role within the family, and familialism scales. (Results were presented in the Measures section.) Univariate odds ratios and multiple logistic regression models were used to examine the relationship between the selected predictors (intention to smoke) and the two stages of smoking (experimentation and regular smoking). Univariate and multivariate logistic models examined the factors affecting respondents' intentions to smoke in the future, trying smoking, and regular smoking. In addition, we examined the role of intention to smoke as a mediator to trying cigarettes and regular smoking. Results of the logistic regression analyses are presented as exponentiated coefficients, that is, odds ratios and 95 percent confidence intervals. A pseudoadjusted R^2 statistic, the Nagelkerke's R^2, interpreted as the proportion of variation explained for discrete models, provided an indicator of the adequacy of the statistical model (Nagelkerke, 1991).

RESULTS

Demographic Characteristics of Respondents

Overall, 58.2 percent of the respondents were classified as never smokers, 33.5 percent as experimenters (tried cigarettes but smoked fewer than one hundred cigarettes in their lifetime), and 8.4 percent as regular smokers. Table 19.1 shows the

Table 19.1. Demographic Characteristics of Latina Adolescents, Los Angeles Family Planning Clinic Patients, by Smoking Stage, 1992–1993

	Overall N (%)	Never Smokers (N = 821, 58.2%)	Triers/ Experimenters[a] (N = 472, 33.5%)	Regular Smokers[b] (N = 118, 8.4%)
Age (NS)				
17 and younger	305 (21.6)	58.4	35.1	6.6
18–19	365 (25.9)	54.5	35.1	10.4
20 and older	741 (52.5)	59.9	32.0	8.1
Education (p < .0001)				
6 years or less	401 (28.4)	69.8	24.7	5.5
7–11	798 (56.6)	54.4	36.7	8.9
12 years or more	212 (15.0)	50.5	37.7	11.8
Marital status (p < .05)				
Not married	959 (68.0)	56.8	33.4	9.8
Married	452 (32.0)	61.1	33.6	5.3
Country of birth (p < .0001)[c]				
Foreign	1,266 (90.6)	60.1	32.9	7.0
United States	132 (9.4)	38.6	40.9	20.5
Income (NS)[c]				
$0–5,000	317 (44.1)	60.3	30.6	9.1
$5,001–7,500	131 (18.2)	58.0	34.4	7.6
$7,501–15,000	215 (29.9)	54.4	36.3	9.3
More than $15,000	56 (7.8)	48.2	44.6	7.1

[a]Triers/experimenters: Respondents who indicated having tried or experimented with cigarette smoking, even a few puffs, but have smoked fewer than one hundred cigarettes.

[b]Regular smokers: Respondents who indicated smoking one hundred cigarettes or more in their lifetime irrespective of current smoking status.

[c]Does not include missing values.

sample demographic characteristics and the percentages of respondents at each smoking level. The sample was almost equally distributed between adolescents (ages 14–19) and young adults (ages 20–24); the average age of the sample was 20 years (S.D. 2.6). Educational attainment (mean 8.5 years; S.D. 2.8) was lower than would be expected for the age of the young women in the sample, with only

15 percent of the respondents reporting twelve or more years of education. The majority of the respondents were not married at the time of the interview (68.0 percent). The vast majority of the respondents (90.6 percent) were foreign born. Among those who reported income, the vast majority (62.3 percent) reported $7,500 or less in annual income. Overall, there were no age differences in the proportion of respondents across the different smoking stages. However, the distribution of smoking stage of respondents was not the same across educational level, marital status, and country of birth. In particular, respondents with a higher education (twelve years or more) were more likely to start smoking than those with six or less years of education (37.7 percent versus 24.7 percent, $p < .0001$) and were more likely to reach a level of regular smoking than those who had completed six grades or less (11.8 percent versus 5.5 percent, $p < .0001$). With respect to marital status, married women were slightly less likely to have tried smoking than women who were never married (61.1 percent versus 56.8 percent, $p < .05$). Foreign-born respondents were more likely to be never smokers than those born in the United States (60.1 percent versus 38.6 percent, $p < .0001$) and were less likely to become regular smokers than U.S.-born respondents (7.0 percent versus 20.5 percent, $p < .0001$).

Table 19.2 presents the overall distribution of each of the indicators and the corresponding unadjusted odds ratios for comparisons of never smokers with triers and regular smokers and, among those who smoke, triers versus regular smokers. With respect to linguistic acculturation, 74 percent of the sample reported having a Spanish orientation. Almost 40 percent (37.2 percent) were classified as having traditional beliefs regarding women's roles within the family and almost 70 percent (67.8 percent) as having strong traditional values about family obligation as measured by the familialism scale. The three cultural indicators were significantly associated with ever having tried cigarettes. In particular, those reporting nontraditional attitudes and English orientation were more likely to have tried cigarettes. However, only linguistic acculturation was positively associated with regular smoking in the univariate models: those with an English orientation were more likely to report being regular smokers.

Nearly one-third (32.2 percent) of respondents indicated that they had at least one parent who smoked, and 63.5 percent of the young women indicated that they had a friend, sibling, or significant other who smoked. All parental and peer smoking behavior variables significantly increased experimentation and regular smoking—with one exception. Respondents having one peer who smokes did not significantly increase the risk of being a regular smoker compared to those with no peers who smoke.

Almost all of the respondents (91.1 percent) reported that their parents would tell them to stop smoking if they found out; however, this proportion decreased to 78.6 percent for siblings' reaction and 44.9 percent for friends' reactions. Siblings' reaction was the only variable associated with ever trying cigarettes

Table 19.2. Univariate Odds Ratios for Two Stages of Cigarette Smoking (95 Percent Confidence Intervals), Los Angeles Family Planning Clinic Patients, 1992–1993

	Total	Never Smokers Versus Triers and Regular Smokers[a] (N = 1,411)	p Value	Triers Versus Regular Smokers[b] (N = 590)	p Value
Socioenvironmental factors					
Cultural indicators					
Linguistic acculturation scale					
Spanish orientation	74.0	1.00		1.00	
English orientation	26.0	2.26 (1.77–2.88)	<.0001	2.03 (1.43–2.89)	<.0001
Familialism scale					
Traditional	67.8	1.00		1.00	
Nontraditional	32.2	1.95 (1.55–2.45)	<.0001	1.22 (0.86–1.73)	.26
Beliefs about women's roles scale					
Traditional	37.2	1.00		1.00	
Nontraditional	62.8	1.79 (1.43–2.25)	<.0001	1.11 (0.76–1.61)	.60
Parental and peer smoking behavior					
Any parent smokes					
No	67.8	1.00		1.00	
Yes	32.2	1.65 (1.32–2.07)	<.0001	1.46 (1.03–2.06)	.03
Peers currently smoke					
None	36.5	1.00		1.00	
One	40.2	1.30 (1.05–1.62)	.02	1.33 (0.94–1.87)	<.10
Two or more	23.3	2.49 (1.93–3.20)	<.0001	1.74 (1.22–2.49)	<.002

	%	OR (95% CI)[a]	p	OR (95% CI)[b]	p
Smoking-related norms					
Parents will tell them to stop					
No	8.9	1.00		1.00	
Yes	91.1	0.75 (0.52–1.08)	.12	0.58 (0.34–0.99)	.05
Siblings will tell them to stop					
No	21.4	1.00		1.00	
Yes	78.6	0.47 (0.36–0.60)	<.0001	0.44 (0.30–0.63)	<.0001
Friends will care if they smoke					
No	55.1	1.00		1.00	
Yes	44.9	0.98 (0.79–1.21)	.84	0.90 (0.64–1.26)	.53
Personal factors					
Risk-taking behaviors					
Ever used drugs					
No	84.9	1.00		1.00	
Yes	15.1	3.70 (2.71–5.05)	<.0001	3.46 (2.35–5.10)	<.0001
Ever used alcohol					
No	59.7	1.00		1.00	
Yes	40.3	4.91 (3.83–6.29)	<.0001	1.65 (1.04–2.61)	.03
General risk taking					
No	81.1	1.00		1.00	
Yes	18.9	2.36 (1.80–3.11)	<.0001	2.00 (1.37–2.92)	.0003
Smoking-related attitudes					
Intention to smoke in the future					
Definitely no intention to smoke	82.5	1.00		1.00	
Some intention to smoke	17.5	8.25 (5.87–11.60)	<.0001	18.96 (12.31–29.21)	<.0001

[a]Never smokers = 0; triers and regular smokers = 1.

[b]Triers = 0; regular smokers = 1.

and subsequent progression to regular smoking. Respondents who perceived siblings would react negatively were less likely to experiment with smoking and less likely to become regular smokers compared to those who perceived siblings would not react negatively. Perceived negative reactions of parents were also significantly related to a decreased likelihood of regular smoking.

With respect to risk-taking behavior, almost 19 percent of the respondents indicated agreement with the statement addressing high-risk behaviors: "I get a kick out of doing things every now and then that are a little dangerous or risky." A small proportion of the women (15.1 percent) reported ever taking a nonlegal substance, and 40.3 percent reported ever drinking alcohol. All the variables were significantly related to both outcome variables: increased substance use, alcohol use, and risk-taking attitude were associated with a greater likelihood of ever trying or progressing to regular smoking.

Finally, 82.5 percent of the respondents indicated that they would definitely not smoke in the future. In the univariate models, intention to smoke in the future was positively related to both ever trying cigarettes and smoking regularly.

Predicting Smoking Stage

Table 19.3 shows results from the multivariate logistic analyses for intention to smoke and the two stages of smoking. The first column shows the relationship between the predictors and intention to smoke in the future. Among the demographic indicators, only those who earned more than $15,000 annually were less likely to report an intention to smoke (OR 0.37, CI 0.15–0.94). Among the socioenvironmental factors, none of the cultural indicators was significantly related to intentions. Both parental and peer smoking-behavior indicators were significantly related to intention to smoke. Respondents with at least one parent who smoked were over one and a half times more likely to report an intention to smoke compared to those whose parents did not smoke (OR 1.59, CI 1.14–2.21). Those with one peer or more who smoked were also significantly more likely to intend to smoke than those with no peers who smoke (OR 1.57, CI 1.32–1.88). Among the norms indicators, respondents who stated that a sibling would tell them to stop smoking were less likely to report an intention to smoke in the future (OR 0.67, CI 0.46–0.96) than those who did not. Among the high-risk behaviors, all indicators were positively associated with intention to smoke in the future. Respondents who reported ever using drugs were three times more likely to report an intention to smoke (OR 2.99, CI 2.00–4.48), those who reported ever using alcohol were one and a half times more likely to report intention to smoke (OR 1.57, CI 1.07–2.29), and those who indicated a high-risk attitude were twice as likely to report intention to smoke in the future (OR 2.14, CI 1.49–3.07).

A second analysis (results displayed in the second and third columns) examined the relationship between the predictors and the two stages of smoking with intention to smoke taken out of the model. None of the demographic indicators was significantly related to ever trying or being a regular smoker except for marital status, with being married decreasing the likelihood of being a regular smoker. Among the socioenvironmental indicators, linguistic acculturation and familialism significantly predicted trying cigarettes. English-oriented respondents who held more nontraditional family values were more likely to have tried cigarettes (OR 1.24, CI 1.05–1.45 and OR 1.35, CI 1.05–1.72, respectively). However, none of the cultural indicators was related to regular smoking. Parental smoking was not significantly related to any of the smoking stages. In contrast, peer smoking independently predicted whether respondents would ever try smoking (OR 1.60, CI 1.38–1.86) or become regular smokers (OR 1.66, CI 1.32–2.10). None of the indicators assessing norms were significantly related to ever trying smoking or regular smoking. Among the risk-taking indicators, all variables were positively associated with ever trying cigarettes. Respondents who reported prior use of drugs or alcohol were over three times more likely to have smoked one hundred cigarettes or more (OR 3.12, CI 2.08–4.69 and OR 3.36, CI 2.55–4.42, respectively). Those who reported a high-risk attitude were almost twice as likely to have ever tried cigarettes (OR 1.90, CI 1.38–2.63) and to have become regular smokers (OR 1.62, CI 1.05–2.50). Alcohol use was not related to regular smoking.

Since intentions play an important role in determining behavior, we included intention to smoke in this third analysis to determine whether the effect of each of the independent variables was mediated by intention to smoke (results displayed in fourth and fifth columns). We examined the change in coefficients for the predictors as compared to the model that did not include intentions. With intentions in the model, acculturation and familialism remained significant predictors of ever trying cigarettes. The effect of peers' smoking remained a significant predictor of both ever trying smoking and regular smoking, although its effect was somewhat diminished (OR 1.60, CI 1.38–1.86 versus OR 1.48, CI 1.27–1.73; and OR 1.66, CI 1.32–2.10 versus OR 1.39, CI 1.05–1.83, respectively). Reported past drug use, alcohol use, and risk-taking attitudes remained significant predictors of ever trying smoking with intention included in the model, but only drug use was significantly related to regular smoking (OR 2.71, CI 1.52–4.83). For regular smokers, risk-taking attitude was no longer a significant predictor after intention to smoke was added to the model. Finally, with respect to intentions, respondents who indicated some possibility of smoking in the future were significantly (almost seven times) more likely to have ever tried cigarettes (OR 7.02, CI 4.61–10.71) and over seventeen times more likely to be associated with regular smoking (OR 17.31, CI 10.52–28.51) compared to those with no intention of smoking.

Table 19.3. Multivariate Logistic Regression for Intentions to Smoke and Two Stages of Cigarette Smoking, Los Angeles Family Planning Clinic Patients, 1992–1993

Predictors	Intention to Smoke in the Future Versus No Intention[a] (n = 1,411)	Intentions to Smoke in the Future Excluded from the Model		Intentions to Smoke in the Future Included in the Model	
		Never Smokers Versus Triers and Regular Smokers[b] (n = 1,411)	Triers vs. Regular Smokers[c] (n = 590)	Never Smokers Versus Triers and Regular Smokers[b] (n = 1,411)	Triers Versus Regular Smokers[c] (n = 590)
Demographic indicators					
Age (continuous, range 12–24)	1.00 (0.94–1.08)	0.97 (0.92–1.02)	1.06 (0.97–1.16)	0.96 (0.91–1.02)	1.06 (0.95–1.18)
Education (continuous, range 0–15)	1.00 (0.93–1.07)	0.99 (0.94–1.05)	0.99 (0.91–1.09)	0.99 (0.94–1.05)	0.94 (0.84–1.04)
Marital status (not married = 0; married = 1)	0.71 (0.48–1.03)	1.01 (0.76–1.33)	0.54 (0.34–0.87)*	1.10 (0.82–1.46)	0.58 (0.32–1.02)
Country of birth (foreign born = 0; United States = 1)	0.87 (0.48–1.55)	0.68 (0.41–1.13)	1.21 (0.62–2.37)	0.67 (0.40–1.15)	1.29 (0.57–2.90)
Income					
$0–5,000	1.00	1.00	1.00	1.00	1.00
$5,001–7,500	0.56 (0.30–1.06)	0.97 (0.60–1.57)	0.81 (0.37–1.75)	1.10 (0.67–1.81)	1.30 (0.51–3.31)
$7,501–15,000	0.66 (0.39–1.11)	1.02 (0.68–1.55)	0.80 (0.42–1.51)	1.15 (0.74–1.78)	1.22 (0.57–2.64)
More than $15,000	0.37 (0.15–0.94)*	0.89 (0.45–1.78)	0.75 (0.28–2.03)	1.04 (0.51–2.13)	1.83 (0.59–5.71)
Unknown	0.82 (0.55–1.22)	1.12 (0.81–1.56)	1.04 (0.62–1.74)	1.21 (0.86–1.72)	1.43 (0.77–2.67)
Socioenvironmental factors					
Cultural indicators					
Linguistic acculturation scale (Spanish orientation = 1 to English orientation = 5)	1.06 (0.87–1.30)	1.24 (1.05–1.45)*	1.10 (0.86–1.39)	1.25 (1.06–1.48)**	1.14 (0.85–1.52)
Familialism scale (traditional = 1 to nontraditional = 3)	1.29 (0.95–1.74)	1.35 (1.05–1.72)*	0.91 (0.63–1.33)	1.30 (1.01–1.68)*	0.74 (0.47–1.15)

Beliefs about women's roles scale (traditional = 1 to nontraditional = 3)	1.03 (0.78–1.37)	1.16 (0.94–1.44)	1.02 (0.72–1.43)	1.17 (0.93–1.46)	1.01 (0.67–1.53)
Parental and peer smoking behavior					
Any parent smokes (0 = none; 1 = at least one)	1.59 (1.14–2.21)**	1.25 (0.96–1.64)	1.08 (0.71–1.62)	1.14 (0.86–1.51)	0.86 (0.52–1.41)
Peers currently smoke (0 to 4)	1.57 (1.32–1.88)***	1.60 (1.38–1.86)***	1.66 (1.32–2.10)***	1.48 (1.27–1.73)***	1.39 (1.05–1.83)*
Smoking-related norms					
Parents will tell them to stop (0 = no; 1 = yes)	0.60 (0.35–1.02)	0.82 (0.50–1.34)	0.61 (0.32–1.16)	0.97 (0.58–1.64)	0.70 (0.32–1.54)
Siblings will tell them to stop (0 = no; 1 = yes)	0.67 (0.46–0.96)*	0.79 (0.57–1.10)	0.68 (0.44–1.06)	0.85 (0.60–1.21)	0.72 (0.43–1.23)
Friends will care if they stop (0 = no; 1 = yes)	1.15 (0.83–1.59)	0.92 (0.71–1.19)	0.95 (0.64–1.41)	0.89 (0.68–1.17)	0.80 (0.49–1.29)
Personal factors					
Risk-taking behaviors					
Ever used drugs (0 = no; 1 = yes)	2.99 (2.00–4.48)***	3.12 (2.08–4.69)***	3.12 (1.94–5.02)***	2.53 (1.65–3.89)***	2.71 (1.52–4.83)***
Ever used alcohol (0 = no; 1 = yes)	1.57 (1.07–2.29)*	3.36 (2.55–4.42)***	0.92 (0.55–1.56)	3.40 (2.55–4.55)***	0.91 (0.48–1.71)
Risk-taking attitude (0 = low risk; 1 = high risk)	2.14 (1.49–3.07)***	1.90 (1.38–2.63)***	1.62 (1.05–2.50)*	1.68 (1.19–2.36)***	1.13 (0.67–1.92)
Smoking-related attitudes					
Intention to smoke in the future (0 = no intention; 1 = some possibility)	—			7.02 (4.61–10.71)***	17.32 (10.52–28.51)***
Nagelkerke R^2		.22	.21	.28	.50

[a]No intentions to smoke = 0, intentions to smoke = 1.

[b]Never smokers = 0; triers and regular smokers = 1.

[c]Triers = 0; regular smokers = 1.

*$p < .05$.

**$p < .01$.

***$p < .001$.

DISCUSSION

We examined the effects of socioenvironmental and personal factors on two key stages of the smoking continuum—trying cigarettes and regular smoking—as well as the effects of these predictors on reported intention to smoke. Among the socioenvironmental factors, we included cultural constructs, smoking behavior of family and peers, and norms. Among the personal indicators were risk-taking behaviors and smoking-related attitudes (specifically, intention to smoke). Results indicate that the five domains included were directly or indirectly related to the stages of smoking with some differences by stage of smoking.

The differences in the predictors of each stage of smoking are of interest. In particular, among the cultural constructs, language acculturation and familialism only predicted whether respondents ever tried smoking and not the transition from trying to regular smoking. This finding suggests that culture and the changes in acculturation have an impact on initiation of high-risk behaviors but not maintenance of them. Once a young woman takes the initial step, her cultural orientation does not affect whether she will continue to smoke; other factors may influence whether she remains an experimenter or advances on the smoking continuum.

Beliefs about women's roles did not independently predict intention to smoke, experimentation, or regular smoking, although it was significant at the univariate level, indicating confounding effects by the other predictors. This finding is supported by similar studies conducted by Waldron and Lye (1990) that found no significant effect of gender role indicators among a predominantly White sample. This appears to be true for Latinas as it is for women of other ethnic groups. Whether young women envision themselves as working outside the home or in the home does not affect their health behavior, particularly as it relates to smoking. Although cultural indicators did not independently predict intention to smoke in the future, they did affect experimentation behavior. It is possible that the effect of acculturation on behavior is mediated by other indicators, such as attitudes toward smoking or other unmeasured indicators. Hanson (1997) reports similar results and concludes that ". . . in a strong family environment, the data suggest that even though the influence of family did not directly affect smoking intention, it did have an effect on the development of the respondent's attitudes toward and perception of control over smoking." Future research should empirically test this possibility.

Parental smoking was an independent predictor of intentions and was significantly related to both smoking stages at the univariate level. However, in multivariate analyses, parental smoking was not independently associated with smoking behavior. These results indicate that the effects of parental smoking may be mediated by other factors in the model. In contrast, peer smoking was a consistent predictor of intentions and both smoking stages. That is, the relationship between peers' smoking and smoking stages remains consistent after including intention to smoke in the model. This suggests that the effect of peers is only partially mediated by intention to smoke and that peer influence exerts an effect independent of intentions. This relationship is consistent with the literature on smoking initiation, particularly as it relates to young Latinos (Landrine, Richardson, Klonoff, and Flay, 1994). Unfortunately, the cross-sectional nature of the data does not allow us to disentangle whether young women who smoke tend to associate more often with other young women who are smokers or if the influence of peer smokers promotes the respondents' risk-taking behavior.

Among the normative indicators, we found that at the univariate level, the perception of siblings' reactions was negatively associated with ever trying a cigarette and being a regular smoker and, independently, affected intention to smoke. However, at the multivariate level, norms did not predict any of the stages of smoking. The lack of significant effects of norms on intentions is consistent with results found in Hanson's analyses (1997) of the Theory of Planned Behavior in a sample of Puerto Rican women. In contrast, other research has found some relationship between parents' approval and ever trying cigarettes (Flay, Hu, and Richardson, 1998). Although the norms of friends have also been identified as important predictors of smoking behavior, these results have not been replicated in this analysis. It is feasible that friends' approval does not play as important a role among young Latinas. Sibling approval is usually not measured, and its importance may be underestimated, particularly for young Latinas, who may perceive siblings not only as peers but also as family role models. Unfortunately, our data do not allow us to determine whether the siblings are older or younger than the respondents or to assess their gender. We can only hypothesize that these factors may have a differential influence on a young woman's behavior.

Among the personal factors, all measures of risk-taking behavior were positively associated with respondents' intentions to smoke and trying cigarettes. This is consistent with studies conducted by Jessor and Jessor that contend that high-risk behaviors tend to cluster and that some young people exhibit a propensity for high-risk behavior (Donovan, Jessor, and Costa, 1988; Johnston, O'Malley, and Bachman, 1992). Drug use and risk-taking attitudes were related to regular smoking in the multivariate model that did not include intention to smoke. After including intentions, the effect of risk-taking attitudes diminished, indicating that the relationship was mediated by reported intention to smoke. Ever using drugs remained significant, although its effect was somewhat diminished, indicating this relationship is partially mediated by intentions. Ever use of alcohol was not directly associated with regular smoking. The data suggest that regular smoking is related to behaviors that involve a higher level of health hazard. It also raises the possibility that factors other than behavioral ones may play a role in the use of addictive substances. In any case, the clustering of high-risk behaviors may be supportive of interventions that target multiple behaviors rather than each behavior in isolation.

Finally, intention to smoke was the single greatest predictor of both smoking stages after controlling for other indicators. The measure of intentions is part of a construct developed by Pierce assessing susceptibility to smoking and has proved to have very strong predictive validity (Pierce and others, 1998). The respondents who indicated some possibility of smoking in the future were significantly (seven times) more likely to have ever tried cigarettes and seventeen times more likely to smoke more than one hundred cigarettes in their lifetime than those who had no intention of smoking. Although the cross-sectional nature of the data do not allow us to examine causality in the relationship between intention and smoking behavior, this finding has implications for clinical practice in the rapid assessment of individual risk. This potential benefit should be assessed in a longitudinal design in which the sequence of intentions and behavior is prospectively assessed. If proven predictive, assessment of intention to smoke could allow for targeting of smoking prevention and cessation interventions to individuals at high risk of initiation and regular smoking.

In summary, the data obtained allow us to identify groups at risk for trying cigarettes and for regular smoking among Latina adolescents. However, these findings should be interpreted with caution. The respondents in this study were recruited from a clinic sample, and, thus, results are not immediately generalizable to the larger Latina population. The data are cross-sectional in nature and therefore limit the interpretation of the results. However, the findings have important implications for smoking prevention programs designed for young Latinas and highlight the importance of separating the different stages of smoking in analyses.

APPENDIX

Women's roles within the family	A woman's place is in the home, not in the office or shop.
	A wife who carries out her full family responsibilities doesn't have time for outside employment.
	The employment of wives leads to more juvenile delinquency.
	It is much better for everyone if the man is the achiever outside the home and the woman takes care of the home and family.
	Women are much happier if they stay at home and take care of their children.

Familialism   Aging parents should live with their relatives.

Much of what a daughter does should be done to please her parents.

One can count on help from his/her relatives to solve most problems.

One should spend most of their free time with relatives.

References

Ajzen, I., and Fishbein, M. *Understanding Attitudes and Predicting Social Behavior.* Upper Saddle River, N.J.: Prentice Hall, 1980.

Alaniz, M. L. "Mexican Farmworker Women's Perspectives on Drinking in a Migrant Community." *International Journal of Addictions,* 1994, *29*(9), 1173–1188.

Barret, M., Joe, G. W., and Simpson, D. D. "Acculturation Influences on Inhalant Use." *Hispanic Journal of Behavioral Sciences,* 1991, *13*(3), 276–296.

Bauman, K. L., Foshee, V. A., Linzer, M. A., and Koch, G. C. "Effect of Parental Smoking Classification on the Association Between Parental and Adolescent Smoking." *Addictive Behaviors,* 1990, *15*, 414–422.

Berman, B. A., and Gritz, E. R. "Women and Smoking: Current Trends and Issues for the 1990s." *Journal of Substance Abuse,* 1991, *3*, 221–238.

Best, J. A., and others. "Preventing Cigarette Smoking Among School Children." *Annual Review of Public Health,* 1988, *9*, 161–201.

Betancourt, H., and Lopez, S. "The Study of Culture, Ethnicity and Race in American Psychology." *American Psychologist,* 1993, *48*(6), 629–637.

Burnam, M. A., Telles, C. A., Hough, R. L., and Escobar, J. I. "Measurement of Acculturation in Community Population of Mexican Americans." *Hispanic Journal of Behavioral Sciences,* 1987, *9*, 105–130.

Burns, D., and Pierce, J. *Tobacco Use in Los Angeles, 1990–1991.* Sacramento: California Department of Health and Human Services, 1992.

Campbell, K., and Kaplan, C. P. "The Relationship Between Language Orientation and Cigarette Smoking Beliefs of Latinas." *American Journal Health Behavior,* 1996, *21*(1), 12–20.

Canino, G. "Alcohol Use and Misuse Among Hispanic Women: Selected Factors, Processes and Studies." *International Journal of the Addictions,* 1994, *29*(9), 1083–1100.

Chassin, L., Presson, C. C., Sherma, S., and Edwards, D. "Four Pathways to Young-Adult Smoking Status: Adolescent Social Psychological Antecedents in a Midwestern Community Sample." *Health Psychology,* 1991, *10*(6), 409–418.

Cuellar, I., Harris, L., and Jasso, R. "An Acculturation Scale for Mexican American Normal and Clinical Populations." *Hispanic Journal of Behavioral Sciences,* 1980, *2*(3), 199–217.

Domino, G., and Acosta, A. "The Relations of Acculturation and Values in Mexican-Americans." *Hispanic Journal of Behavioral Sciences,* 1987, *9,* 131–150.

Donovan, J. E., Jessor, R., and Costa, F. "Syndrome of Problem Behavior in Adolescence: A Replication." *Journal of Consulting and Clinical Psychology,* 1988, *56*(5), 1–4.

Donovan, J. E., Jessor, R., and Costa, F. "Adolescent Health Behavior and Conventionality-Unconventionality: An Extension of Problem Behavior Theory." *American Journal of Public Health,* 1991, *73,* 543–551.

Epstein, J., Botvin, G. J., and Diaz, T. "Linguistic Acculturation and Gender Effects on Smoking Among Hispanic Youth." *Preventive Medicine,* 1998, *27*(4), 583–589.

Ernster, V. "Mixed Messages for Women. A Social History of Cigarette Smoking and Advertising." *New York State Journal of Medicine,* 1985, *85*(7), 335–340.

Escobedo, L. G., and Remington, R. L. "Birth Cohort Analysis of Prevalence of Cigarette Smoking Among Hispanics in the United States." *JAMA,* 1989, *261,* 66–69.

Flay, B. R., Hu, F. B., and Richardson, J. "Psychosocial Predictors of Different Stages of Cigarette Smoking Among High School Students." *Preventive Medicine,* 1998, *27,* A9–A18.

Flay, B. R., Ockene, J., and Tager, I. B. "Smoking: Epidemiology, Cessation and Prevention." *Chest,* 1992, *102*(3), 277s–301s.

Flay, B. R., and others. "Cigarette Smoking: Why Young People Do It and Ways to Prevent It." In P. McGrath and P. Firestone (eds.), *Pediatric Adolescent Behavioral Medicine: Issues and Treatment.* New York: Springer, 1983.

Garza, R. T., and Gallegos, P. I. "Environmental Influences and Personal Choice: A Humanistic Perspective on Acculturation." *Hispanic Journal of Behavioral Sciences,* 1985, *7,* 365–379.

Gerber, R. W., Newman, I. M., and Martin, G. L. "Applying the Theory of Reasoned Action to Early Adolescent Tobacco Chewing." *Journal of School Health,* 1988, *58*(10), 410–413.

Glynn, T. J., Anderson, D. M., and Schwartz, L. "Tobacco-Use Reduction Among High-Risk Youth: Recommendations of a National Cancer Institute Advisory Panel." *Preventive Medicine,* 1991, *20,* 279–291.

Gritz, E. R. "Cigarette Smoking by Adolescent Females: Implications for Health and Behavior." *Women Health,* 1984, *9,* 103–115.

Guendelman, S., and Abrams, B. "Dietary Intake Among Mexican American Women: Generational Differences and a Comparison with White Non-Hispanic Women." *American Journal of Public Health,* 1995, *85,* 20–25.

Hanson, M. J. "The Theory of Planned Behavior Applied to Cigarette Smoking in African American, Puerto Rican, and Non-Hispanic White Teenage Females." *Nursing Research,* 1997, *46*(3), 155–162.

Jessor, R., and Jessor, S. *Problem Behavior and Psychosocial Development: A Longitudinal Study of Youth.* Orlando, Fla.: Academic Press, 1977.

Johnston, L. D., O'Malley, P. M., and Bachman, J. G. *Smoking, Drinking, and Illicit Drug Use Among American Secondary School Students, College Students, and Young Adults, 1975–1991*. Washington, D.C.: National Institute on Drug Abuse, U.S. Department of Health and Human Services, Public Health Service, National Institutes of Health, 1992.

Kaplan, C. P., and Tanjasiri, S. P. "Smoking Prevalence Among Young Latina Women: Assessment of Two Interview Methodologies." *Drug Use and Misuse*, 1996, *31*(8), 947–963.

Keefe, S. "Acculturation and the Extended Family Among Urban Mexican-Americans." In A. M. Padilla (Ed.), *Acculturation, Theory, Models and Some New Findings*. Boulder, Colo.: Westview Press, 1980.

Landrine, H., Richardson, J. L., Klonoff, E. A., and Flay, B. "Cultural Diversity in the Predictors of Adolescent Smoking: The Relative Influence of Peers." *Journal of Behavioral Medicine*, 1994, *17*(3), 331–346.

Leventhal, H., and Cleary, P. D. "The Smoking Problem: A Review of the Research and Theory in Behavioral Risk Modification." *Psychological Bulletin*, 1980, *88*, 370–405.

Lovato, C. Y., and others. "Cigarette and Alcohol Use Among Migrant Hispanic Adolescents." *Community Health*, 1994, *16*(4), 18–31.

Marin, G., and others. "The Role of Acculturation in the Attitudes, Norms and Expectancies of Hispanic Smokers." *Journal of Cross-Cultural Psychology*, 1989, *20*(4), 399–415.

Markides, K. S., and Coreil, J. "The Health of Hispanics in the Southwestern United States: An Epidemiologic Paradox." *Public Health Reports*, 1986, *101*, 253–265.

Markides, K. S., Coreil, J., and Ray, L. A. "Smoking Among Mexican-Americans: A Three Generation Study." *American Journal of Public Health*, 1987, *77*(6), 708–711.

Moore, J. W. *Mexican-American*. Upper Saddle River, N.J.: Prentice Hall, 1970.

Moreno, C., and others. "Parental Influences to Smoke in Latino Youth." *Preventive Medicine*, 1994, *23*, 48–53.

Nagelkerke, N.J.D. "A Note on a General Definition of the Coefficient of Determination." *Biometrika*, 1991, *78*, 691–692.

Otero-Sabogal, R., Sabogal, F., and Pérez-Stable, E. "Psychosocial Correlates of Smoking Among Immigrant Latina Adolescents." *Journal of the National Cancer Institute Monographs*, 1995, *18*, 65–71.

Pierce, J. P., and others. *Tobacco Use in California: An Evaluation of the Tobacco Control Program, 1989–1993*. La Jolla: University of California, San Diego, 1994.

Pierce, J. P., and others. *Tobacco Control in California: Who's Winning the War? An Evaluation of the Tobacco Control Program, 1989–1996*. La Jolla: University of California, San Diego, 1998.

Sabogal, F., Otero-Sabogal, R., Pérez-Stable, E. J., and Marin, B. V. "Perceived Self-Efficacy to Avoid Cigarette Smoking and Addiction: Differences Between Hispanics and Non-Hispanic Whites." *Hispanic Journal of Behavioral Science*, 1989, *11*, 13–147.

Sabogal, F., and others. "Hispanic Families and Acculturation: What Changes and What Doesn't?" *Hispanic Journal of Behavioral Sciences*, 1987, *9*(4), 397–412.

Sallis, J. F., and others. "Parenting Prompting of Smoking Among Adolescents in Tijuana, Mexico." *International Journal of Behavioral Medicine*, 1994, *1*(2), 122–136.

Scribner, R. "Paradox as Paradigm—The Health Outcomes of Mexican Americans." *American Journal of Public Health*, 1996, *86*, 303–304.

Stern, R. A., Prochaska, J. O., Velicer, W. F., and Elder, J. P. "Stages of Adolescent Cigarette Smoking Acquisition: Measurement and Sample Profiles." *Addictive Behavior*, 1987, *12*, 19–329.

U.S. Department of Health and Human Services. *Preventing Tobacco Use Among Young People: A Report of the Surgeon General.* Washington, D.C.: Center for Disease Control and Prevention, National Center for Chronic Disease Prevention and Health Promotion, Office on Smoking and Health Preventing, 1994.

Vega, W., and others. "Risk Factors for Early Adolescent Use in Four Ethnic and Racial Groups." *American Journal of Public Health*, 1993, *83*(2), 185–189.

Waldron, I., and Lye, D. "Relationships Between Teenage Smoking and Attitudes Towards Women's Rights, Sex Roles, Marriage, Sex and Family." *Women and Health*, 1990, *16*(3/4), 23–46.

Wolff, C. B., and Portis, M. "Smoking, Acculturation, and Pregnancy Outcome Among Mexican Americans." *Health Care for Women International*, 1996, *17*, 563–573.

CHAPTER TWENTY

The Role of Intergenerational Discrepancy of Cultural Orientation in Drug Use Among Latina Adolescents

María Félix-Ortiz de la Garza
Alicia Fernandez
Michael D. Newcomb

This chapter reviews the literature and analyzes the findings that explain the influence of intergenerational discrepancy, family support, culture, and environmental factors on smoking, alcohol, and drug usage among Latina adolescents.

The available data suggest that the rates of drug use among Latino populations may be increasing and highlight the need for focused efforts to better understand the etiology of drug use in these populations (Hunsaker, 1985; Maddahian, Newcomb, and Bentler, 1985; Schinke and others, 1988). For example, among adult Latinos, there is a dramatic gender difference in alcohol and drug use prevalence rates: women tend to abstain, and men tend to be high-quantity/high-frequency users of alcohol (Caetano, 1986; Canino, Burnam, and Caetano, 1992). However, this trend is not apparent among some Latino adolescents: Mexican American girls did not differ substantially from their male counterparts in their drug use (Félix-Ortiz, Muñoz, and Newcomb, 1994).

Understanding how imputed "protective" influences may mitigate risk for drug use may be important in preventing a drug use epidemic among Latino youth. Recent attempts to understand drug use etiology have included a consideration of both "risk" and "protective" factors. Using this approach, drug use is hypothesized to be associated with an increasing number of risk factors rather than being associated with a specific type of risk factor, and "protective factors" are examined to determine how these may reduce risk. Exposure to more risk factors not only is a reliable correlate of drug use but increases drug use over time, implying a true etiological role (Newcomb and Félix-Ortiz, 1992; Newcomb, Maddahian, and Bentler, 1986; Scheier and Newcomb, 1991). For example, Moncher, Holden, and Trimble (1990) demonstrated that a multiple risk factor index was linearly related to reported prevalence of using beer or wine, inhalants, marijuana, and cocaine among a sample of Native American youth. "Protective factors" have been defined as influences that prevent, limit, or reduce drug use and that may counter, buffer, neutralize, and interact with risk factors within or across time (Brook, Nomura, and Cohen, 1989a, 1989b; Newcomb, 1992). However, "protective" and "risk" factors have often been conceptualized as representing opposite ends of the same continuum so that the absence of risk is equivalent to protection. If this is true, then protection should not provide any unique, direct effect on predicting drug use independent of risk. However, recent work demonstrates that the imputed protection appears to function in a manner similar to risk and can be operationalized as a multiple factor index (Félix-Ortiz and Newcomb, 1992, 1997; Newcomb and Félix-Ortiz, 1992). In these studies, it was found that a multiple protective factor index was also associated with the frequency and quantity of drug use among teenagers and improved the prediction of drug use beyond that accounted for by a risk factor index alone. Protection was also found to be a construct distinct from risk, and its influence on drug use had both direct and moderator effects. The main or direct effect of protection was to predict less drug use, while the direct effect of risk was to predict increased drug involvement. Moreover, for high levels of risk in the presence of low levels of protection, certain types of drug use were elevated, and for high levels of risk in the presence of higher levels of protection, certain types of drug use were relatively reduced.

However, risk and protective factors for drug and alcohol involvement among Latina adolescents have not been examined sufficiently. An understanding of such factors and how they interact would inform the implementation and development of effective drug use prevention programs for Latina youths that differ from those used with Latino youth or with older Latinas. In this study, we examine the role of familial and cultural factors in drug use among a predominantly Mexican American sample of adolescent girls. Specifically, the primary aims of this study are to examine how a difference between a Latina adolescent's cultural orientation and her family's cultural orientation (that is intergenerational discrepancy) are related to drug use. Moreover, if intergenerational discrepancy influences drug use, does family support moderate the influence of intergenerational discrepancy on drug use?

REVIEW OF THE LITERATURE

See Table 20.1 for a summary of details for the studies reviewed.

Table 20.1. Adolescents at Risk for Substance Use: Selected Parameters, Processes, and Studies

Independent Variables	Author(s)	N	Type of Participants	Ethnicities of Participants	Method	Results	Strengths and Limitations
				Family and Parental Influences			
Parent personality, adolescent personality, parent-adolescent relationship, family, and ecological measures	Brook and others (1990)	649 and 429	College students and fathers, mother–child pairs	White American, diverse income and location	Cross-sectional, longitudinal; questionnaires	Multivariate techniques; conflict-free parent–child attachment and child's identification with parent led to affiliation with peers who did not use drugs	+Cross-sectional data and longitudinal data, inclusion of father–child as well as mother–child relationship −Self-report measures
Affection, child centeredness, communication, conflict, identification of adolescent with mother, satisfaction with adolescent, time spent with adolescent, and pregnancy and early childhood variables	Brook, Nomura, and Cohen (1989a)	638	Mother–child pairs followed to adolescence	White American, diverse income and location	Longitudinal, three points across 10 years; interview and questionnaire	Multiple regression analyses; early risk of unwanted pregnancy and major illness were associated with cigarettes, alcohol, and marijuana use but not illicit drug use	+Consideration of distal early childhood variables as well as proximal parenting variables −Did not control for different stages of adolescence; early childhood data based on self-report

(Continued)

Table 20.1. Adolescents at Risk for Substance Use: Selected Parameters, Processes, and Studies (Continued)

Independent Variables	Author(s)	N	Type of Participants	Ethnicities of Participants	Method	Results	Strengths and Limitations
				Family and Parental Influences			
School environment, neighborhood environment, family relations, and peer association variables	Brook, Nomura, and Cohen (1989b)	518	Adolescents and their mothers	White American, diverse income	Longitudinal across 2 years	Regression analyses; family and peer variables had a direct impact on adolescent drug involvement	+Consideration of the interrelationship of neighborhood, school, peer, and family variables in drug involvement −Paid participants and used a predominantly White sample for collection of data. Also did not quantify drug use
Personality and social environment variables	Donovan, Jessor, and Costa (1988)	388	Eleventh- and twelfth-grade boys and girls	White, Hispanic, Native American, Asian American	Longitudinal, questionnaire	Maximum likelihood factor analyses; support the concept of problem behavior in adolescence	+Assessed problem behaviors longitudinally −Based on school sample so may not represent all adolescents
Community contact and individual-level familial and child variables	Simcha-Fagan, Gersten, and Langner (1986)	553	Adolescent males	White and Black urban American	Questionnaire, official record, severe self-recorded delinquency	Structural constraints characteristic of a community are associated with the nature of the community's organizational base, which in turn affects delinquency directly and indirectly by social bonds to key socializing institutions	+Used both self-reported and officially recorded reporting of delinquency −Sample is not representative of whole population

Variables	Author (Year)	N	Sample	Ethnicity	Design	Results	Comments
Mother's rejection of the child, limit setting, inconsistency, parental conflict, parental concern	Vicary and Lerner (1986)	133	Adolescents and their families	White middle-class American	Longitudinal, four time points across 30 years; interviews with parent and child	Discriminant function analysis showed that parental conflict in child-rearing practices, inconsistent discipline, and maternal rejection were associated with alcohol and marijuana use in older adolescents	+Assessed drug use longitudinally −Assessed marijuana, tobacco, and alcohol use only using a global measure
Cohesion, flexibility, parent–child relationship, stressful events and changes, and four interpersonal and six intrapersonal variables	Needle and others (1988)	508	Adolescents and their families; normal and clinical sample	White middle-class American	Retrospective case-control and prospective longitudinal design spanning 6 years	Multivariate analysis of variance with repeated measures design; clinical adolescents and nonclinical drug users reported lower family cohesion, lower family flexibility, more frequent stressful events and changes in the family, and more strain with parents than did adolescents who did not use drugs	+Used both clinical and nonclinical drug users as well as normal adolescents −Measured only infrequency of drug use; did not assess relationship between independent variables (for example, moderator/mediators)

(Continued)

Table 20.1. Adolescents at Risk for Substance Use: Selected Parameters, Processes, and Studies (Continued)

Independent Variables	Author(s)	N	Type of Participants	Ethnicities of Participants	Method	Results	Strengths and Limitations
				Family and Parental Influences			
Number of problems, parent–child relationship, peer relationship, reactive coping, and personal satisfaction variables	Labouvie (1986)	617	Boys and girls of 15 and 18 years of age	Predominantly White American	Telephone interview, face-to-face interview	Correlational and cross-sectional analyses showed that the experience of strained social relationships and a heightened sense of powerlessness/helplessness may induce adolescents to rely more heavily on substance use as a means of emotional self-regulation that requires little effort and ability, promises instant effects, and provides a sense of control	+ Assessed alcohol and drug use in a correlational and cross-sectional analyses − Decrease in sample size during face-to-face interview, overrepresentation of higher socioeconomic levels
Family and school involvement, perceived sanctions against deviant behavior, and five other intra- and interpersonal variables	Rodriguez and Weisburd (1991)	1,077	Adolescent males, aged 12 to 19 years	Lowest-income Puerto Rican American	Longitudinal two time points; self-reported face-to-face interview	Integrated Social Control model. Among Puerto Rican American adolescents, family bonding is a more important influence on delinquency, whereas peer bonding is less important than is the case in the national sample of more affluent White youths	+ Analyses replicated Elliott, Huizinga, and Ageton's analytical model of delinquency based on an integration of social control, social learning, and strain theories − Loss of original sample size may have possible influence of cohort differences on obtained results because the two studies were conducted 10 years apart

Family Cultural Orientation

Variables	Study	N	Sample	Cultural Orientation	Design	Findings	+/−
Maladjustment (particularly drug misuse) child's acculturation, and family's acculturation	Szapocznik and Kurtines (1980)	55	Families referred to a family clinic	Cuban	Cross-sectional; interview and questionnaire	Analyses of variance revealed that families with drug-using boys had larger intergenerational acculturation gaps	+A consideration of family–child cultural dynamics and their influence on child's behavior −Type of gap not specified, sample limited to boys
Psychosocial variables, acculturation variables, and family protective variables	Vega and others (1993)	1,843	Sixth- and seventh-grade boys and girls	Cuban descent	Longitudinal design questionnaires	Hierarchical multiple regression analyses; family protective effects decrease delinquent behavior indirectly by decreasing disposition to deviance. Family factors are related to the development of attitudes favoring deviance, whereas acculturation conflicts are associated with delinquent behavior	+Used both boys and girls in this clinical sample −Relied on self-report and based on school sample so may not represent all adolescents
Child's personality, behavior, development, child-rearing techniques, family structure, family health and demographics	Brook, Whiteman, Gordon, and Cohen (1986)	356	Youngsters and their mothers	White American	Longitudinal, two time points; interview and questionnaire	Existence of personality risk factors in childhood had an impact on the existence of personality risk factors in adolescence, which then resulted in higher stages of drug use	+Consideration of personality changes across time −Did not quantify or state frequency of drug use and relied on self-report

(Continued)

Table 20.1. Adolescents at Risk for Substance Use: Selected Parameters, Processes, and Studies (Continued)

Independent Variables	Author(s)	N	Type of Participants	Ethnicities of Participants	Method	Results	Strengths and Limitations
				Family Cultural Orientation			
Supportive home relationships, perceived sanctions against drug use, and twelve other intra- and interpersonal variables	Newcomb and Félix-Ortiz (1992)	1,634	Adolescent students (oversampling of low socioeconomic status)	Hispanic, Black, Asian, and White American	Longitudinal, two time points; questionnaire	Bivariate, multivariate analyses, and structural equations modeling; these factors were among five others that were identified as protective (that is, associated with reduced drug use)	+Use of sophisticated analyses, consideration of frequency and quantity of many types of drug used −Relied on self-report and based on school sample so may not represent all adolescents
				Latina Alcohol and Drug Use/Misuse			
Religious participation, religiosity, peer associations, family support/communication variables	Brownfield and Sorenson (1991)	800	Male high school students	White American	Secondary analyses from a large-scale project assessing the validity and reliability of self-reported delinquent behavior	Latent class analyses; measures of religious participation and religiosity are strong negative correlates of drug use	+Used three populations of adolescents to assess for drug use −Used a school sample that may not be representative of all adolescents

Variables	Study	N	Sample	Population	Method	Findings	Notes
Acculturation variables	Caetano (1987)	1453	Men and women	U.S. Hispanic population	Questionnaire	Multistage probability analysis; more acculturated individuals have more liberal attitudes toward drinking, allowing more drinking, especially for women	+Assessed drinking attitudes using a multistage probability sample −Acculturation was assessed unidimensionally
Consumption of alcoholic beverage and nine other intra- and interpersonal variables	Holck, Warren, Smith, and Rochat (1984)	2031	Women aged 15–44	Mexican, Mexican American, White American; residing along the U.S.-Mexico border	Survey interview	The level of alcohol consumption increased markedly with the years of education completed. Almost all of the overall ethnic differences observed could be accounted for by the generally lower level of education among the Mexican Americans	+Assessed level of alcohol consumption of Mexican American and of Anglo women and of two subgroups of Mexican Americans: Mexicana and Chicana −Did not control for differences in length of time in mainstream society

Perceived Family Support

Although a variety of family and parental factors have been associated with adolescent problem behaviors in general (Donovan, Jessor, and Costa, 1988), these factors are also specifically associated with adolescent drug use. Poor parenting practices, high levels of conflict in the family, and poor parent–child relationships increase the risk for adolescent drug use (Brook, Nomura, and Cohen, 1989a, 1989b; Brook and others, 1990; Vicary and Lerner, 1986). Lower family cohesion, flexibility, and more frequent stressful events and changes in the family characterized families of drug users and misusers (Needle and others, 1988). Furthermore, Labouvie (1986) suggests that "the experience of strained social relationships and a heightened sense of powerlessness/helplessness may induce adolescents to rely more heavily on substance use as a means of emotional self-regulation which requires little effort and ability, promises instant effects, and provides a sense of control" (p. 333). For example, in a study of 617 15- and 18-year-olds, Labouvie (1986) found that environments unable to provide social support mechanisms tended to foster these feelings of powerlessness and helplessness and that this lack of personal control was conducive to the development of a relatively strong link between substance use and emotional self-regulation in adolescence. Unfortunately, Labouvie's study was correlational and cross-sectional in nature, thus limiting the confidence with which one can assert causal relationships. Kagan (1991) has also hypothesized that anxiety- or anger-inducing family environments place a child at risk for problem behaviors. These investigators highlight the contributions of a negatively charged family environment to adolescent alcohol and drug use, but are particularly relevant to the case of ethnic minority children and their families because of the second-class status of such individuals in U.S. society.

Family Cultural Orientation

Because we live in a multicultural environment, it is essential to focus attention on the cultural orientation of the family and its potential effects on a child's mental health. A difference between the cultural orientation of the family and the cultural identity of the Latino child may increase the imputed child's vulnerability to deviant behavior. More specifically, immigrant families tend to develop a family struggle in which the younger family members struggle to autonomy (that is, American value) and the older family members struggle for family connectedness (Latino value). This intergenerational discrepancy appears to be associated with adolescent problem behaviors (Szapocznik and Kurtines, 1993). For example, in a study conducted by Szapocznik and Kurtines (1980) with Miami's Cuban immigrant population, families of adolescents who used drugs had exaggerated intergenerational acculturation gaps where the substance-using Cuban boy was more acculturated than the older family members, suggesting that drug use was associated with the acculturation process in both family and child (Szapocznik and Kurtines, 1980). The earlier a person immigrates to the host culture, the more quickly acculturation occurs, which may result in large intergenerational differences and account for family and behavioral disorders in adolescence, particularly if the intergenerational differences are between adolescent male youths and their mothers (Szapocznik and Kurtines, 1980). In their study the intergenerational discrepancy was operationalized as a significant difference between the parents' score and the boy's score on the acculturation scale.

However, in a study of delinquent behavior among Cuban American adolescents, Vega and others (1993) found that family variables (such as parental support and family cohesion) rather than acculturative stressors (such as intergenerational discrepancy in cultural orientation) were more important in predicting deviant behavior. Family protective influences appeared to create a vulnerability to adolescent conduct problems, whereas acculturative stresses appeared to trigger the problem, thereby playing a less important role in the etiology of the problem behavior. Among Latinos, family variables are seen as both theoretically important and culturally salient because Latinos have been found to be highly familistic (Vega, 1990).

Protective Factors as Moderators of Risk

Among Latino adolescents, not only are problems in acculturation associated with deviance, but high levels of family acceptance and support are correlated with low levels of deviant behavior (Rodriguez and Weisburd, 1991). In this case, family acceptance and support function as protective factors. For example, in a study of a sample of mostly White U.S. American adolescents, Newcomb and Félix-Ortiz (1992) found that supportive home relationships and perceived sanctions against drug use were factors that were strongly associated with reduced drug use. "Protection" was also found to be a construct distinct from "risk," and its influence on drug use had both direct and moderator effects. Substantively, the main or direct effect of protection is to predict less drug use, while the direct effect of risk is to predict increased drug involvement. The moderator or interaction effect of protection can buffer the relationship between risk and drug use as well as have a direct effect on drug use (Baron and Kenny, 1986). A limitation of these studies is that the number of factors considered was limited to a small, finite number, thus possibly omitting distal and proximal contextual influences or other conditions that might influence the operation of these imputed risks and protective factors. The number of possible protective and risk factors is probably infinite given that these are likely to vary across different demographic subgroups.

Latina Alcohol and Drug Misuse

Although Latino cultures probably vary with class and environment, certain aspects of the traditional culture appear to be consistently associated with less drug and alcohol use among Latinas. For example, high education is associated with higher alcohol use, while marriage and being a housewife is associated with low alcohol use (Caetano, 1987; Holck, Warren, Smith, and Rochat, 1984). Gilbert (1987) found that abstinence from alcohol use was more prevalent among immigrant Latina women, while moderate- to high-quantity/high-frequency drinking was reported by younger, American-born Latina women. Frequent church attendance and religious affirmation appear to buffer Latinas against drug use (Brownfield and Sorenson, 1991).

Feminism is a belief system that stands in contrast to the traditional stereotypic roles that women are expected to fulfill within our society. Yet, feminism is an unusual concept in the Latino culture due to the clear separation of roles taken by men and women in that culture. The marianismo and machismo roles are deeply rooted in the Latino culture. Machismo demands that men are responsible for providing for the welfare and honor of the family. Marianismo holds that women are to be self-sacrificing for the benefit of their children and family, and model virgin purity and motherhood as did the Virgin Mary in the Catholic religion (Comas-Diaz, 1987). The Latino culture sets the standard for both sexes early in childhood. Boys are given greater freedom, encouraged to be sexually aggressive, and are not restricted to household responsibilities, while the girls are taught to be passive, obedient, and responsible for the household duties of the family (Comas-Diaz, 1987). Adult Latinas may be caught in a double bind when they want to maintain their Latino family obligations while also acculturating into the mainstream society by adopting more feminist values. For example, some data suggest that Latinas have found themselves in the situation of either suffering guilt over failing to fulfill familial demands or failing to achieve an educational goal because of their need to fulfill traditional expectations (Young, 1992). As a result, Latina women may lose their family support systems, become more vulnerable to stress, and resort to alcohol and drug use to cope with stress and isolation (Gibson, 1983).

LIMITATIONS OF THE RESEARCH

These studies of Latino and Latina drug use have typically suffered from several problems. Age, gender, and the influence of cultural identity have not received sufficient attention in analyses of substance misuse among Latinas. Although some investigators have examined how acculturation influences drug use, the specific manner in which familial and cultural variables interact to influence Latina alcohol and drug use are not well understood and have not received sufficient attention in the research literature. Further, few studies focus specifically on alcohol and drug use among young Latina adolescents or examine the protective factors that may mitigate substance misuse in this group. Instead, many studies have utilized a between-group design to compare drug use prevalence rates between Latin women and men and have not tested for moderators or mediators of the relationship between certain independent variables and drug use (Canino, Burnam, and Caetano, 1992). In some research the focus has been on a clinical sample (Szapocznik and Kurtines, 1980), which may limit the generalizability of the results. In other research, a distinction between conflict related to intergenerational discrepancy and conflict due to generic family issues and unrelated to uniquely Latino family processes is not made clearly. In the study by Vega and others (1993), the Family Protective Factor includes two indicators named Family Respect and Family Pride. These two indicators may have unique significance or meaning when applied to Latino families given their ethnic minority status in the United States and therefore may not be adequate indicators of generic family processes.

THIS STUDY

In this study, we examine the role of intergenerational cultural orientation discrepancy in the etiology of drug use among Latina adolescents. A young Latina endorsing feminism, a value more characteristic of American-identified youth, in the context of a traditionally oriented family may be "vulnerable" to drug use because of the intergenerational discrepancy of cultural values between her and her family. This discrepancy may generate family–child conflict and stress the Latina adolescent. If the young Latina also perceives a lack of family support (conflict in the family is not tolerated and she is sanctioned by the family), she may cope with her stress through drug use. Therefore, the primary aims of this research are to examine the generalizability of Szapocznik and Kurtines's model (1980) to Latina adolescents. If intergenerational discrepancy is related to Latina adolescent drug use, we will extend their model by examining whether family social support moderates the relationship between intergenerational discrepancy and drug use among Latinas. Intergenerational discrepancy will be operationalized as a discrepancy between the language that is used at home (whether Spanish is spoken at home) and the level of feminism endorsed by the Latina adolescent (high or low feminism). As suggested by Baron and Kenny (1986), a 2 × 2 analysis of variance will be conducted to examine this latter relationship.

METHOD

Recruitment of Participants

In 1991, survey data regarding drug use and its possible correlates (psychological and environmental influences) were collected by the first author from 516 ninth- and tenth-grade students of Latino descent for use in another study

(Félix-Ortiz, Newcomb, and Myers, 1994). The students represent four schools in the Los Angeles area: two schools east of Los Angeles, where much of the Los Angeles County Latino and Mexican American population is concentrated as per census estimates, one near downtown Los Angeles, and one in the West Los Angeles area, areas where many Central Americans reside. Although these schools were all located in densely populated urban-suburban areas and despite the high rate of community violence in Los Angeles County (high rate of homicide), no violence was observed on any high school campus. Each school was well maintained and secure, teachers were fairly involved with the students, and classrooms were under the teacher's control. Due to the sensitivity of the data being requested and the difficulty enlisting school participation, a non-random sample was used. Approximately 1,266 students of all ethnicities were invited to participate, and about half ($n = 688$, 54 percent) actually participated. The high response rate is attributed to a preparticipation orientation conducted on the first visit. If parents consented, the vast majority of students assented and participated, but a specific count was not documented.

Data collection involved two on-site visits to present the research project and obtain assent and administer questionnaires during a class at each school. The first author visited with students in their class to inform them about the study and explain the consent and assent forms in the first visit. Before the first author informed them about the study, she used two strategies to engage student participation in the research: she described what drug use was like when she was an adolescent (for example, popular drugs, modes of uses, availability), and she led a discussion on the reasons students use drugs, a discussion that elicited a great diversity of responses. Teachers collected parent consent forms. A week later, after obtaining informed assent from the students whose parents consented, the questionnaires were administered. Students were allowed to decline participation even if their parents consented to participation, as stipulated by the American Psychological Association ethical code (American Psychological Association, 1992). Student consent was obtained for students who were not minors (under the age of 18).

Confidentiality of participant identity and the data was ensured by collecting assent forms separately from questionnaires and careful, secure storage of consent and assent forms. The consent and assent forms were stored in a secure location separate from the questionnaires and were accessible only by the first author. Questionnaires were accessed only by research assistants. No school personnel, parents, or high school students had access to any of the data.

Sample Characteristics

Table 20.2 presents sample characteristics for the total sample of 295 Latina adolescent high school students; the table is divided into those that were assessed as having low feminist values, high feminist values, and the total sample. Most

Table 20.2. Sample Characteristics of Latina High School Students

Variable	Low Feminists N	Low Feminists %	High Feminists N	High Feminists %	Total N	Total %
Age						
14 or less	23	7.8	28	9.5	51	17.3
15	44	14.9	66	22.4	110	37.3
16	46	15.6	36	12.2	82	27.8
17	21	7.1	18	6.1	38	13.2
18	9	3.1	2	0.7	11	3.7
19	1	0.3	1	0.3	2	0.7
Mean[a]		15.7		15.4		
Average overall grade						
Mostly A's	24	8.2	27	9.1	51	17.3
Mostly B's	62	20.9	68	23.1	130	44.0
Mostly C's	22	7.2	28	9.5	50	17.0
Mostly C's or less	36	12.2	28	9.5	64	21.7
Mean[b]	2.5		2.4			
Educational aspiration						
Diploma	37	12.5	24	8.1	61	20.7
Associate	34	13.2	32	11.9	66	25.1
Bachelor's	42	12.5	44	13.9	86	26.4
Graduate degree	31	10.5	51	17.3	82	27.8
Parents' education						
No diplomas	83	28.1	79	26.8	162	54.9
One diploma	32	10.8	27	9.2	59	20.0
Two diplomas	17	5.8	20	6.8	37	12.5
No diploma/degree	4	1.4	7	2.4	11	3.7
Diploma/degree	3	1.0	10	3.4	13	4.4
Degree/degree	5	1.7	8	2.7	13	4.4

[a]Mean age for low feminists is 15 to 16 years old. The mean age for high feminists is 15 years old.

[b]Mean grades for low feminists are between B's and C's. Mean grades for high feminists is mostly B's.

of the Latina adolescent participants were of Mexican descent (over 80 percent), 15 or 16 years old (65 percent), and first generation (that is, born in the United States: 93 percent), and many were raised by parents without a high school diploma (55 percent). Most were "B" students (44 percent), and most aspired to some college degree (80 percent).

The majority of the sample were raised by parents neither of whom had a high school diploma (55 percent). Another 32.5 percent had one parent with a high school diploma, and 12.5 percent were from families where at least one parent had a college degree. The majority of the sample reported an average overall grade of B in their classes (42 percent). While there was no mean difference in educational achievement (average grade was "mostly B's with some C's"), there was a significant difference in the educational aspirations between high-feminist Latina students and low-feminist Latina students. More high-feminist Latina students (17.3 percent) aspired to postundergraduate degrees than did low-feminist Latina students (10.5 percent; $p \leq .055$). Over three-quarters of the Latina students aspired to some college degree (79.3 percent), while 20.7 percent did not plan to pursue formal education beyond the high school diploma. Over half of the sample (54 percent) aspired to a bachelor's degree or higher.

Measures

Table 20.3 presents a summary of details regarding the measures.

Drug Use. Frequency of use was assessed for the past six months on 7-point anchored scales ranging from (1) "never" to (7) "more than once a day." One item captured cigarettes, one measured alcohol use (beer, wine, and illicit liquor), one measured marijuana use, and one was a general measure for "other" illicit drug use. Illicit drug use was captured by collapsing four items measuring crack, cocaine, PCP, and an item measuring "other illicit" drugs (for example, heroin, LSD, barbiturates, amphetamines) into one item. These drugs were collapsed into a general measure of illicit drug use because less than 5 percent of the sample had used cocaine, crack, and PCP any time during the past six months (alpha = .49). In addition, since no major differences emerged between different types of alcohol use, these measures were also collapsed into a general frequency of alcohol use measure to simplify analyses (alpha = .66). These scales of alcohol use, marijuana use, and illicit drug use have been used successfully with diverse samples in the past (Newcomb and Bentler, 1988).

Three quantity-of-drug-use measures for cigarettes, alcohol, and marijuana use were rated on 7-point scales ranging from no ingestion to high quantity use. Cigarettes smoked in one day ranged from (1) "no cigarettes" to (7) "more than 40 cigarettes (more than 2 packs a day)." The average daily amount of alcohol consumed for the past six months was reflected by the number of "bottles of beer, glasses of wine, or mixed drinks on a typical day" and ranged from (1) "none" to (7) "six or more." Amount of marijuana used was measured as the number of marijuana "joints" or cigarettes personally consumed in a day and ranged from (1) "none" to (7) "six or more."

Intergenerational Discrepancy. This variable was created from existing data about the Latina adolescent's level of feminism (high or low) and another variable, Spanish spoken at home (mostly Spanish spoken or mostly English spoken).

Table 20.3. Measures

Measure	Type	Number of Items	Studies in Which the Measure Has Been Used	Samples Used
Frequency of drug use	7-point Likert scale: (1) never to (7) more than once a day	Three items: cigarettes, alcohol, marijuana, and one item for five other types of illicit drugs	Newcomb, Bentler, and Collins (1986), Stacy, Newcomb, and Bentler (1991), Newcomb and Bentler (1988)	Adolescents and young adults (approximately 60 percent White)
Quantity of drug use	7-point Likert scale: (1) no ingestion to (7) forty cigarettes, or six drinks, or six marijuana cigarettes	Three items: cigarettes, alcohol, marijuana	Newcomb, Bentler, and Collins (1986), Stacy, Newcomb, and Bentler. (1991), Newcomb and Bentler (1988)	Adolescents and young adults (approximately 60 percent White)
Cultural orientation of the Latina: Feminism	5-point Likert scale: (1) strongly disagree to (5) strongly agree	Three items	Félix-Ortiz and Newcomb (1995), Félix-Ortiz, Newcomb, and Myers (1994)	Latino adults and adolescents
Cultural orientation of the family: Spanish spoken at home	5-point Likert scale: (1) mostly Spanish to (5) mostly English	One item	Félix-Ortiz and Newcomb (1995), Félix-Ortiz, Newcomb, and Myers (1994), Marin and others (1987)	Primarily Mexican American adults and adolescents
Intergenerational discrepancy (feminism/Spanish spoken at home)	Dichotomous, yes and no	One item	(See above scales/items)	(See above scales/items)
Parent/family support	5-point Likert scale: (1) strongly disagree to (5) strongly agree	Eight items	Newcomb and Bentler (1986, 1988)	Adolescents and young adults (approximately 60 percent White)

Feminism, assessed as a value of egalitarianism in family and household roles, was measured using a three-item 5-point Likert scale (alpha = .81). The scale has been used successfully in other studies (Félix-Ortiz, Newcomb, and Myers, 1994). Because the distribution for feminism was skewed in the positive direction toward many girls endorsing high feminism, the distribution for this scale was divided into two categories to reflect high feminist values (upper 51.2 percent of the distribution) and low feminist values (lower 48.8 percent of the distribution). The cultural orientation of the family was assessed by dividing the distribution of one 5-point Likert scale item, Spanish spoken at home, into two categories representing high Latino orientation (mostly Spanish spoken at home; 57 percent), and American orientation (mostly English spoken at home; 43 percent).

These two dichotomous variables (low versus high feminism and Spanish versus English spoken at home) were combined to yield a new dichotomous variable, intergenerational discrepancy. If the Latina adolescent had high feminist values and the family spoke Spanish at home, or if she endorsed few feminist values and her family spoke English at home, then this was taken to signify that intergenerational discrepancy between the girl and her family's cultural values existed. If, however, the Latina adolescent had high feminist values and spoke English at home, or if she endorsed low feminist values and her family spoke Spanish at home, then this was taken to signify that no intergenerational discrepancy between the girl and her family's cultural values existed.

Parent/Family Support. This measure was an eight-item 5-point Likert scale that evaluated the relationship with parents and family (alpha = .86). These items evaluated the amount of support, communication, affection, and inclusion experienced in each of these types of relationships and has been used successfully in other studies (Newcomb and Bentler, 1988). For example, one item states, "My parents don't think my ideas are much." Another states, "My family really understands me." This variable was hypothesized to function as a moderator of the relationship between the discrepancy variable and drug use. To simplify analysis for the identification of a moderator effect, the parent/family support variable was transformed into a dichotomous variable to represent low parent/family support (the lower 50 percent of the distribution) and high parent/family support (the upper 50 percent of the distribution).

RESULTS

Mean Drug Use

Table 20.4 presents a mean drug use for high- and low-feminist Latinas. Trimmed means are presented. A separate t-value was used if homoscedasticity was violated. For every measure of drug use except frequency of marijuana use,

Table 20.4. Mean Drug Use Among Low- and High-Feminist Latina Adolescents
in the Past Six Months

Variable	Low Feminist	High Feminist	t
	Frequency of drug use		
Cigarettes	1.48 (1.27)	2.05 (1.68)	3.29***
Alcohol	4.50 (2.50)	5.11 (2.41)	2.21*
Marijuana	1.21 (0.78)	1.38 (1.09)	1.52
Other illicit drugs	4.05 (0.39)	4.20 (1.20)	2.00*
	Quantity of drug use		
Cigarettes	0.23 (0.71)	0.41 (0.98)	1.95*
Alcohol	1.32 (1.87)	1.82 (1.90)	2.25*
Marijuana	0.13 (0.50)	0.32 (0.95)	20.8*

Note: Standard deviations are presented in parentheses following means. *$p \leq .05$; **$p \leq .01$; ***$p \leq .001$. Values represent the following categories: (1) never; (2) once or twice. The exceptions are alcohol frequency, which is a composite of three drug categories, and other illicit drugs, which is a composite of four drug categories.

high-feminist Latinas used drugs more frequently and used a higher quantity of drugs than did low-feminist Latinas. This difference between the two groups may not be as alarming as it initially appears since most Latina adolescents did not use or used only once or twice in the past six months. The greatest difference was for frequency of alcohol use (4.50 for low feminists versus 5.11 for high feminists; $p \leq .05$).

Inergenerational Discrepancy and Drug Use

t-tests comparing mean drug use (cigarettes, alcohol, marijuana, and illicit drugs) for two groups, Latina adolescents experiencing intergenerational discrepancy and those who did not, and point biserial correlations between intergenerational discrepancy and drug use were calculated. For this analysis, no distinction was made between type of intergenerational discrepancy (for example, a Latina who is Latino oriented in the context of an American-oriented family). Trimmed means are presented. A separate t-value was used if homoscedasticity was violated. No significant differences were obtained except for a relationship observed between frequency of cigarette use and intergenerational discrepancy in which the presence of a discrepancy was associated with more frequent cigarette use [$\bar{x} = 1.97$ (SD = 1.66) for discrepancy versus $\bar{x} = 1.61$ (SD = 1.38) for no discrepancy; $p \leq .05$].

Table 20.5 presents t-tests comparing mean drug use (cigarettes, alcohol, marijuana, and illicit drugs) for two groups: Latina adolescents from Latino-oriented families experiencing intergenerational discrepancy and those who

Table 20.5. Mean Drug Use for Latino-Oriented Girls (No ID) and American-Oriented Girls (ID) of Latino-Oriented Families and Point Biserial Correlations

Drug Use	No ID	ID	t	rpb
Frequency of use over the past six months				
Cigarettes	1.46 (1.32)	2.03 (1.74)	2.81**	.18
Alcohol	4.47 (2.26)	5.08 (2.54)	1.99*	.13
Marijuana	1.17 (0.69)	1.32 (1.04)	1.32	.08
Other illicit drugs	4.06 (0.41)	4.14 (1.26)	1.01	.06
Quantity of drug use				
Cigarettes	0.20 (0.72)	0.36 (0.94)	1.71	.11
Alcohol	1.30 (1.86)	1.78 (1.89)	1.93*	.12
Marijuana	0.11 (0.45)	0.27 (0.96)	1.67	.11

Note: Standard deviations are presented in parentheses following means. $*p \leq .05$; $**p \leq .01$; $***p \leq .001$. Values represent the following categories: (1) never; (2) once or twice. The exceptions are alcohol frequency, which is a composite of three drug categories, and other illicit drugs, which is a composite of four drug categories. rpb = point biserial correlations. ID = intergenerational discrepancy.

did not, and point biserial correlations between intergenerational discrepancy and drug use were calculated. Trimmed means are presented. A separate *t*-value was used if homoscedasticity was violated. Latino-oriented girls of Latino-oriented families used cigarettes ($p \leq .01$) and alcohol ($p \leq .05$) less frequently than American-oriented girls of Latino-oriented families. Latino-oriented girls of Latino-oriented families also used a lesser quantity of alcohol than American-oriented girls of Latino-oriented families ($p \leq .05$). In comparing Latino-oriented girls and American-oriented girls of American-oriented families, there were no significant differences in mean drug use. Because the effect of intergenerational discrepancy on drug use was specific to girls in Latino-oriented families, the remaining analyses were conducted using only these girls from Latino-oriented families.

Moderating Effect of Parent/Family Support

Baron and Kenny (1986) clarified the difference between mediating and moderating variables and proposed several ways of testing for these effects depending on the type of variables (continuous or dichotomous). A moderator is a third variable that affects the strength or direction of a relationship between two other variables depending on the level of the moderator, and it is always an independent variable. A mediator, in contrast, can (1) reduce a relationship between two variables to zero (the relationship between the two variables holds for *every* level of the mediator), (2) can be either an independent variable or a dependent variable, and (3) must temporally follow the independent variable and temporally precede the dependent variable. Since this last criterion was not met by a concurrent assessment of the variables used in this study, we tested for moderating effects. Furthermore, when both hypothesized moderator and independent variable are dichotomous, a simple 2 × 2 analysis of variance can be used in lieu of a multiple regression analysis to test for a moderating effect. An interaction between the independent variable and the putative moderator suggests the presence of moderation.

Table 20.6 presents 2 × 2 analyses of variance to test for the moderating effect of parent/family support on the relationship between intergenerational discrepancy and drug use for girls from Latino-oriented families. A main effect of intergenerational discrepancy was observed for frequency of cigarette and alcohol use and for quantity of alcohol and marijuana use ($p \leq .05$). A main effect of parent/family support was found for all measures of drug use except illicit drug use; in every case, Latinas experiencing higher parent/family support reported less frequency of drug use. However, parent/family support did not moderate the relationship between intergenerational discrepancy and drug use as evidenced by the absence of an interaction between parent/family support and intergenerational discrepancy.

DISCUSSION

In this study, part of a model of "vulnerability" and "resistance" to substance use was tested on a sample of Latina high school girls, and the specific contributions of intergenerational discrepancy between child and family cultural orientation were investigated. A specific type of intergenerational discrepancy where the family is traditionally Latino and the girl is feminist (American oriented) was associated with increased frequency of cigarette use, alcohol use, and increased quantity of alcohol use. However, the effect of intergenerational discrepancy on drug use was limited to this specific type of intergenerational discrepancy and to specific types of drug use, thereby failing to completely support results of Szapocznik and Kurtines's study (1980) that found intergenerational discrepancy to be associated with drug use in Cuban American boys. Furthermore, to expand on their model, we examined family support as a possible moderating variable in the relationship between intergenerational discrepancy and drug use. Family support had a main effect of lowering drug use but did not moderate the relationship between intergenerational discrepancy and drug use.

The results support both Szapocznik and Kurtines's (1980) model and Vega and others' model (1993). Szapocznik and Kurtines's (1980) model attributes conduct problems including drug use to the intergenerational discrepancies that surface as a result of the acculturation process within the family. However, for girls, this effect is limited to the case of an American-oriented girl in a

Table 20.6. Two-Way Analysis of Variance for Moderating Effect of Parent/Family Support

Drug Use	Latino-Oriented Girls		American-Oriented Girls		F-Value		
	Low PFS	High PFS	Low PFS	High PFS	ID	PFS	ID × PFS
Frequency of drug use							
Cigarettes	1.70 (1.51)	1.13 (0.77)	2.32 (1.83)	1.69 (1.56)	8.90**	9.20**	0.02
Alcohol	4.94 (2.48)	3.83 (1.59)	5.53 (2.60)	4.57 (2.38)	4.61*	11.38***	0.06
Marijuana	1.31 (0.85)	1.00 (0)	1.46 (1.08)	1.22 (0.98)	2.78	5.79*	0.09
Other illicit drugs	4.12 (0.51)	4.00 (0)	4.26 (1.48)	4.20 (0.87)	1.99	0.56	0.08
Quantity of drug use							
Cigarettes	0.31 (0.61)	0.13 (0.88)	0.52 (1.11)	0.24 (0.60)	2.34	4.49*	0.20
Alcohol	1.60 (1.92)	0.87 (1.68)	2.08 (1.98)	1.39 (1.69)	4.29*	8.50**	0.00
Marijuana	0.20 (0.56)	0.01 (0.04)	0.43 (1.14)	0.14 (0.58)	3.82*	6.37**	0.27

Note: Standard deviations are presented in parentheses following means. *$p \leq .05$; **$p \leq .01$; ***$p \leq .001$. Values represent the following categories: (1) never; (2) once or twice. The exceptions are alcohol frequency, which is a composite of three drug categories, and other illicit drugs, which is a composite of four drug categories. ID = intergenerational discrepancy. PFS = parent/family support.

Latino-oriented family and limited to specific types of drug use, alcohol, and cigarettes. It may be that the effect is limited to cigarettes and alcohol because these young women are not frequent users of any substance and, due to their young age and gender expectations, they have not progressed to harder illicit drug use. However, it may also be the case that intergenerational discrepancy is not associated at all with illicit drug use. It may be that a complete alienation from the family rather than family conflict alone is associated with illicit drug use.

Vega and others' model (1993) holds that child–parent conflicts are an important factor in creating vulnerability for drug use and that the presence of an intergenerational gap in acculturation is what triggers drug use. Our study only partially supports that model. When examining the effects of family support, a generic family protective influence, there was a significant main effect of family support on all drug use measures except for frequency of illicit drug use. However, family support did not reduce the effect of intergenerational discrepancy on frequency of cigarette and alcohol use among Latinas. Therefore, family support is not a moderator of the relationship between intergenerational discrepancy and drug use in this nonclinical sample of Latina youth, but it did have a main effect of reducing drug use and appeared to exert a broader influence, decreasing most types of drug use.

Although we provide some evidence for the possibility that intergenerational discrepancy in cultural orientation may be a risk factor for some types of drug use among Latina youth, it may be premature to conclude that all intergenerational discrepancies in cultural orientation generate family conflict in every case and that this conflict inevitably leads to conduct problems. For example, in our data, there was no relationship between intergenerational discrepancy and drug use among Latinas who were Latino oriented in the context of an American-oriented family. It may be, however, that (1) this type of intergenerational discrepancy does not generate family conflict because an "autonomous connectedness" (S. Einstein, personal communication, Jan. 17, 1997) is encouraged by American-oriented families, or (2) that some family process other than family conflict may account for the relationship between intergenerational discrepancy and drug use. For example, it may be that some Latina adolescents were more vulnerable to drug use for reasons unrelated to family functioning such as neighborhood or other societal influences. Many Latino families in Los Angeles live in low-income neighborhoods in which one can find many local liquor stores and cigarette and alcohol billboards but few public libraries or parks. Peer influences may interact with parent influences and reduce the protective effect of a positive parent influence. It may also be possible that gender influences this vulnerability somehow (that boys are more sensitive to certain types of family conflicts than are girls). These relationships may be difficult to fully capture in a single model because cultural and societal variables tend to be dynamic in nature (versus linear and continuous), but are usually assessed using measures which assume a stable, linear process. This type of shortcoming in assessment is likely to be reflected in less effective treatment. In the future, it may be useful to replicate this type of research using nonlinear artificial science paradigms that are sensitive to complex, dynamic phenomenon. (S. Einstein, personal communication, Jan. 17, 1997). The limited cross-sectional nature of this study did not allow for the exploration of a larger or developmental model.

The trend toward higher drug use among Latina feminists may not be as alarming as it initially appears: most Latinas did not use or used only once or twice in the past six months. Furthermore, for Latinas, familiarity with other aspects of American culture may actually offer some additional protection against drug use (Félix-Ortiz and Newcomb, 1995). Familiarity with American culture, for example, may allow for increased opportunities for involvement and the mainstream culture may include empowering knowledge of important social and behavioral skills, and greater perceived rewards, all of which are important protective factors as identified by the social development model (Hawkins and Weis, 1985).

Although this study is intriguing in its implications, it is only an initial foray into this area and is not without some limitations. The assessment of intergenerational discrepancy was limited to an indirect and dichotomous measure; in future studies, this should be assessed by questioning the adolescent directly about perceived intergenerational discrepancy and understanding how various levels of this variable are related to drug use. It will also be important to obtain fuller measures of family process based on continuous variables. Because cultural identity is a multidimensional construct more precisely defined by at least four domains—language, familiarity with culture, behavior, and attitudes (Félix-Ortiz, Newcomb, and Myers, 1994)—a more detailed assessment of cultural identity for the adolescent and each family member may have yielded different results. For example, for some youth, there are both "risk-inducing" and "protective" components of cultural identity that are related to drug use (Félix-Ortiz and Newcomb, 1995). Also, it will be important to explicitly establish that conflict mediates the relationship between intergenerational discrepancy and conduct problems. In this study, a secondary analysis of a database, no data on family conflict were available. In the future, other important influences on drug use among Latino youth should be explored; familism is only one of many values important to Latino mental health. It is also important to ensure that cultural influences are isolated from more generic family processes. In this study, we assessed one family process, family support, to compare against cultural factors. However, it is arguable that it is impossible to separate family and culture, that the family creates a culture of its own. Furthermore, because self-reports were used to obtain these data, they may be influenced by social desirability, resulting in underreporting or overreporting of drug use. Finally, these results may not be generalizable to the intergenerational discrepancy in other cultures or to other Latino subcultures and may be specific to Mexican Americans, most of whom comprised our sample.

In traditional efforts to educate teens on the dangers of drug use, programs have solely directed their efforts on the teens themselves, without incorporating the involvement of the whole family. While these strategies may have some effectiveness, these data indicate that drug education programs must involve the whole family, primarily the parents, and attend to cultural differences that may exist within the family. In addition, prevention efforts might be tailored to address issues unique to Latina adolescents (such as high rates of teen pregnancy) in addition to issues of cultural identity and identity development (such as feminism).

References

American Psychological Association. "Ethical Principles of Psychologists and Code of Conduct." *American Psychologist*, 1992, *47*, 1597–1611.

Baron, R. M., and Kenny, D. A. "The Moderator-Mediator Variable Distinction in Social Psychological Research: Conceptual, Strategic, and Statistical Considerations." *Journal of Personality and Social Psychology*, 1986, *51*, 1173–1181.

Brook, J. S., Nomura, C., and Cohen, P. "A Network of Influences on Adolescent Drug Involvement: Neighborhood, School, Peer, and Family." *Genetics, Social, and General Psychology Monographs*, 1989a, *115*, 125–145.

Brook, J. S., Nomura, C., and Cohen, P. "Prenatal, Perinatal, and Early Childhood Risk Factors and Drug Involvement in Adolescence." *Genetics, Social, and General Psychology Monographs*, 1989b, *115*, 223–241.

Brook, J. S., Whiteman, M., Gordon, A. S., and Cohen, P. "Some Models and Mechanisms for Explaining the Impact of Maternal and Adolescent Characteristics on Adolescent Stage of Drug Use." *Developmental Psychology*, 1986, *22*(4), 460–467.

Brook, J. S., and others. "The Psychosocial Etiology of Adolescent Drug Use: A Family Interactional Approach." *Genetics, Social, and General Psychology Monographs*, 1990, *116*.

Brownfield, D., and Sorenson, A. M. "Religion and Drug Use Among Adolescents: A Social Support Conceptualization and Interpretation." *Deviant Behavior*, 1991, *12*, 259–276.

Caetano, R. "Patterns and Problems of Drinking Among U.S. Hispanics." In T. E. Malone (ed.), *Report of the Secretary's Task Force on Black and Minority Health: Vol. 7. Chemical Dependency and Diabetes*. Washington, D.C.: Government Printing Office, 1986.

Caetano, R. "Acculturation and Attitudes Toward Appropriate Drinking Among US Hispanics." *Alcohol*, 1987, *22*, 427–433.

Canino, G., Burnam, A., and Caetano, R. "The Prevalence of Alcohol Abuse and/or Dependence in Two Hispanic Communities." In J. Helzer and G. Canino (eds.), *Alcoholism in North America, Europe, and Asia.* New York: Oxford University Press, 1992.

Comas-Diaz, L. "Feminist Therapy with Mainland Puerto Rican Women." *Psychology of Women Quarterly,* 1987, *11,* 461–474.

Donovan, J. E., Jessor, R., and Costa, F. M. "Syndrome of Problem Behavior in Adolescence: A Replication." *Journal of Consulting and Clinical Psychology,* 1988, *56,* 762–765.

Félix-Ortiz, M., Muñoz, R., and Newcomb, M. D. "The Role of Emotional Distress in Drug Use Among Latino Adolescents." *Journal of Child and Adolescent Substance Abuse,* 1994, *3,* 1–22.

Félix-Ortiz, M., and Newcomb, M. D. "Risk and Protective Factors for Drug Use Among Latino and White Adolescents." *Hispanic Journal of Behavioral Sciences,* 1992, *14,* 291–309.

Félix-Ortiz, M., and Newcomb, M. D. "Cultural Identity and Drug Use Among Latino and Latina Adolescents." In G. J. Botvin, S. Schinke, and M. A. Orlandi (eds.), *Drug Abuse Prevention with Multiethnic Youth.* Thousand Oaks, Calif.: Sage, 1995.

Félix-Ortiz, M., and Newcomb, M. D. "Vulnerability for Drug Use Among Latino Adolescents." Manuscript submitted for publication, 1997.

Félix-Ortiz, M., Newcomb, M. D., and Myers, H. "A Multidimensional Scale of Cultural Identity for Latino and Latina Adolescents." *Hispanic Journal of Behavioral Sciences,* 1994, *16*(2), 99–115.

Gibson, G. "Hispanic Women: Stress and Mental Health Issues." In J. H. Robbins and R. J. Josefowitz (eds.), *Women Changing Therapy: New Assessments, Values, and Strategies.* New York: Hawthorne Press, 1983.

Gilbert, J. "Alcohol Consumption Patterns in Immigrant and Later Generation Mexican American Women." *Hispanic Journal of Behavioral Sciences,* 1987, *9,* 299–313.

Hawkins, J. D., and Weis, J. G. "The Social Developmental Model: An Integrated Approach to Delinquency Prevention." *Journal of Primary Prevention,* 1985, *6,* 73–97.

Holck, S. E., Warren, C. W., Smith, J. C., and Rochat, R. W. "Alcohol Consumption Among Mexican American and Anglo Women: Results of a Survey Along the U.S.-Mexico Border." *Journal of Studies of Alcohol,* 1984, *45,* 149–154.

Hunsaker, A. C. "Chicano Drug Abuse Patterns: Using Archival Data to Test Hypotheses." *Hispanic Journal of Behavioral Sciences,* 1985, *7*(1), 93–104.

Kagan, J. "Etiologies of Adolescents at Risk." *Journal of Adolescent Health,* 1991, *12,* 591–596.

Labouvie, E. W. "Alcohol and Marijuana Use in Relation to Adolescent Stress." *International Journal of the Addictions,* 1986, *21,* 333–345.

Maddahian, E., Newcomb, M. D., and Bentler, P. M. "Single and Multiple Patterns of Adolescent Substance Use: Longitudinal Comparisons of Four Ethnic Groups." *Journal of Drug Education,* 1985, *15,* 311–326.

Marin, G., and others. "Development of a Short Acculturation Scale for Hispanics." *Hispanic Journal of Behavioral Sciences*, 1987, *9*, 183–205.

Moncher, M. S., Holden, G. W., and Trimble, J. E. "Substance Abuse Among Native American Youth." *Journal of Consulting and Clinical Psychology*, 1990, *58*, 408–415.

Needle, R., and others. "Familial, Interpersonal, and Intrapersonal Correlates of Drug Use: A Longitudinal Comparison of Adolescents in Treatment, Drug-Using Adolescents Not in Treatment, and Non-Drug-Using Adolescents." *International Journal of the Addictions*, 1988, *23*, 1211–1240.

Newcomb, M. D. "Understanding the Multidimensional Nature of Drug Use and Abuse: The Role of Consumption, Risk Factors, and Protective Factors." In M. D. Glantz and R. Pickens (eds.), *Vulnerability to Drug Abuse*. Washington, D.C.: American Psychological Association, 1992.

Newcomb, M. D., and Bentler, P. M. "Loneliness and Social Support: A Confirmatory Hierarchical Analysis." *Personality and Social Psychology Bulletin*, 1986, *12*, 520–535.

Newcomb, M. D., and Bentler, P. M. *Consequences of Adolescent Drug Use: Impact on the Lives of Young Adults*. Thousand Oaks, Calif.: Sage, 1988.

Newcomb, M. D., Bentler, P. M., and Collins, C. "Alcohol Use and Dissatisfaction with Self and Life: A Longitudinal Analysis of Young Adults." *Journal of Drug Issues*, 1986, *16*, 479–494.

Newcomb, M. D., and Félix-Ortiz, M. "Multiple Protective and Risk Factors for Drug Use and Abuse: Cross-Sectional and Prospective Findings." *Journal of Personality and Social Psychology*, 1992, *63*, 280–296.

Newcomb, M. D., Maddahian, E., and Bentler, P. M. "Risk Factors for Drug Use Among Adolescents: Concurrent and Longitudinal Analyses." *American Journal of Public Health*, 1986, *76*, 525–531.

Rodriguez, O., and Weisburd, D. "The Integrated Social Control Model and Ethnicity: The Case of Puerto Rican American Delinquency." *Criminal Justice Behavior*, 1991, *18*, 464–479.

Scheier, L. M., and Newcomb, M. D. "Psychosocial Predictors of Drug Use Initiation and Escalation: An Expansion of the Multiple Risk Factors Hypothesis Using Longitudinal Data." *Contemporary Drug Problems*, 1991, *18*, 31–73.

Schinke, S. P., and others. "Hispanic Youth, Substance Abuse, and Stress: Implications for Prevention Research." *International Journal of the Addictions*, 1988, *23*, 809–826.

Simcha-Fagan, O., Gersten, J. C., and Langner, T. S. "Early Precursors and Concurrent Correlates of Pattern of Illicit Drug Use in Adolescence." *Journal of Drug Issues*, 1986, *16*, 7–28.

Stacy, A. W., Newcomb, M. D., and Bentler, P. M. "Personality, Problem Drinking, and Drunk Driving: Mediating, Moderating, and Direct-Effect Models." *Journal of Personality and Social Psychology*, 1991, *60*, 795–811.

Szapocznik, J., and Kurtines, W. M. "Acculturation, Biculturalism and Adjustment Among Cuban Americans." In A. M. Padilla (ed.), *Theory, Models and Some New Findings*. Boulder, Colo.: Westview Press, 1980.

Szapocznik, J., and Kurtines, W. M. "Family Psychology and Cultural Diversity: Opportunities for Theory, Research and Application." *American Psychologist*, 1993, *48*, 400–407.

Vega, W. A. "Hispanic Families in the 1980s: A Decade of Research." *Journal of Marriage and the Family*, 1990, *52*, 1015–1024.

Vega, W. A., and others. "Acculturation and Delinquent Behavior Among Cuban American Adolescents: Toward an Empirical Model." *American Journal of Community Psychology*, 1993, *21*, 113–125.

Vicary, J. R., and Lerner, J. V. "Parental Attributes and Adolescent Drug Use." *Journal of Adolescence*, 1986, *9*, 115–122.

Young, G. "Chicana College Students on the Texas-Mexico Border: Tradition and Transformation." *Hispanic Journal of Behavioral Sciences*, 1992, *14*(3), 341–352.

Depressive Symptoms and Suicidal Ideation Among Mexican-Origin and Anglo Adolescents

Robert E. Roberts
Yuan-Who Chen

This chapter represents an important step for understanding a problem of major proportion within the Latino community that the mental health profession often neglects: suicidal ideation among Latino adolescents. Although the study focuses primarily on Mexican-origin adolescents in La Cruces, New Mexico, the sample size of 1,350 Latinos (half of whom are Latinas) and 925 Whites offers important information not obtained in other studies on this subject. This work, which provides insight into the factors that distinguish Latinos from non-Latinos, reports that Latinas had higher prevalence rates of symptoms of depression and thoughts of suicide than their White counterparts.

Thisarticle addresses a topic much neglected by mental health researchers: the experience of depression and suicide among minority youth. More specifically, we investigate the relation between depressive symptomatology and suicidal ideation, comparing adolescents from two ethnocultural groups—those of Mexican origin and non-Hispanic Whites or Anglos. The rationale for our focus is straightforward: there are virtually no data on depression and suicidal behavior among minority children and adolescents. An indication of the paucity of information is that three recent comprehensive reviews of the literature cite not a single study of depression and suicide among Hispanic youth (Feldman and Elliott, 1990; Fleming and Offord, 1990; Stiffman and Davis, 1990). The dearth of data on minority adolescents is not surprising, given the

This research was supported in part by grants MH44214 and MH44773 from the National Institute of Mental Health, the Hogg Foundation for Mental Health, and the Center for Cross-Cultural Research.

This article was adapted from a presentation at the annual meeting of the American Academy of Child and Adolescent Psychiatry, October 1993.

lack of data on adolescent depression and suicide in general. For example, there have been few community-based epidemiological studies of adolescent depression. Perusing the studies that have been done, it is difficult to identify a coherent empirical pattern due to the great diversity in research designs, study populations, and methods of case ascertainment. For example, Fleming and Offord (1990) identified nine epidemiological studies of clinical depression and report that prevalence of current depression ranged from 0.4 to 5.7 percent in the five studies reporting such data. The mean prevalence of current major depression was 3.6 percent. Subsequent to that review, several other articles have appeared. Lewinsohn, Rohde, and Seeley (1993) report data from a large sample of high school students indicating a point prevalence for DSM-III-R major depression of 2.6 percent. Garrison and others (1992) report one-year prevalence rates of approximately 9 percent for DSM-III major depressive disorder in a large sample of middle school students. There is equal diversity in studies that focus on depressive symptoms. Five school-based studies using the Beck Depression Inventory report mean scores ranging from 6.0 to 10.3; the average was 8.6 (Baron and Parron, 1986; Doerfler and others, 1988; Gibbs, 1985; Kaplan, Hong, and Weinhold, 1984; Teri, 1982). Seven studies, all school based, have used the Center for Epidemiologic Studies Depression Scale (CES-D) (Doerfler and others, 1988; Garrison and others, 1990; Manson and others, 1990; Roberts, Andrews, Lewinsohn, and Hops, 1990; Schoenbach, Kaplan, Grimson, and Wagner, 1982; Swanson and others, 1992; Tolor and Murphy, 1985). These studies report mean scores for the CES-D in the range of 16 to 20, with a mean of approximately 17. Prevalence of depressive symptoms using the standard CES-D caseness criterion of 16 or greater is in the range of 45 to 55 percent.

Given the limited number of epidemiological studies of adolescent depression in general, it is not surprising that there have been few studies published focusing on race or ethnic status. Again, even among this small subset of studies, the findings are not cohesive. While some studies find no evidence of ethnic differences in adolescent depression (Doerfler and others, 1988; Garrison and others, 1990; Kandel and Davies, 1982; Manson and others, 1990), others report that minority adolescents report greater levels of depressive symptoms (Emslie and others, 1990; Schoenbach, Kaplan, Grimson, and Wagner, 1982) and others that minority youth have lower levels of depression (Doerfler and others, 1988). But again, it is difficult to draw any firm conclusions concerning ethnic status and risk of depression from these studies, because they use different measures of depression and they also focus on different ethnic minority adolescents (for example, African American, Hispanic American, or Native American).

Four published studies have included adolescents of Mexican origin. Weinberg and Emslie (1987) report that in their sample of high school students, Anglos had the lowest rates of depression on both the Beck Depression Inventory and the

Weinberg Screening Affective Scale, African Americans were intermediate, and Mexican Americans had the highest rates.

Roberts and Sobhan (1992) analyzed data from a national survey of persons 12 through 17 years of age ($n = 2,200$), comparing symptom levels of Anglo American, African American, Mexican-origin, and other Hispanic Americans using a twelve-item version of the CES-D. Males of Mexican origin reported more depressive symptoms than other males, and the same was true for females of Mexican origin, although to a lesser extent. Roberts (forthcoming) examined depression rates among 2,614 Mexican-origin and Anglo adolescents sampled from middle schools in Las Cruces, New Mexico. The minority youth had significantly higher rates of depressive symptoms on both the standard twenty-item CES-D and the Weinberg Screening Affective Scale.

Only one article has focused on both depression and suicide among youth of Mexican origin. Swanson and his colleagues (1992) conducted a school-based survey in three cities in Texas and three in Mexico along the U.S.-Mexico border. The U.S. sample, composed of more than 95 percent Mexican-origin adolescents, had a prevalence of 48 percent using the score of 16 or more on the CES-D, while 23 percent reported that they had thought about killing themselves during the past week.

Studies of children and adolescents also have reported a strong relation between depression and suicidal behaviors (Andrews and Lewinsohn, 1992; Garrison and others, 1991a, 1991b; Kashani, Goddard, and Reid, 1989; Kovacs, Goldstein, and Gatsonis, 1993; Lewinsohn, Rohde, and Seeley, 1993; Velez and Cohen, 1988; Weiner and Pfeffer, 1986). In general, youth evidencing suicidal ideation and suicide attempts, as well as those who commit suicide, are all reported to have elevated rates of depression.

Suicidal behaviors (ideation and attempts) in community samples suggest that such behaviors are not uncommon and constitute a significant public health problem (Kashani, Goddard, and Reid, 1989) Recent community-based, epidemiological studies report prevalence of suicidal ideation ranging from about 2 percent to as high as 60 percent (Garrison and others, 1991b). The prevalence of suicide attempts tends to be much lower, with lifetime prevalence for adolescents ranging from 3.5 percent to 11 percent (see Lewinsohn, Rohde, and Seeley, 1993). In general, race or ethnicity has been little studied in relation to suicidal behaviors. Results from the few studies that have examined ethnic or racial differences have been equivocal, with several studies reporting no differences between white and black adolescent suicidal behaviors (Dubow and others, 1989; Garrison and others, 1991b) and several reporting higher suicidal behaviors among black adolescents (Garrison and others, 1991a; Harkavy Friedman, Asnis, Boeck, and DiFiore, 1987). Lester and Anderson (1992), using data from a very small school-based sample in New Jersey, report that Hispanic students had higher scores on both depression and suicidal ideation than did

African American students. Given the location, we presume most of the Hispanic students were of Puerto Rican origin.

Vega, Gil, Zimmerman, and Warheit (1993), using data from a large school-based survey of Cuban, Nicaraguan, other Hispanic, African American, and Anglo American males in grades 6 and 7, report that African Americans had the highest prevalence of suicidal ideation in the previous six months. Nicaraguans and other Hispanics had the highest levels of lifetime suicide attempts.

Given the equivocal results thus far on the role of ethnicity, and the dearth of data on Hispanics in general and Mexican-origin youth in particular, our purpose here is to further explore ethnic differentials in adolescent depressive symptoms and suicidal ideation, contrasting non-Hispanic whites (Anglos) with Mexican-Americans.

METHOD

The data presented are from a school-based survey conducted in Las Cruces, New Mexico, in the 1990–1991 school year. Las Cruces is a community with a population of approximately 100,000 in southern New Mexico. The economy is mixed, primarily agriculture and light industry. The second largest college in the state is located there. With nearly 20,000 students, the district is the second largest public school system in the state. The district is 41 percent Anglo, 56 percent Hispanic (virtually all Mexican origin), and 3 percent other. This composition closely reflects the demography of New Mexico. Approximately half of the students (49 percent) are from families with incomes below the poverty level.

Surveys were done in the three largest middle schools (grades 6 through 8). Completed questionnaires were obtained from 2,614 subjects. Of these, 924 were Anglo and 1,354 were Mexican American. The remainder were American Indian, African American, from other Hispanic groups, or of mixed ancestry. All of these individual categories consisted of small numbers of subjects. Passive parental and active student consent procedures were used. Nonparticipants (13.1 percent) consisted of those who refused consent and those who were absent on the day of the surveys. In addition, some questionnaires (5.4 percent) were returned incomplete. Usable questionnaires numbered 2,614, or 81.5 percent. Total enrollment in the three schools was 3,206. The questionnaires were in English only.

A number of mental health measures from the Oregon Adolescent Depression Project (Hops, Lewinsohn, Andrews, and Roberts, 1990; Roberts, Andrews, Lewinsohn, and Hops, 1990) were included: the CES-D, four suicide items, eight loneliness items, and five anxiety items.

The primary measure of depression was the standard twenty-item version of the CES-D. The reliability and validity of the CES-D scale have been assessed on adult clinic populations (Craig and Van Natta, 1973; Roberts, Vernon, and Rhoades, 1989; Weissman and others, 1977) and on adult respondents from a number of community studies (Comstock and Helsing, 1976; Radloff, 1977; Roberts, 1980). There have been fewer studies involving adolescents. However, the available data indicate that the CES-D exhibits similar operating characteristics with adolescents as with older populations in terms of reliability, dimensionality, and efficacy in detecting clinical depression (Roberts, Andrews, Lewinsohn, and Hops, 1990; Roberts, Lewinsohn, and Seeley, 1991; Schoenbach, Kaplan, Grimson, and Wagner, 1982; Wells, Klerman, and Deykin, 1987).

Also included in the analyses are two additional measures that are correlated with depression: suicidal ideation and loneliness. The suicide measure consists of four items, formatted exactly like the items in the CES-D. These items, used initially in the Oregon study, had an alpha reliability of .85. The items are "thoughts about death"; "family and friends better off if I were dead"; "thought about killing myself"; and "would kill myself if I knew a way." The eight loneliness items were adapted from the UCLA loneliness measure (Russell, Peplau, and Cutrona, 1980) by the first author and also included in the Oregon survey. The items exhibited good reliability (alpha = .78) and demonstrated good construct validity in the Oregon study (Roberts, Lewinsohn, and Seeley, 1993). The scale is called the Roberts version of the UCLA Loneliness Scale, or RULS-8.

Ethnic status was ascertained by an item that asked: "What is your racial/ ethnic background?" The response categories were (1) White, non-Hispanic; (2) Black or African American; (3) Hispanic (Mexican, Cuban, Puerto Rican, or other American); (4) American Indian/Eskimo/Aleut; (5) Asian/Pacific Islander; and (6) other. Here, the contrast of interest is White, non-Hispanic, and Mexican American.

Other variables from the survey included for purposes of these analyses were age (in years), gender, household composition, and English use. Preliminary analyses (not shown) suggested that the most salient aspect of household composition was whether the adolescent lived in a two-parent household versus "other," and that is the measure used here. Following Vega, Gil, Zimmerman, and Warheit (1993), we employ language use as an indicator of relative level of acculturation.

Subject characteristics are presented in Table 21.1. Two points are worth noting. First, questions about educational level of parents were not successful, as can be seen. A large proportion of adolescents did not know their parents' educational level. Second, the overwhelming majority of youths were bilingual or English dominant. In fact, only 57 students of Mexican origin reported being Spanish dominant. Cognizant of this fact, the schools had recommended conducting the survey in English. Although we had reservations about this strategy, we reluctantly agreed to do so to maintain our collaborative relation with the schools.

Table 21.1. Distribution of Selected Demographic Variables, by Ethnicity

	Anglo (%)	Mexican Origin (%)
Overall	920	1,297
Gender		
Male	456 (49.6)	617 (47.6)
Female	464 (50.4)	680 (52.4)
Age		
11 years or less	192 (20.9)	268 (20.7)
12 years	312 (33.9)	342 (26.6)
13 years	288 (31.3)	408 (31.5)
14 years or over	128 (13.9)	276 (21.3)
Language use		
Mostly/only English	910 (98.9)	779 (60.1)
Both equally	10 (1.1)	518 (39.9)
Father's education		
Less than high school	38 (4.1)	186 (14.3)
High school graduate	126 (13.7)	243 (18.7)
Less than 4 years of college	126 (13.7)	128 (9.9)
4 years of college or more	339 (36.9)	121 (9.4)
Missing or not applicable	291 (31.6)	619 (47.7)
Household structure		
Two-parent household	690 (75.0)	873 (67.3)
Other	230 (25.0)	424 (32.7)

RESULTS

The CES-D exhibited good internal consistency reliability across groups, with alpha values of .92 for Anglo and .93 for Mexican-origin adolescents. The four suicide items also showed good internal consistency, with alpha values of .88 for Anglo adolescents and .92 for their Mexican-origin counterparts. The alpha values for the loneliness items were .90 for Anglos and .88 for Mexican Americans. We also contrasted alpha reliability values for those adolescents of Mexican origin who spoke mostly or only English versus those who spoke English and Spanish equally. The internal consistency for the contrasted groups was similar and very good. For example, alpha on the CES-D was .93 for the former and .94 for the latter. For the suicide items, alpha was .93 for the first group and .90 for the second. There were fifty-seven subjects of Mexican origin who reported speaking "mostly Spanish." However, only thirteen completed all twenty CES-D

Table 21.2. Prevalence and Mean Scores on the Center for Epidemiologic Studies Depression Scale (CES-D), by Ethnicity, Gender, and Age

	CES-D Scores							
	Percentage 16+		Percentage 24+		Percentage 31+		Mean	
	Anglo	Mexican Origin	Anglo	Mexican Origin	Anglo	Mexican Origin	Anglo	Mexican Origin
Overall	35.7***	47.5	19.9**	29.8	12.3***	18.0	14.4***	17.7
Gender								
Male	32.7**	41.6	18.1**	24.8	9.3**	14.1	13.1***	15.6
Female	38.5***	52.8	21.6***	34.2	15.2**	21.6	15.8**	19.5
Age								
11 years or less	37.7**	50.2	21.5*	31.4	11.5*	18.0	14.9**	18.6
12 years	32.5***	46.4	17.0***	29.3	11.3**	17.7	13.5***	17.2
13 years	36.1**	46.6	18.9**	28.4	10.5**	18.5	14.4***	17.3
14 years or more	39.4	47.6	26.8	30.8	19.7	18.0	16.0	17.8

Note: The asterisks indicate a significant difference between ethnic groups.

*$p < .05$; **$p < .01$; ***$p < .001$.

items. The alpha reliability values for this small group were .93 for the CES-D and .93 for suicidal ideation.

Table 21.2 presents mean scores and prevalence rates for the CES-D by ethnic status, age, and gender. Prevalence rates were calculated using the generally accepted "caseness" criteria of 16 or greater as well as 24 or greater and 31 or greater. The 24+ criterion is based on earlier research (Roberts, Lewinsohn, and Seeley, 1991), which indicated a score of 24+ proved the most efficient screen for DSM-III-R clinical depression among adolescents in that study. In that article, we classified adolescent depression as mild, moderate, or severe on the basis of CES-D scores of 16+, 21+, and 31+ following the suggestion of Barnes and Prosen (1985). Using receiver operating curve analyses, we also found in previous work that the optimal caseness screening score was 24 for girls, 22 for boys, and 24 overall. In the interest of parsimony, we present data using 16+, 24+, and 31+ here. Although it is questionable how useful 16+ is as a caseness score, since it was derived with data on adults, we use it because most other researchers also have used it as at least one measure with adolescents.

As can be seen, regardless of the scoring procedure used, the adolescents of Mexican origin reported significantly more depression on the CES-D than did the Anglo adolescents (approximately 50 percent more by the criteria of 24+ or 31+).

Table 21.3. Prevalence and Mean Scores on Suicidal Ideation, by Ethnicity, Gender, and Age

| | Suicidal Ideation | | | |
| | Percentage 5+ | | Mean | |
	Anglo	Mexican Origin	Anglo	Mexican Origin
Overall	14.1***	25.2	1.8***	2.9
Gender				
Male	13.1**	21.6	1.7***	2.5
Female	15.0***	28.5	1.8***	3.2
Age				
11 years or less	13.9***	27.8	1.7***	3.1
12 years	12.0***	22.8	1.5***	2.7
13 years	13.0***	26.9	1.8**	3.1
14 years or more	22.0	23.4	2.3	2.6

Note: The asterisks indicate a significant difference between ethnic groups.

**p* < .01; ****p* < .001.

As is often the case in published research, females reported more depressive symptoms than males. Females of Mexican origin were clearly most likely to report depressive symptoms. Overall, there were no age effects within each ethnic group.

Similar data on suicidal ideation are presented in Table 21.3. Again, the overall pattern is one in which adolescents of Mexican origin reported more thoughts of suicide than their Anglo counterparts. With higher prevalence defined as a score of 5 or greater (5+), approximately 50 percent more adolescents of Mexican origin reported suicidal ideation. Females reported more ideation than males, with the more dramatic differences occurring among minority adolescents. Those 14 years of age had about twice the rate of those younger than 14. However, for the age subcategories, there were significant differences of ethnic effects for both prevalence and mean scores up through age 13, but not for ages 14 or older. The rates also were much higher for those 14 and older.

Given the often-reported association between depression and suicide (Kovacs, Goldstein, and Gatsonis, 1993; Lewinsohn, Rohde, and Seeley, 1993), we also assessed this relation. For example, the correlation between the CES-D (which contains no items on suicide) and the four-item suicide scale was quite high: .70 overall, .68 for Anglos, and .71 for Mexican Americans (data not shown). Among those with CES-D scores of 24 or greater, 37 percent of the Anglo and 36 percent of the Mexican American youth scored high (5 or more) on suicidal ideation.

Table 21.4. Crude and Adjusted Odds Ratios for Depression by Demographic
and Mental Health Variables (n = 2,065)

	Crude Odds Ratios			Adjusted Odds Ratios		
	OR	(95% CI)	p	OR	(95% CI)	p
Race[a]	1.7	(1.4, 2.1)	.001		NS	
Gender[b]	1.5	(1.2, 1.8)	.001		NS	
Age[c]	1.1	(0.9, 1.3)	.468		NS	
Speaking English[d]	2.0	(1.6, 2.4)	.001	1.4	(1.0, 1.8)	.028
Two parents[e]	1.4	(1.1, 1.7)	.003		NS	
Suicidal ideation[f]	15.2	(11.8, 19.5)	.001	10.9	(8.3, 14.4)	.001
Loneliness[f]	7.7	(6.2, 9.6)	.001	5.8	(4.5, 7.5)	.001

Note: Depression was measured using a score of 24 or greater on the Center for Epidemiologic Studies Depression Scale. Suicidal ideation was measured using a score of 5 or greater. Loneliness was measured using a score of 9 or greater on the Roberts version of the UCLA Loneliness Scale. Zero indicates the reference group in the calculation of odds ratio. OR = odds ratio; CI = confidence interval; NS = not significant.

[a]0 = Anglo; 1 = Mexican American.

[b]0 = male; 1 = female.

[c]0 = younger than 13 years; 1 = 13 or older.

[d]0 = most or only English; 1 = both equally.

[e]0 = two parents; 1 = otherwise.

[f]0 = negative; 1 = positive.

Among those youth scoring 5 or more on suicidal ideation, 84 percent of the Anglos and 81 percent of the Mexican Americans scored high on depression (24+). None of these ethnic differences were statistically significant (data not shown).

In Table 21.4, we present the results of logistic regression analyses in which we estimated the odds ratios (ORs) for each of seven factors. In these analyses, the small group of students who reported speaking mostly Spanish is excluded from the analyses, rather than include them in the both equally or bilingual group. The subsample was too small for meaningful analyses. Using crude prevalence, all but age were significant correlates of depression. The strongest associations were for suicidal ideation (OR = 15.2) and loneliness (7.7). The OR for ethnic status indicates that adolescents of Mexican origin had approximately 1.7 times the risk of depressive symptoms as their Anglo counterparts. We then examined the ORs for each factor's association with the outcome, CES-D caseness score, controlling for the effects of all other factors in each analysis (Hosmer and Lemeshow, 1989). Thus, in the case of ethnic status, its association with depression was calculated, controlling for the effects of gender, age, language, number of parents in household, suicidal ideation, loneliness, and so

Table 21.5. Crude and Adjusted Odds Ratios for Suicidal Ideation by Demographic and Mental Health Variables (n = 2,065)

	Crude Odds Ratios			Adjusted Odds Ratios		
	OR	(95% CI)	p	OR	(95% CI)	p
Race[a]	2.1	(1.6, 2.6)	.001	1.6	(1.2, 2.1)	.005
Gender[b]	1.4	(1.1, 1.7)	.005		NS	
Age[c]	1.2	(0.9, 1.4)	.167		NS	
Speaking English[d]	2.2	(1.7, 2.7)	.001	1.4	(1.0, 1.9)	.044
Two parents[e]	1.6	(1.3, 2.0)	.001	1.4	(1.1, 1.9)	.012
Depression[f]	15.2	(11.8, 19.5)	.001	10.6	(8.1, 14.0)	.001
Loneliness[f]	5.0	(4.0, 6.3)	.001	2.1	(1.6, 2.8)	.001

Note: Depression was measured using a score of 24 or greater on the Center for Epidemiologic Studies Depression Scale. Suicidal ideation was measured using a score of 5 or greater. Loneliness was measured using a score of 9 or greater on the Roberts version of the UCLA Loneliness Scale. Zero indicates the reference group in the calculation of odds ratio. OR = odds ratio; CI = confidence interval; NS = not significant.

[a]0 = Anglo; 1 = Mexican American.

[b]0 = male; 1 = female.

[c]0 = younger than 13 years; 1 = 13 or older.

[d]0 = most or only English; 1 = both equally.

[e]0 = two parents; 1 = otherwise.

[f]0 = negative; 1 = positive.

on. The adjusted OR values indicate that three factors remain significant: suicidal ideation, loneliness, and English use, in that order. Ethnic status is no longer statistically significant.

Similar data are presented for prevalence of suicidal ideation in Table 21.5. Crude ORs indicate that ethnic status (OR = 2.1) and five of the other six factors (excluding age) are significantly related to risk of suicidal ideation. Depression (OR = 15.2) is by far the most significant correlate of suicidal ideation, followed by loneliness (OR = 5.0). The adjusted ORs reveal that ethnic status (OR = 1.6), living in other than a two-parent household, English use, depression, and loneliness remain significant. Depression remains the most powerful risk factor for suicidal ideation (OR = 10.6).

In earlier logistic regression analyses of these data, we included education of head of household as a measure of socioeconomic status. There was no significant effect of parental education on either depression or suicidal ideation. This was unexpected, given that social class variables are typically the most powerful predictors of mental health status (Roberts and Vernon, 1984). Our findings may be attributable in part to the large numbers of students (34 percent) who did not report parental education. Other analyses indicated a strong association between parental education and English language use reported by students (gamma = .76, $p <$ .001). In view of the large sample loss and reduced representativeness generated by missing data on parental education, the high association between parental education and language use, and the fact that the ORs for other risk factors were very similar with and without parental education in the equations, we elected to present the latter results in Table 21.4 and Table 21.5. (The results including parental education are available from the authors.)

DISCUSSION

To recapitulate briefly, depressive symptoms were prevalent among both Anglo and Mexican-origin middle school students. By the standard caseness score of 16 or more on the CES-D, more than a third of the Anglo and almost half of the minority adolescents were depressed. These rates are comparable to rates reported in other surveys using the CES-D. Even with a more stringent criterion of 24 or more, one-fifth of the Anglos and three in ten of the Mexican Americans were depressed. Approximately 10 percent of majority and 15 percent of minority youth reported high levels of suicidal ideation. As might be expected, the correlation between symptoms of depression and thoughts of suicide was quite high in both groups (.68, .71). More than a third of both groups who scored 24 or greater on the CES-D also scored high on suicidal ideation. The rate was even more dramatic for those with high scores on suicidal ideation: more than 80 percent of both groups scored above the caseness criterion on depression. Clearly, on the basis of crude rates, depression appears to be a powerful risk factor (correlate) for suicidal ideation in both ethnic groups.

The findings on ethnic status and gender among adolescents in Las Cruces corroborate those from other studies of this age group (Emslie and others, 1990; Garrison and others, 1990; Roberts, Andrews, Lewinsohn, and Hops, 1990; Roberts, Lewinsohn, and Seeley, 1991). The data from middle school students in Las Cruces are congruent with those from the 1985 national survey by the National Institute on Drug Abuse (Roberts and Sobhan, 1992). In that study, crude prevalence rates were higher among females and Mexican Americans. The latter were at least one and a half times more likely to report depressive symptoms than Anglos, adjusting for the effects of age, gender, perceived health, and socioeconomic status. In the only other published study comparing Anglo, African, and Mexican American adolescents on depression, Emslie and others (1990) also found females and Mexican Americans to be at greater risk in terms of crude rates.

Given the limited community-based prevalence data available for children and adolescents, how do our rates of 10 percent for Anglos and 15 percent for Mexican-origin youths compare with other studies of suicidal ideation? The most direct comparison is the study by Garrison and others (1991a), who report that 20.9 percent of middle school students reported some ideation and 10 percent reported moderate to high ideation. Their measure was very similar to ours. Dubow and others (1989) report that 12 percent of junior high and high school subjects reported suicidal ideation that was "somewhat troubling" and 7 percent ideation that was "extremely troubling." Pfeffer and others (1984) report that approximately 12 percent of youth 6 through 12 years of age reported some suicide ideation. Andrews and Lewinsohn (1992) report lifetime rates of 21 percent for suicidal ideation among high school students and a one-year prevalence of almost 5 percent. Their rates are derived from clinical interviews using the K-SADS rather than self-administered questionnaires. In view of the results of these studies, rates of suicidal ideation among adolescents appear to be in the range of 10 to 20 percent.

Logistic regression analyses of a very limited set of putative risk factors or, more properly, correlates of depression and suicidal ideation further confirmed the strong relation between these two indicators of mental health status. Controlling for the effects of ethnic status, gender, age, language, number of parents in household, and loneliness, suicidal ideation was by far the most powerful predictor of depression. The OR was 10.9 ($p < .001$). Loneliness also was a strong correlate (OR = 5.8, $p < .001$). The same analysis with suicidal ideation as the outcome, adjusting for the other six correlates, yielded an OR of 10.6 for depression. These same analyses suggest that adolescents of Mexican origin are at greater risk of suicidal ideation than their Anglo counterparts, even after controlling for a number of possibly confounding factors. The same was not true for depression; multivariate logistic regression analyses indicated minority status was not a significant risk factor for depression.

Our results on the relation between suicidal ideation and depression among both majority and minority youth corroborate a growing body of evidence that some psychiatric disorders, particularly depression, constitute important risk factors for suicidal behaviors (Andrews and Lewinsohn, 1992; Garrison and others, 1991a, 1991b; Kashani, Goddard, and Reid, 1989; Kovacs, Goldstein, and Gatsonis, 1993; Lewinsohn, Rohde, and Seeley, 1993; Velez and Cohen, 1988).

To our knowledge, only one study (Swanson and others, 1992) has reported data on depression and suicidal ideation among youth of Mexican origin. How do our results compare with their findings? Table 21.6 presents data from the two studies, with depression and suicidal ideation scored using the same procedures. For depression, prevalence is scored as the proportion scoring 16 or greater on the CES-D, and for suicidal ideation, it is the proportion reporting that during the past week they had thought about killing themselves on one or more days. We used 16+ as the definition of caseness because it allowed us to make a direct comparison with the results of Swanson and others (1992). As can be seen, results from the two studies are in many respects quite similar. On both depressive symptoms and suicidal ideation, the Mexican-origin adolescents

Table 21.6. Comparison of Las Cruces Data with Those of Swanson and Others (1992)

	Las Cruces		Swanson and Others (1992)	
	Anglo	Mexican Origin	Texas	Mexico
Depression	13.5	47.3	48.1	39.4
Suicidal ideation	14.1	25.2	23.4	11.6

Note: Values are percentages. Depression was measured using a score of 16 or greater on the Center for Epidemiologic Studies Depression Scale.

in Texas and New Mexico have similar rates, and the Anglos and the Mexican adolescents have similar rates, suggesting that minority status may be one plausible explanation. The data also provide evidence for the validity of both the CES-D and the suicide items used in the studies. Prevalence rates are virtually identical for Mexican-origin adolescents in southern Texas and New Mexico.

In the only community-based study to date of psychiatric disorder, suicidal ideation, and suicide attempts, Sorenson and Golding (1988) used the Epidemiologic Catchment Area (ECA) data from Los Angeles to contrast Anglos and Hispanics. The latter reported less lifetime suicidal ideation and fewer attempts, almost half the rates for Anglos. Women reported higher rates of ideation and attempts in both ethnic groups, about twice as high as men. Why the ethnic differential for adults in the ECA survey is the opposite of that observed for adolescents in New Mexico is unclear. Many factors could account for the observed differences, including differences in time, place, age of respondents, and measurement. We used a symptom scale in Las Cruces; in Los Angeles, they used structured psychiatric interviews and obtained data on lifetime episodes. As Simon and Vonkorff (1992) have demonstrated, lifetime reports in the ECA study appear to have substantial error. Whether this error differs by ethnicity is unclear. Clearly this is an area in need of further study.

The Las Cruces survey collected data on relatively few factors known or hypothesized to increase the risk for depression (Hops, Lewinsohn, Andrews, and Roberts, 1990; Kovacs, 1989; Lewinsohn, Hoberman, Teri, and Hautzinger, 1985; Paykel, 1982; Roberts, 1987; Rutter, Tizard, and Read, 1986) among both adults and adolescents, or for suicidal behaviors (Dubow and others, 1989; Garrison and others, 1991b; Kashani, Goddard, and Reid, 1989; Kovacs, Goldstein, and Gatsonis, 1993; Lewinsohn, Rohde, and Seeley, 1993; Nelson, 1987; Rich and Bonner, 1987). Thus, in the case of the findings we presented here indicating more depression and suicidal ideation among Mexican American adolescents, we are unable to explore whether this difference is due, for example, to differential exposure to stress or to differential vulnerability (see, for example, Ulbrich, Warheit, and Zimmerman, 1989).

One fruitful line of investigation on the relation of ethnicity to mental health may be the construct of ethnic identity. As Alba (1990) has noted, traditional manifestations of ethnicity in ethnic social structures organized around national origin, religion, occupation, politics, and geographic location are decreasingly important in defining ethnicity (see also Trimble, 1990–1991). One consequence has been increasing primacy of ethnic identity, the subjective orientation toward ethnic origins. Although many writers have noted that ethnic identity is crucial to self-concept and to psychological functioning of ethnic group members, to date there has been little empirical research on ethnic identity among children and adolescents, and essentially none on whether ethnic identity increases or decreases risk for psychiatric disorder (Phinney, 1990; Rotheram-Borus, 1990).

Ethnic status per se has not provided much explanatory power (Roberts and Vernon, 1984; Trimble, 1990–1991). Clearly, this is so here as well. Although we found ethnic differentials in crude rates (ORs) of depression and suicidal ideation, statistical controls for possibly confounding factors eliminated ethnic differentials in depression and attenuated those for suicidal ideation.

Perhaps reconceptualizing our epidemiological models to include ethnic identity as a putative risk factor for child and adolescent disorders, specifying conditions under which ethnic identity operates as a stressor or resource (Ensel and Lin, 1991) may provide a better understanding of the mental health effects of ethnicity, in particular minority status. Recent developments in measurement of the construct of ethnic identity make such a line of investigation more feasible than in the past (Alba, 1990; Phinney, 1992). The only dimension of ethnicity we included other than ethnic status was language use. The logistic regression analyses clearly indicate that increasing acculturation (use of English) greatly decreased the risk of depression and suicidal ideation among adolescents of Mexican origin. For example, among youths of Mexican origin, the CES-D prevalence rates by language group were 26.3 for mostly or only English, 36.0 for both equally, and 46.4 for mostly Spanish ($p < .001$), using 24+ as the criterion. Similar differences were observed using 16+. For suicidal ideation, the prevalence rates were 22.1 for mostly or only English, 30.9 for both equally, and 36.0 for mostly Spanish ($p < .01$). Vega, Gil, Zimmerman, and Warheit (1993) found higher levels of suicide attempts with higher acculturation among their Hispanic subsamples (Cuban, Nicaraguan, other). No data were reported on acculturation and ideation.

Our results, while interesting overall and generally consistent with other findings, are limited in some respects because of the nature of our measures of depression and suicidal behavior. Our measure of depression is a brief symptom scale, and our measure of suicide is a four-item scale of suicidal ideation. Essentially all studies of ethnic status and psychological disorder among adolescents have relied on nonclinical or nondiagnostic measures of dysfunction, to the exclusion of clinical disorder (for an exception, see Bird and others, 1988).

Symptoms of depression are highly prevalent among adolescents in general, and they are the source of considerable suffering. A better understanding of their etiology and consequences is needed. However, absence of a measure of clinical depression omits the more serious forms of depressive illness. From an epidemiological perspective, the differences in prevalence are substantial. For example, studies indicate that the prevalence of clinical depression among adolescents is perhaps 3 to 4 percent (Fleming and Offord, 1990; Roberts, Lewinsohn, and Seeley, 1991). In the only study of clinical depression among Hispanic youth, Bird and others (1988) report the six-month prevalence of depression/dysthymia in Puerto Rico was 2.8 percent. Whether nonclinical and clinical depression differ in etiology and consequences is an important epidemiological question, and one for which as yet we have no empirical data.

We chose the CES-D as one of our measures of depression because it had been widely used in other studies of adults and adolescents, including Mexican Americans, and data were available on its operating characteristics, including its relation to putative risk factors for depression. It clearly is not a measure of clinical depression (Roberts, Lewinsohn, and Seeley, 1991). However, internal consistency reliability, prevalence rates, and correlation with hypothesized risk factors are closely comparable to those found in other studies, suggesting that the CES-D operates in the same fashion for our Mexican-origin adolescents as for other groups.

The same is true for suicidal behaviors. Essentially all of our data on minority youth are for suicidal ideation. A suicide attempt is much more serious and a less prevalent form of suicidal behavior, as recent studies have shown (Dubow and others, 1989; Garrison and others, 1991a; Kovacs, Goldstein, and Gatsonis, 1993; Lewinsohn, Rohde, and Seeley, 1993; Velez and Cohen, 1988). At this juncture, we do not know the prevalence of more serious forms of suicidal behavior among Mexican-origin or other minority children and adolescents, nor do we know for minority or majority youth whether there are important epidemiological differences between ideators and attempters.

Given the results reported here, and the limited data on the mental health of minority adolescents generally, more comparative research is needed, both of suicidal behaviors and depression as well as other psychiatric disorders and whether and how ethnocultural background constitutes a risk factor for such problems.

References

Alba, R. D. *Ethnic Identity: The Transformation of White America.* New Haven, Conn.: Yale University Press, 1990.

Andrews, J. A., and Lewinsohn, P. M. "Suicidal Attempts Among Older Adolescents: Prevalence and Co-Occurrence with Psychiatric Disorders." *Journal of the American Academy of Child and Adolescent Psychiatry,* 1992, *32,* 655–662.

Barnes, G. E., and Prosen, H. "Parental Death and Depression." *Journal of Abnormal Psychology,* 1985, *94,* 64–69.

Baron, P., and Parron, L. M. "Sex Differences in the Beck Depression Inventory Scores of Adolescents." *Journal of Youth and Adolescence,* 1986, *15,* 165–171.

Bird, H. R., and others. "Estimates of the Prevalence of Childhood Maladjustment in a Community Survey in Puerto Rico. The Use of Combined Measures." *Archives of General Psychiatry,* 1988, *45,* 1120–1126.

Comstock, G. W., and Helsing, K. J. "Symptoms of Depression in Two Communities." *Psychological Medicine,* 1976, *6,* 551–563.

Craig, T. J., and Van Natta, P. "Validation of the Community Mental Health Assessment Interview Instrument Among Psychiatric Inpatients." Working Paper. Washington, D.C.: National Institute of Mental Health, 1973.

Doerfler, L. A., and others. "Depression in Children and Adolescents: A Comparative Analysis of the Utility and Construct Validity of Two Assessment Measures." *Journal of Consulting and Clinical Psychology,* 1988, *56,* 769–772.

Dubow, E. F., and others. "Correlates of Suicidal Ideation and Attempts in a Community Sample of Junior High and High School Students." *Journal of Clinical Child Psychology,* 1989, *18,* 158–166.

Emslie, G. J., and others. "Depressive Symptoms by Self-Report in Adolescence: Phase I of the Development of a Questionnaire for Depression by Self-Report." *Journal of Child Neurology,* 1990, *5,* 114–121.

Ensel, W. M., and Lin, N. "The Life Stress Paradigm and Psychological Distress." *Journal of Health and Social Behavior,* 1991, *32,* 321–341.

Feldman, S. S., and Elliott, G. R. *At the Threshold: The Developing Adolescent.* Cambridge, Mass.: Harvard University Press, 1990.

Fleming, J. E., and Offord, D. R. "Epidemiology of Childhood Depressive Disorders: A Critical Review." *Journal of the American Academy of Child and Adolescent Psychiatry,* 1990, *29,* 571–580.

Garrison, C. Z., and others. "A Longitudinal Study of Depressive Symptomatology in Young Adolescents." *Journal of the American Academy of Child and Adolescent Psychiatry,* 1990, *29,* 581–585.

Garrison, C. Z., and others. "A Longitudinal Study of Suicidal Ideation in Young Adolescents." *Journal of the American Academy of Child and Adolescent Psychiatry,* 1991a, *30,* 597–603.

Garrison, C. Z., and others. "Suicidal Behaviors in Young Adolescents." *American Journal of Epidemiology,* 1991b, *133,* 1005–1014.

Garrison, C. Z., and others. "Major Depressive Disorder and Dysthymia in Young Adolescents." *American Journal of Epidemiology,* 1992, *135,* 792–802.

Gibbs, J. T. "Psychological Factors Associated with Depression in Urban Adolescent Females: Implications for Assessment." *Journal of Youth and Adolescence,* 1985, *14,* 47–60.

Harkavy Friedman, J.M.N., Asnis, G. M., Boeck, M., and DiFiore, J. "Prevalence of Specific Suicidal Behaviors in a High School Sample." *American Journal of Psychiatry,* 1987, *144,* 1203–1206.

Hops, H., Lewinsohn, P. M., Andrews, J. A., and Roberts, R. E. "Psychological Correlates of Depressive Symptomatology Among High School Students." *Journal of Clinical and Child Psychology,* 1990, *19,* 211–220.

Hosmer, D. W., and Lemeshow, S. *Applied Logistic Regression.* New York: Wiley, 1989.

Kandel, D. B., and Davies, M. "Epidemiology of Depressive Mood in Adolescents." *Archives of General Psychiatry,* 1982, *39,* 1205–1212.

Kaplan, G. A., Hong, G. K., and Weinhold, C. "Epidemiology of Depressive Symptomatology in Adolescents." *Journal of the American Academy of Child and Adolescent Psychiatry,* 1984, *23,* 91–98.

Kashani, J. H., Goddard, P., and Reid, J. C. "Correlates of Suicidal Ideation in a Community Sample of Children and Adolescents." *Journal of the American Academy of Child and Adolescent Psychiatry,* 1989, *28,* 912–917.

Kovacs, M. "Affective Disorders in Children and Adolescents." *American Psychologist,* 1989, *44,* 209–215.

Kovacs, M., Goldstein, D., and Gatsonis, C. "Suicidal Behaviors and Childhood-Onset Depressive Disorders: A Longitudinal Investigation." *Journal of the American Academy of Child and Adolescent Psychiatry,* 1993, *32,* 8–20.

Lester, D., and Anderson, D. "Depression and Suicidal Ideation in African-American and Hispanic American High School Students." *Psychological Reports,* 1992, *71,* 618.

Lewinsohn, P. M., Hoberman, H., Teri, L., and Hautzinger, M. "An Integrative Theory of Depression." In S. Reiss and R. Bootzin (eds.), *Theoretical Issues in Behavior Therapy.* Orlando, Fla.: Academic Press, 1985.

Lewinsohn, P. M., Rohde, P., and Seeley, J. R. "Psychosocial Characteristics of Adolescents with a History of Suicide Attempt." *Journal of the American Academy of Child and Adolescent Psychiatry,* 1993, *32,* 60–68.

Manson, S. M., and others. "Depressive Symptoms Among American Indian Adolescents: Psychometric Characteristics of the CES-D Psychological Assessment." *Journal of Consulting and Clinical Psychology,* 1990, *2,* 231–237.

Nelson, F. L. "Evaluation of a Youth Suicide Prevention Program." *Adolescence,* 1987, *22,* 813–825.

Paykel, E. *Handbook of Affective Disorders.* New York: Guilford Press, 1982.

Pfeffer, C. R., and others. "Suicidal Behavior in Normal School Children: A Comparison with Child Psychiatric Inpatients." *Journal of the American Academy of Child and Adolescent Psychiatry,* 1984, *23,* 416–423.

Phinney, J. S. "Ethnic Identity in Adolescents and Adults: Review of Research." *Psychological Bulletin,* 1990, *108,* 499–514.

Phinney, J. S. "The Multigroup Ethnic Identity Measure: A New Scale for Use with Diverse Groups." *Journal of Adolescent Research,* 1992, *7,* 156–176.

Radloff, L. S. "The CES-D Scale: A Self-Report Depression Scale for Research in the General Population." *Applied Psychological Measurement,* 1977, *1,* 385–401.

Rich, A., and Bonner, R. L. "Concurrent Validity of a Stress-Vulnerability Model of Suicidal Ideation and Behavior: A Follow-Up Study." *Suicide Life-Threatening Behavior,* 1987, *17,* 265–271.

Roberts, R. E. "Reliability of the CES-D Scale in Different Ethnic Contexts." *Psychiatry Research,* 1980, *2,* 125–134.

Roberts, R. E. "Epidemiological Issues in Measuring Preventive Effects." In R. F. Munoz (ed.), *The Prevention of Depression: Research Directions.* Washington, D.C.: Hemisphere, 1987.

Roberts, R. E. "An Exploration of Depression Among Mexican Origin and Anglo Adolescents." In R. Malgady and O. Rodriguez (eds.), *Theoretical and Conceptual Issues in Hispanic Mental Health Research.* Melbourne, Fla.: Krieger, forthcoming.

Roberts, R. E., Andrews, J. A., Lewinsohn, P. M., and Hops, H. "Assessment of Depression in Adolescents Using the Center for Epidemiologic Studies Depression Scale." *Psychological Assessment,* 1990, *2,* 122–128.

Roberts, R. E., Lewinsohn, P. M., and Seeley, J. R. "Screening for Adolescent Depression: A Comparison of the CES-D and BDI." *Journal of the American Academy of Child and Adolescent Psychiatry,* 1991, *30,* 58–66.

Roberts, R. E., Lewinsohn, P. M., and Seeley, J. R. "A Brief Measure of Loneliness Suitable for Use with Adolescents." *Psychological Reports,* 1993, *72,* 1379–1391.

Roberts, R. E., and Sobhan, M. "Symptoms of Depression in Adolescence: A Comparison of Anglo, African, and Hispanic Americans." *Journal of Youth and Adolescence,* 1992, *21,* 639–651.

Roberts, R. E., and Vernon, S. W. "Minority Status and Psychological Distress Reexamined: The Case of Mexican Americans." In J. R. Greenley (ed.), *Research in Community and Mental Health.* Greenwich, Conn.: JAI Press, 1984.

Roberts, R. E., Vernon, S. W., and Rhoades, H. M. "The Effects of Language and Ethnic Status on Reliability and Validity of the CES-D Scale with Psychiatric Patients." *Journal of Nervous and Mental Disorders,* 1989, *177,* 581–592.

Rotheram-Borus, M. J. "Adolescents' Reference-Group Choices, Self-Esteem, and Adjustment." *Journal of Personality and Social Psychology,* 1990, *59,* 1075–1081.

Russell, D., Peplau, A., and Cutrona, C. "The Revised UCLA Loneliness Scale: Concurrent and Discriminant Validity Evidence." *Journal of Personality and Social Psychology,* 1980, *39,* 471–480.

Rutter, M., Tizard, C. E., and Read, P. B. *Depression in Young People.* New York: Guilford Press, 1986.

Schoenbach, V. J., Kaplan, B. H., Grimson, R. C., and Wagner, E. H. "Use of a Symptom Scale to Study the Prevalence of a Depressive Syndrome in Young Adolescents." *American Journal of Epidemiology,* 1982, *116,* 791–800.

Simon, G. B., and Vonkorff, M. "Reevaluation of Secular Trends in Depression Rates." *American Journal of Epidemiology,* 1992, *135,* 1411–1422.

Sorenson, S. B., and Golding, J. M. "Suicide Ideation and Attempts in Hispanics and Non-Hispanic Whites: Demographic and Psychiatric Disorder Issues." *Suicide and Life-Threatening Behavior,* 1988, *18,* 205–218.

Stiffman, A. R., and Davis, L. E. *Ethnic Issues in Adolescent Mental Health.* Thousand Oaks, Calif.: Sage, 1990.

Swanson, J. W., and others. "A Binational School Survey of Depressive Symptoms, Drug Use, and Suicidal Ideation." *Journal of the American Academy of Child and Adolescent Psychiatry,* 1992, *31,* 669–678.

Teri, L. "The Use of the Beck Depression Inventory with Adolescents." *Journal of Abnormal Child Psychology,* 1982, *10,* 277–284.

Tolor, A., and Murphy, V. M. "Stress and Depression in High School Students." *Psychological Reports,* 1985, *57,* 535–541.

Trimble, J. E. "Ethnic Specification, Validation Prospects, and the Future of Drug Use Research." *International Journal of the Addictions,* 1990–1991, *25,* 149–170.

Ulbrich, P. A., Warheit, G. J., and Zimmerman, R. S. "Race, Socioeconomic Status, and Psychological Distress: An Examination of Differential Vulnerability." *Journal of Health and Social Behavior,* 1989, *30,* 131–146.

Vega, W. A., Gil, A. G., Zimmerman, R. S., and Warheit, W. J. "Risk Factors for Suicidal Behavior Among Hispanic, African American, and Non-Hispanic White Boys in Early Adolescence." *Ethnicity and Disease,* 1993, *3,* 229–241.

Velez, C. N., and Cohen, P. "Suicidal Behavior and Ideation in a Community Sample of Children: Maternal and Youth Reports." *Journal of the American Academy of Child and Adolescent Psychiatry,* 1988, *27,* 349–356.

Weinberg, W. A., and Emslie, G. J. "Depression and Suicide in Adolescents." *International Pediatrics,* 1987, *2,* 154–159.

Weiner, A. S., and Pfeffer, C. "Suicidal Status, Depression, and Intellectual Functioning in Preadolescent Psychiatry Inpatients." *Comparative Psychiatry,* 1986, *27,* 372–380.

Weissman, M. M., and others. "Assessing Depressive Symptoms in Five Psychiatric Populations: A Validation Study." *American Journal of Epidemiology,* 1977, *106,* 203–214.

Wells, V. E., Klerman, G. L., and Deykin, E. Y. "The Prevalence of Depressive Symptoms in College Students." *Social Psychiatry,* 1987, *22,* 20–28.

PART EIGHT

RURAL AND MIGRANT FARMWORKER LATINAS

CHAPTER TWENTY-TWO

Cancer-Screening Determinants Among Hispanic Women Using Migrant Health Clinics

Tracy L. Skaer
Linda M. Robison
David A. Sclar
Gary H. Harding

This chapter describes one of the few studies on cancer-preventive practices of low-income and foreign-born Latina farmworkers, predominantly from Mexico, who are among the most marginal of women in the workforce and whose social isolation makes access to primary and preventive services limited at best. The authors focus on Papanicolaou smear, mammography, and breast self-examination behaviors and identify strategies for increasing cancer-preventive practices among these women. The study examined here provides the foundation on which to build further investigations into preventive health behaviors of Latina farmworkers and to advance the development of strategies to increase their cancer screening behaviors.

Between 1987 and 1992, breast and cervical cancer screening rates among the general U.S. Hispanic population revealed an encouraging upward trend (Anderson and May, 1995). Reported use of mammography in "the past three years" among Hispanic women 50 years of age or older increased from 17.7 percent to 44.7 percent; Papanicolaou (Pap) smear use increased from 57.1 percent to 62.6 percent during this same time interval among Hispanic women 18 years of age or older (Anderson and May, 1995). In spite of these

This project was supported by Research Grant 20904 from the Robert Wood Johnson Foundation. The authors wish to acknowledge the directors and staff of the Columbia Basin Health Association, Othello, Washington; Columbia Valley Community Health Services, Wenatchee, Washington; Moses Lake Community Health Center, Moses Lake, Washington; and Yakima Valley Farm Workers Clinic at Yakima, Toppenish, and Grandview, Washington, for their assistance with data collection.

gains, Hispanic women are less likely than are African Americans or Whites to report prior breast or cervical cancer screening (Anderson and May, 1995; Vernon and others, 1992; Calle and others, 1993; Suarez, 1994). In addition, Hispanics are at greater risk for late-stage breast and cervical cancer diagnosis and mortality (McCoy and others, 1994; Richardson and others, 1987; Novello, Wise, and Kleinman, 1991; Morris and others, 1989; Whitman and others, 1991; U.S. Department of Health and Human Services, 1986; De la Rosa, 1989; Longman, Saint-Germain, and Modiano, 1992). Low screening rates may account for these differences, and differences may vary among Hispanic socio-demographic subgroups. However, subgroup differences among Hispanics have generally been ignored (Delgado and Estrada, 1993).

Beyond ethnicity, a number of factors deterring breast and cervical cancer screening are well established, including being older, less educated, having an income below the national U.S. poverty level, and residing in a rural area as compared with an urban area (Anderson and May, 1995). Other commonly reported barriers include lack of knowledge of preventive procedures (Costanza, 1994; Elnicki, Morris, and Shockcor, 1995; Yancey and Walden, 1994), language (Woloshin and others, 1995; Stein and Fox, 1990; Harlan, Bernstein, and Kessler, 1991; Marks and others, 1887; Solis and others, 1990), lack of recommendation by a health care provider (Costanza, 1994; "Screening Mammography," 1990; Fulton and others, 1991), and concern for cost of a mammogram (Vernon and others, 1992; Elnicki, Morris, and Shockcor, 1995; Bastani, Marcus, and Hollatz-Brown, 1991; Halabi and others, 1993; Harper, 1993; Kiefe and others, 1994; Lerman and others, 1990; Stein, Fox, and Murata, 1991; Weinberger and others 1991; Vogel and others, 1993). To plan effective screening interventions within specific cultural and sociodemographic subgroups, one must obtain current and accurate information regarding baseline screening rates and gain an understanding of barriers specific to the target population (Bastani and others, 1995).

Among the goals of the Public Health Service's Healthy People 2000 initiative is to increase the use of mammography among all women and to place special emphasis on Hispanic women (U.S. Public Health Service, 1990). Another objective is to increase to at least 95 percent the proportion of Hispanic women who have ever received a Pap smear and increase to at least 80 percent the proportion who have received a Pap smear within the preceding three years (U.S. Public Health Service, 1994). Criteria for establishing these goals were based on Hispanic health data generated from general population samples, which overrepresent women with more years of education, higher family income, and telephone access (Bastani, Marcus, and Hollatz-Brown, 1991; Texidor del Portillo, 1987; Espino, Burge, and Moreno, 1991; Rust, 1990). General population samples may underestimate the true magnitude of the problem and mask barriers that need to be identified for successful cancer screening intervention programs among those most difficult to reach.

This study identifies a high-risk subgroup of foreign-born Hispanic women in eastern Washington State, as evidenced by their low utilization patterns and knowledge of cancer screening. Screening determinants within this rural population are presented, along with implications for the development of interventions focused on those most in need.

METHODS

Within the state of Washington, a network of twenty-three migrant health clinics provide medical care to low-income and migrant populations. This study was conducted in six of these clinics located throughout, and representative of, rural, eastern Washington State (Grandview, Moses Lake, Othello, Toppenish, Wenatchee, and Yakima). All six of the clinics are private, nonprofit corporations with an informal interagency referral system. Clinics were selected as data collection sites to obtain a requisite sample size across age categories of interest and to overcome logistical difficulties previously encountered in survey research involving migrant and low-income populations (Aday, Chiu, and Andersen, 1980; Howard and others, 1983; Hazuda and others, 1986). Traditional survey methods such as random digit dialing and mailings remain inappropriate because of low literacy rates and because many of these individuals do not maintain telephone access.

All foreign-born Hispanic women, 20 years of age or older, with no history of breast or cervical cancer who attended any one of the six migrant health clinics were eligible to participate in the study. On the basis of a questionnaire used by the National Cancer Institute Breast Cancer Screening Consortium ("Screening Mammography," 1990; Zapka and others, 1991), a survey instrument was developed to obtain self-reported sociodemographic characteristics; frequency of health service utilization; settled-in versus seasonal residency status; and knowledge and use of Pap smear, mammography, and breast self-examination (BSE) practices. Questions regarding mammography were asked only of those women 40 years of age or older. Visual aids included hand cards to assist in ascertaining categorical responses to scaled questions.

The questionnaire was translated into Spanish, pretested, and refined to match colloquial usage within the study population. The migrant health clinics' directors and medical staff assessed the cultural appropriateness and sensitivity of the survey instrument and authorized its use.

Bilingual female medical assistants and nurses were hired from within each clinic and trained as interviewers. Specific interviewing days were established within each clinic. Women with a scheduled or walk-in appointment who fit the study criteria were approached by the interviewer and informed of the purpose of the study, after which informed consent was obtained. All interviews were conducted face-to-face with the women before their scheduled appointments. Subjects chose their preference to respond to the survey in either Spanish or English. Interviews lasted between ten and fifteen minutes. All interviews were conducted in the spring of 1994.

The study was designed to interview an equal number of women from within each of the six clinics and within four age categories: 20 to 29 years old, 30 to 39 years old, 40 to 49 years old, and 50 or more years old. Women were interviewed consecutively until all age strata were completed. Some of the clinics exceeded the minimum sample size requirements. A total of 515 women were approached for an interview; 512 (99.4 percent) provided consent and completed the interview.

Data were entered on a mainframe computer with dual entry verification. Statistical analyses were conducted using the Statistical Analysis System version 6.10. Descriptive statistics were used to characterize the study population and cancer-screening utilization patterns by age-specific categories. Odds ratios (ORs) and 95 percent confidence intervals (CIs) were generated using logistic regression to discern the influence of independent factors on Hispanic women's use or nonuse of Pap smear, BSE, and mammography. In the logistic regression models, age, number of years of formal education, number of children, and the number of years residing in the United States were treated as continuous variables. All other variables were categorized dichotomously. Marital status was collapsed as married or single, with married being defined as either married or living as married; single was defined as divorced, widowed, separated, or never married. Concern for direct expense of a mammogram was categorized as either a low concern or high concern. Low concern included such responses to a Likert-type scale as "not at all concerned" or "somewhat concerned" about cost; high concern included those responding as "quite concerned" or "extremely concerned" about cost.

A significant number of women reported having never heard of a Pap smear (14.7 percent). We therefore hypothesized that if a woman had never heard of a Pap smear, she was unlikely to have ever received a Pap smear. Therefore, logistic regression models were discerned for two cohorts of women: (1) all women in the study population and (2) only those women who reported to have heard of a Pap smear. Thirty-eight percent of women reported having never heard of a mammogram. In turn, we hypothesized that if a woman had never heard of a mammogram, she was unlikely to have ever received one. Therefore, as with Pap smear, logistic regression models were discerned for two cohorts of women: (1) all women in the study population (40 years of age and older), including those who had never heard of a mammogram and were therefore assumed to have never received one, and (2) only those women who reported to have heard of a mammogram (40 years of age and older). Thus, the construct of cost as an independent factor influencing a woman's decision to pursue mammography was evaluated solely among women who reported having heard of the procedure.

RESULTS

Characteristics of the study population are detailed in Table 22.1. Nearly all of the women were born in Mexico (96.7 percent). On average, the women had

Table 22.1. Characteristics of Hispanic Women Using Migrant Health Clinics (n = 512)

Characteristic	Number of Respondents	(Percentage)
Age in years		
20–29	151	(29.5)
30–39	142	(27.7)
40–49	111	(21.7)
50 or more	108	(21.1)
Country of birth		
Mexico	494	(96.7)
Other	17	(3.3)
Number of years lived in the		
United States		
Less than 11	50	(10.0)
1–3	110	(22.0)
4–10	171	(34.3)
More than 10	168	(33.7)
Language preference		
English	75	(14.6)
Spanish	437	(85.4)
Years of education		
None	55	(11.2)
1–6	271	(55.0)
7–11	105	(21.3)
12	44	(8.9)
More than 12	18	(3.6)
Total family income		
Less than $5,000	177	(35.5)
$5,000–15,000	245	(49.2)
More than $15,000	76	(15.3)

(Continued)

Table 22.1. Characteristics of Hispanic Women Using Migrant Health Clinics ($n = 512$) (Continued)

Characteristic	Number of Respondents	(Percentage)
Current employment status		
Full time	91	(17.8)
Part time	45	(8.8)
Work occasionally	70	(13.7)
Unemployed	127	(24.9)
Homemaker	144	(28.2)
Other	33	(6.5)
Marital status		
Married	361	(70.5)
Living as married	57	(11.1)
Divorced	24	(4.7)
Separated	29	(5.7)
Widowed	23	(4.5)
Never married	18	(3.5)
Number of children		
None	24	(4.7)
1–2	145	(28.4)
3–4	122	(23.9)
5–6	98	(19.2)
More than 6	121	(23.7)
Involved in farm labor		
Yes	343	(67.1)
No	168	(32.9)
Moved in the past two years to find work		
Yes	201	(39.6)
No	307	(60.4)
Distance to see a physician (miles)		
Less than 1	94	(18.4)
1–10	230	(45.1)
11–25	113	(22.2)
More than 25	73	(14.3)
Ever been to this health clinic before		
Yes	437	(85.7)
No	73	(14.3)
Telephone in the home		
Yes	354	(69.3)
No	157	(30.7)

lived in the United States for 9.6 years, with a range from 1 month to 61 years. Spanish was the language of preference, chosen by 85.4 percent of the women, in which to respond to the questionnaire. The mean years of education was 5.5 years; 11.2 percent of the participants had no formal education. Approximately 85 percent of the women had a total family income of $15,000 or less per year, with 35.5 percent having a family income of less than $5,000. Sixty-seven percent reported being involved in some form of farm labor.

Table 22.2 presents a summary of the knowledge of procedures and utilization patterns for Pap smear, BSE, and mammography by ten-year age-specific categories, except for the open-ended age category of 50 and older where women ranged from 50 to 81 years of age, with a mean age of 57.7 years. Overall, 14.7 percent of the study population had never heard of a Pap smear, whereas 78.1 percent reported ever having received at least one Pap smear. This compares unfavorably with 91 percent of all U.S. women and 83 percent of Hispanic women reporting ever having received a Pap smear (U.S. Public Health Service, 1994). Study participants 50 years of age or older were the least knowledgeable of Pap smears (26.2 percent had never heard of one), exhibited the lowest utilization rate (60.7 percent ever having received one), and were the least likely to have received a Pap smear within the preceding year (24.3 percent compared with 44.5 percent overall).

Only 72.6 percent of women had been taught BSE, and 62.2 percent had ever performed BSE (as compared with over three-fourths of U.S. women; Dawson and Thompson, 1987). Moreover, only 40.9 percent of women had performed BSE within the past month. Again, women 50 years of age or older were found to be the least likely to have been taught BSE (59.3 percent), the least likely to perform BSE (42.6 percent), and by far the least likely to have performed BSE within the past month (25.0 percent compared with 40.9 percent overall).

Sixty-two percent of women 40 years of age or older had ever heard of a mammogram and 38 percent had ever received a mammogram, with 21.2 percent having received one in the previous year and only 30.2 percent in the previous two years. Little difference was seen by age group (40–49 years of age; 50 or more years of age). These findings differ markedly from national studies, which document that 57.7 percent of U.S. women and 46.7 percent of Hispanic women 40 years of age or older have ever received a mammogram for routine screening (Rakowski, Rimer, and Bryant, 1993).

Results of the logistic regression analyses are reported in Table 22.3 (Pap smear), Table 22.4 (BSE), and Table 22.5 (mammography). Table 22.3 presents the Pap smear model inclusive of all women in the study, predicated on the hypothesis that if a woman had never heard of a Pap smear, she had never received a Pap smear. The ORs indicate that marital status, income, education, and number of years residing in the United States are significant independent factors influencing whether one receives a Pap smear. Married women were over

Table 22.2. Knowledge and Use of Pap Smear, Breast Self-Examination, and Mammography Among Hispanic Women Attending Migrant Health Clinics by Age-Specific Categories

Screening Procedure Use	20–29 Years		30–39 Years		40–49 Years		50 or More Years		Total	
	Number	(Percentage)	Number	(Percentage)	Number	(Percentage)	Number	(Percentage)	Number	(Percentage)
Pap smear (n = 510)										
Ever heard of	123	(82.0)	131	(92.3)	102	(91.9)	79	(73.8)	435	(85.3)
Ever received[a]	110	(73.3)	127	(89.4)	95	(87.2)	65	(60.7)	397	(78.1)
Received in past year	79	(53.0)	70	(49.3)	50	(46.3)	26	(24.3)	225	(44.5)
Breast self-examination (n = 511)										
Ever been taught	107	(70.9)	113	(79.6)	87	(79.1)	64	(59.3)	371	(72.6)
Ever performed	95	(62.9)	101	(71.1)	76	(69.1)	46	(42.6)	318	(62.2)
Performed in past month	59	(39.6)	63	(45.3)	58	(52.7)	27	(25.0)	207	(40.9)
Mammography (n = 213)										
Ever heard of	—	—	—	—	68	(63.6)	65	(61.3)	133	(62.4)
Ever received[a]	—	—	—	—	40	(37.4)	41	(38.7)	81	(38.0)
Received in past year	—	—	—	—	22	(20.6)	23	(21.9)	45	(21.2)
Received in past two years	—	—	—	—	30	(28.0)	34	(32.4)	64	(30.2)

[a]Assumes women who have never heard of procedure have never received procedure.

Table 22.3. Logistic Regression-Derived Odds Ratio (ORs) and 95 Percent Confidence Intervals (CIs) for Factors Influencing Whether a Woman Has Ever Received a Pap Smear

Variables in Model	All Women[a] N = 467[b] OR (CI)	Restricted to Women Who Have Heard of a Pap Smear[c] n = 398[d] OR (CI)
Marital status	2.54*	3.36*
0 = single	(1.34–4.80)	(1.37–8.25)
1 = married		
Total family income in past year	2.13*	1.28
0 = Less than $5,000	(1.26–3.59)	(0.56–2.91)
1 = $5,000 or more		
Number of years of education	1.13*	1.14*
	(1.03–1.23)	(1.00–1.30)
Number of years living in United States	1.07*	1.07*
	(1.03–1.11)	(1.01–1.13)
Language of preference	1.06	2.20
0 = English	(0.49–2.29)	(0.80–6.03)
1 = Spanish		
Age in years	1.00	0.99
	(0.98–1.03)	(0.96–1.03)
Moved in prior two years to find employment	0.96	0.94
0 = no	(0.58–1.59)	(0.43–2.05)
1 = yes		
Number of children	0.93	0.98
	(0.85–1.02)	(0.87–1.12)

[a]Model chi square 76.52 with 8 *df*, $p = 0.0001$.

[b]Forty-five subjects were removed from the logistic regression model because of missing data.

[c]Model chi square 29.28 with 8 *df*, $p = 0.0003$.

[d]Thirty-seven subjects were removed from the logistic regression model because of missing data.

*$p \leq 0.05$.

two and one-half times more likely (OR = 2.54, 95 percent CI = 1.34–4.80) than single women to have ever received a Pap smear. Women with family incomes of $5,000 or more were more than twice as likely (OR = 2.13, 95 percent CI = 1.26–3.59) to have received a Pap smear as women with family incomes of less than $5,000. For each additional year of education, the likelihood of receiving a Pap smear increased 13 percent (OR = 1.13, 95 percent CI = 1.03–1.23), and for each additional year of residence in the United States, the likelihood of having ever received a Pap smear increased approximately 7 percent (OR = 1.07, 95 percent CI = 1.03–1.11). Restricting the model to only women who had heard of a Pap smear yielded similar results. Again, married women were significantly more likely (OR = 3.36, 95 percent CI = 1.37–8.25) than single women to have ever received a Pap smear; for each additional year of education, the likelihood of receiving a Pap smear increased 14 percent (OR = 1.14, 95 percent CI = 1.00–1.30); and for each additional year of residence in the United States, the likelihood of having ever received a Pap smear increased approximately 7 percent (OR = 1.07, 95 percent CI = 1.01–1.13).

Table 22.4 indicates that women who had been taught how to perform BSE were over nine times more likely (OR = 9.28, 95 percent CI = 5.59–15.40) to

Table 22.4. Logistic Regression-Derived Odds Ratios and 95 Percent Confidence Intervals for Factors Influencing Whether a Woman Performs Breast Self-Examination (n = 468)

Variables in Model[a]	Odds Ratio	Confidence Interval
Ever been taught breast self-examination 0 = no 1 = yes	9.28*	(5.59–15.40)
Total family income in past year 0 = Less than $5,000 1 = $5,000 or more	2.07*	(1.26–3.41)
Marital status 0 = single 1 = married	0.66	(0.35–1.25)
Number of years of education	1.06	(0.99–1.14)
Number of years living in United States	1.00	(0.98–1.03)
Language of preference 0 = English 1 = Spanish	1.88	(0.98–3.61)
Age in years	0.98	(0.96–1.01)
Moved in prior two years to find employment 0 = no 1 = yes	0.94	(0.60–1.50)
Number of children	1.03	(0.95–1.13)

Note: Forty-four subjects were removed from the logistic regression model because of missing data.
[b]Model chi square 126.92 with 9 df, p = 0.0001.

*p ≤ 0.05.

perform the procedure than those who had not been taught and twice as likely (OR = 2.07, 95 percent CI = 1.26–3.41) if their family income was more than, or equal to, $5,000 per year.

Table 22.5 presents the mammography model inclusive of all women 40 years old or older, based on the hypothesis that if a woman had never heard of a

Table 22.5. Logistic Regression-Derived Odds Ratios (ORs) and 95 Percent Confidence Intervals (CIs) for Factors Influencing Whether a Woman Forty Years Old or Older Has Ever Received a Mammogram

Variables in Model	All Women[a] N = 188[b] OR (CI)	Restricted to Women Who Have Heard of a Mammogram[c] n = 114[d] OR (CI)
Direct expense of mammogram	—	6.73*
0 = high concern		(2.47–18.39)
1 = low concern		
Number of years living in	1.05*	1.04*
United States	(1.02–1.09)	(1.00–1.08)
Number of years of education	1.18*	1.06
	(1.06–1.30)	(0.92–1.21)
Age in years	1.06	1.04
	(0.99–1.11)	(0.98–1.11)
Marital status	1.44	2.48
0 = single	(0.64–3.21)	(0.83–7.38)
1 = married		
Total family income in past year	1.27	1.35
0 = Less than $5,000	(0.56–2.87)	(0.47–3.86)
1 = $5,000 or more		
Language of preference	1.37	1.24
0 = English	(0.54–3.45)	(0.36–4.32)
1 = Spanish		
Moved in prior two years to	0.96	1.21
find employment		
0 = no	(0.46–1.98)	(0.47–3.12)
1 = yes		

[a]Model chi square 34.14 with 7 *df, p* = 0.0001.

[b]Thirty-one subjects were removed from the logistic regression model because of missing data.

[c]Model chi square 32.45 with 8 *df, p* = 0.0001.

[d]Nineteen subjects were removed from the logistic regression model because of missing data.

*$p \leq 0.05$.

mammogram, she had never received one. The ORs indicate that years residing in the United States and education were significant independent factors influencing whether a woman obtains a mammogram. For each additional year of residence in the United States, the likelihood of having ever received a mammogram increased approximately 5 percent (OR = 1.05, 95 percent CI = 1.02–1.09). For each additional year of education, the likelihood of having ever received a mammogram increased 18 percent (OR = 1.18, 95 percent CI = 1.06–1.30).

It was hypothesized that the cost of a mammogram would represent a major deterrent to seeking this procedure because of the low family incomes reported by the study population. The issue of cost as a barrier to accessing mammography was therefore addressed solely among women who had heard of the procedure and thereby were potentially aware of the expense involved. A model restricted to women who had heard of the procedure, inclusive of the independent variable concern for direct expense of a mammogram, is presented in Table 22.5. Women who reported a "low concern" for cost were nearly seven times more likely (OR = 6.73, 95 percent CI = 2.47–18.39) to have ever received a mammogram than those reporting a "high concern" for cost. Number of years residing in the United States was a significant independent determinant for ever having received a mammogram, with each additional year of residency increasing the likelihood by 4 percent (OR = 1.04, 95 percent CI = 1.00–1.08).

DISCUSSION

Hispanics are the fastest growing minority in the United States and will become our largest minority group by the year 2000 ("Hispanic Health in the United States," 1991; Furino and Munoz, 1991). Hispanics are currently Washington State's largest minority (Cook, 1991). While the Hispanic population in the United States increased 53 percent between 1980 and 1990, Washington State experienced a 78 percent increase during the same time period (U.S. Bureau of the Census, 1983a, 1983b, 1992a, 1992b). Findings from this study depict a subgroup of Hispanic women with a low level of awareness regarding, and utilization patterns for, breast and cervical cancer screening as compared with general population samples of Hispanics. Women participating in this study were all seeking and obtaining medical care as demonstrated by their interaction with migrant health clinics. Because of this, the collected sample may not be representative of those individuals exhibiting the lowest rate of utilization for preventive health services. If this were the case, then results stemming from this inquiry would represent a conservative estimate as to the true magnitude of the problems examined and may thereby overestimate actual utilization rates.

A preliminary analysis comparing whether one had ever heard of a Pap smear by income category (less than $5,000 or $5,000 and above) revealed that two-thirds of the women who had never heard of the procedure (and thereby hypothesized as never having received a Pap smear) had family incomes below $5,000 ($p \leq 0.001$). Multivariate models inclusive of all women participating in the study documented a direct relationship between family income, marital status, educational attainment, and years of residence in the United States with receipt of a Pap smear. Socioeconomic status has been reported to be a primary determinant to accessing, and thereby benefiting from, the health care delivery system (McCoy and others, 1994; Fulton, Rakowski, and Jones, 1995; Roetzheim and others, 1993). Low educational attainment has been correlated with an under-use of cancer-screening procedures in the general U.S. population (Anderson and May, 1995; Calle and others, 1993), the general Hispanic population (Anderson and May, 1995; Breen and Kessler, 1994), as well as older Hispanic women (Fox and Roetzheim, 1994), and subgroups of the poor (Harper, 1993). We are aware of no other studies that have examined length of residency in the United States as a determinant for the use of cancer-screening procedures among foreign-born Hispanics. Length of residence may represent an indirect measure of acculturation, a factor previously reported to be a significant determinant for the use of cancer-screening procedures among Hispanics (Harlan, Bernstein, and Kessler, 1991; Solis and others, 1990; Elder and others, 1991). Fox and Roetzheim (1994) argue that to arrive at comparable screening rates across racial/ethnic groups, national programming efforts will need to focus on strategies that acculturate Hispanics by removing the barrier of information asymmetry.

Multivariate models inclusive solely of women who had heard of a Pap smear revealed a direct relationship between marital status, educational attainment, and years of residence in the United States with receipt of a Pap smear and a nonsignificant finding with regard to family income. Thus, an improvement in financial status, albeit marginal relative to national standards, correlated with a women's increased awareness as to the existence of the Pap smear, yet failed to influence receipt of the procedure. However, factors associated with learned insight and acculturation (educational attainment and years of residence in the United States) were again seen to mediate a woman's receipt of a Pap smear.

Univariate findings indicate that financial status, a primary determinant for accessing the health care delivery system, was correlated with having been taught how to perform BSE ($p \leq 0.001$), and multivariate models established that these two variables determined use of the procedure. As was the case with having received a Pap smear, women's knowledge—and thereby performance of cancer-screening procedures—was directly mediated by socioeconomic status. Given these findings and the fact that once taught how to perform BSE, women used the technique, health care professionals need to redouble efforts to ensure the provision of educational programming for BSE at every opportunity.

Among all study participants 40 years of age or older, the probability for receipt of a mammogram increased with years of residence in the United States and years of education. Restricting the inquiry to women who had heard of a mammogram (68 percent of women 40 years of age or older) revealed that there existed an increasing probability for receipt of the procedure with years of residence in the United States and a low level of concern relative to direct expense. Cost has been extensively documented as a barrier to screening mammography, especially among rural and low-income women (Vernon and others, 1992; Harper, 1993; Kiefe and others, 1994; Stein, Fox, and Murata, 1991). However, until now, empirical evidence as to the magnitude of the effect on utilization has been limited (Urban, Anderson, and Peacock, 1994). Health insurance programs that partially subsidize screening mammography, such as Medicare, have not been successful in increasing the rate of utilization among low-income beneficiaries (Kiefe and others, 1994). Complete subsidization for screening mammography among low-income women may represent a cost-effective approach for the allocation of financial resources given the utilization of health care services, and thus expenditures, involved in late-stage diagnosis and treatment of breast cancer (Zavertnik, 1993; Skaer and others, 1996). Finally, there exists an extensive body of literature as to the positive influence of a physician's recommendation on receipt of screening mammography. In this study, the vast majority of women (101/131 = 77.1 percent) who had heard of a mammogram had been advised by a physician to obtain the procedure. Of the women who reported receipt of a mammogram, all but one indicated they had been advised to do so by a physician (78/79 = 98.7 percent). Because of this finding, it was not permissible to incorporate a dichotomous variable examining the influence of physician recommendation to obtain a screening mammogram into our multivariate models. The effect of physician recommendation in concert with length of residence in the United States and degree of concern regarding direct expense for mammography on women's use of the procedure requires further investigation.

Determinants identified in this study may serve as the basis for the development of tailored cancer-screening interventions among Hispanic migrants to the United States. Programming efforts must aspire to engender an understanding of the importance of performing BSE and that receipt of a Pap smear or mammogram must occur at recommended intervals (Morrison, 1985). Therefore, it is recommended that educational efforts use elements of both "outreach" and "inreach" strategies (Fulton and others, 1991). Community-based outreach efforts should strive to identify and empower those individuals exhibiting the lowest utilization patterns for cancer-screening procedures. Our findings indicate there exists an inverse relationship between a woman's age and receipt of a Pap smear or the performance of BSE, and the rate of mammography screening among women 40 years of age or older remains significantly lower than that found in general population samples of Hispanics. These data may imply that once the childbearing years have ended, many of the women within the study population do not undertake preventive health care measures or access health care services only when it is deemed medically necessary.

Outreach efforts will enhance the number of at-risk women initiating cancer-screening procedures; inreach is essential if women are to remain in compliance with recommended schedules for BSE, Pap smears, and mammograms. The migrant health clinics participating in this study appear to be ideal settings for inreach intervention, as results indicate they have successfully negated a primary barrier to cancer screening as cited in previous research: language (Woloshin and others, 1995). Studies have routinely found English-speaking Hispanics to be far more likely to have received preventive health care services (Stein and Fox, 1990; Harlan, Bernstein, and Kessler, 1991; Marks and others, 1987; "Screening Mammography," 1990; Fox and Stein, 1991; Johnson and Meischke, 1994). Although 85 percent of women in this study chose Spanish as their language of preference, multivariate findings indicate that language was not a deterrent to performing BSE or to receipt of either a Pap smear or a mammogram. All of the migrant health clinics participating in this study employed bilingual health care professionals and translators and thereby appear to have mitigated the effect of language as a barrier to the performance or receipt of cancer-screening procedures. Sensitivity to cultural beliefs and language proficiency is essential if programming efforts are to achieve their stated objectives.

CONCLUSION

Given the projected growth of the Hispanic population, breast and cervical cancer mortality rates will remain high, and actual numbers of deaths per year from these cancers will increase unless barriers for those most at risk for underusing screening procedures are further identified and culturally sensitive interventions are implemented.

References

Aday, L. A., Chiu, G. Y., and Andersen, R. "Methodologic Issues in Health Care Surveys of the Spanish Heritage Population." *American Journal of Public Health,* 1980, *70*(4), 367–374.

Anderson, L. M., and May, D. S. "Has the Use of Cervical, Breast, and Colorectal Cancer Screening Increased in the United States?" *American Journal of Public Health,* 1995, *85*(6), 840–842.

Bastani, R., Marcus, A. C., and Hollatz-Brown, A. "Screening Mammography Rates and Barriers to Use: A Los Angeles County Survey." *Preventive Medicine,* 1991, *20*(3), 350–363.

Bastani, R., and others. "Initial and Repeat Mammography Screening in a Low-Income Multi-Ethnic Population in Los Angeles." *Cancer Epidemiology Biomarkers and Prevention,* 1995, *4*(2), 161–167.

Breen, N., and Kessler, L. "Changes in the Use of Screening Mammography: Evidence from the 1987 and 1990 National Health Interview Surveys." *American Journal of Public Health,* 1994, *84*(1), 62–67.

Calle, E. E., and others. "Demographic Predictors of Mammography and Pap Smear Screening in U.S. Women." *American Journal of Public Health,* 1993, *83*(1), 53–60.

Cook, A. K. Increasing Racial and Ethnic Diversity in Washington." *Washington Counts,* 1991, *2,* 1–13.

Costanza, M. E. "The Extent of Breast Cancer Screening in Older Women." *Cancer,* 1994, *74*(7 Suppl.), 2046–2050.

Dawson, D. A., and Thompson, G. B. *Breast Cancer Risk Factors and Screening: United States, 1987.* Bethesda, Md.: National Center for Health Statistics, 1987.

De la Rosa, M. "Health Care Needs of Hispanic Americans and the Responsiveness of the Health Care System." *Health Social Work,* 1989, *14*(2), 104–113.

Delgado, J. L., and Estrada, L. "Improving Data Collection Strategies." *Public Health Reports,* 1993, *108*(5), 540–545.

Elder, J. P., and others. "Differences in Cancer-Risk-Related Behaviors in Latino and Anglo Adults." *Preventive Medicine,* 1991, *20*(6), 751–763.

Elnicki, D. M., Morris, D. K., and Shockcor, W. T. "Patient-Perceived Barriers to Preventive Health Care Among Indigent, Rural Appalachian Patients." *Archives of Internal Medicine,* 1995, *155*(4), 421–424.

Espino, D. V., Burge, S. K., and Moreno, C. A. "The Prevalence of Selected Chronic Diseases Among the Mexican-American Elderly: Data from the 1982–1984 Hispanic Health and Nutrition Examination Survey." *Journal of the American Board of Family Practice,* 1991, *4*(4), 217–222.

Fox, S. A., and Roetzheim, R. G. "Screening Mammography and Older Hispanic Women: Current Status and Issues." *Cancer,* 1994, *74*(7 Suppl.), 2028–2033.

Fox, S. A., and Stein, J. A. "The Effect of Physician-Patient Communication on Mammography Utilization by Different Ethnic Groups." *Medical Care,* 1991, *29*(11), 1065–1082.

Fulton, J. P., Rakowski, W., and Jones, A. C. "Determinants of Breast Cancer Screening Among Inner-City Hispanic Women in Comparison with Other Inner-City Women." *Public Health Reports,* 1995, *110*(4), 476–482.

Fulton, J. P., and others. "A Study Guided by the Health Belief Model of the Predictors of Breast Cancer Screening of Women Ages 40 and Older." *Public Health Reports,* 1991, *106*(4), 410–420.

Furino, A., and Munoz, E. "Health Status Among Hispanics: Major Themes and New Priorities." *JAMA,* 1991, *265*(2), 255–257.

Halabi, S., and others. "Recruiting Older Women for Screening Mammography." *Cancer Detection and Prevention*, 1993, *17*(3), 359–365.

Harlan, L. C., Bernstein, A. B., and Kessler, L. G. "Cervical Cancer Screening: Who Is Not Screened and Why?" *American Journal of Public Health*, 1991, *81*(7), 885–890.

Harper, A. P. "Mammography Utilization in the Poor and Medically Underserved." *Cancer*, 1993, *72*(4 Suppl.), 1478–1482.

Hazuda, H. P, and others. "A Comparison of Three Indicators for Identifying Mexican Americans in Epidemiologic Research: Methodological Findings from the San Antonio Heart Study." *American Journal of Epidemiology*, 1986, *123*(1), 96–112.

"Hispanic Health in the United States: Council of Scientific Affairs." *JAMA*, 1991, *265*(2), 248–252.

Howard, C. A., and others. "Survey Research in New Mexico Hispanics: Some Methodological Issues." *American Journal of Epidemiology*, 1983, *117*(1), 27–34.

Johnson, J. D., and Meischke, H. "Factors Associated with Adoption of Mammography Screening: Results of a Cross-Sectional and Longitudinal Study." *American Women's Health*, 1994, *3*(2), 97–105.

Kiefe, C. I., and others. "Is Cost a Barrier to Screening Mammography for Low-Income Women Receiving Medicare Benefits? A Randomized Trial." *Archives of Internal Medicine*, 1994, *154*(11) 1217–1224.

Lerman, C., and others. "Factors Associated with Repeat Adherence to Breast Cancer Screening." *Preventive Medicine*, 1990, *19*(3), 279–290.

Longman, A. J., Saint-Germain, M. A., and Modiano, M. "Use of Breast Cancer Screening by Older Hispanic Women." *Public Health Nursing*, 1992, *9*(2), 118–124.

Marks, G., and others. "Health Behavior of Elderly Hispanic Women: Does Cultural Assimilation Make a Difference?" *American Journal of Public Health*, 1987, *77*(10), 1315–1319.

McCoy, C. B., and others. "Increasing the Cancer Screening of the Medically Underserved in South Florida." *Cancer*, 1991, *67*(6 Suppl.), 1808–1913.

McCoy, C. B., and others. "Breast Cancer Screening of the Medically Underserved: Results and Implications." *Cancer Practice*, 1994, *2*(4), 267–274.

Morris, D. L., and others. "Cervical Cancer, a Major Killer of Hispanic Women: Implications for Health Education." *Health Education*, 1989, *20*(5), 23–28.

Morrison, A. S. *Screening in Chronic Disease.* New York: Oxford University Press, 1985.

Novello, A. C., Wise, P. H., and Kleinman, D. V. "Hispanic Health: Time for Data, Time for Action." *JAMA*, 1991, *265*(2), 253–255.

Rakowski, W., Rimer, B. K., and Bryant, S. A. "Integrating Behavior and Intention Regarding Mammography by Respondents in the 1990 National Health Interview Survey of Health Promotion and Disease Prevention." *Public Health Reports*, 1993, *108*(5), 605–624.

Richardson, J. L., and others. "Frequency and Adequacy of Breast Cancer Screening Among Elderly Hispanic Women." *Preventive Medicine*, 1987, *16*(6), 761–774.

Roetzheim, R. G., and others. "Barriers to Screening Among Participants of a Media-Promoted Breast Cancer Screening Project." *Cancer Detection and Prevention*, 1993, *17*(3), 367–377.

Rust, G. S. "Health Status of Migrant Farmworkers: A Literature Review and Commentary." *American Journal of Public Health*, 1990, *80*(10), 1213–1217.

"Screening Mammography: A Missed Clinical Opportunity? Results of the NCI Breast Cancer Screening Consortium and National Health Interview Survey Studies." *JAMA*, 1990, *264*(1) 54–58.

Skaer, T. L., and others. "Financial Incentive and the Use of Mammography Among Hispanic Migrants to the U.S." *Health Care for Women International*, 1996, *17*(4), 281–291.

Solis, J. M., and others. "Acculturation, Access to Care, and Use of Preventive Services by Hispanics: Findings from HHANES 1982–84." *American Journal of Public Health*, 1990, *80*(Suppl.), 11–19.

Stein, J. A., and Fox, S. A. "Language Preference as an Indicator of Mammography Use Among Hispanic Women." *American National Cancer Institute*, 1990, 7, *82*(21), 1715–1716.

Stein, J. A., Fox, S. A., and Murata, P. J. "The Influence of Ethnicity, Socioeconomic Status, and Psychological Barriers on Use of Mammography." *Journal of Health and Social Behavior*, 1991, *32*(2), 101–113.

Suarez, L. "Pap Smear and Mammogram Screening in Mexican-American Women: The Effects of Acculturation." *American Journal of Public Health*, 1994, *84*(5), 742–746.

Texidor del Portillo, C. "Poverty, Self-Concept, and Health: Experience of Latinas." *Women Health*, 1987, *12*(3–4), 229–242.

U.S. Bureau of the Census. *1980 Census of Population, General Social and Economic Characteristics, Part 1; United States Summary.* Washington, D.C.: U.S. Government Printing Office, 1983a.

U.S. Bureau of the Census. *1980 Census of Population, General Social and Economic Characteristics, Part 49; Washington Summary.* Washington, D.C.: U.S. Government Printing Office, 1983b.

U.S. Bureau of the Census. *1990 Census of Population, General Population Characteristics. Washington.* Washington, D.C.: U.S. Government Printing Office, 1992a.

U.S. Bureau of the Census. *1990 Census of Population, General Population Characteristics. United States.* Washington, D.C.: U.S. Government Printing Office, 1992b.

U.S. Department of Health and Human Services. *Cancer Among Blacks and Other Minorities: A Statistical Profile.* Bethesda, Md.: National Institutes of Health, 1986.

U.S. Public Health Service. Healthy People 2000: *National Health Promotion and Disease Prevention Objectives.* Washington, D.C.: U.S. Government Printing Office, 1990.

U.S. Public Health Service. *Healthy People 2000 Review, 1993.* Washington, D.C.: U.S. Government Printing Office, 1994.

Urban, N., Anderson, G. L., and Peacock, S. "Mammography Screening: How Important Is Cost as a Barrier to Use?" *American Journal of Public Health,* 1994, *84*(1), 50–55.

Vernon, S. W., and others. "Breast Cancer Screening Behaviors and Attitudes in Three Racial/Ethnic Groups." *Cancer,* 1992, *69*(1), 165–174.

Vogel, V. G., and others. "The Texas Breast Screening Project: Part II. Demographics, Risk Profiles, and Health Practices of Participants." *Southern Medical Journal,* 1993, *86*(4), 391–396.

Weinberger, M., and others. "Breast Cancer Screening in Older Women: Practices and Barriers Reported by Primary Care Physicians." *Journal of the American Geriatric Society,* 1991, *39*(1), 22–29.

Whitman, S., and others. "Patterns of Breast and Cervical Cancer Screening at Three Public Health Centers in an Inner-City Urban Area." *American Journal of Public Health,* 1991, *81*(12), 1651–1653.

Woloshin, S., and others. "Language Barriers in Medicine in the United States." *JAMA,* 1995, *273*(9), 724–728.

Yancey, A. K., and Walden, L. "Stimulating Cancer Screening Among Latinas and African-American Women: A Community Case Study." *Journal of Cancer Education,* 1994, *9*(1), 46–52.

Zapka, J. G., and others. "Interval Adherence to Mammography Screening Guidelines." *Medical Care,* 1991, *29*(8), 697–707.

Zavertnik, J. J. "Strategies for Reaching Poor Blacks and Hispanics in Dade County, Florida." *Cancer,* 1993, *72*(3 Suppl.), 1088–1092.

CHAPTER TWENTY-THREE

Lifetime Prevalence of and Risk Factors for Psychiatric Disorders Among Mexican Migrant Farmworkers in California

Ethel Alderete
William A. Vega
Bohdan Kolody
Sergio Aguilar-Gaxiola

The findings reported in this chapter represent the first comparative study of mental health among Latino men and women (of Mexican descent) migrant farmworkers. In addition, the authors establish the impact of acculturation on the mental health of their cohort. Among Latinas, migrant farmworkers are among the most underdocumented in the literature but also among those with the greatest needs. This study makes an important contribution to the literature in that it is the first to provide prevalence rates of twelve major lifetime psychiatric diagnoses as defined in the Diagnostic and Statistical Manual of Mental Disorders, *Third Edition, Revised (DSM-III-R).*

Migrant farmworkers constitute almost half (42 percent) of the population employed in seasonal agricultural work in the United States (Gabbard, Mines, and Boccalandro, 1994; Vincent, 1996). The majority of farmworkers (70 percent) are foreign born, and of those, 90 percent are Mexican. In California, about half of the estimated 1 million farmworkers are migrants, and

E. Alderete planned the study and analyzed the data. W. A. Vega assisted in the conceptualization of the study and the writing and editing of the chapter. B. Kolody supervised the statistical analyses, and S. Aguilar-Gaxiola provided assistance in constructing and estimating psychiatric diagnoses.

This study was supported by grant MH51192 from the National Institute of Mental Health.

The views expressed in this chapter are solely those of the authors and do not necessarily represent the views of the funding agency or of the University of California, Berkeley, where the research was conducted.

as many as 98 percent are Mexican (Vincent, 1996). From Texas, Florida, and California, farmworkers follow well-established migration routes through the eastern, central, and western agricultural states. According to the National Agricultural Workers Survey (Mines, Gabbard, and Steirman, 1997), the farmworker population in the United States is predominantly (80 percent) male and young (two-thirds are younger than 35 years). However, most farmworkers are married and have children. They are also poor, with a median personal income between $2,500 and $5,000, but despite these meager earnings few use publicly assisted social services.

In recent years, an increasingly diverse farm labor pool has come to California from Latin America and Asia (Gabbard, Mines, and Boccalandro, 1993). Among these are indigenous people, such as the Hmong from Southeast Asia, the Mixtec and Zapotec from Mexico, and the Maya from Guatemala. Here we report our findings about the mental health status of migrant workers from Mexico, both Indian and non-Indian, working in California agriculture. This is the first study to provide prevalence rates of twelve major lifetime psychiatric diagnoses as defined in the *Diagnostic and Statistical Manual of Mental Disorders, Third Edition, Revised* (DSM-III-R; 1987), for U.S. migrant farmworkers by sex and ethnic group.

THE MENTAL HEALTH OF MIGRANT FARMWORKERS IN THE UNITED STATES

Few studies have been conducted on the mental health of migrant farmworkers in the United States. Vega, Warheit, and Palacio (1985) used the Health Opinion Survey (MacMillan, 1957) to assess the mental health status of farmworkers in Fresno County, California. The rate of "caseness," defined as a presumptive need for treatment, was 20 percent. Studies have also been conducted in New York State, where an estimated 30,000 to 40,000 farmworkers are seasonally employed. Chi (1986) surveyed 218 Black migrant farmworkers, using the index of general well-being, and found that subjective well-being was associated with lifestyle, social support, housing conditions, age, sex, and education. Also in New York State, White-Means (1991) found a significant positive association between mental health and weekly wages.

Three studies have presented data on substance use among migrant farmworkers in the eastern United States. Watson and others (1985) interviewed African American and Haitian workers in labor camps in New York State. Approximately one-fourth of these workers consumed alcohol frequently and in large quantities; about 22 percent reported consuming five or more drinks at a single sitting. Social isolation was considered the main risk factor related to alcohol consumption (Watson and others, 1985). In another multiethnic study conducted in

New York State, binge drinking (drinking more than a six-pack at one sitting) was reported by 25 percent of the workers (Chi and McClain, 1992). Those who were married and had family members present in the camp were less likely to be regular drinkers. Lafferty, Foulk, and Ryan (1990–1991) reported that 2.6 percent of a sample of 378 Hispanic farmworkers self-injected recreational drugs.

THE MENTAL HEALTH OF MIGRANT WORKERS IN EUROPE

Another pertinent set of literature consists of research on the mental health of migrant or "guest workers" in Europe. Friessem (1975) found Turks in Germany to be more affected than the local population by neurosis, personality disorders, psychosomatic disturbances, and abnormal reactions. Increased depressive symptomatology has been reported in the Netherlands among Yugoslav (Dosen, 1983) and Moroccan workers (Van der Meer, 1984). Simoes and Binder (1980) found that migrant Portuguese workers did not differ significantly in their mental health status from the local Swiss population. Furthermore, such workers fared better in terms of mental health status than the general population of Portugal (Simoes and Binder, 1980). Migrant laborers in Western Europe also had lower rates of mental illness than did the general population (Ramon, Shanin, and Strimpel, 1977).

The epidemiologic evidence points to the complexity and multiplicity of factors that affect migrant workers' living conditions and social environment (Vega, Warheit, and Palacio, 1985; Fabrega, 1969; Portes and Rumbaut, 1990). Migrant farm laborers endure difficult working conditions, low pay, and precarious living situations. On the other hand, psychiatric morbidity rates in their countries of origin may be lower than the prevalence rates in the host society. Thus, it is possible that migrant farmworkers do have better mental health status than the general population, owing to the presence of protective factors inherent in the sending society and its culture.

METHODS

Research Site

The research site, Fresno County, has an area of approximately six thousand square miles. Despite the fact that it contains the cities of Fresno and contiguous Clovis, it is primarily a low-density agricultural region with scattered hamlets, small towns, and expanses of unincorporated land devoted to agricultural production. According to a 1996 estimate, the population of the county is 748,686, with 463,600 living in the Fresno–Clovis metropolitan area. Hispanics, almost all of whom are of Mexican origin, constitute 38.3 percent (286,747) of the total county population (*Vision 20/20,* 1996). Thirty percent of Mexican-origin families living in Fresno are considered to be living in poverty, and much higher levels of poverty are found among farmworkers.

Sampling

The Mexican American Prevalence and Services Survey (MAPSS) included resident and migrant samples of the Mexican-origin population in Fresno County, California. Methods of sampling residents have been described in detail elsewhere (Vega and others, 1998). The 3,012 resident participants were selected under a fully probabilistic, stratified, multistage cluster sampling design. The two hundred primary sampling units in each stratum were census blocks or block aggregates selected with a probability proportionate to the size of their Hispanic population. In the second sampling stage, a quota of five households was randomly selected in each primary sampling unit. In the final stage, one person per household was randomly selected. Enumerators generated a full numbered list of eligible persons in order of age within each household. Random digits attached to the enumeration form dictated which person on the list would become the study subject. The refusal and nonresponse rate for the resident sample was 10 percent.

The migrant sampling strategy was designed to maximize representativeness. The high mobility and seasonal migration of farmworkers make it impossible to accurately estimate the size of the entire population or to draw a true probability sample. To a large extent, farmworkers do not dwell in conventional housing during their stay in the county. Living arrangements include farm labor camps, trailers, and outbuildings. Inasmuch as no list of migrant workers exists, an area cluster sampling procedure was devised to ensure geographic representation.

The county was divided into map grids that formed the clusters or primary sampling units. Within the selected grids, locations occupied by migrants were exhaustively enumerated. Individuals aged 18 to 59 years were systematically sampled from these grids, in proportion to the estimated subpopulation of migrants in that cluster. When immediate relatives were found in a housing unit, only one was randomly selected. Since the survey instrument was available only in English and Spanish, our sample did not include the less acculturated Indians who spoke only their native language. The refusal and noncompletion rate was 4.7 percent. A total of 500 men and 501 women were interviewed. The data were collected in 1996.

Instrumentation

In this study, psychiatric diagnoses were based on a modified version of the Composite International Diagnostic Interview (CIDI; Robins and others, 1988). The CIDI is a fully structured clinical interview developed jointly by the World Health

Organization (WHO) and the former U.S. Alcohol, Drug Abuse, and Mental Health Administration as the instrument of choice for large-scale international psychiatric epidemiologic research. The CIDI has undergone comprehensive field trials with both clinical (Wittchen, 1994) and general population samples, including clinical reappraisal using the Structural Clinical Interview for DSM-III-R (SCID) semistructured interviews. Positive predictive values between the CIDI and the SCID were 0.60, based on a sample of clinical respondents, and 0.65, based on the National Comorbidity Survey results (Kessler and others, 1994, 1998).

While it is certainly true that all diagnostic field instruments have important limitations, the results of these methodological studies show good performance for the University of Michigan (UM) CIDI, the instrument used in the National Cormorbidity Study, which was used as the template for caseness criteria in the Fresno survey. The primary difference between the UM-CIDI and other CIDI versions is that the UM-CIDI uses techniques to increase the likelihood that respondents understand the intent of the key questions about age at onset and to vastly improve respondents' ability to provide accurate information about distant and possibly painful life events. For example, key screening questions for disorders are placed at the beginning of the interview to avoid respondents' "learning the instrument" or having memory problems owing to mental fatigue. We believe these key differences in memory prompts found in the UM-CIDI are especially useful for low-income respondents such as those found in the Fresno survey (Wittchen and others, 1984).

The questionnaire is available in English and Spanish and was specifically adapted for use with respondents of Mexican origin. It incorporates culturally and linguistically sensitive elements and includes probes for respondent's idiomatic expressions of psychological distress. Translation into Spanish was accomplished by the translation and back-translation method. A panel of bilingual experts conducted an item-by-item review of the translation, paying special attention to cultural and linguistic adaptations appropriate for use with Mexican-origin populations. A computer-assisted personal interview version was developed for instrument administration. The average face-to-face administration time for this version was eighty-six minutes for respondents without extensive psychiatric histories. Respondents who met case criteria for multiple psychiatric disorders took two hours or longer to complete the interview.

The modified CIDI used in this study provides lifetime, twelve-month, six-month, and one-month prevalence estimates for fourteen specific DSM-III-R diagnoses: mood disorders (major depressive episode, manic episode, dysthymia); anxiety disorders (panic disorder, agoraphobia, social phobia, simple phobia); substance use disorders (alcohol abuse, alcohol dependence, drug abuse, drug dependence); nonaffective psychosis; somatization disorder; and antisocial personality disorder. Rates of nonaffective psychosis and somatization disorder are not reported here. Diagnoses from the modified CIDI are generated by algorithms based on the diagnostic criteria of DSM-III-R and the *International Classification of Diseases, 10th Revision,* and the WHO-CIDI's version 1.1 format ("Mental Health and Behavioral Disorders," 1991).

The questionnaire includes questions on sociodemographics, employment, migration history, gender roles and family dynamics, instrumental and emotional social support, acculturation and acculturation stress, self-rated physical and mental health status, and physical health problems. Indian respondents were identified by asking whether they themselves, their parents, or their grandparents could speak a native language (for example, Mixtec, Zapotec, Nahuatl).

The seven-item acculturation measure was adapted from the scale by Cuellar, Harris, and Jasso (1980) and had been validated and used with Latinos in a previous study (Vega and others, 1993). Acculturation is characterized as a transition from patterns of behaviors of the culture of origin to those of the host cultural environment (Berry and Annis, 1988; Szapocznik, Scopetta, and Kurtines, 1978; Padilla, 1980). Self-identification, country of birth and generational status, ethnicity of acquaintances, and specific ethnic practices are other elements usually included in acculturation scales (Cuellar, Harris, and Jasso, 1980). However, for Mexican Americans, language use in diverse social contexts explains most of the variance in these scales (Cobas and others, 1996; Vega and Gil, 1998). The unidimensional seven-item scale used in this survey measures use of Spanish or a native language versus English in different social contexts (for example, work, home, with friends). Each item has a range of five responses that indicate, in a Likert format, a preference for using Spanish or a native language versus English. Therefore, a grand mean score of 1 indicates minimal acculturation and a score of 5 indicates very high acculturation. Acculturation categories were defined by the distribution of the data as low (1.000–1.001), medium (1.002–1.430), and high (1.431–5.000). The Cronbach alpha was 0.83.

Data Analysis

SAS version 6.11 was used for data analysis. The distribution of demographic and acculturation variables, as well as the prevalence of DSM-III-R lifetime mood, anxiety, and antisocial personality disorders and substance abuse/dependence, was calculated across ethnic groups and sexes. Chi-square tests were also calculated. Prevalence rates and standard errors were adjusted to the age–sex distribution of the total migrant sample. The five-year intervals employed by the U.S. Census Bureau were used for age adjustment. Logistic regression models were used to test the adjusted effects of demographic and acculturation variables on outcomes of interest. The diagnostic categories were (1) lifetime affective disorders, (2) anxiety disorders, (3) alcohol abuse or dependence, and (4) drug abuse or dependence. Sex, age, ethnicity (Indian versus non-Indian), marital status, income, education, main country of residence (Mexico or the United States), and acculturation were included as categorical covariates.

Prevalence rates in the migrant sample were compared with those in the MAPSS resident sample and with those in two large field surveys that used the CIDI for ascertainment of DSM-III-R disorders: the National Comorbidity Survey, which represents U.S. national rates, and a field survey conducted in Mexico City by researchers from the Mexican Institute of Psychiatry. In the MAPSS sample, length of time in the United States was examined by means of a trichotomous variable: less than thirteen years' residence (the median) in the United States, thirteen or more years' residence in the United States, and birth in the United States. Because these three studies examined different age ranges, for comparison purposes, the age range was restricted to 18 through 54 years. Further, because the age distributions differ among the four studies, survey data were adjusted to the age–sex distribution of the National Comorbidity Survey (Vega and others, 1998).

RESULTS

Comparative Demographic Characteristics

In our sample of migrant workers, women were more likely than men to be married and to be U.S. residents. More women than men reported having an annual family income of more than US $9,000 and having more than 6 years of education (Table 23.1).

Indian respondents constituted 11 percent of the sample. Indians in the sample were younger than non-Indians, and more Indians than non-Indians reported having an annual family income of less than $9,000. The mean annual family income for Indians ($7,821) fell below the 1996 federal poverty level of $7,740 for a one-person household, and 83 percent of Indian respondents had annual family incomes below the poverty level for a two-person household ($10,360) (Table 23.1). On the other hand, the mean income for non-Indians ($11,529) was above these poverty levels. The acculturation scale distribution was skewed, with a mean of 1.4. Acculturation levels did not differ significantly between men and women. However, the majority (54 percent) of Indians had a medium to high preference for English over Spanish or their native language, compared with only 28 percent of the non-Indian respondents.

Prevalence of DSM-III-R Psychiatric Disorders

In this sample, the lifetime rate of any psychiatric disorder was lower for women (16.3 percent) than for men (27.6 percent). Rates of alcohol dependence were nine times higher among men than among women, and rates of drug dependence were five times higher (Table 23.2). Migrant men and women had similar rates of mood disorders (men = 7.2 percent; women = 6.7 percent) and anxiety disorders (men = 15.1 percent, women = 12.9 percent). The most prevalent

Table 23.1. Demographic and Acculturation Characteristics, by Ethnicity and Sex: Migrant Farmworkers from Mexico in Fresno County, California, 1996 (in percent)

	Non-Indians			Indians			Total		
	Men (n = 426)	Women (n = 468)	Total (n = 894)	Men (n = 74)	Women (n = 33)	Total (n = 107)	Men (n = 500)	Women (n = 501)	Total (n = 1001)
Age (years)									
18–25	34.0	29.9	31.9	36.5	31.3	34.6	34.4	29.9	32.2
26–39	44.0	45.6	44.9	44.6	56.3	45.8	44.0	45.7	44.9
40–59	22.0	24.5	23.3	18.9	12.5	19.6	21.6	24.4	23.0
Marital status									
Not married	31.5	14.9	22.8	29.7	21.2	25.2	31.2	15.4	23.3[b]
Married	61.3	75.1	68.4	56.8	75.8	63.6	60.8	75.0	67.9
Widowed/divorced	7.3	10.0	8.7	13.5	3.0	11.2	8.0	9.6	8.8
Income									
$9,000 or below	69.7	56.5	62.8	87.8	72.7	83.2[a]	72.0	57.3	64.7[b]
More than $9,000	30.3	43.5	37.2	12.2	27.3	16.8	28.0	42.7	35.3
Education (years)									
0–6	66.9	56.3	61.4	63.5	65.6	64.5	61.3	57.0	60.3[b]
More than 6	33.1	43.7	38.6	36.5	34.4	35.5	38.7	43.0	39.7
Country of residence									
Mexico	59.4	31.8	45.5	53.4	30.0	47.6	58.7	32.2	45.9[b]
United States	40.6	68.2	54.5	46.6	60.0	52.4	41.3	67.8	54.1
Acculturation									
Low	73.2	71.8	72.5	48.6	42.4	46.2[a]	69.2	70.1	69.6
Medium	25.6	22.6	24.0	25.7	30.3	25.5	25.6	22.8	24.2
High	1.2	5.6	3.5	25.7	27.3	28.3	5.2	7.2	6.2

[a]Chi-square test comparing male versus female, $p < .05$.

[b]Chi-square test comparing non-Indian versus Indian, $p < .05$.

Table 23.2. Lifetime Prevalence of Psychiatric Disorders, by Ethnicity and Sex: Migrant Farmworkers from Mexico in Fresno County, California, 1996

	Non-Indians			Indians			Total		
	Men (n = 426)	Women (n = 468)	Total (n = 894)	Men (n = 74)	Women (n = 33)	Total (n = 107)	Men (n = 500)	Women (n = 501)	Total (n = 1001)
Major depressive episode	0.2 (0.7)	4.9 (0.9)	3.6 (0.6)	0.4 (0.2)	0.8 (4.9)	6.2 (2.6)	3.3 (1.4)	5.1 (1.0)	3.8 (0.6)
Manic episode	0.5 (0.3)	0.2 (0.2)	0.3 (0.2)	1.5 (1.5)	0.0	1.3 (1.3)	0.8 (0.7)	0.2 (0.2)	0.4 (0.2)
Dysthymia	1.7 (0.6)	2.1 (0.7)	1.9 (0.5)	3.5 (2.6)	0.0	2.1 (1.6)	3.1 (1.4)	2.0 (0.6)	1.9 (0.4)
Any mood disorder	4.3 (1.0)	6.6 (1.1)	5.5 (0.8)	7.4 (3.4)	8.4 (4.9)	8.3 (3.0)	7.2 (2.0)	6.7 (1.1)	5.7 (0.7)
Panic disorder	1.2 (0.5)	0.8 (0.4)	1.0 (0.3)	0.0	0.0	0.0	0.3 (0.1)	0.8 (0.4)	0.9 (0.3)
Agoraphobia without panic disorder	4.0 (1.0)	7.5 (1.2)	5.8 (0.8)	7.7 (3.0)	0.0	5.3 (2.2)	5.9 (1.8)	6.9 (1.1)	5.8 (0.7)
Social phobia	5.9 (1.1)	5.5 (1.1)	5.7 (0.8)	6.7 (3.1)	4.9 (3.6)	5.7 (2.2)	8.2 (2.1)	5.6 (1.0)	5.8 (0.7)
Simple phobia	6.0 (1.2)	6.4 (1.1)	6.2 (0.8)	6.2 (2.7)	6.3 (4.4)	6.2 (2.3)	8.2 (2.1)	6.4 (1.1)	6.2 (0.7)
Any anxiety disorder	11.4 (1.6)	13.0 (1.6)	12.3 (1.1)	16.1 (4.4)	11.1 (5.6)	14.0 (3.4)	15.1 (2.7)	12.9 (1.5)	12.5 (1.1)

Alcohol abuse	1.8	0.4	1.1	0.0	0.0	0.0	0.5	0.4	1.0
	(0.6)	(0.3)	(0.3)				(1.2)	(0.3)	(0.3)
Alcohol dependence	12.2	0.9	6.2	12.9	1.7	9.9	8.9	1.0	6.6
	(1.6)	(0.4)	(0.8)	(4.2)	(1.7)	(3.2)	(2.0)	(0.5)	(0.8)
Drug abuse	0.7	0.2	0.4	1.0	0.0	0.6	0.9	0.2	0.5
	(0.4)	(0.2)	(0.2)	(1.0)		(0.6)	(0.7)	(0.2)	(0.2)
Drug dependence	2.6	0.6	1.6	4.9	0.0	3.9	3.0	0.6	3.0
	(0.8)	(0.3)	(0.4)	(2.5)		(2.0)	(0.8)	(0.3)	(0.6)
Any substance abuse/ dependence	15.4	1.9	8.3	15.3	1.7	11.9	11.8	2.0	8.7
	(1.7)	(0.6)	(0.9)	(4.4)	(1.7)	(3.4)	(2.2)	(0.6)	(0.9)
Antisocial personality disorder	0.2	0.2	0.2	0.0	0.0	0.0	0.1	0.2	0.2
	(0.2)	(0.2)	(0.2)				(0.1)	(0.2)	(0.1)
Any disorder	24.1	16.5	20.1	30.4	14.6	26.0	26.7	16.8	20.6
	(2.1)	(1.7)	(1.3)	(5.6)	(6.4)	(4.5)	(3.3)	(1.7)	(1.3)

Note: Numbers in table represent the percentage of the sample who had ever been diagnosed with the disorder. Standard errors are shown in parentheses.

disorder among women was agoraphobia (6.9 percent); the most prevalent disorder among men was alcohol dependence (8.9 percent). The lifetime prevalence of any psychiatric disorder differed significantly between Indians and non-Indians. Among non-Indians, the most prevalent disorders were simple phobia (6.2 percent) and alcohol dependence (6.2 percent); the most prevalent disorder among Indians was alcohol dependence (9.9 percent).

Risk for Psychiatric Outcomes

In logistic regression models, the risk of lifetime mood or anxiety disorders was similar for male and female migrant workers (Table 23.3). Women had a significantly lower risk for lifetime alcohol abuse or dependence than did men (adjusted odds ratio [OR] = 0.10; 95 percent confidence interval [CI] = 0.04, 0.22). The point estimate of women's risk of drug abuse or dependence was low (adjusted OR = 0.32), but it did not reach statistical significance. The likelihood of lifetime alcohol abuse or dependence was higher among those aged 26 to 39 years (adjusted OR = 3.50; 95 percent CI = 1.54, 7.96) and those aged 40 to 59 years (adjusted OR = 7.93; 95 percent CI = 2.93, 21.41) than among younger migrant workers. No significant effects were found for marital status or income.

Respondents with more than six years of education had a higher risk of alcohol abuse or dependence (adjusted OR = 1.89; 95 percent CI = 1.05, 3.40) and drugs (adjusted OR = 3.83; 95 percent CI = 1.16, 12.60) than did respondents with fewer years of education. Acculturation increased the likelihood of mood disorders (adjusted OR = 3.80; 95 percent CI = 1.28, 11.27) and of drug abuse or dependence (adjusted OR = 10.94; 95 percent CI = 1.56, 76.57). In comparison with those whose main country of residence was the United States, respondents who were primarily residents of Mexico had less than half the risk of alcohol (adjusted OR = 0.40; 95 percent CI = 0.22, 0.73) or drug (adjusted OR = 0.27; 95 percent CI = 0.08, 0.93) abuse or dependence.

Table 23.4 shows lifetime prevalence rates for psychiatric disorders among Mexican migrant farmworkers in the Fresno County sample and among respondents in local, national, and international samples. The lifetime prevalence rate among Fresno County migrants (21.1 percent) was similar to that of recent immigrant residents in the county (18.4 percent) and to rates found in Mexico City (23.4 percent); however, it was less than half the rate for U.S.-born Mexican Americans (48.7 percent) or for the U.S. Hispanic population as a whole (51.4 percent). The past-year prevalence rate for any psychiatric disorder (not shown in Table 23.4) was 10.5 percent for migrants, 9.5 percent for immigrants with less than thirteen years in the United States, 19.7 percent for immigrants with thirteen years or more in the United States, and 27.7 percent for those born in the United States.

Table 23.3. Adjusted Odds Ratios (from Logistic Regression) for Lifetime Psychiatric Disorders, by Demographic and Acculturation Characteristics: Migrant Farmworkers from Mexico in Fresno County, California, 1996

	Adjusted OR (95% CI)			
	Mood Disorders	Anxiety Disorders	Alcohol Abuse or Dependence	Drug Abuse or Dependence
Sex (reference: male)				
Female	1.27 (0.68, 2.37)	1.35 (0.89, 2.07)	0.10 (0.04, 0.22)	0.34 (0.10, 1.08)
Age, years (reference: 18–25)				
26–39	1.33 (0.65, 2.72)	0.78 (0.46, 1.32)	3.48 (1.51, 7.98)	2.15 (0.60, 7.71)
40–59	1.81 (0.73, 4.47)	0.96 (0.49, 1.87)	7.94 (2.91, 21.65)	2.38 (0.38, 14.97)
Marital status (reference: never married)				
Married	0.77 (0.36, 1.66)	0.69 (0.40, 1.20)	0.56 (0.26, 1.22)	1.42 (0.39, 5.19)
Widowed/divorced	2.04 (0.77, 5.37)	1.57 (0.75, 3.28)	0.58 (0.17, 1.93)	3.99 (1.00, 15.88)
Income (reference: $9,000 or less)				
More than $9,000	1.17 (0.63, 2.20)	0.65 (0.40, 1.04)	1.07 (0.59, 1.95)	0.87 (0.26, 2.87)
Education, years (reference: 0–6)				
More than 6	1.43 (0.75, 2.74)	1.27 (0.81, 1.97)	1.86 (1.04, 3.33)	3.50 (1.06, 11.50)
Main country of residence (reference: United States)				
Mexico	0.95 (0.51, 1.78)	0.80 (0.51, 1.25)	0.40 (0.22, 0.73)	0.28 (0.08, 0.96)
Ethnicity (reference: non-Indian)				
Indian	1.10 (0.42, 2.85)	1.07 (0.55, 2.08)	0.79 (0.32, 1.98)	0.82 (0.16, 4.11)
Acculturation (reference: low)				
Medium	1.02 (0.49, 2.10)	1.10 (0.68, 1.78)	1.39 (0.74, 2.62)	2.79 (0.82, 9.42)
High	3.72 (1.26, 11.02)	1.41 (0.58, 3.44)	2.64 (0.70, 9.96)	10.00 (1.40, 1.06)

Note: OR = odds ratio; CI = confidence interval.

Table 23.4. Lifetime Prevalence of Psychiatric Disorders Among Migrant Workers and Residents in the Mexican American Prevalence and Services Survey, Among Residents of Mexico City, and Among Respondents to the National Comorbidity Survey

	Mexican American Prevalence and Services Survey Respondents, % (SE)			Mexico City Respondents % (SE)	National Comorbidity Survey Respondents, % (SE)	
	Migrant Workers	Immigrants Less Than Thirteen Years in the United States	Immigrants More Than Thirteen Years in the United States	U.S. Born		Hispanics	Total Sample
Any mood disorder	5.9 (0.8)	5.9 (1.4)	10.8 (2.0)	18.5 (1.7)	9.0 (1.1)	20.4 (2.8)	19.5 (0.6)
Any anxiety disorder	12.1 (1.1)	7.6 (1.2)	17.1 (2.1)	24.1 (2.0)	8.3 (0.8)	28.0 (2.5)	25.0 (0.8)
Any drug abuse or dependence	10.0 (1.1)	9.7 (2.6)	14.3 (1.9)	29.3 (2.0)	11.8 (0.8)	24.7 (2.7)	28.2 (1.0)
Any disorder	21.1 (1.5)	18.4 (2.7)	32.3 (2.6)	48.7 (2.3)	24.7 (51.4)	51.4 (2.7)	48.6 (1.0)

Note: All prevalence rates are adjusted to National Comorbidity Survey total age–sex distribution and are for persons aged 18 to 54 years.

DISCUSSION

Epidemiologic studies of the U.S. population have found no significant differences in overall prevalence of psychiatric disorders between men and women (Vega and others, 1998; Kessler and others, 1994; Robins and Reiger, 1991). However, in our migrant sample, women had lower lifetime prevalence rates of psychiatric disorders than did men. In contrast to the findings of these resident-population studies (Vega and others, 1998; Kessler and others, 1994; Robins and Reiger, 1991), we found that migrant women had mood disorder rates similar to those of migrant men. In addition, men's odds ratios for substance abuse or dependence were higher than those of women. Sex-specific patterns of psychiatric disorders merit further study to elucidate differential effects of stressors in men and women as well as protective factors associated with the living and working conditions of migrant populations.

The similarity in rates of psychiatric disorders between residents of Mexico and migrants and recent immigrants in the United States argues against selective migration of healthy individuals. To address the issue of time order in the onset of psychiatric disorders, we calculated past-year rates in addition to lifetime rates. The patterns of past-year prevalence rates were similar to those of lifetime rates. Collectively, these results suggest an increase in onset rates of psychiatric disorders with increased length of residence in the United States.

The paradox of better health outcomes among low-income immigrants in the United States, a high-risk group, has been attributed to protective sociocultural factors that may weaken as immigrants become established within the host society. Regional differences in patterns of mental health problems have been reported for indigenous people (Jones and Horne, 1973; Bignault and Ryder, 1977; Kelly, 1973; Fleming, Watson, McDonald, and Alexander, 1991; Al-Issa and Tousignant, 1997; Al-Issa, 1995). Ethnicity-specific cultural factors may be protective of both Indian and non-Indian immigrants' mental health, countering the potentially detrimental effects of their low socioeconomic attainment and minority status (Al-Issa, 1995; Vega and Rumbaut, 1991). Among the Latino population, protective sociocultural factors mentioned in the literature include social support, strong family ties, and group identity (Vega and Gil, 1998; Portes and Weeks, 1996; Vega and Amaro, 1994). Among indigenous peoples, a variety of factors have been associated with mental health problems, namely, low family support and decimated family structure, deculturation, loss of cultural coping styles, social stress and discrimination, and factors associated with Westernization and other modernization, such as social and geographic mobility (King, Beals, Manson, and Trimble, 1992; Kraus and Buffler, 1997; Young and French, 1996; Larse, 1980; Khan, 1982; Raphael and Swan, 1997). These mental health risk factors may affect indigenous people who migrate from other countries as their exposure to American society increases.

CONCLUSION

These findings on the prevalence of major psychiatric disorders among Mexican migrant farmworkers in the United States are based on a unique database. They hold significant implications for evaluating and planning for mental health needs in this high-risk population, particularly since these data permit sex- and ethnicity-specific assessments. The evidence presented here of an association between acculturation and prolonged U.S. residence and an increased risk of psychiatric disorders underscores the potential for progressive deterioration of migrant farmworkers' mental health as they extend their contact with the host society or become permanent settlers in the United States. Such deterioration may affect subsequent generations of migrant farmworkers as well. Special attention should be paid to facilitating access to culturally appropriate mental health services and to planning interventions to address the social adjustment problems of migrant farmworkers and their children.

References

Al-Issa, I. (ed.). *Handbook of Culture and Mental Illness: An International Perspective.* Madison, Conn.: International Universities Press, 1995.

Al-Issa, I., and Tousignant, M. (eds.). *Ethnicity, Immigration and Psychopathology.* New York: Plenum Press, 1997.

American Psychiatric Association. *Diagnostic and Statistical Manual of Mental Disorders* (rev. 3rd ed.). Washington, D.C.: American Psychiatric Association, 1987.

Berry, J. W., and Annis, R. C. (eds.). *Ethnic Psychology: Research and Practice with Immigrants, Refugees, Native Peoples, Ethnic Groups and Sojourners.* Lisse, Netherlands: Swets & Zeitlinger, 1988.

Bignault, I., and Ryder, C. "Abstinence and Alcohol Use Among Urban Aborigines in Western Australia." *Drug and Alcohol Review,* 1977, *16,* 365–371.

Chi, P. S. "Variation in Subjective Well-Being Among Black Migrant Farm Workers in New York." *Rural Sociology,* 1986, *51,* 183–198.

Chi, P. S., and McClain, J. "Drinking, Farm and Camp Life: A Study of Drinking Behavior in Migrant Camps in New York State." *Journal of Rural Health,* 1992, *7,* 45–51.

Cobas, J. A., and others. "Acculturation and Low-Birthweight Infants Among Latino Women: A Reanalysis of HHANES Data with Structural Equation Models." *American Journal of Public Health,* 1996, *86,* 394–396.

Cuellar, I., Harris, L. C., and Jasso, R. "An Acculturation Scale for Mexican Normal and Clinical Populations." *Hispanic Journal of Behavioral Sciences,* 1980, *2,* 199–217.

Dosen, A. "Het gastarbeider syndroom. Een onderzoek bij Joegoslavische migranten." *Maandblad Geestelijke Volksgezondheid,* 1983, *4,* 387–395.

Fabrega, H. "Social Psychiatric Aspects of Acculturation and Migration: A General Statement." *Comparative Psychiatry*, 1969, *10*, 314–326.

Fleming, J., Watson, C., McDonald, D., and Alexander, K. "Drug Use Patterns in Northern Territory Aboriginal Communities, 1986–1987." *Drug and Alcohol Review*, 1991, *10*(4), 367–380.

Friessem, D. H. "Travailleurs étrangers en République Fédérale d'Allemagne. Quelques résultats et réflexions dans une optique médico-sociale et psychiatrique." *L'Information Psychiatrique*, 1975, *51*, 283–291.

Gabbard, S., Mines, R., and Boccalandro, B. *Mixtec Migrants in California Agriculture.* Davis: California Institute for Rural Studies, 1993.

Gabbard, S., Mines, R., and Boccalandro, B. *Migrant Farmworkers: Pursuing Security in an Unstable Labor Market.* Washington, D.C.: Office of Program Economics, Office of the Assistant Secretary for Policy, U.S. Department of Labor, 1994.

Jones, I. H., and Horne, D. J. "Psychiatric Disorders Among Aborigines of the Australian Western Desert." *Social Science and Medicine*, 1973, *7*, 219–228.

Kelly, R. "Mental Illness in the Maori Population of New Zealand." *Acta Psychiatrica Scandinavica*, 1973, *49*, 722–734.

Kessler, R. C., and others. "Lifetime and 12-Month Prevalence of DSM-III-R Psychiatric Disorders in the United States." *Archives of General Psychiatry*, 1994, *51*, 8–19.

Kessler, R. C., and others. "Methodological Studies of the Composite International Diagnostic Interview (CIDI) and the US National Comorbidity Survey." *International Journal of Methods in Psychiatric Research*, 1998, *7*, 33–55.

Khan, M. W. "Cultural Clash and Psychopathology in Three Aboriginal Cultures." *Academic Psychology Bulletin*, 1982, *4*, 553–561.

King, J., Beals, J., Manson, S. M., and Trimble, J. E. "A Structural Equation Model of Factors Related to Substance Use Among American Indian Adolescents." *Drugs and Society*, 1992, *6*, 253–368.

Kraus, R. F., and Buffler, P. A. "Sociocultural Stress and the American Native in Alaska: An Analysis of Changing Patterns of Psychiatric Illness and Alcohol Abuse Among Alaska Natives." *Culture, Medicine, and Psychiatry*, 1997, *3*, 111–151.

Lafferty, J., Foulk, D., and Ryan, R. "Needle Sharing for the Use of Therapeutic Drugs as a Potential AIDS Risk Behavior Among Migrant Hispanic Farm Workers in the Eastern Stream." *International Quarterly of Community Health Education*, 1990–1991, *11*, 135–143.

Larse, K. S. "Aboriginal Group Identification and Problem Drinking." *Australian Psychologist*, 1980, *15*, 385–392.

MacMillan, A. "The Health Opinion Survey: Technique for Estimating Prevalence of Psychoneurotic and Related Types of Disorders in Communities." *Psychological Reports*, 1957, *3*(Suppl. 7), 325–329.

"Mental Health and Behavioral Disorders (Including Disorders of Psychological Development)." In *International Classification of Diseases—10th Revision.* Geneva, Switzerland: World Health Organization, 1991.

Mines, R., Gabbard, S., and Steirman, A. *A Profile of US Farmworkers: Demographics, Household Composition, Income and Use of Services.* Washington, D.C.: Office of Program Economics, Office of the Assistant Secretary for Policy, U.S. Department of Labor, 1997.

Padilla, A. M. (ed.). *Acculturation.* Boulder, Colo.: Westview Press, 1980.

Portes, A., and Rumbaut, R. *Immigrant America: A Portrait.* Berkeley: University of California Press, 1990.

Portes, R. G., and Weeks, J. R. "Unraveling a Public Health Enigma: Why Do Immigrants Experience Superior Perinatal Health Outcomes?" *Research in the Sociology of Health Care,* 1996, *13,* 337–391.

Ramon, S., Shanin, T., and Strimpel, J. "The Peasant Connection: Social Background and Mental Health of Migrant Workers in Western Europe." *Mental Health Sociology,* 1977, *4,* 270–290.

Raphael, B., and Swan, P. "The Mental Health of Aboriginal and Torres Strait Islander People." *International Journal of Mental Health,* 1997, *26,* 9–22.

Robins, L. N., and Reiger, D. A. (eds.). *Psychiatric Disorders in America: The Epidemiologic Catchment Area Study.* New York: Free Press, 1991.

Robins, L. N., and others. "The Composite International Diagnostic Interview: An Epidemiologic Instrument Suitable for Use in Conjunction with Different Diagnostic Systems and in Different Cultures." *Archives of General Psychiatry,* 1988, *45,* 1069–1077.

Simoes, M., and Binder, J. "A Socio-Psychiatric Field Study Among Portuguese Emigrants in Switzerland." *Social Psychiatry,* 1980, *15,* 1–7.

Szapocznik, J., Scopetta, M., and Kurtines, W. "Theory and Measurement of Acculturation." *American Journal of Psychology,* 1978, *12,* 113–130.

Van der Meer, P. J. *Uiting van depressie bij Marokkanen. Symposiumverslag Depressie bij etnische minderheden.* Nijmegen, Netherlands: Ciba/Geigy, 1984.

Vega, W. A., and Amaro, H. "Latino Outlook: Good Health, Uncertain Prognosis." *Annual Review of Public Health,* 1994, *15,* 39–67.

Vega, W. A., and Gil, A. G. *Drug Use and Ethnicity in Early Adolescence.* New York: Plenum Press, 1998.

Vega, W. A., and Rumbaut, R. G. "Ethnic Minorities and Mental Health." *Annual Review of Sociology,* 1991, *17,* 351–383.

Vega, W. A., Warheit, G., and Palacio, R. "Psychiatric Symptomatology Among Mexican American Farm Workers." *Social Science and Medicine,* 1985, *20,* 39–45.

Vega, W. A., and others. "Acculturative Strain Theory: Its Application in Explaining Drug Use Behavior Among Cuban and Non-Cuban Hispanic Youth." In M. De La Rosa (ed.), *Drug Abuse Among Minority Youth: Advances in Research and Methodology.* Rockville, Md.: National Institute on Drug Abuse, 1993.

Vega, W. A., and others. "Lifetime Prevalence of DSM-III-R Psychiatric Disorders Among Urban and Rural Mexican Americans in California." *Archives of General Psychiatry,* 1998, *55,* 771–778.

Vincent, K. "Redefining Poverty in California: Public Policy and the Mexican Rural Poor." *U.C. Mexus News,* 1996, *32*(1), 4–6.

Vision 20/20. Snapshot of Fresno County. Fresno, Calif.: New United Way, 1996.

Watson, J., and others. "Alcohol Use Among Migrant Laborers in Western New York." *Journal of Studies on Alcohol,* 1985, *46,* 403–411.

White-Means, S. "The Economic Returns from Investments in Physical and Mental Health: A Case Study of Migrant Farmworkers in Rural New York." *Journal of Health and Social Policy,* 1991, *2*(3), 39–51.

Wittchen, H.-U. "Reliability and Validity Studies of the WHO–Composite International Diagnostic Interview (CIDI): A Critical Review." *Journal of Psychiatric Research,* 1994, *28,* 57–84.

Wittchen, H.-U., and others. "Cross-Cultural Feasibility, Reliability and Sources of Variance of the Composite International Diagnostic Interview (CIDI)." *British Journal of Psychiatry,* 1984, *159,* 645–653.

Young, T., and French, L. A. "Suicide and Homicide Rates Among US Indian Health Service Areas: The Income Inequality Hypothesis." *Social Behavior and Personality,* 1996, *24*(4), 365–366.

Intimate Victimization
of Latina Farmworkers

A Research Summary

Joe Gorton
Nikki R. Van Hightower

Although the issue of physical and sexual abuse against women has only recently been addressed within the public health sector, Latinas who are poor and part of the farmworker community receive little, if any, attention when it comes to abuse. They are geographically and socially isolated and thus often far from the attention of the health and social welfare communities. For these reasons, this chapter makes a significant contribution to the literature in a study that covers nine states with large representations of agricultural workers. The authors identify determinants that contribute to increased abuse among Latina farmworkers and offer a great deal of insight into the special needs of these women and how they might be addressed.

In response to concerns voiced by migrant health clinicians about domestic violence injuries among migrant and seasonal farmworker women, the Migrant Clinicians Network (MCN) in 1994 documented the extent of domestic violence among farmworker women in Michigan, New York, Colorado, Wisconsin, Pennsylvania, Iowa, Washington, Texas, and North Carolina. (Migrant Clinicians Network provides networking, education, accreditation, and research services to clinics that serve migrant and seasonal farmworkers.) Our analysis used the MCN data to examine the prevalence of victimization among Latina farmworkers and the degree to which various social and demographic factors predicted intimate violence against these women.

This research was supported in part by grants from the Bureau of Primary Health Care and the Agency for Health Care Policy Research of the U.S. Department of Health and Human Services and a grant from the Texas A&M University School of Rural Public Health. The authors gratefully acknowledge the assistance of the Migrant Clinicians Network, the migrant health clinics, and their patients who participated in the study.

LITERATURE REVIEW

Previous researchers have found that domestic violence occurs among all racial, ethnic, and socioeconomic groups (Centerwall, 1984; Straus, Gelles, and Steinmetz, 1980; Walker, 1984). Despite these findings, few researchers have attempted to analyze factors that contribute to domestic violence among impoverished minorities and residents of rural areas (Pinn and Chunko, 1997; Websdale, 1997). Pinn and Chunko's recent study (1997) of culturally sensitive interventions in domestic abuse cases suggests that low-income women and those who live in isolated conditions (for example, do not own telephones, reside in remote areas, do not speak English) are at highest risk for all types of violence. Hogeland and Rosen's analysis (1991) of immigrant women in California found that 25 to 35 percent had been victims of domestic abuse.

Anderson's analysis (1993) of victimization among immigrant Latinas in the Washington, D.C., area revealed that domestic violence against them increased after they immigrated to the United States. Additionally, Anderson found that the rate of battering was highest among undocumented or conditional resident Latinas who were married to citizens of the United States or lawful permanent residents.

METHOD

A sample of 820 Latina farmworkers completed a domestic violence survey instrument. Respondents' ages ranged from 18 to 72, with a mean age of 30 ($SD = 11.2$). Ethnicity was determined by interviewees' responses to an opened-ended question that enabled respondents to designate their ethnic origin. Of the respondents, 77 percent ($n = 637$) identified themselves as Hispanic, 21 percent ($n = 172$) as Mexican, 1 percent ($n = 8$) as Puerto Rican, and 0.4 percent ($n = 3$) as Guatemalan. Of the sample, 57 percent ($n = 469$) were pregnant, 37 percent ($n = 302$) were not pregnant, and 6 percent ($n = 49$) did not respond to the survey item concerning pregnancy. Most of the women in the study, 68 percent ($n = 561$), were legally married or cohabiting with a male partner; 28 percent ($n = 233$) were single, widowed, divorced, or separated, and 3 percent ($n = 26$) did not report their marital status. Of the sample, 35 percent ($n = 287$) reported that they were migrant farmworkers, and 38 percent ($n = 312$) reported that they were seasonal workers (that is, permanent residents within the local area). Twenty-seven percent of the sample ($n = 221$) did not identify themselves as either migrant or seasonal workers.

Because the dependent variable in this study is a dichotomous measure of spousal abuse, logistic regression analysis was used to predict the likelihood of respondents' being victimized. The significance of the contribution of each independent variable may be seen in the Wald statistic (the ratio of the regression coefficient B to an estimate of its standard error). Regression coefficients were considered statistically significant if $p < .05$ or if the Wald statistic exceeded a critical value of 2. The Exp (B) for each logistic regression coefficient gives the logs-odds ratio for the predictor variables. Odds ratios greater than one indicate an increase in the odds of being abused, and odds ratios less than one indicate a decrease in the odds of being abused.

RESULTS

Among the 820 Latina farmworkers, 17.4 percent ($n = 143$) reported that they had been physically or sexually abused during the past year. During the year in question, the number of abuse incidents experienced by respondents who were abused ranged from 1 to 70, and the average number of incidents per abused respondent was 11.5.

Table 24.1 presents the results of the logistic regression analysis in which abuse is the dependent variable. The model fit well (Model chi square = 93.77, $df = 6$, $p < .000$) and correctly classified 82.12 percent of the cases. After controlling for migrant status, age, martial status, and whether the respondent had children, two variables were significantly related to the probability that the respondents had been abused during the preceding twelve months. The logs-odds ratio for drug and/or alcohol use shows that women with husbands, boyfriends, or companions who used drugs and/or alcohol were approximately eight times more likely to be victimized than women with spouses, boyfriends, or companions who abstained from drug and/or alcohol use ($p < .0000$). In contrast to drug and/or alcohol use, pregnancy reduced the probability of victimization. By a factor of .42, or 58 percent ($p < .0036$), pregnancy decreased

Table 24.1. Logistic Regression Predicting Spousal Abuse

Predictor Variable	B	Wald	Significance	R	Exp(B)
Drug and/or alcohol use	2.12	58.90	.0000	.34	8.32
Pregnancy	−0.86	8.45	.0036	−.12	0.42
Age	0.02	0.96	.3263	.000	1.02
Children	0.70	1.45	.2283	.000	2.01
Migrant/seasonal	0.27	1.06	.3042	.030	0.76
Marital status	−0.18	0.39	.5286	.000	0.83
Model chi-square	93.77		.000		
Degrees of freedom	6				

respondents' chances of being abused. Measures of statistical significance for the influence of migrant status, age, whether the respondent had children, and marital status indicate that these variables did not significantly affect the likelihood that the respondents would be abused.

DISCUSSION AND CONCLUSIONS

This study examined the prevalence of domestic abuse experienced by Latina farmworkers and the influence of various factors on the intimate victimization of these women. Among the study participants, approximately 17 percent had been physically or sexually abused by a husband, boyfriend, or companion. The strongest predictors of domestic abuse of Latina farmworkers included in this analysis were drug and/or alcohol use by respondent's partner and whether the respondent was pregnant.

Women in this study with intimate partners who used drugs and/or alcohol were significantly more likely to be abused than respondents whose intimate partners were abstainers. The direct influence of drug and/or alcohol use on spousal abuse was present regardless of respondents' marital status, age, race, migrant status, whether they were pregnant, or had children. These findings are consistent with a large volume of research that documents the positive relationship between drug and/or alcohol use and domestic violence (Conner and Ackerley, 1994).

Our analysis shows that Latina farmworker women who were pregnant were less likely to be victims of domestic violence than those who were not pregnant. Given the paucity of research pertaining to the influence of pregnancy and non-pregnancy on partner violence (as opposed to research focusing on prevalence of abuse among pregnant women), we can only speculate about possible relationships between pregnancy and abuse. Because the regression model used in our analysis does not specify a temporal ordering of pregnancy and abuse, there are two contrasting possibilities. First, becoming pregnant might actually lessen the probability of victimization of farmworker women. This could occur if abusers have internalized pronatalist values that mediate against victimizing women who are pregnant. Second, a rational actor model would suggest that farmworker women who have experienced abuse might choose to avoid pregnancy. In other words, being free from abuse might have a positive influence on the decision of farmworker women to become pregnant, whereas experiencing abuse would have the opposite effect. This outcome would contribute to our finding of a negative relationship between pregnancy and abuse.

Among the sample population included in this study, domestic violence was an equal opportunity scourge in terms of age, marital status, fertility, and migrant status. Although violent victimizations by intimate partners are generally more likely to be targeted against younger women (Bachman, 1994), the domestic violence victims in this study were not clustered within a particular age group. Likewise, migrant status did not have a statistically significant effect on the probability of victimization. Respondents who were married or cohabiting were not significantly more likely to be victimized than women who were single, divorced, separated, or widowed. Similarly, the likelihood of being abused was not significantly influenced by whether respondents had children.

References

Anderson, M. J. "A License to Abuse: The Impact of Conditional Status on Female Immigrants." *Yale Law Journal,* 1993, *102,* 1401–1430.

Bachman, R. *Violence Against Women: A National Crime Victimization Survey Report.* Washington, D.C.: Department of Justice, Bureau of Justice Statistics, 1994.

Centerwall, B. S. "Race, Socioeconomic Status and Domestic Homicide, Atlanta, 1971–72." *American Journal of Public Health,* 1984, *74,* 813–815.

Conner, K. R., and Ackerley, G. D. "Alcohol-Related Battering: Developing Treatment Strategies." *Journal of Family Violence,* 1994, *9,* 143–155.

Hogeland, C., and Rosen, K. *Dreams Lost, Dreams Found: Undocumented Women in the Land of Opportunity.* San Francisco: Coalition for Immigrant and Refugee Rights and Services, 1991.

Pinn, V. W., and Chunko, M. T. "The Diverse Faces of Violence: Minority Women and Domestic Abuse." *Academic Medicine Supplement,* 1997, *72,* 65–71.

Straus, M. A., Gelles, R. J., and Steinmetz, S. D. *Behind Closed Doors: Violence in the American Family.* New York: Doubleday, 1980.

Walker, L. *The Battered Woman Syndrome.* New York: Springer, 1984.

Websdale, N. *Rural Woman Battering and the Justice System: An Ethnography.* Thousand Oaks, Calif.: Sage, 1997.

PART NINE

SPECIAL ISSUES

Relation of Demographic and Lifestyle Factors to Symptoms in a Multiracial/Ethnic Population of Women Forty- to Fifty-Five Years of Age

Ellen B. Gold

Barbara Sternfeld

Jennifer L. Kelsey

Charlotte Brown

Charles Mouton

Nancy Reame

Loran Salamone

Rebecca Stellato

This chapter addresses menopause and related issues of midlife among women of color, a topic largely missing from the literature. The sample of 16,065 participants includes Latinas (Central Americans, Cubans, Dominicans, Mexicans, and Puerto Ricans), Japanese, Chinese, African American, and White women. The special significance of this study is the inclusion of Latinas with other women of color and the comparisons that it enables. The chapter represents a milestone and useful beginning toward building an understanding of Latinas in this life stage.

By the year 2025, the number of postmenopausal women in the United States is projected to double from the mid-1990s (Gist and Velkoff, 1997) with half a million women added annually to the midlife population for the rest of this decade (Skolnick, 1992). An estimated $3 to $5 billion will be spent

---

The Study of Women's Health Across the Nation (SWAN) was funded by the National Institute on Aging, the National Institute of Nursing Research, and the Office of Research on Women's Health

annually by the year 2005 for hormone replacement and physician monitoring alone (Weinstein and Tosteson, 1990). However, relatively little is known about the prevalence of symptoms in women in their fifth and sixth decades of life, and much of what is known is derived from studies of White women. Developing preventive strategies for such women who are undergoing social and physiologic transition requires understanding multiple factors that affect symptom reporting in women from different socioeconomic and racial/ethnic backgrounds.

In this study, we investigated the relation of sociodemographic and lifestyle factors to a number of specific symptoms or conditions in a large, multiethnic, community-based sample of women from across the United States who participated in the first phase of the Study of Women's Health Across the Nation (SWAN). We hypothesized that: (1) vasomotor and other estrogen-related symptoms would be more frequently associated with factors that result in decreased production of estrogen, such as surgical menopause, smoking, reduced body mass, and physical activity; (2) prevalence of non-estrogen-related symptoms would increase with age, independent of menopausal status; and (3) factors resulting in physiologic, economic, or social stress (lower education, being unmarried, difficulty paying for basics, and unemployment) would be associated with increased symptomatology but that the prevalence of specific symptoms would differ by race/ethnicity.

---

of the National Institutes of Health. Supplemental funding from the National Institute of Mental Health, the National Institute on Child Health and Human Development, the National Center on Complementary and Alternative Medicine, the Office of Minority Health, and the Office of AIDS Research is also gratefully acknowledged.

Participating institutions and principal staff were as follows. *Clinical Centers:* University of Michigan, Ann Arbor (grant U01 NR04061; MaryFran Sowers, Principal Investigator); Massachusetts General Hospital, Boston (grant U01 AG12531; Robert Neer, Principal Investigator, 1994–1999; Joel Finkelstein, Principal Investigator, current); Rush University, Rush-Presbyterian–St. Luke's Medical Center, Chicago (grant U01 AG12505; Lynda Powell, Principal Investigator); University of California, Davis/Kaiser (grant U01 AG12554; Ellen Gold, Principal Investigator); University of California, Los Angeles (grant U01 A12539; Gail Greendale, Principal Investigator); University of Medicine and Dentistry–New Jersey Medical School, Newark (grant U01 AG12535; Gerson Weiss, Principal Investigator); and the University of Pittsburgh, Pittsburgh (grant U01 AG12546; Karen Matthews, Principal Investigator). *Central Laboratory:* University of Michigan, Ann Arbor (grant U01 AG12495; Central Ligand Assay Satellite Services, Rees Midgley, Principal Investigator). *Coordinating Center:* New England Research Institutes, Watertown, Massachusetts (grant U01 AG12553; Sonja McKinlay, Principal Investigator). *Project Officers:* Taylor Harden, Carol Hudgings, Marcia Ory, and Sheryl Sherman. *Steering Committee Chair:* Christopher Gallagher (1994–1996); Jennifer L. Kelsey (currently).

The authors thank the study staff at each site and all of the women who participated in SWAN. They also gratefully acknowledge the statistical programming assistance of Yan Luo and Marianne O'Neill Rasor.

The manuscript was reviewed by the Publications and Presentations Committee of SWAN and has its endorsement.

MATERIALS AND METHODS

Study Population

The first phase of SWAN consisted of a cross-sectional survey conducted from 1995 through 1997 of 16,065 women from seven geographic areas in the United States (Boston, Chicago, Detroit, Los Angeles, Newark, Oakland, and Pittsburgh). The purpose of the survey was twofold: (1) to screen women for eligibility for enrollment into a longitudinal study of premenopausal women and (2) to investigate cross-sectional relations of a limited number of risk factors and health outcomes. Each site screened one minority population (African Americans in Pittsburgh, Boston, the Detroit area, and Chicago; Japanese in Los Angeles; Chinese in the Oakland area of California; and Hispanics in New Jersey) in addition to a Caucasian population. Community-based sampling, using established lists of populations at five sites and random digit dialing combined with a "snowball" approach at two sites (Neugarten and Kraines, 1965) (those with the Hispanic and Japanese minority samples), was used to sample women aged 40 to 55 years, who resided in the area surrounding each clinical site. In the snowball technique, women first identified by a list-based or random digit dialing technique were asked for the names and contact information of other women who would meet the eligibility criteria, and these women in turn were contacted, screened for eligibility, and asked for the names of other appropriate women. This process continued until a sufficient number of eligible women was identified. Women were included who spoke English, Spanish, Cantonese, or Japanese at the respective sites where these languages were used and who identified themselves as Caucasian, African American, Hispanic, Japanese, or Chinese, depending on the site-specific population screened.

Data Collection

Ascertainment of Symptoms. Since the cross-sectional survey had to be brief, the presence of vasomotor, psychologic, and physical symptoms during the previous two weeks was determined from self-reported (yes/no) responses to closed-ended questions. Most interviews were computer-assisted telephone interviews, with about half being in-person at two sites. The specific symptoms included were based primarily on previous epidemiologic work on Caucasian women (Neugarten and Kraines, 1965; Matthews and others, 1994; Avis and McKinlay, 1991) and included the following: difficulty sleeping, night sweats, headaches, hot flushes or flashes, forgetfulness, vaginal dryness, leaking urine, feeling tense or nervous, feeling blue or depressed, and irritability or grouchiness. In addition, symptoms such as stiffness or soreness in joints, neck, or shoulders and heart pounding or racing were included, based on previous anthropologic work in the different race/ethnic groups (Lock, Kaufert, and Gilbert, 1988; Lock, 1991). Symptoms thought to be associated with menopause, such as hot flashes, night sweats, and vaginal dryness, were interspersed with other symptoms to minimize bias from stereotypic thinking about menopause (Kaufert, 1996). The relation of demographic and lifestyle variables to the psychologic symptoms is addressed elsewhere, while the relations to physical symptoms are addressed here (Bromberger and others, 2001).

Assessment of Independent Variables. Independent variables of interest were self-reported current status related to demographic factors (age, race/ethnicity, educational attainment, employment, marital status, number of children, and ability to pay for basics), lifestyle factors (smoking, physical activity), height and weight, and menopausal status.

Race/ethnicity was self-defined as Black or African American, non-Hispanic Caucasian, Chinese or Chinese American, Japanese or Japanese American, or Hispanic (Central American, Cuban or Cuban American, Dominican, Mexican or Mexican American, Puerto Rican, South American or Spanish, or other Hispanic). In addition, respondents could specify a race/ethnicity other than the defined categories or indicate mixed or no primary affiliation. Since most extant literature is based on non-Hispanic Caucasians, this was the reference group. Questions about smoking were modified from those of the American Thoracic Society (Ferris, 1978). Physical activity was assessed with one question about activity level relative to other women of the respondent's age. The body mass index was calculated from self-reported height and weight and equals weight $(kg)/height (m)^2$.

Menopausal status was based on menstrual characteristics as: *surgical,* indicating menses had stopped as a result of hysterectomy and/or oophorectomy (thus not necessarily representing cessation of hormonal cycling); *postmenopausal,* indicating menses had stopped for at least twelve months without surgery; *late perimenopausal,* indicating menses had occurred in the past twelve months but not in the last three months; *early perimenopausal,* indicating menses had occurred in the past three months but had become less predictable; and *premenopausal,* indicating menses had occurred in the past three months with no decrease in predictability. Women whose menstrual periods had stopped because of medication, radiotherapy, pregnancy or lactation, or extreme weight change ($n = 311$), who reported use of exogenous female hormones in the past three months (since such use might reflect greater symptom prevalence or reduced symptom reporting and thus be uninterpretable, $n = 1,635$), or who reported their race/ethnicity as mixed/other (since this was a very nonhomogeneous group, $n = 1,694$) were excluded, for a total of 12,425 included in the present analyses.

Data Analyses

Crude prevalence odds ratios for the association between the selected characteristics and each symptom were computed. Multiple logistic regression was used to adjust prevalence odds ratios simultaneously for site and demographic, lifestyle, and reproductive characteristics (SAS Institute, 1989). As a result of factor analyses (Avis and others, forthcoming), we combined hot flashes and night sweats into one outcome variable of hot flashes and/or night sweats. The odds ratios for the symptoms "difficulty sleeping," "forgetful," and "heart pounding or racing" were also adjusted for reporting irritability, feeling tense, or feeling anxious or depressed. Initial exploratory adjustment for diagnosis or treatment of arthritis was made for the symptom "stiffness or soreness in joints, neck, or shoulders," but this did not modify the results. Exploratory adjustment for language in which the interview was conducted, as an indicator of acculturation, also did not modify the results.

Parity was treated as a continuous variable. Four-year age groups and body mass index (Manson and others, 1995) were treated as categorical variables, since they were not linearly related to the prevalence of most of the symptoms. All categorical variables were treated as dummy variables in the logistic regression, thus assuming no particular ordering. Goodness of fit of models was tested by the Hosmer and Lemeshow procedure (Hosmer and Lemeshow, 1989). Because sites were not randomly selected and because sampling procedures varied by site to accommodate the difficulties in attaining adequate numbers of each racial/ethnic minority (formal representative sampling procedures were not exclusively used at two sites), use of estimation procedures based on formal sampling methods was inappropriate. The variance estimates used in the confidence intervals shown here were thus based on simple random sampling, but they should be interpreted with caution for these reasons.

Interactions of race/ethnicity or menstrual status with the association of each factor and symptom were first examined by stratifying on race/ethnicity or menstrual status to determine if the stratum-specific natural logarithms of the odds ratios differed from each other or from the unstratified natural logarithm odds ratio by more than two times the standard error for the unstratified effect. If so, the statistical significance of interaction terms was examined in the multiple logistic regression model.

RESULTS

Characteristics of the Study Population

Age distributions were generally similar by race/ethnic group, although a higher proportion of Chinese women were aged 40 to 43 years and a lower proportion were aged 52 to 55 years compared with other race/ethnic groups (Table 25.1).

Table 25.1. Distributions of Study Population by Race/Ethnicity and Selected Characteristics, SWAN, 1995–1997

	African American		Non-Hispanic Caucasian		Japanese		Chinese		Hispanic	
	(No.)	(%)	(No.)	(%)	(No.)	(%)	(No.)	(%)	(No.)	(%)
Age (years)										
40–43	904	24.6	1,732	30.0	189	26.6	172	31.5	506	29.4
44–47	1,134	30.8	1,764	30.6	240	33.8	206	37.7	517	30.1
48–51	933	25.4	1,358	23.5	172	24.2	122	22.3	404	23.5
52–55	705	19.2	920	15.9	110	15.5	46	8.4	291	16.9
Education										
Less than high school	319	8.8	277	4.8	5	0.7	97	17.8	619	36.2
High school/equivalent	1,023	28.1	1,574	27.3	138	19.4	96	17.6	470	27.5
Some college	1,450	39.8	1,668	29.0	261	36.8	123	22.5	377	22.0
College graduate	412	11.3	1,063	18.5	212	29.9	136	24.9	179	10.5
Postgraduate	437	12.0	1,177	20.4	94	13.2	94	17.2	66	3.9
Difficulty paying for basics										
Very hard	480	13.1	492	8.6	24	3.4	34	6.3	526	30.8
Somewhat hard	1,321	36.1	1,746	30.3	192	27.1	147	27.2	799	46.7
Not at all hard	1,859	50.8	3,518	61.1	492	69.5	360	66.5	385	22.5
Marital status										
Never married	751	20.5	693	12.0	37	5.2	39	7.1	126	7.4
Married/living as	1,630	44.4	3,904	67.7	595	83.7	448	82.0	1,123	65.6
Separated	284	7.7	170	3.0	24	3.4	4	0.7	174	10.2
Widowed	206	5.6	171	3.0	11	1.6	10	1.8	85	5.0
Divorced	799	21.8	825	14.3	44	6.2	45	8.2	205	12.0

	n	%	n	%	n	%	n	%	n	%
Parity										
0	322	8.8	1,254	21.7	102	14.4	76	13.9	136	7.9
1	641	17.4	953	16.5	107	15.0	85	15.6	284	16.6
2	1,039	28.3	1,869	32.4	320	45.0	256	46.9	541	31.6
3	800	21.8	1,044	18.1	147	20.7	97	17.8	427	24.9
4 or more	872	23.7	649	11.2	35	4.9	32	5.9	326	19.0
Menstrual status										
Surgical	976	26.6	673	11.7	53	7.4	13	2.4	273	15.9
Postmenopausal	484	13.2	802	13.9	75	10.6	63	11.4	334	19.4
Late perimenopausal	169	4.6	317	5.5	30	4.2	19	3.5	78	4.5
Early perimenopausal	1,018	27.7	1,801	31.2	183	25.7	158	28.9	396	23.0
Premenopausal	1,029	28.0	2,181	37.8	370	52.0	294	53.8	637	37.1
Body mass index (weight (kg)/height (m)^2)										
Below 19	158	4.3	342	5.9	67	9.4	61	11.2	164	9.6
19–26.9	1,273	34.9	3,350	58.2	565	79.6	433	79.3	893	52.1
27–31.9	1,037	28.4	1,100	19.1	64	9.0	40	7.3	420	24.5
32 or more	1,180	32.4	962	16.7	14	2.0	12	2.2	236	13.8
Smoking										
Never	1,822	49.7	2,687	46.6	497	70.1	463	94.7	1,117	65.2
Past	803	21.9	1,630	28.3	139	19.6	16	3.3	289	16.9
Current	1,044	28.4	1,450	25.1	73	10.3	10	2.0	306	17.9
Physical activity										
Much less	274	7.7	282	5.0	40	5.7	22	4.6	108	6.6
Somewhat less	649	18.3	828	14.6	103	14.8	69	14.3	196	12.0
Same	1,331	37.5	2,185	38.6	277	39.7	227	46.9	822	50.2
Somewhat more	753	21.2	1,572	27.8	181	25.9	94	19.4	261	15.9
Much more	544	15.3	795	14.0	97	13.9	72	14.9	251	15.3

Most women were premenopausal or in the early perimenopause; the proportion of women who had had surgical menopause was higher in African Americans, and the proportion who were postmenopausal was higher in Hispanics than in other race/ethnic groups. Hispanics had the lowest and Caucasians the highest educational attainment, while Japanese and Chinese women reported the least difficulty paying for basics. African American and Hispanic women had higher parity, and African Americans had higher body mass index than did women in the other race/ethnic groups. Smoking rates were lower in Japanese and Chinese women. The perception of amount of physical activity compared with other women of the same age did not differ greatly by race/ethnic group.

Unadjusted Relation of Sociodemographic, Health, and Lifestyle Factors to Symptom Prevalence

Increased age, lower educational level, difficulty paying for basics, race/ethnicity, increased parity, and employment were related to the prevalence of most symptoms (Table 25.2). Virtually all symptoms, except stiffness and soreness in joints, neck, and shoulders, were less frequently reported in Japanese and Chinese women, while vasomotor symptoms (hot flashes or night sweats) were most frequently reported by African American or Hispanic women. Urine leakage, vaginal dryness, and heart pounding or racing were more frequently reported by Hispanic women. The prevalence of most symptoms varied by site, thus warranting inclusion of site in multivariate logistic regression analyses.

Vasomotor symptoms were much more frequently reported by women in the late perimenopause or by women who were surgically or naturally postmenopausal compared with premenopausal women Table 25.2). Most other symptoms were also more frequent in women who were peri- or postmenopausal, but the differences were not as large. Prior to adjustment for other covariates, the prevalences of hot flashes or night sweats increased with age in most menstrual status categories, except for postmenopausal women in whom it declined (data not shown). However, the prevalence of most symptoms varied more by menstrual status than by age. Heart pounding or racing and difficulty sleeping were not independently related to age (data not shown). Reporting of all other symptoms increased with age, although not in a monotonic trend. Current smoking, engaging in less physical activity than other women of the same age, and increased body mass index were associated with increased prevalence of almost every symptom, although the trends were not monotonic.

Multivariate Adjusted Associations of Risk Factors to Symptoms

Age. After adjustment for the other covariates in Table 25.1, vasomotor symptoms and urine leakage were not related to age in postmenopausal and late perimenopausal women (data not shown).

Table 25.2. Crude Percentage of Women with Each Symptom (of Those Reporting) by Demographic and Health Characteristics, SWAN, 1995–1997

	Symptom (%)						
Characteristics[a]	Hot Flashes/ Night Sweats[b] (n = 3,963)	Urine Leakage (n = 2,135)	Vaginal Dryness (n = 1,629)	Difficult Sleep (n = 4,632)	Stiff/Sore (n = 6,620)	Heart Pounding (n = 2,315)	Forgetfulness (n = 4,843)
Age (years)							
40–43 (n = 3,493; 28.3%)	25.2	14.8	8.6	37.0	50.9	18.2	33.1
44–47 (n = 3,834; 31.0%)	31.2	17.0	11.3	35.8	52.0	19.0	39.2
48–51 (n = 2,965; 24.0%)	42.7	19.6	16.7	39.9	56.1	17.4	43.7
52–55 (n = 2,066; 16.7%)	46.4	19.3	19.8	39.1	56.1	20.8	42.4
Education							
Less than 8 years (n = 376; 3.1%)	41.0	22.9	23.7	41.5	56.1	34.3	52.9
8–11 years (n = 935; 7.6%)	41.5	22.8	18.6	45.0	55.6	29.9	52.1
12 years high school (n = 3,285; 26.7%)	39.7	17.8	14.1	37.5	53.5	20.6	40.7
Some college (n = 3,857; 31.4%)	36.6	17.3	13.0	38.3	54.6	18.2	38.5
College graduate (n = 1,992; 16.2%)	11.8	14.6	10.1	33.7	50.8	14.6	33.2
Postgraduate/professional (n = 1,855; 15.1%)	25.2	15.3	10.1	35.7	52.4	12.1	34.7

(Continued)

Table 25.2. Crude Percentage of Women with Each Symptom (of Those Reporting) by Demographic and Health Characteristics, SWAN, 1995–1997 (Continued)

	Symptom (%)						
Characteristics[a]	Hot Flashes/ Night Sweats (n = 3,963)[b]	Urine Leakage (n = 2,135)	Vaginal Dryness (n = 1,629)	Difficult Sleep (n = 4,632)	Stiff/Sore (n = 6,620)	Heart Pounding (n = 2,315)	Forgetfulness (n = 4,843)
Difficulty paying for basics							
Very hard (n = 1,544; 12.6%)	45.8	24.8	19.6	53.5	63.9	33.7	54.6
Somewhat hard (n = 4,184; 34.0%)	37.4	18.5	13.7	40.4	54.6	20.7	43.0
Not at all hard (n = 6,579; 53.5%)	30.6	14.9	11.5	32.2	50.2	13.9	33.0
Race/ethnicity							
African American (n = 3,650; 29.5%)	45.6	16.7	14.8	34.9	55.7	19.2	43.0
Caucasian (n = 5,746; 46.5%)	31.2	18.2	11.2	40.6	54.6	17.0	35.2
Japanese (n = 707; 5.7%)	17.6	12.6	6.7	29.1	50.3	10.3	33.0
Chinese (n = 542; 4.4%)	20.5	11.0	10.2	31.9	48.2	14.1	40.5
Hispanic (n = 1,712; 13.8%)	35.4	19.7	20.4	38.6	47.1	28.1	46.0
Menstrual status							
Surgical (n = 1,988; 16.0%)	46.9	22.1	19.4	43.5	59.4	23.7	43.8
Postmenopausal (n = 1,753; 14.2%)	48.8	17.7	21.2	40.4	54.8	19.5	42.0

Late perimenopausal (n = 611; 4.9%)	56.8	19.6	18.2	43.9	58.4	20.7	44.8
Early perimenopausal (n = 3,547; 28.6%)	36.9	20.6	12.9	40.6	57.9	20.1	44.0
Premenopausal (n = 4,497; 36.3%)	19.4	12.3	7.1	30.9	45.8	14.7	31.2
Marital status							
Single (n = 1,646; 13.3%)	34.7	14.5	9.9	37.8	54.5	18.9	36.2
Married/living as (n = 7,700; 62.1%)	33.0	16.9	14.0	35.5	52.0	17.2	37.9
Separated/divorced (n = 2,574; 20.8%)	39.2	27.2	12.7	42.8	56.3	21.9	39.2
Widowed (n = 483; 3.9%)	40.8	19.9	12.4	41.0	54.9	23.6	44.1
Parity							
0 (n = 1,890; 15.2%)	29.2	12.4	10.0	37.2	53.1	14.0	30.2
1 (n = 2,070; 16.7%)	34.2	16.6	12.4	38.6	54.5	17.4	37.0
2 (n = 4,025; 35.4%)	34.5	16.7	13.4	36.1	52.6	17.2	39.0
≥3 (n = 4,429; 35.7%)	37.9	20.0	14.5	37.7	53.5	22.6	43.7
Body mass index (kg/m^2)							
Below 19 (n = 792; 6.4%)	30.6	14.9	12.7	40.6	53.4	18.2	40.1
19–26.9 (n = 6,514; 42.7%)	29.9	13.3	12.1	35.2	48.7	16.6	35.7
27–31.9 (n = 2,661; 21.5%)	39.5	18.8	13.8	37.3	54.9	19.7	41.9
32 or more (n = 2,404; 19.4%)	43.8	27.5	15.8	43.4	64.5	23.0	44.4

(Continued)

Table 25.2. Crude Percentage of Women with Each Symptom (of Those Reporting) by Demographic and Health Characteristics, SWAN, 1995–1997 (Continued)

	Symptom (%)						
Characteristics[a]	Hot Flashes/ Night Sweats[b] (n = 3,963)	Urine Leakage (n = 2,135)	Vaginal Dryness (n = 1,629)	Difficult Sleep (n = 4,632)	Stiff/Sore (n = 6,620)	Heart Pounding (n = 2,315)	Forgetfulness (n = 4,843)
Smoking							
Never (n = 6,566; 53.3%)	30.0	15.8	13.0	34.6	50.4	16.3	37.6
Past (n = 2,872; 23.3%)	35.5	19.2	13.7	38.0	56.7	19.7	42.0
Current (n = 2,875; 23.4%)	45.5	19.4	13.5	44.6	56.9	23.3	39.6
Physical activity							
Much less (n = 717; 6.0%)	52.5	29.8	21.6	60.8	73.1	35.6	56.9
Some less (n = 1,831; 15.3%)	42.2	22.9	15.2	50.1	65.1	25.1	47.0
Same (n = 4,822; 40.3%)	32.3	16.3	12.8	34.3	50.8	17.0	38.6
Some more (n = 2,853; 23.8%)	31.4	14.8	11.5	33.9	49.6	14.9	33.2
Much more (n = 1,752; 14.6%)	32.6	13.6	11.9	31.2	46.8	15.8	33.5

[a]Numbers are after exclusions and include those who had missing information for some variables, since for any cell, the proportion missing was less than 2 percent.
[b]Numbers indicate those reporting yes.

Menstrual Status. Menstrual status had the largest adjusted prevalence odds ratios of any risk factor for most symptoms, particularly vasomotor (Table 25.3). All symptoms were more frequent in women who were not premenopausal. Vasomotor symptoms were particularly frequent in women who were in the late perimenopause, although the numbers in this category were relatively small.

Sociodemographic Factors. Adjusted prevalence odds ratios for vasomotor symptoms and heart pounding or racing generally increased with decreasing level of educational attainment (Table 25.3). The prevalences of vaginal dryness and forgetfulness were elevated only in women with less than a high school education. All symptoms were increased in women who reported difficulty paying for basics, and prevalence increased with greater difficulty. Heart pounding or racing, forgetfulness, and difficulty sleeping increased in women who were not employed full time. Vasomotor symptoms, urine leakage, and vaginal dryness were reported less frequently among never married, widowed, or divorced than currently married women (data not shown).

Race/Ethnicity. All symptoms, except heart pounding and forgetfulness, were reported less frequently by Japanese and Chinese women compared with non-Hispanic Caucasians. This finding persisted after adjustment for language as a measure of acculturation (data not shown). Urine leakage and difficulty sleeping were reported significantly less often, but vasomotor symptoms and vaginal dryness were reported significantly more frequently by African American than by Caucasian women. Hispanic women reported urine leakage, vaginal dryness, heart pounding or racing, and forgetfulness more frequently than did non-Hispanic Caucasian women. All minority ethnic groups reported difficulty sleeping significantly less frequently than did Caucasians after adjusting for other covariates. No marked interaction of race/ethnicity with prevalence odds ratios for risk factors and symptoms was observed.

Body Mass Index. Hot flashes or night sweats, urine leakage, and stiffness or soreness in joints, neck, or shoulders were reported more frequently in women with a body mass index of 27 kg/m^2 or greater compared with women with a body mass index of 19 to 26.9 kg/m^2 (or less). This relation was particularly marked for urine leakage, for which prevalence increased more than twofold for women with a body mass index of 32 kg/m^2 or greater. However, hot flashes or night sweats were not associated with an increased body mass index in postmenopausal and late perimenopausal women (data not shown).

Smoking. Past smoking and current smoking were related to prevalence of most symptoms, except vaginal dryness and forgetfulness (the latter being positively

Table 25.3. Adjusted Prevalence Odds Ratios for Each Symptom by Selected Characteristics, SWAN, 1995–1997

Characteristic	Hot Flashes/Night Sweats (n = 4,324) (OR)[b]	(95% CI)[b]	Urine Leakage (n = 2,135) (OR)	(95% CI)	Vaginal Dryness (n = 1,629) (OR)	(95% CI)	Stiff/Sore (n = 6,620) (OR)	(95% CI)	Heart Pounding[a] (n = 2,315) (OR)	(95% CI)	Forgetful[a] (n = 4,843) (OR)	(95% CI)	Difficulty Sleeping[a] (n = 4,632) (OR)	(95% CI)
Age (years)														
40–43[c]	1.00		1.00		1.00		1.00		1.00		1.00		1.00	
44–47	1.26	1.13, 1.41	1.13	0.99, 1.29	1.26	1.08, 1.48	1.01	0.92, 1.11	1.07	0.94, 1.21	1.33	1.20, 1.48	0.94	0.84, 1.04
48–51	1.68	1.49, 1.89	1.27	1.10, 1.46	1.65	1.40, 1.95	1.12	1.00, 1.24	0.91	0.79, 1.06	1.62	1.44, 1.83	1.08	0.96, 1.21
52 or over	1.49	1.27, 1.72	1.17	0.98, 1.39	1.63	1.34, 1.98	1.07	0.94, 1.23	1.11	0.92, 1.33	1.52	1.31, 1.76	1.00	0.86, 1.17
Education														
Less than 12 years	1.76	1.45, 2.13	1.10	0.88, 1.38	1.25	0.97, 1.60	1.04	0.87, 1.23	1.69	1.33, 2.15	1.25	1.03, 1.50	0.92	0.76, 1.12
12/GED[b]	1.76	1.45, 2.13	0.92	0.78, 1.12	1.09	0.88, 1.35	0.92	0.80, 1.05	1.48	1.21, 1.82	1.00	0.92, 1.25	0.84	0.72, 0.98
Some college	1.54	1.32, 1.80	0.97	0.81, 1.16	1.09	0.89, 1.34	0.98	0.86, 1.11	1.33	1.09, 1.63	0.98	0.85, 1.13	0.96	0.83, 1.11
College graduate	1.15	0.98, 1.35	0.98	0.81, 1.19	0.97	0.78, 1.22	1.02	0.89, 1.16	1.26	1.02, 1.55	0.92	0.79, 1.07	0.88	0.76, 1.03
Postgraduate/professional[c]	1.00		1.00		1.00		1.00		1.00		1.00		1.00	
Employed														
No	1.09	0.97, 1.22	1.11	0.96, 1.27	1.04	0.89, 1.22	0.97	0.88, 1.08	1.10	0.95, 1.26	1.12	1.00, 1.26	1.06	0.95, 1.19
Part time	1.06	0.97, 1.22	1.04	0.93, 1.18	1.03	0.90, 1.17	0.96	0.88, 1.06	1.12	0.99, 1.26	1.08	0.98, 1.20	1.22	1.05, 1.30
Full time[c]	1.00		1.00		1.00		1.00		1.00		1.00		1.00	
Difficulty paying for basics														
Very hard	1.47	1.29, 1.68	1.52	1.30, 1.77	1.48	1.24, 1.75	1.77	1.56, 2.02	1.38	1.18, 1.61	1.51	1.32, 173	1.52	1.32, 1.74
Somewhat hard	1.21	1.10, 1.32	1.19	1.06, 1.27	1.12	0.99, 1.27	1.23	1.13, 1.33	1.09	0.97, 1.22	1.26	1.14, 1.38	1.20	1.09, 1.31
Not at all hard[c]	1.00		1.00		1.00		1.00		1.00		1.00		1.00	

Race/ethnicity														
African American	1.56	1.39, 1.75	0.64	0.55, 0.73	1.17	1.00, 1.37	0.84	0.75, 0.93	1.10	0.95, 1.27	1.42	1.27, 1.60	0.70	0.62, 0.79
Japanese	0.63	0.49, 0.82	0.84	0.62, 1.16	0.70	0.47, 1.02	0.96	0.78, 1.18	1.07	0.77, 1.48	1.50	1.19, 1.89	0.71	0.56, 0.91
Chinese	0.65	0.49, 0.87	0.56	0.40, 0.79	0.80	0.54, 1.17	0.84	0.66, 1.08	1.22	0.86, 1.73	1.63	1.24, 2.12	0.80	0.61, 1.05
Hispanic	1.10	0.93, 1.31	1.26	1.02, 1.56	1.85	1.48, 2.33	0.81	0.69, 0.95	1.43	1.17, 1.74	1.50	1.26, 1.78	0.76	0.63, 0.90
Caucasian[c]	1.00		1.00		1.00		1.00		1.00		1.00		1.00	
Marital status														
Never married	0.84	0.74, 0.96	0.82	0.69, 0.96	0.62	0.52, 0.75	0.97	0.86, 1.09	1.13	0.96, 1.33	0.95	0.83, 1.08	1.04	0.91, 1.18
Married/living as[c]	1.00		1.00		1.00		1.00		1.00		1.00		1.00	
Separated	1.11	0.91, 1.30	1.24	1.01, 1.52	0.90	0.72, 1.13	1.12	0.94, 1.33	1.16	0.94, 1.42	0.91	0.76, 1.09	1.30	1.08, 1.56
Widowed	0.76	0.62, 0.93	0.96	0.75, 1.22	0.54	0.40, 0.72	0.93	0.77, 1.13	1.16	0.91, 1.48	1.02	0.83, 1.25	1.09	0.88, 1.34
Divorced	0.85	0.76, 0.96	0.97	0.84, 1.11	0.62	0.53, 0.74	1.00	0.90, 1.12	1.07	0.92, 1.22	1.11	0.98, 1.24	1.07	0.95, 1.21
Parity (per child)	0.98	0.95, 1.01	1.07	1.03, 1.10	1.00	0.96, 1.04	0.98	0.96, 1.01	1.08	1.04, 1.12	1.06	1.03, 1.09	0.97	0.94, 1.00
Menstrual status														
Surgical	2.40	2.11, 2.73	1.64	1.41, 1.92	2.39	2.00, 2.85	1.50	1.33, 1.69	1.43	1.22, 1.68	1.27	1.11, 1.44	1.52	1.33, 1.74
Postmenopausal	2.81	2.43, 3.24	1.24	1.04, 1.49	2.57	2.12, 3.12	1.31	1.14, 1.50	1.17	0.97, 1.40	1.28	1.11, 1.49	1.37	1.18, 1.60
Late perimenopausal	4.32	3.58, 5.21	1.42	1.12, 1.79	2.30	1.80, 2.96	1.48	1.24, 1.78	1.29	1.20, 1.64	1.43	1.18, 1.74	1.48	1.22, 1.80
Early perimenopausal	2.06	1.86, 2.29	1.67	1.48, 1.90	1.77	1.52, 2.07	1.48	1.35, 1.62	1.19	1.05, 1.35	1.44	1.30, 1.59	1.25	1.13, 1.38
Premenopausal[c]	1.00		1.00		1.00		1.00		1.00		1.00		1.00	
Body mass index (kg/m^2)														
Below–19	0.94	0.79, 1.12	1.04	0.84, 1.29	0.90	0.71, 1.14	1.14	0.98, 1.32	0.98	0.80, 1.21	1.08	0.91, 1.28	1.19	1.00, 1.41
19–26.9[c]	1.0		1.0		1.0		1.0		1.0		1.0		1.0	
27–31.9	1.15	1.04, 1.28	1.42	1.25, 1.62	0.93	0.81, 1.07	1.19	1.08, 1.31	1.01	0.89, 1.15	1.08	0.97, 1.20	0.97	0.87, 1.08
32 or more	1.18	1.05, 1.32	2.18	1.92, 2.48	1.01	0.87, 1.17	1.53	1.38, 1.70	1.05	0.92, 1.21	0.99	0.88, 1.11	1.05	0.93, 1.17

(Continued)

Table 25.3. Adjusted Prevalence Odds Ratios for Each Symptom by Selected Characteristics, SWAN, 1995–1997 (Continued)

Characteristic	Hot Flashes/ Night Sweats (n = 4,324) (OR)[b]	(95% CI)[b]	Urine Leakage (n = 2,135) (OR)	(95% CI)	Vaginal Dryness (n = 1,629) (OR)	(95% CI)	Stiff/Sore (n = 6,620) (OR)	(95% CI)	Heart Pounding[a] (n = 2,315) (OR)	(95% CI)	Forgetful[a] (n = 4,843) (OR)	(95% CI)	Difficulty Sleeping[a] (n = 4,632) (OR)	(95% CI)
Smoking														
Never[c]	1.0		1.0		1.0		1.0		1.0		1.0		1.0	
Past	1.24	1.12, 1.37	1.21	1.08, 1.37	1.07	0.93, 1.22	1.24	1.13, 1.36	1.25	1.11, 1.52	1.18	1.07, 1.31	1.04	0.94, 1.16
Current														
Less than 10 cigarettes/ day	1.50	1.28, 1.76	0.97	0.78, 1.20	0.85	0.67, 1.07	1.16	0.99, 1.35	1.23	1.00, 1.50	0.76	0.64, 0.91	1.19	1.01, 1.41
10–19/day	1.65	1.42, 1.92	1.15	0.95, 1.39	1.04	0.85, 1.29	1.15	0.99, 1.33	1.14	0.95, 1.37	0.82	0.70, 0.96	1.23	1.05, 1.44
20 or more cigarettes/ day	1.68	1.46, 1.94	1.50	1.27, 1.77	0.96	0.79, 1.18	1.23	1.07, 1.41	1.16	0.98, 1.38	0.92	0.79, 1.06	1.17	1.01, 1.35
Physical activity														
Much less	1.71	1.42, 2.07	1.66	1.34, 2.06	1.64	1.29, 2.08	2.33	1.92, 2.82	1.65	1.33, 2.05	1.51	1.24, 1.84	2.00	1.64, 2.43
Somewhat less	1.33	1.16, 1.54	1.36	1.14, 1.61	1.24	1.02, 1.50	1.78	1.56, 2.03	1.34	1.13, 1.59	1.30	1.13, 1.51	1.65	1.43, 1.91
Same	0.96	0.85, 1.08	1.03	0.88, 1.18	1.02	0.87, 1.20	1.12	1.00, 1.23	1.00	0.86, 1.16	1.12	1.00, 1.26	1.06	0.94, 1.20
Some more	1.02	0.90, 1.16	1.03	0.88, 1.21	1.03	0.86, 1.24	1.09	0.97, 1.22	0.97	0.82, 1.15	0.96	0.84, 1.09	1.09	0.96, 1.24
Much more[c]	1.0		1.0		1.0		1.0		1.0		1.0		1.0	

Note: Each covariate adjusted for all others as well as for site; with parity, adjusted as a continuous variable.

[a]Forgetful and heart pounding/racing also adjusted for irritability, depression, and tense/anxious; difficulty sleeping adjusted for these and any other symptoms.

[b]OR, odds ratio; CI, confidence interval; GED, high school equivalency.

[c]Referent category.

related only to past smoking). No clear trends with amount currently smoked were observed.

Physical Activity. All symptoms (particularly stiffness or soreness, heart pounding or racing, forgetfulness, and difficulty sleeping) were more frequent among women who reported getting less physical activity compared with women who reported getting much more or somewhat more physical activity than women of the same age. A trend appeared of increasing prevalence of these symptoms with decreasing physical activity.

DISCUSSION

The SWAN cross-sectional study is one of the largest multiethnic studies of demographic and lifestyle factors associated with symptom reporting in midlife women, and the findings have potentially important preventive implications. We found significant independent effects of age, educational level, difficulty paying for basics, race/ethnicity, body mass, smoking, physical activity, and menstrual status on the prevalence of vasomotor and other physical symptoms.

Despite the use of quite varied methodologies, in numerous cross-sectional studies of clinical, psychosocial, and sociodemographic factors associated with the menopausal transition in Caucasian women, a few major findings have emerged. First, vasomotor symptoms, such as hot flashes or flushes and night sweats, are unequivocally linked to hormonal changes (Wilbur and others, 1998; Greene, 1992; World Health Organization, 1981). Longitudinal studies have largely confirmed the relation between vasomotor symptoms and the climacteric (Matthews and others, 1994; World Health Organization, 1981; Holte, 1992; Hunter, 1992; McKinlay, Brambilla, and Posner, 1992), and reports of vasomotor symptoms at peri- or postmenopause have been found to be inversely related to the level of serum estrogens (Matthews and others, 1994; Wilbur and others, 1998). Menopause and reduction in endogenous estrogen levels result in atrophic changes of epithelial tissues including the skin and vaginal wall (Jaszman, 1973). Other symptoms, such as sleep difficulties, are less consistently associated with menopausal status (Hunter, Battersby, and Whitehead, 1986; Kuh, Wadsworth, and Hardy, 1997; McKinlay and Jeffreys, 1974; Sharma and Saxena, 1981; Thompson, Hart, and Durno, 1973). Further, a subset of women with low socioeconomic status who experience difficulties with personal and social functioning during the climacteric may report more symptoms (Greene, 1992).

Menstrual Status and Age

The results from our study indicate that over half of late perimenopausal women report hot flashes or night sweats. This estimate is in agreement with other studies showing that the occurrence of hot flashes increases with irregularity in menses, peaking at 50 percent just prior to menopause, and later declining in the postmenopause (Avis and McKinlay, 1995). The prevalence of hot flashes in perimenopausal women of Anglo-European origin is reported to be 50 to 85 percent (McKinlay and Jeffreys, 1974; Thompson, Hart, and Durno, 1973).

The prevalence of vaginal dryness in the present study was 13.1 percent, in agreement with several studies (Hagstad and Janson, 1986; Hammar, Berg, and Lindgren, 1990; O'Connor, and others, 1995; Oldenhave, Jaszman, and Haspels, 1993). However, in a cross-sectional study of 5,990 Swedish women, aged 46 to 62 years, the prevalence of vaginal dryness was 21 percent, with prevalence increasing with age to about 34 percent in 62-year-old women (Stadberg, Mattsson, and Milsom, 1997). Wilbur and others (1998) noted a higher prevalence (29 percent in women aged 35 to 69 years), with the wider age range than our population possibly accounting for the higher prevalence. Another limitation of previous work, however, is using age as a surrogate for menstrual status, whereas this study used reported bleeding patterns.

Socioeconomic Status

In this study, lower educational attainment and greater difficulty paying for basics were related to increased symptom prevalence. In addition, lack of full-time employment was associated with heart pounding or racing, forgetfulness, and difficulty sleeping. These findings are consistent with those of a number of others (Wilbur and others, 1998; Kuh, Wadsworth, and Hardy, 1997; Schwingl, Hulka, and Harlow, 1994; Avis, Crawford, and McKinlay, 1997).

Race/Ethnicity

The prevalence of vasomotor symptoms in developed countries in largely Caucasian populations has previously been examined in cross-sectional (Jaszman, 1973; McKinlay and Jeffreys, 1974; Oldenhave, Jaszman, and Haspels, 1993; Stadberg, Mattsson, and Milsom, 1997; Lindgren and others, 1993) and prospective (Hunter, 1992; McKinlay, Brambilla, and Posner, 1992) studies, with considerable variability in results. The finding in this study that more African American women reported hot flashes or night sweats than Caucasian women (37 percent versus 24 percent) is of interest. In a study of Caucasian and African American women from a population-based study of reproductive cancers, 71 percent of participants reported experiencing hot flashes at menopause, with no racial differences in prevalence (Schwingl, Hulka, and Harlow, 1994). Our finding of increased reporting of vaginal dryness in African-American women also differs from recent unadjusted findings by Wilbur and others (1998), which also indicate an increased risk of urine leakage in African American women, while we found a reduced prevalence of this symptom in this group compared with Caucasians. Also of interest in this study, Hispanic women reported the highest prevalence of vaginal dryness. Asian women (Lock, 1991; Lindgren and others, 1993; Chompootweep and others, 1993; Goodman, Stewart, and Gilbert, 1997; Haines, Chung, and Leung, 1994) report fewer hot flashes than do Caucasian women. Because of simultaneous adjustment of multiple variables in this study, differences among race/ethnic groups in these other variables (for example, body mass index or smoking) do not account for differences in symptom reporting among the groups.

Body Mass Index

In this study, women with a body mass index of at least 32 kg/m^2 had a greater prevalence of hot flashes or night sweats (43.8 percent) than did those having a body mass index of less than 19 kg/m^2 (30.6 percent). A higher body mass index has been associated with increased symptom reporting during the menopausal transition in one study (DenTonkelaar, Seidell, and vanNoord, 1996) and with fewer hot flashes in other studies (Schwingl, Hulka, and Harlow, 1994; Campagnoli and others, 1981; Erlik, Meldrum, and Judd, 1982). Since adrenal androgens are converted to estrogen in adipose tissue (Hershcopf and Bradlow, 1987), and since vasomotor symptoms are thought to be related to reduced estrogen levels, a lower prevalence of vasomotor symptoms is expected in heavier women. The reasons for the findings are unclear. Possibly the rate (and steepness) of the decline in or the widely fluctuating levels of estradiol (Santoro and others, 1996) may affect symptoms more than absolute levels (which would be associated with body weight). Differences in study design (cross-sectional versus prospective), sample size, methods in ascertaining body mass index (self-report versus direct measurement), and simultaneous control of covariates (especially smoking) may also account for discrepant findings.

Smoking

Past smoking and current smoking were positively associated in this study with prevalence of vasomotor symptoms, in agreement with most but not all (Schwingl, Hulka, and Harlow, 1994) others (Dennerstein and others, 1993; Hunter, 1993; Leidy, 1990; Hart and others, 1976). Women who smoke would be expected to have a higher prevalence of vasomotor symptoms because of the antiestrogenic effects of smoking (Lindquist and Bengtsson, 1979; Michnovicz and others, 1986; Guthrie and others, 1995); however, the lack of association of smoking with vaginal dryness is thus unexpected, suggesting that other factors may be more important in the occurrence of vaginal dryness. We did observe that vaginal dryness was significantly less often reported among never married, widowed, or divorced women compared with married women, suggesting that opportunity for sexual activity may be related to reporting of vaginal dryness.

Physical Activity

In contrast to this study, previous cross-sectional surveys have generally failed to find any association between physical activity and vasomotor symptoms (Hunter, 1993; Slaven and Lee, 1997; Sternfeld, Quesenberry, and Husson, 1999; Wilbur and others, 1990; Wilbur, Holm, and Dan, 1992). One study reported a lower prevalence of hot flashes among regularly active perimenopausal women compared with population controls whose activity level was not determined (Hammar, Berg, and Lindgren, 1990). The inconsistency between the present findings and those of previous investigations may be due in part to the assessment method. This study asked about the respondent's perception of activity level but not what she actually did. This may predispose women who are having more symptoms to perceive themselves as less active than their peers. Alternatively, previous studies, with more limited sample sizes, may not have had the statistical power of this study to detect significant relations between activity and vasomotor symptoms. Most cross-sectional surveys have observed fewer somatic symptoms (Slaven and Lee, 1997) and better health status (Sternfeld, Quesenberry, and Husson, 1999; Wilbur, Holm, and Dan, 1992) in active women compared with sedentary women. Given the cross-sectional design of all of these studies, it is not possible to determine whether women feel better because they are active or are less active because they are symptomatic.

Limitations of This Study

This study was cross-sectional. Thus, for certain variables, such as body mass index and physical activity, we could not be certain that the factor actually preceded and thus predisposed to the occurrence of symptoms. However, a number of the factors (for example, education, parity, and smoking) were unlikely to have changed recently for most women and thus were likely to have preceded symptom reporting. Nonetheless, the temporal sequence of these associations will be better established in the next phase of SWAN, the longitudinal study.

Another limitation is self-reporting, particularly of symptoms, body mass index, and menstrual status. The use of standard questions for these items enhances the comparability of these results with those of prior studies. Again, however, these assessments will be improved in longitudinal assessment and correlation with biologic measures of endocrine status in the next phase of SWAN.

A third limitation is the varied sampling methods used among sites, necessitated by difficulties in achieving needed sample size of minority populations, making use of formal estimation procedures inappropriate. Thus, the confidence intervals reported here should be interpreted with caution.

A final limitation is the potential for inadequate detail on variables of interest and inadequate control of potential confounding factors. In this limited interview, it was not possible to examine all such potential factors. In particular, more detailed questions could not be asked about both symptoms (for example, nature of headaches and difficulty with sleep) and additional risk factors, such as diet, nature of occupation, income, pack-years of smoking, and nature and intensity of physical activity. Thus, uncontrolled confounding and insufficient detail are potential limitations that will be better addressed in the SWAN longitudinal study.

Strengths of This Study

This is the first study to have large numbers of women at various stages of the menopausal transition and from five race/ethnic groups. Women were selected to be generally representative of their racial/ethnic group in their geographic area and came from several geographic areas in the United States. Thus, these results should apply to a large segment of women in this age group in this country. In addition, the use of standardized methods of data collection over several geographic areas is an important strength. Finally, the effects of each variable were examined while controlling for many others.

The results of the SWAN cross-sectional survey indicate that a number of potentially modifiable factors affect symptom reporting. Thus, for women for whom medical treatment is contraindicated, undesired, or not tolerated, alternatives may be offered in lifestyle changes. In particular, smoking cessation was associated with lower prevalence than in current smokers of vasomotor symptoms and difficulty sleeping. Increased physical activity was associated with lower prevalence of virtually all symptoms. Overweight was associated with hot flashes/night sweats, urine leakage, and stiffness or soreness. All of these factors are, of course, also associated with a number of other adverse health effects. Our results also provide guidance to health care providers in assessing symptoms by increasing their sensitivity to differences in symptom-reporting patterns by race/ethnicity and menstrual status. Importantly, our results also show that most indicators of low socioeconomic status, particularly low educational level and difficulty paying for basics, were associated with significantly increased reporting of almost all symptoms.

References

Avis, N. E., Crawford, S., and McKinlay, S. "Psychosocial, Behavioral, and Health Factors Related to Menopause Symptomatology." *Journal of Women's Health*, 1997, *3*, 103–120.

Avis, N. E., and McKinlay, S. M. "A Longitudinal Analysis of Women's Attitudes Toward the Menopause: Results from the Massachusetts Women's Health Study." *Maturitas*, 1991, *13*, 65–79.

Avis, N. E., and McKinlay, S. M. "The Massachusetts Women's Health Study: An Epidemiologic Investigation of the Menopause." *Journal of the American Women's Medical Society,* 1995, *50,* 45–49.

Avis, N. E., and others. "Is There a Menopausal Syndrome? Menopausal Status and Symptoms Across Ethnic Groups." *Social Science and Medicine,* forthcoming.

Bromberger, J. T., and others. "Psychologic Distress and Natural Menopause: A Multiethnic Community Study." *American Journal of Public Health,* 2001, *91*(9), 1435–1442.

Campagnoli, C., and others. "Climacteric Symptoms According to Body Weight in Women of Different Socio-Economic Groups." *Maturitas,* 1981, *3,* 279–287.

Chompootweep, S., and others. "The Menopausal Age and Climacteric Complaints in Thai Women in Bangkok." *Maturitas,* 1993, *17,* 63–71.

Dennerstein, L., and others. "Menopausal Symptoms in Australian Women." *Medical Journal of Australia,* 1993, *159,* 232–236.

DenTonkelaar, I., Seidell, J., and vanNoord, P. "Obesity and Fat Distribution in Relation to Hot Flashes in Dutch Women from the DOM Project." *Maturitas,* 1996, *23,* 301–305.

Erlik, Y., Meldrum, D. R., and Judd, H. L. "Estrogen Levels in Postmenopausal Women with Hot Flashes." *Obstetrics and Gynecology,* 1982, *59,* 403–407.

Ferris, B. G. "Epidemiology Standardization Project (American Thoracic Society)." American Review of Respiratory *Diseases,* 1978, *118,* 1–120.

Gist, Y. J., and Velkoff, V. A. *Gender and Aging. Demographic Dimensions.* Washington, D.C.: U.S. Department of Commerce, Economics and Statistics Administration, 1997.

Goodman, M. J., Stewart, C. J., and Gilbert, F. "Patterns of Menopause: A Study of Certain Medical and Physiological Variables Among Caucasian and Japanese Women Living in Hawaii." *Journal of Gerontology,* 1997, *32,* 291–298.

Greene, J. G. "The Cross-Sectional Legacy: An Introduction to Longitudinal Studies of the Climacteric." *Maturitas,* 1992, *14,* 95–101.

Guthrie, J. R., and others. "Physical Activity and the Menopause Experience: A Cross-Sectional Study." *Maturitas,* 1995, *20,* 71–80.

Hagstad, A., and Janson, P. O. "The Epidemiology of Climacteric Symptoms." *Acta Obstetrica et Gynecologica Scandinavica,* 1986, *134,* 59–65.

Haines, C. J., Chung, T. K., and Leung, D. H. "A Prospective Study of the Frequency of Acute Menopausal Symptoms in Hong Kong Chinese Women." *Maturitas,* 1994, *18,* 175–181.

Hammar, M., Berg, G., and Lindgren, R. "Does Physical Exercise Influence the Frequency of Postmenopausal Hot Flushes?" *Acta Obstetrica et Gynecologica Scandinavica,* 1990, *69,* 409–412.

Hart, P., and others. "Enhanced Drug Metabolism in Cigarette Smokers." *British Medical Journal,* 1976, *2,* 147–149.

Hershcopf, R., and Bradlow, H. L. "Obesity, Diet, Endogenous Estrogens, and the Risk of Hormone-Sensitive Cancer." *American Journal of Clinical Nutrition,* 1987, *45*(Suppl.), 283–289.

Holte, A. "Influences of Natural Menopause on Health Complaints: A Prospective Study of Healthy Norwegian Women." *Maturitas,* 1992, *14,* 127–141.

Hosmer, D. W., and Lemeshow, S. *Applied Logistic Regression.* New York: Wiley, 1989.

Hunter, M. "The South-East England Longitudinal Study of the Climacteric and Post-menopause." *Maturitas,* 1992, *14,* 117–126.

Hunter, M. S. "Predictors of Menopausal Symptoms: Psychosocial Aspects." *Baillieres Clinical Endocrinology and Metabolism,* 1993, *7,* 33–45.

Hunter, M., Battersby, R., and Whitehead, M. "Relationships Between Psychological Symptoms, Somatic Complaints, and Menopausal Status." *Maturitas,* 1986, *8,* 217–228.

Jaszman, L. "Epidemiology of Climacteric and Post-Climacteric Complaints: Ageing and Estrogens." *Front Hormone Research,* 1973, *2,* 22–34.

Kaufert, P. A. "The Social and Cultural Context of Menopause." *Maturitas,* 1996, *23,* 169–180.

Kuh, D. L., Wadsworth, M., and Hardy, R. "Women's Health in Midlife: The Influence of the Menopause, Social Factors and Health in Earlier Life." *British Journal of Obstetrics and Gynaecology,* 1997, *104,* 923–933.

Leidy, L. "Comparison of Body Size and Age of Menopause Between Mexican-American and White American Women." *Annals of the New York Academy of Science,* 1990, *592,* 443–444.

Lindgren, R., and others. "Hormonal Replacement Therapy and Sexuality in a Population of Swedish Postmenopausal Women." *Acta Obstetrica et Gynecologica Scandinavica,* 1993, *72,* 292–297.

Lindquist, O., and Bengtsson, C. "Menopausal Age in Relation to Smoking." *Acta Medical Scandinavica,* 1979, *205,* 73–77.

Lock, M. "Contested Meanings of the Menopause." *Lancet,* 1991, *337,* 1270–1272.

Lock, M., Kaufert, P., and Gilbert, P. "Cultural Construction of the Menopausal Syndrome: The Japanese Case." *Maturitas,* 1988, *10,* 317–322.

Manson, J. E., and others. "Body Weight and Mortality Among Women." *New England Journal of Medicine,* 1995, *333,* 677–685.

Matthews, K. A., and others. "Influence of the Peri-Menopause on Cardiovascular Risk Factors and Symptoms of Middle-Aged Healthy Women." *Archives of Internal Medicine,* 1994, *154,* 2349–2355.

McKinlay, S. M., Brambilla, D. J., and Posner, J. G. "The Normal Menopause Transition." *American Journal of Human Biology,* 1992, *4,* 37–46.

McKinlay, S. M., and Jeffreys, M. "The Menopausal Syndrome." *British Journal of Preventive Social Medicine,* 1974, *28,* 108–115.

Michnovicz, J., and others. "Increased 2-Hydroxylation of Estradiol as a Possible Mechanism for the Anti-Estrogenic Effect of Cigarette Smoking." *New England Journal of Medicine,* 1986, *315,* 1305–1309.

Neugarten, B. L., and Kraines, R. J. "Menopausal Symptoms in Women of Various Ages." *Psychosomatic Medicine,* 1965, *2,* 266–273.

O'Connor, V. M., and others. "Do Psychosocial Factors Contribute More to Symptom Reporting by Middle-Aged Women Than Hormonal Status?" *Maturitas*, 1995, *20*, 63–69.

Oldenhave, A., Jaszman, L. J., and Haspels, A. A. "Impact of Climacteric on Well-Being: A Survey Based on 5213 Women, 39 to 60 Years Old." *American Journal of Obstetrics and Gynecology*, 1993, *168*, 772–780.

Santoro, N., and others. "Characterization of Reproductive Hormone Dynamics in the Perimenopause." *Journal of Clinical Epidemiology and Metabolism*, 1996, *81*, 1495–501.

SAS Institute. SAS proprietary software, release 6.07 ed. Cary, N.C.: SAS Institute, 1989.

Schwingl, P. J., Hulka, B. S., and Harlow, S. D. "Risk Factors for Menopausal Hot Flashes." *Obstetrics and Gynecology*, 1994, *84*, 29–34.

Sharma, V., and Saxena, M. "Climacteric Symptoms." *Maturitas*, 1981, *3*, 11–20.

Skolnick, A. A. "At Third Meeting, Menopause Experts Make the Most of Insufficient Data." *JAMA*, 1992, *268*, 2483–2485.

Slaven, L., and Lee, C. "Mood and Symptom Reporting Among Middle-Aged Women: The Relationship Between Menopausal Status, Hormone Replacement Therapy, and Exercise Participation." *Health Psychology*, 1997, *16*, 203–208.

Sowers, M. F., and others. "SWAN: A Multi-Center, Multi-Ethnic, Community-Based Cohort Study of Women and the Menopausal Transition." In R. A. Lobos, J. Kelsey, and R. Marcus (eds.), *Menopause: Biology and Pathobiology*. Orlando, Fla.: Academic Press, 2000.

Stadberg, E., Mattsson, L. A., and Milsom, I. "The Prevalence and Severity of Climacteric Symptoms and the Use of Different Treatment Regimens in a Swedish Population." *Acta Obstetrica et Gynecologica Scandinavica*, 1997, *76*, 442–448.

Sternfeld, B., Quesenberry, C. P., Jr., and Husson, G. "Habitual Physical Activity and Menopausal Symptoms: A Case-Control Study." *Journal of Women's Health*, 1999, *8*, 115–123.

Thompson, B., Hart, S. A., and Durno, D. "Menopausal Age and Symptomatology in a General Practice." *Journal of Biosocial Science*, 1973, *5*, 71–82.

Weinstein, M. C., and Tosteson, A. N. "Cost-Effectiveness of Hormone Replacement." *Annals of the New York Academy of Science*, 1990, *592*, 162–172.

Wilbur, J., Holm, K., and Dan, A. "The Relationship of Energy Expenditure to Physical and Psychologic Symptoms in Women at Midlife." *Nursing Outlook*, 1992, *40*, 269–276.

Wilbur, J., and others. "The Relationship Among Menopausal Status, Menopausal Symptoms, and Physical Activity in Midlife Women." *Family and Community Health*, 1990, *13*, 67–78.

Wilbur, J. E., and others. "Socio-Demographic Characteristics, Biological Factors, and Symptom Reporting in Midlife Women. Menopause." *Journal of the North American Menopause Society*, 1998, *5*, 43–51.

World Health Organization. *Research on the Menopause*. Geneva, Switzerland: World Health Organization, 1981.

CHAPTER TWENTY-SIX

Lesbian Women of Color

Triple Jeopardy

Beverly Greene

This well-conceived overview addresses a topic that is all but absent from the literature and the attention of researchers and service providers. Based on an in-depth review of the literature, the author presents and describes a variety of cultural factors that affect the lives of lesbian women of color: African American, Black American of Caribbean descent, Latina, Asian American, Native American, and South Asian. She discusses the special problems and unique challenges that these women face and identifies approaches to treating lesbian women of color.

The professional literature on mental health has in recent years significantly expanded its inquiry into the roles of culture, ethnicity, gender, and sexual orientation in mental health, and the delivery of psychological services to women. This inquiry has included closer scrutiny into the impact of racism, sexism, heterocentric bias, and the factors associated with them on the psychological development of women of color, and thus on the process of assessment and treatment. The literature of professional psychology in these areas has slowly begun to reflect the appropriate exploration of the effects of membership in institutionally oppressed and disparaged groups on the development of both psychological resilience and psychological vulnerability, and has done so from a wide range of perspectives (Greene, 1990a). Lesbian women of color, however, often still find themselves and their concerns invisible in the scholarly research of both women of color and of lesbians.

The author thanks Nancy Boyd-Franklin, Connie Chan, Lillian Comas-Diaz, Vickie Sears, and Judith White for their helpful comments and discussions during the preparation of this chapter. This work is dedicated to the memory of Dr. F. Kitch Childs (1937–1993) and Andre Lorde (1934–1992).

This chapter includes African American, Black American of Caribbean descent, Latina, Asian American, Native American, and Indian women in the designation "women of color." Those who consider that their primary romantic and sexual attractions are to women are considered lesbian. Hence, women from the aforementioned ethnic minority groups who consider themselves lesbians will be the group referred to in this chapter as lesbian women of color. Clearly, there are lesbians from other ethnic minority groups who could also be considered lesbian women of color and to whom many of the statements made in this chapter could apply. The observations made here, however, are limited in their generalizability to the groups mentioned. The absence of specific mention of the others is not intended to suggest that their concerns are of lesser significance; rather, I have limited this discussion to those groups about whom there are clinical, empirical, or anecdotal studies available.

The vast majority of clinical and empirical research on or with lesbians is conducted with overwhelmingly White, middle-class respondents (Amaro, 1978; Chan, 1989, 1992; Gock, 1985, 1992; Greene, 1996; Mays and Cochran, 1988; Mays, Cochran, and Rhue, forthcoming; Morales, 1989; Tremble, Schneider, and Appathurai, 1989; Wooden, Kawasaki, and Mayeda, 1983). Similarly, the scant research on women of color rarely, if ever, acknowledges that not all of the groups' members are heterosexual. Hence, there is no exploration of the complex interaction between sexual orientation and ethnic and gender identity development. Nor does the literature take into account the realistic and social psychological tasks and stressors that are a component of lesbian identity formation for women who are members of visible ethnic minority groups. An exploration of the vicissitudes of racism, sexism, homophobia, same-gender socialization, and their effects on the couple relationships of lesbians of color is another important but neglected area of scrutiny.

Empirical and clinical research on lesbians and on women of color rarely states that their generalizability is limited to heterosexual women of color and lesbians who are White. This practice can inadvertently lead readers of these studies to assume that findings that are applicable to women in these groups are equally applicable to lesbians of color or that the concerns of lesbians of color do not warrant specific attention in the mental health literature. Such narrow clinical and research perspectives leave us with a limited understanding of the diversity of women of color and of lesbians as a group. Another more serious consequence of such omissions is that practitioners are left ill equipped to address, in culturally sensitive and literate ways, the clinical needs of lesbians who are also stigmatized by their racial or ethnic identity.

A note of caution: broad descriptions of cultural practices or values in this chapter should not be applied with uniformity to all lesbian women of color or to all lesbians in any specific cultural or ethnic group. There are significant differences between the experiences and realities of lesbians of color and their

White counterparts, but there is also great diversity within groups of lesbians from specific cultures and races. Clients should not be made to fit arbitrarily into preconceived notions of what all of the women of a group must be like. For example, lesbians who are Latina come from many different countries, with different languages and often many different cultural norms. Asian lesbians come from similarly diverse geographical regions and cultural backgrounds and speak different languages, as do their Indian and Native American counterparts. In these examples, the group's label conceals many different subgroups and distinct cultures. Furthermore, within each subgroup, distinctive differences may be found between lesbians from rural and urban environments as well as between lesbians from various socioeconomic and educational backgrounds within an ethnic culture.

Just as the experience of sexism is "colored" by the lens of race and ethnicity for women of color, so is the experience of heterosexism similarly filtered for lesbian women of color. This chapter provides practitioners with a framework from which to begin looking at lesbians and women of color from a more diverse perspective and at lesbians of color with greater cultural sensitivity. Its aim is to assist in sensitizing practitioners to cultural factors bearing significantly on the ways that lesbian women of color perceive the world, the unique tasks and stressors they must manage on a routine basis, and mental health and therapy issues. It is necessary, however, for practitioners to explore every client's plight with an understanding of the client's own unique perspective of her cultural heritage, sexual orientation, and the respective significance of these in her life.

THE CONDITIONS OF TRIPLE JEOPARDY

The underpinnings of traditional approaches to psychology are riddled with androcentric, heterocentric, and ethnocentric biases (Garnets and Kimmel, 1991; Glassgold, 1992; Greene, 1993a), thus reinforcing the triple discrimination lesbians of color face in the world at large. Heterocentric thinking often leads both professional and lay persons to make a range of inaccurate and unexamined but commonly held assumptions about lesbians. These assumptions are maintained to varying extents within ethnic minority groups as much as they are in the dominant culture. Among many commonly accepted and fallacious notions is that women who are lesbians want to be men, are "mannish" in appearance (Taylor, 1983), are unattractive or less attractive than heterosexual women (Dew, 1985), are less extroverted (Kite, 1994), are unable to get a man, have had traumatic relationships with men that presumably "turned" them against men, or are defective females (Christian, 1985; Collins, 1990; Greene, 1994; Kite, 1994). Members of ethnic minority groups, like their counterparts in the dominant culture, believe that sexual attraction to men is embedded in the definition of what it means to be a normal woman. Acceptance of this assumption often leads to a range of equally inaccurate conclusions. One is that reproductive sexuality is the only form of sexual expression that is psychologically normal and morally correct (Garnets and Kimmel, 1991; Glassgold, 1992). Another incorrect assumption is that there is a direct relationship between sexual orientation and a woman's conformity or lack thereof to traditional gender roles and physical appearance within the culture (Kite and Deaux, 1987; Newman, 1989; Whitley, 1987). The mistaken conclusions that follow are twofold. One is that women who do not conform to traditional gender-role stereotypes must be lesbian. The equally mistaken corollary to this is that those who do conform to such stereotypes must be heterosexual. These assumptions are used in many cultures to threaten women with the stigma of being labeled lesbian if they fail to adhere to traditional gender-role stereotypes in which males are dominant and females are submissive (Collins, 1990; Gomez and Smith, 1990; Smith, 1982).

The fear of being labeled a lesbian can be used to prevent women who fear it, whether they are lesbian or not, from seeking nontraditional roles or engaging in nontraditional behaviors. Shockley (1979) suggests that the fear of being labeled lesbian has been strong enough to have deterred Black women writers from examining lesbian themes in their writing. In an atmosphere of tenacious homophobia within ethnic minority groups as well as within the dominant culture, some scholars who are also women of color feel that simply writing about or acknowledging such themes will raise questions about their own sexual orientation (Clarke, 1991). In a patriarchal society, in which male dominance and female subordination has been viewed as normative, threats of being labeled lesbian, fears of that label, and its realistic negative social consequences may be used in the service of maintaining inequitable patterns in the distribution of power.

ASSESSMENT OF RELEVANT CULTURAL FACTORS

A range of factors should be considered in determining the impact of ethnic identity, gender, lesbian sexual orientation, and the ongoing dynamic interaction of these with one another in the course of a woman's development. An understanding of the meaning and the reality of being a woman of color who is lesbian requires a careful exploration and understanding of these factors. These factors include the nature and importance of the culture's traditional gender-role stereotypes and their relative fluidity or rigidity, the role and importance of family and community, and the role of religion and spirituality in the culture. Other important factors include the role of racial and ethnic stereotypes, the prevalence of sexism within their minority culture, racism and ethnic discrimination from the larger culture, and the contribution of these to the ethnosexual mythology applied to these women.

For members of some oppressed groups, specifically African Americans and Native Americans, reproductive sexuality is given even greater importance than it is given by other groups because it is the way of continuing the group's presence in the world, when that presence has been historically endangered by racist, genocidal practices. Hence, sexual practice that is not reproductive may be viewed by persons of color as yet another instrument of an oppressive system designed to limit the growth of these groups or to eliminate them altogether. Kanuha (1990) refers to such beliefs as "fears of extinction" (p. 176) and posits that they are used in the service of scapegoating lesbians of color as if they were responsible for threats to the group's survival. It is interesting to note that such fears do not attend to the reality that a lesbian sexual orientation is not synonymous with a disinclination toward having children, particularly among lesbians of color. This does not mean that fears of extinction among persons of color are unwarranted, rather that it is the institutional racism of the dominant culture that places the survival of persons of color at risk, not lesbians or heterosexual women of color who choose not to reproduce. Nonetheless, the internalization of this view can make it more difficult for a lesbian of color to accept affirmatively her sexual orientation. When this internalization occurs, addressing it must be considered a part of the therapeutic work.

In therapy with lesbian clients of color, the family context, that is, the role and expectations of parents in the lives of their children, is an important factor to consider. For example, the extent to which the parents or family of origin may continue to control or influence children, even when they are adults, and the importance of the family as a source of economic and emotional support warrants understanding (Mays and Cochran, 1988). Other factors to consider include the importance of procreation and the continuation of the family line, the importance of ties to the ethnic community, the degree of acculturation or assimilation of the individual client, significant differences between the degree of acculturation of family members and the individual, and the history of discrimination or oppression that the particular group has experienced from individuals and institutions of the dominant culture. When examining the history of discrimination of an ethnic group, it is imperative that group members' own understandings of their oppression and their strategies for coping with discrimination be incorporated into any analysis. A cursory review of only the dominant culture's perspectives on lesbians or women carries the danger of perpetuating ethnocentric, heterocentric, and androcentric biases.

Another important dimension that must be considered is that of sexuality. Sexuality and its meaning is contextual. Therefore, what it means to be a lesbian will be related to the meaning assigned to both gender and sexuality in the individual's culture. Espín (1984) suggests that in most cultures, a range of sexual behaviors is tolerated and that range varies from culture to culture. It is important for the clinician to determine where the client's behavior fits within the spectrum for her particular culture (Espín, 1984). The therapist must also explore the range of sexuality that is sanctioned, in what forms it may be expressed and by whom, as well as the consequences for those who deviate from or conform to such norms. In exploring the range of sexuality tolerated by the woman's culture, it is helpful to determine if there are sexual practices that are formally forbidden but tolerated as long as they are not discussed and not labeled.

It is also important to determine the ethnosexual mythology that has been part of a woman of color's upbringing and its relationship to her understanding of a lesbian sexual orientation. This mythology may include the sexual myths the dominant culture has generated and holds about women of color. Such myths and stereotypes often represent a complex combination of racial and sexual stereotypes designed to objectify women of color, set them apart from their idealized White counterparts, and facilitate their sexual exploitation and control (Collins, 1990; Greene, 1993a; hooks, 1981). The symbolism of these stereotypes and its interaction with stereotypes held about lesbians are important areas of inquiry.

CULTURAL FACTORS IN THE LIVES OF LESBIANS OF COLOR

Immigration and Acculturation

Espín (1987) suggests that the time of and reasons for immigration are important factors in the treatment of Latina lesbians in the United States. In my experience, these factors are also relevant for Black lesbians from the West Indies and Caribbean islands, as well as for other lesbians of color who are members of immigrant groups. In her discussion, Espín (1987) addresses the effect of separation from one's homeland. Such separation often involved leaving significant family members behind (or even perhaps having been left behind for a time) as well as other major changes in the family's lifestyle. A mourning process associated with this type of loss may be normative. Even when entire families immigrate, many persons of color continue to have intense attachment to their birthplace or homeland, often for many years after leaving. Lesbian women of color are no exception. Departures from the country they consider home may be painful in ways that a therapist who is born and raised in the United States, particularly if she or he is a member of the dominant culture, may have difficulty appreciating. Furthermore, just because immigration is voluntary—such as when the client is escaping an oppressive political regime, seeking a place where she may have greater freedom to be open as a lesbian, or seeking work that is unobtainable in her native country—this does not eradicate significant ties to the homeland itself.

If immigration is recent, the lesbian woman of color may have a significant dependence on her family members and members of her ethnic community for emotional and perhaps economic support. This may complicate issues involved in "coming out" or being open about a lesbian sexual orientation. It is particularly problematic if the family, community, or traditional cultural values are perceived or selectively interpreted as rejecting lesbian sexual orientation. New immigrants, if not acculturated, may not yet have contact with a broader lesbian community, or even with lesbians of their own communities. Chan (1989, 1992) writes that the latter tend to be invisible, if they exist at all in Asian and some other ethnic minority communities (Garnets and Kimmel, 1991; H., 1989). Some lesbians from the West Indies and other Caribbean islands have left their native lands because they believe that their sexual orientation will be easier to be open about in the heterogeneity of the United States than it is on small islands with smaller interconnected communities. In such a setting, anonymity is nearly impossible, and discovery is difficult to avoid. Silvera's essay (1991) effectively describes the shroud of secrecy around the existence of lesbians in her native home, Jamaica, as well as the contempt with which they are regarded.

Language

Espín (1984) writes that a bilingual woman's first language may be laden with affective meanings that are not captured in translating the words themselves. Since a language reflects a culture's values, it may contain few or no words for lesbian that are not negative if the culture views lesbian sexual orientations negatively. Espín (1984) suggests that shifts between first (native) and second languages may represent attempts at distancing and estrangement around certain topics in therapy. Espín (1984) observes that a lesbian's second language may be used to express feelings or impulses that are culturally forbidden and that many women would not dare verbalize in their native tongue, which allows them to distance themselves from these feelings. The concept of sexuality is considerably laden with cultural values, and as such it may be revealing if a client shifts from speaking in one language to the other during discussions of this material. It is also worth noting that in cultures where English is spoken fluently by the majority of the population, such as India, some Caribbean islands, and for Native Americans, the second language is not always processed or understood similarly, and the same words do not necessarily have the meaning they do in mainstream America (Tafoya and Rowell, 1988).

Family and Gender Roles

Lesbian women of color (and their heterosexual counterparts) see the family as the primary social unit and as a major source of emotional and material support. The family and the ethnic community provide women of color with an additional and important support, functioning as a refuge and buffer against racism in the dominant culture. Lesbians feel separation and rejection by family and community keenly, and many women will not jeopardize their connections to their families and communities by forming alliances with the broader lesbian community or even by simply divulging the fact that they are lesbians. These observations are true for Latina, African American/Caribbean, Asian American, Indian, South Asian, and Native American lesbians (Allen, 1984, 1986; Amaro, 1978; Boyd-Franklin, 1990; Espín, 1984, 1987; Gock, 1992; Greene, 1986, 1993a; Hidalgo and Hidalgo-Christensen, 1976; Icard, 1986; Mays and Cochran, 1988; Morales, 1989, 1992; Moses and Hawkins, 1982; Vasquez, 1979). The boundaries of the family in many ethnic cultures go beyond that of the nuclear family in Western culture; they extend to persons who are not related by blood but are experienced as though they were. These persons are considered extended family. The complex networks of interdependence and support in these families that include lesbian members should not be seen as undifferentiated by a culturally naïve therapist.

I will discuss characteristic features of negotiating a lesbian sexual orientation within the family and the ethnic community, complicated by the strong family ties that are common in most ethnic cultures. Lesbian women of color tend to perceive that their ethnic communities not only reject lesbian sexual orientations and are antagonistic to women who overtly label themselves as lesbian, but also that they are more tenaciously antagonistic than the dominant culture (Allen, 1984, 1986; Chan, 1987; Croom, 1993; Espín, 1987; Folayan, 1992; Greene, 1990b, 1993a, 1996; Mays and Cochran, 1988; Morales, 1989; Namjoshi, 1992; Poussaint, 1990; Ratti, 1993; Weston, 1991). The perception that antagonism toward lesbians is greater in the ethnic than in the dominant culture is based only on anecdotal reports of lesbians of color about their respective communities. There are no empirical studies to date that systematically assess attitudes toward lesbian sexual orientation in any of these groups.

It is also important to distinguish same-gender sexual behavior that may be known and accepted within a culture from a lesbian identity. Chan (personal communication, Nov. 1992), Espín (1984), Comas-Diaz (personal communication, Jan. 1993) and Jayakar (1994) note that same-gender sexual behavior is known to occur in India, Asian, and Latin cultures between males, but that it is not accompanied by a self-identification as homosexual. It is noteworthy that in same-gender sexual behavior between Latino men, it is the role of the passive or female-identified recipient that is devalued.

In many cultures, same-gender sexual behavior between women may not be defined or adopted by those who engage in such behavior or relationships as lesbian sexual orientation. This may be particularly so in cultures where lesbians are not tolerated, but the behavior is tolerated as long as it is not accompanied by such a label. There may be a sense that the stigmatized identity would only result from adopting the label; such relationships or behavior can be engaged in other ways. This type of strategy may also represent a culturally prescribed way of managing a potential conflict indirectly rather than in direct confrontation with it. This phenomenon can be problematic for the clinician in attempts to determine whether the avoidance of the label has its origins in culturally prescribed methods of managing potential conflicts, culturally distinct or different concepts about what constitutes a lesbian identity, a reflection of internalized homophobia, or all of these elements. Attention to the client's personal history and a familiarity with her cultural norms will be crucial to making such determinations accurately. In many cultures, openly adopting the identity of lesbian or declaring a sexual preference for persons of the same gender is what is most problematic for and unacceptable to family members and heterosexual ethnic peers.

LESBIAN WOMEN OF COLOR: DISTINCT POPULATIONS

African American Lesbians

The legacy of sexual racism plays a role in the response of many African Americans to lesbians in their families and as visible members of their communities. Generally, the African American community is perceived by many of its lesbian members as extremely homophobic and rejecting of lesbians (Croom, 1993; Mays and Cochran, 1988). This rejection increases the pressure on lesbians to remain in the closet and hence invisible in their communities (Clarke, 1983; Collins, 1990; Croom, 1993; Gomez and Smith, 1990; Greene, 1993b, 1996; Icard, 1986; Mays and Cochran, 1988; Mays, Cochran, and Rhue, forthcoming; Poussaint, 1990; Smith, 1982).

Gender roles in African American families have been somewhat more flexible than in those of their White and many of their ethnic minority counterparts. This flexibility is explained in part as a derivative of the value of interdependence among group members and the more egalitarian nature of many pre-colonial African tribes. It is also a function of the need to adapt to racism in the United States. The question then is, How did this homophobia—and particularly that directed toward lesbian sexuality—develop?

African Americans are a diverse group of persons. Their ancestors were unwilling participants in their immigration, as they were the primary objects of the U.S. slave trade (Greene, 1992, 1993a, 1993b, 1996). The roles of African American women, as women, were as pieces of property; forced sexual relationships with African males and White slavemasters were the norm for them. African American women of Caribbean but not Latin descent come from diverse backgrounds in Caribbean islands that were colonized by Great Britain and France; their cultural values and practices may be significantly different from those of African Americans, reflecting the culture of the country responsible for their colonization.

Ethnosexual stereotypes about African American women have their roots in images created by a White society struggling to reconcile a range of contradictions. An elaboration of those contradictions is beyond the scope of this chapter. hooks (1981) proposes that the image of women as castrating was promulgated by psychoanalysis in the 1950s to stigmatize any woman who wanted to work outside the home or cross the gender-role barriers of a patriarchal culture. Because the history of racism had not conferred on African American women the feminine role of homemaker nearly to the degree White women held this role, these women were already working outside the home in greater proportion than White women. Popular images of these women as castrating therefore developed as part of an arrangement of social power in which African American men and women were subordinate to Whites and women were subordinate to men. Hence, today's stereotypes are riddled with a legacy of ethnosexual myths that depict African American women as not sufficiently subordinate to African American men, inherently sexually promiscuous, morally loose, independent, strong, assertive, matriarchal, and castrating masculinized females when compared to their White counterparts (Christian, 1985; Clarke, 1983; Collins, 1990; Greene, 1986, 1990a, 1990b, 1993a; hooks, 1981; Icard, 1986; Silvera, 1991). African American women clearly did not fit the traditional stereotypes of women as fragile, weak, and dependent, since they were never allowed to be that way. They came to be defined as all of the things that normal women were not supposed to be. Stereotypes that depict lesbians as masculinized women poignantly intersect with stereotypes of African American and African Caribbean women in this regard. They suggest that both lesbians and African American women are defective females who want to be or act like men and are sexually promiscuous. It is important to understand the history of institutional racism and the significant role it has had in the development of a legacy of myths and distortions regarding the sexuality of lesbians from these groups.

Additionally, racism and sexism come together in attempts to present African American women as the cause of failures in family functioning, suggesting that a lack of male dominance and female subordination has prevented African Americans from being truly emancipated. Males in the culture are encouraged to believe that strong women, and not racist institutions, are responsible for their oppression. Many African American women, including those who are lesbians, have internalized these myths. When internalized, such distortions of the sexuality of African American women, which is treated as if it were depraved, can intensify the negative psychological effects on African American lesbians and further compromise their ability to obtain support from the larger African American community (Clarke, 1983; Collins, 1990).

The African American family has functioned as a necessary and important protective barrier, a survival tool against and refuge from the racism of the dominant culture. Villarosa (quoted in Brownworth, 1993) observes that the status of the African American family and community as central tools for survival and a safe haven makes the process of "coming out" for African American lesbians significantly different from that of their White counterparts:

> It is harder for us to consider being rejected by our families . . . all we have is our families, our community. When the whole world is racist and against you, your family and your community are the only people who accept you and love you even though you are black. So you don't know what will happen if you lose them . . . and many black lesbians (and gay men) are afraid that's what will happen [p. 18].

Because of the strength of family ties, lesbian family members may not be automatically rejected, although there is an undisputed rejection of a lesbian sexual orientation. Villarosa observes that in African American families, they do not throw a lesbian out because of the importance of family members to one another; rather, they "keep you around to talk you out of it" (Brownworth, 1993, p. 18).

A clinician should not infer from this "tolerance" that the family approves of its member being a lesbian (Acosta, 1979). Tolerance is usually contingent on silence about one's lesbian sexual orientation. Serious conflicts between family members may in fact erupt if a family member openly discloses, labels herself, or discusses being a lesbian.

Homophobia among African Americans and many African Caribbeans can be explained as a function of many different determinants. One is the significant presence of Western Christian religiosity, which is often an exaggerated expression of the strong religious and spiritual orientation of these cultures. In this context, selective interpretations of biblical scripture are used to reinforce homophobic attitudes (Claybourne, 1978; Greene, 1996; Icard, 1986; Moses and Hawkins, 1982). Silvera (1991) writes that when she was 27 years old, her grandmother discovered that she was a lesbian, sat her down with Bible in hand, and explained that "this was a thing only people of mixed blood was involved in" (p. 16).

Clarke (1983), Silvera (1991), and Smith (1982) cite heterosexual privilege as another determinant of homophobia among African American women. Because of the rampant sexism in both the dominant and African American cultures and racism in the dominant culture, African American women often find themselves at the bottom of the racial and gender hierarchies heap. Hence, being heterosexual is the only privileged status they may possess.

Internalized racism may be seen as another determinant of homophobia among African Americans and African Caribbeans. For those who have internalized negative stereotypes of people of African and Caribbean descent as they are constructed and held by the dominant culture, the notion that one mistake is a negative reflection on all African Americans is a common idea (Greene, 1996; Poussaint, 1990).

Sexuality has always been an emotionally charged issue, intensified by pejorative ethnosexual myths and stereotypes about African American men and women (Wyatt, Strayer, and Lobitz, 1976). One reaction to negative stereotypes previously mentioned is that of avoiding any behavior that might conform to or resemble those stereotypes. Hence, there may be an exaggerated need to demonstrate "normalcy" and fit into the dominant culture's depiction of what people are supposed to be (Clarke, 1983; deMonteflores, 1986; Gomez, 1983; Greene, 1986, 1996; Wyatt, Strayer, and Lobitz, 1976). As a result, acceptance of a lesbian sexual orientation can be thought of as contradicting the dominant culture's ideal. Hence, lesbians may be experienced by persons who strongly identify with the dominant culture as an embarrassment to them (Poussaint, 1990). Indeed, the only names for lesbians in the African American community are derogatory: "funny women" or "bulldagger women" (Jeffries, 1992, p. 44; Omosupe, 1991). Silvera (1991) writes of her childhood in Jamaica,

> The words used to describe many of these women would be "Man royal" and/or "Sodomite." Dread words. So dread that women dare not use these words to name themselves. The act of loving someone from the same sex was sinful, abnormal—something to hide [pp. 15–16].

She explains that the word *sodomite,* derived from the Old Testament, is peculiar to Jamaica in its use to describe lesbians as well as any strong, independent woman. She continues, "Things are different now in Jamaica. Now all you have to do is not respond to a man's call to you and dem call you sodomite or lesbian" (p. 17).

Clarke (1983) and Jeffries (1992) observe that there was a period of quiet tolerance for gay men and lesbians in some poor African American communities in the 1940s through the 1950s. Clarke explains this as "seizing the opportunity to spite the White man" by tolerating members of a group that the dominant culture devalues. Jeffries attributes this "tolerance" to the empathy of African Americans as oppressed people for the plight of another oppressed group. The recent heightened visibility of lesbians in the dominant culture in general and the higher visibility of African American lesbians in African American communities may ultimately remove the denial of lesbian orientation that has heretofore been required for "tolerance."

Bell and Weinberg (1978), Bass-Hass (1968), Croom (1993), Mays and Cochran (1988), and Mays, Cochran, and Rhue (forthcoming) are among the few studies made up exclusively or that include significant numbers of African American lesbian respondents. Among the findings of these studies are that

African American lesbians are more likely to maintain strong involvements with their families; more likely to have children; and to depend to a greater extent on family members or other African American lesbians for support than their White counterparts. The findings also indicate that they are likely to have more continued contact with men and with heterosexual peers than their White counterparts. The studies found a greater likelihood that African American lesbians will experience tension and loneliness but are less likely to seek professional help. This may contribute to a delay in the seeking of help during a crisis or a condition and may leave African American lesbians more vulnerable to negative psychological outcomes.

Despite the acknowledged homophobia in the African American community, African American lesbians claim a strong attachment to their cultural heritage and to their communities, and cite their identity as African Americans as primary (Acosta, 1979; Croom, 1993; Mays, Cochran, and Rhue, forthcoming). They also cite a sense of conflicting loyalties between the African American community and the mainstream lesbian community, particularly when confronted with homophobia in the African American community (Dyne, 1980; Greene, 1990b, 1996; Icard, 1986; Mays and Cochran, 1988).

Native American Lesbians

Allen (1986) writes, "The lesbian is to the American Indian what the Indian is to the American—invisible" (p. 245). In her brilliant treatise on the role of women in American Native traditions, Allen explains that the written history of Native Americans is a selective one. Those portions of this written history that would establish (1) that the primary social order of native cultures were gynocentric prior to 1800, and (2) that in such systems women held important positions and had the authority to make decisions on all tribal levels—that essentially contradicted a Western, patriarchal worldview—were almost completely deleted. The existence and tolerance of Native American lesbians, who in fact played an integral part of tribal life, had to be obliterated to serve patriarchal interests, resulting in their contemporary invisibility (Allen, 1984, 1986; Tafoya, 1992).

Allen (1986) and Williams (1986) note that in precolonial Native American tribes, physical anatomy was not inextricably linked to gender roles and that mixed, third-gender, or alternative-gender roles were at one time accepted and integrated into tribal life. LaFromboise, Heyle, and Ozer (1990) examine important differences between Western and Native communities' understandings of the world, as well as important differences within the immense numbers of different tribes. Tafoya (1992) suggests that Native people may have a more "sophisticated taxonomy which addresses spirituality and function rather than appearance" (p. 254) and that these elements are understood as they appear situationally in relation to something else, not as absolute entities in and of themselves. Within such a paradigm, dichotomous or mutually exclusive categories such as male and female or lesbian and heterosexual may not accurately capture the Native person's understanding of sexuality and gender (Allen, 1984, 1986; Tafoya, 1992).

While there were divisions of roles by gender, they were divided in ways allowing men and women to assume them irrespective of their gender. For example, women who would be considered lesbians by today's standards would have assumed roles usually occupied by men and would have been considered men in some tribes (Allen, 1986). Persons whom we might consider androgynous or lesbian by today's standards were valued and in some tribes were accorded special respect and honor (Allen, 1986; Grahn, 1984; Weinrich and Williams, 1991). They were also often viewed as people who combined aspects of masculine and feminine styles in one person spiritually, reflected in the roles they assumed (Weinrich and Williams, 1991). Allen (1986) observes that in gynocratic systems, people assume roles within the social order by virtue of the realities of the human constitution, rather than on "denial based social fictions" (p. 3) that force people into arbitrary categories determined by powerful and privileged persons within that society.

Jacobs (cited in Grahn, 1984) found eighty-eight tribes whose documented cultural characteristics mention gayness, and twenty-two of those include specific references to lesbians, with specific names for lesbians in each tribe (Allen, 1986). The eleven tribes who denied, to White anthropologists, the existence of lesbians were observed to come from territories where the most intense and severe puritanical influence from Whites was felt. Allen (1986), Tafoya (1992), and Williams (1986) observe that from the outset, Native American people learned not to discuss matters of gender and sexuality with European settlers since the latter groups viewed tribal customs and rituals with contempt, quickly seeking to eradicate them.

It is important to understand the devastating effect of the colonization of Native Americans on tribal life, values, and practices and its role in current attitudes toward lesbians. The degree of acceptance of a gay or lesbian sexual orientation may also be a function of the religious group that was involved in colonizing a particular tribe (V. L. Sears, personal communication, May 1992). Allen (1986) asserts that colonization resulted in a shift from a gynocentric, egalitarian, ritual-based social system to a secular system that more closely resembles European patriarchy. In the course of this shift, women, lesbians, and leaders who observed tribal customs and rituals have suffered the most severe losses of power, status, and leadership (Allen, 1984, 1986; Tafoya, 1992). Colonizers who came from patriarchal cultures could not tolerate groups who allowed women to be powerful and sought to "discredit" the status of women, as well as the tolerance for lesbians and gay men by the deliberate destruction of both records and lives (Allen, 1986). Williams (1986) writes that the stark homophobia of White recorders of tribal life, reflected in their negative judgments of same-gender sexual relationships, stands in stark contrast to the recorded history of easy acceptance of lesbians and gay men among Native Americans themselves. The colonizers' ultimate goal was to present patriarchy as the best alternative (Allen, 1986). This trend is linked to the growth of homophobia, once a rare phenomenon in many tribes. Allen (1986) cites highly acculturated and Christianized Native Americans as those who are most likely to express "fear and loathing" for lesbians, as for any other aspects of traditional tribal life (p. 199).

Tafoya (1992) suggests that the concept of "two-spirited people" (p. 256) is more relevant to Native American people than English-defined categories of lesbian or heterosexual. A two-spirited person possesses a male and female spirit, regardless of his or her biological gender. In this paradigm, an individual's sexuality is viewed on a continuum, and a wide range of sexual behaviors are deemed acceptable. The dichotomous notions of heterosexuality and homosexuality are of little use in such a continuum model, where less stigma is attached to women whose behavior is "masculine" or to men whose behavior is "feminine" (Tafoya, 1992).

In Blumstein and Schwarz's (cited in Tafoya and Rowell, 1988) research with over two hundred interracial same-sex couples, a higher rate of bisexual behavior was found among Native American respondents than among any other ethnic group in the United States. Additional findings reveal that self-identified Native American lesbians had higher reported rates of heterosexual experiences than their other ethnic counterparts (Tafoya, 1992). In this context, a Native American lesbian might assume more masculine or feminine behavior depending on her partner and the context (Tafoya and Rowell, 1988). This observation supports the assumption of a more fluid concept of gender relations and sexual expression among Native American people than in both their White and other ethnic counterparts.

Despite these findings, contemporary Native Americans, particularly those who reside on reservations, are less accepting of lesbian sexual orientation than their ancestors. This is explained as a function of colonization, genocide, internalized oppression, and a loss of contact with traditional values (Allen, 1986; V. L. Sears, personal communication, May 1992; Tafoya, 1992; Williams, 1986). Hence, Native American lesbians may experience more pressure to be closeted if they live on reservations than not, prompting many to move to larger, urban areas (V. L. Sears, personal communication, May 1992; Williams, 1986). Obliteration of Native American history and lingering fears about acknowledging practices that were once ridiculed and severely punished result in the continued invisibility of Native American lesbians on reservations. Tafoya (1992) notes that many younger lesbians may even assume that they must leave the reservation to find other lesbians.

Family and community assume as significant a level of importance to Native American lesbians as they do for their other ethnic counterparts, and for similar reasons. This country's legacy of pervasive, disparaging media depictions of

Native Americans are often as deeply embedded in the psyche of lesbians in the mainstream as they are in that of the rest of the dominant culture. Hence, the mainstream lesbian community, while it provides a safer place to explore a nontraditional sexual orientation, is not free of the same racism that Native American lesbians experience in other parts of society. The move away from the reservation into the lesbian community may result in the experience of loss of culture and support from family and Native American community. This loss is significant and can precipitate feelings of isolation and depression (V. L. Sears, personal communication, May 1992). Tafoya and Rowell (1988) note that ethnic identity may be primary to Native American lesbians. They may be less likely to present themselves to Native American counseling agencies, out of fear that their sexual orientation will be viewed more negatively by other Native Americans (the same is often true of Asian lesbians, as discussed below).

Tafoya and Rowell (1988) suggest that family therapies are most useful in reintegrating a lesbian member back into the family, and thus they support the culturally syntonic value of reestablishing connectiveness. While there may not be great pressure to marry, the family is often most concerned that a lesbian sexual orientation is synonymous with being childless. Motherhood is an important role for Native American women, since children are seen as the future of the tribe. However, given the higher rates of heterosexual relations of Native American women, this may be less of a realistic concern for them than for their other lesbians of color (Tafoya and Rowell, 1988). Sears (personal communication, May 1992) reports that it is not uncommon for lesbians, including those on reservations, to have children.

Despite these findings, clinicians may encounter Native American lesbians who know nothing of these traditions or concepts and may believe, as do many lesbians on first acknowledging their sexual orientation, that there is no one else like them (Ratti, 1993; Tafoya, 1992).

Asian American Lesbians

Asian Americans lesbians come from a number of different ethnic groups, which makes any generalizations about them potentially inaccurate. For the purposes of this discussion, the category of Asian American lesbians will comprise lesbians of Japanese or Chinese ancestry only, because it is with these groups that most research has been done.

A salient feature of Asian American families is the expectation of obedience to one's parents and their demand for conformity. This is consistent with the respect accorded elders, and the sharp delineation of gender roles (Bradshaw, 1990; Chan, 1989, 1992; Garnets and Kimmel, 1991; Gock, 1985; H., 1989). Women are expected to derive status from their roles of dutiful daughter and ultimately wife and mother, passively deferring to men, to whom they are deemed inferior (Chan, 1992; H., 1989).

Pamela H. (1989) observes that for Asian women, a problem in the development of an identity as a lesbian lies in their devalued identity as women in the culture. In her analysis, women are discouraged from developing any sense of basic self-worth or identity beyond their preordained roles in the family.

In the role of mother, they are responsible for socializing children appropriately and are thus considered responsible by family and peers if children do not conform. Hence, mothers, perhaps more than other family members, are likely to be blamed if a daughter strays from the predetermined truth and declares that she is a lesbian (C. Chan, personal communication, Nov. 1992).

Heterosexual marital relationships are seen as somewhat inevitable, not as something that occurs between two people, but rather between two families for the good of the families. It may be difficult in this context for family members to view a lesbian family member as anything but selfish, in that she has deliberately made her own sexual preference and therefore her own feelings the most important variable in selecting a mate and planning her life.

The development of any sexual identity is also complicated by the taboo against open discussions about sex, which is considered a shameful topic (Chan, 1992; H., 1989). Discussions about sexuality, when they occur, focus on its biological aspects and do not explore nontraditional sexual orientations (H., 1989). Chan (personal communication, Nov. 1992) notes that sex is presumed to be unimportant to women. Asian women are depicted in stereotyped media images in the United States as "passive, quiet, servile" (H., 1989, p. 286) and either "exotically sexy or totally asexual" (p. 293). These images contribute to the ethnosexual mythology that members of the dominant culture hold about Asian women and that some Asian women internalize themselves. Racism in the mainstream lesbian community may be expressed in the expectations of other lesbians that Asian American lesbians actually fit those stereotypes. (Gock, 1992, has reported that this racism is also reflected in the practices of bars, dances, discos, and the like in the mainstream lesbian community, which require more types of identification from Asian American lesbians than from their White counterparts.)

Pamela H. (1989) appropriately reminds us that the media images of lesbians in American films are usually dominated by White women. The tendency for Asian parents to view lesbian sexual orientation as a "Western concept" (p. 284), a product of too much assimilation or a function of losing touch with Asian heritage, may have some of its origins in the invisibility of Asian lesbians in American media depictions of lesbians (Pamela H., 1989). Pamela H. further notes that many Asian parents may be quite "oblivious" to the existence of Asian lesbians and notes that there is no word for "lesbian" in most Asian languages. A declaration of a lesbian sexual orientation may be regarded as an act of open rebellion as well as a blatant rejection of Asian heritage. The declaration of the desire for same-gender relationships may also be regarded as a temporary disorder that the parents hope or just assume their daughter will outgrow. At the other extreme, a lesbian daughter may be thought of by parents as a source of shame to the entire family (Chan, 1992; Pamela H., 1989). Lesbian sexual orientation is viewed as volitional and is presumed to represent a conscious desire to tarnish the family honor. Parents may express the feeling that they can no longer face friends or community.

Because lesbians are incorrectly presumed to be disinterested in becoming parents, a daughter's open disclosure that she is lesbian may be interpreted as a rejection of the role of mother and therefore of her most important role culturally (Chan, 1992; Garnets and Kimmel, 1991; Wooden, Kawasaki, and Mayeda, 1983).

Openly adopting a lesbian sexual orientation will generally be met with disapproval, although individual reactions will of course vary (C. Chan, personal communication, Nov. 1992). The maintenance of outward roles and conformity is an important and distinctive cultural expectation. The fear of negative reactions to disclosure contributes significantly to the pressure to remain closeted within the Asian American community or move away from it to avoid discovery. Chan (1989) noted that over 75 percent of Asian American lesbians (and gay men) surveyed expressed concerns about revealing their sexual orientation to other Asians because of what they perceived as the potential for rejection and stigmatization. This may have relevant implications for choice of therapist. More research is required to determine if Asian American or other lesbians of color deem sexual orientation or a familiarity with such issues a more important variable in therapist selection than the race or ethnicity of the therapist. If lesbians of color experience members of their own ethnic group as more homophobic than members of the dominant culture, this assumption may also apply to their perception of therapists who are members of the same ethnic group. Croom (1993) provides some support for this notion in her study on African American lesbians. Chan (1992) notes that invisibility leads to the absence of Asian American lesbians who might serve as role models for young women struggling with questions about their sexual identity.

Asian American lesbians, like their other ethnic counterparts, frequently report feeling a pressure to choose between these two communities and subsequently declare the aspect of their identity that is primary. In her 1989 study of Asian American gay men and lesbians, Chan found that most respondents saw their primary identification as a gay man or lesbian rather than Asian American. This study noted, however, that the primacy of sexual orientation and ethnicity shifts during development, depending on which stages of ethnic identity development and sexual orientation identity formation the individual fits at that time. Identification may also vary depending on the need at the time. Gock (1992) proposes a detailed descriptive analysis of the identity integration process of

Asian Pacific American lesbians and gay men. Lee (1991) writes of her rejection of her cultural identity,

> For most of my life, I belonged to the "don't wanna be" tribe, being ashamed and embarrassed of my Asian background, rejecting it. . . . My father tried his best to jam "Chineseness" down my throat, . . . [he] warned, "If you marry a White we'll cut you out of our will." . . . With my father's wish for my aware-ness of cultural identity came his expectation that I grow up to be a "nice Chinese girl." This meant I should be a submissive . . . obedient, morally impec-cable puppet who would spend the rest of her life deferring to and selflessly appeasing her husband. . . . He wanted me to become all that was against my nature, and so I rebelled with a fury, rejecting and denying everything remotely associated with Chinese culture. . . . Becoming a lesbian challenged everything in my upbringing and confirmed the fact that I was not a nice, ladylike pam-perer of men [pp. 116, 117].

Similar intricate and complex conflicts of loyalty are also observed in lesbians of color from other ethnic groups.

Unlike gay and lesbian members of other ethnic groups, who report feeling more discrimination for their race than sexual orientation, the Asian American gay male sample in this study reported experiencing more discrimination because they were gay than because they were Asian (Chan, 1989). This find-ing underscores the importance of exploring subtle gender differences in the experience and meaning of certain phenomena, even within the same culture.

Pamela H. (1989) writes that the persistent invisibility of lesbians within Asian American communities is slowly changing, with the development in the early 1980s of Asian American lesbian support and social groups within those communities. Such groups have developed in part in reaction to experiences of invisibility and racial discrimination in the broader lesbian communities, which are predominantly White and often offer little contact with other ethnic lesbians (Noda, Tsui, and Wong, 1979).

Indian and South Asian American Lesbians

Lesbians who identify with the cultures of Bhutan, Bangladesh, India, the Maldives, Nepal, Pakistan, and Sri Lanka are considered South Asian. Although they find themselves confronted with psychological tasks that are similar to other visibly ethnic lesbians (Ratti, 1993), they are virtually absent in the psy-chological literature. The lesbians of these cultures and countries are markedly heterogeneous. They do not necessarily identify with African American lesbians or other women of color, nor do they necessarily consider themselves persons of color at all. Vaid (cited in Meera, 1993) observes that many Indians view Great Britain as their mother country and for that reason may more closely iden-tify with Whites. Hence, clinicians must consider the psychological demands made of lesbians who may be viewed as women of color because of their skin color, but who do not experience themselves as ethnic minorities in the same way that lesbians of color who have been raised in the United States may. They must also consider the conundrum of identifications, alliances, and expectations lesbians of color often have of one another based on assumptions about the meaning of skin color as well as sexual orientation in different parts of the world (see Jayakar, 1994).

Bearing some similarity to broader Asian cultures, gender roles in Indian and South Asian societies are clearly delineated, in a patriarchal social organization. Strict obedience to parents, even among adult children, is expected, as is conformity to social expectations. Among those expectations is that of marriage, which is still frequently arranged by parents or families, and having children. The pressure to marry and have children is quite explicit and may be quite intense. As it is in most other patriarchal societies, women are considered inferior and of less importance than men.

Ratti (1993) and Jayakar (1994) observe India and South Asia as lands of contradiction. Jayakar notes in particular that the open discussion or expression of sexuality is taboo, in the same land that produced the Kama Sutra, the world's first literary classic on sexual matters (AIDS Bhedbar Virodhi Andolan [AIDS BVA], 1993; Ratti, 1993). This makes the discussion of lesbian sexual orientation even less likely and more difficult. Despite a history of sexual behavior between women, reflected in art, literature, sculpture, and painting, as well as sexual and emotional involvement that is self-identified as lesbian, contemporary mainstream Indians view lesbians in much the same way as their other ethnic counterparts, as a social or psychological aberration (AIDS BVA, 1993); as a Western phenomenon or disease that is alien to Indian culture (Bannerji, 1993; Heske, Khayal, and Utsa, 1986; Ratti, 1993).

Generally, the existence of lesbians is not acknowledged in these cultures, but this was not always the case. Heske, Khayal, and Utsa (1986) write that a history of tolerance of same-gender sexual behavior, particularly in India, was punished and then suppressed by British colonization. Utsa (in Heske, Khayal, and Utsa, 1986) notes that despite (or because of) the patriarchal context of Indian society, there is significant emotional bonding and warmth between women. It would be natural, in a society that is segregated on the basis of gender in many arenas, that women who develop in great proximity to one another and apart from men would have more opportunities for close and intimate relationships among them.

The imposition of British morals and values influenced the creation of repressive Indian laws in 1861 (based on British law) that forbid homosexual behavior (Heske, Khayal, and Utsa, 1986). As of 1986, homosexuality was still an illegal offense under Section 377 of the Indian penal code, punishable with prison sentences ranging from ten years to life (Heske, Khayal, and Utsa, 1986).

Kim (1993) observes that gay men and lesbians in India do not make themselves as visible as their White counterparts in the United States, out of a pragmatic fear of the backlash of homophobia that would accompany it.

Ratti (1993) notes that the intense pressure for women to marry—usually in arranged marriages—and raise a family makes it extremely difficult for women who are lesbians to build a life with another woman. This forces many into unhappy heterosexual marriages. Some of these women have secret liaisons with women lovers but maintain a heterosexual marriage. Another significant factor mitigating against such relationships is the economic dependence of women in India. Leaving the country and moving to the United States or Great Britain is often an alternative only for a well-educated or financially secure minority (Heske, Khayal, and Utsa, 1986). Of course, some women come to the United States to study, but they are usually not from the poorer classes or rural areas. Hence, many Indian lesbians encountered in treatment settings in the United States are from more economically or educationally privileged backgrounds.

Ratti (1993) estimates that there are 80 million gay men and lesbians in India (based on an estimate of 10 percent of the general population). But these large numbers of lesbians in India are spread over a vast country. There are no organized, vocal lesbian movements or communities within the country, and few if any magazines or clubs similar to those in the United States. Heske, Khayal, and Utsa (1986) observe that with the exception of small isolated groups that meet individually and informally, it is difficult to know who is lesbian and who is not and thus even to meet other lesbians. Isolation is therefore a significant issue.

In the United States, Indian and South Asian lesbians report that while the broader lesbian community affords them the opportunity to meet other lesbians in a less stigmatized environment, there remains a significant sense of isolation and invisibility (Bannerji, 1993; Heske, Khayal, and Utsa, 1986; Ratti, 1993). Ratti (1993) attributes this invisibility to scarcity and neglect of the concerns of Indian and South Asian lesbians in the lesbian movement in the United States, as well as the expectation that lesbians fit a generic lesbian mold, one that is usually articulated from a majority perspective. This expectation overlooks important cultural differences, which Indian lesbians are left to negotiate. Heske, Khayal, and Utsa (1986) write that for some Indian lesbians, public displays of affection between lesbians in the United States and the transitory nature of some relationships is at variance with their culture's emphasis on public propriety and longstanding monogamy. Utsa (in Heske, Khayal, and Utsa, 1986) states, "I come from a culture where people have very deep, longstanding bonds with each other. . . . For me to look at relationships and friendships in such a short-term fashion is very hard" (p. 143).

Jayakar (1994) notes that Indian women are socialized to deny directly both their sexuality and any sexual knowledge. The clinician may not assume that Indian lesbians would be any more comfortable with direct discussions of sexual matters than their heterosexual counterparts, even in the private context of therapy. Such discussions must be handled with particular sensitivity.

Another challenge confronting lesbians in these groups is that of racism and ethnocentrism in the broader lesbian community in the United States. Khayal (in Heske, Khayal, and Utsa, 1986) characterizes White women as narrow minded in their concepts of lesbianism in other societies. Heske (in Heske, Khayal, and Utsa, 1986) offers an example in reporting her own surprise in finding that an Indian woman dressed in traditional Indian clothing who she had recently met was a lesbian, and that there was a large population of Indian women who were lesbian as well. This phenomenon may also be a reflection of the invisibility of Indian lesbians in India and the absence of their images in the popular media depictions of lesbians in the United States. Each phenomenon may then circularly reinforce the other.

Like lesbians from other groups discussed here, Indian American lesbians are faced with marginalization and racism in the broader lesbian community (Bannerji, 1993; Heske, Khayal, and Utsa, 1986; Khush, 1993; Ratti, 1993). Reports of being treated like strange, exotic creatures are not uncommon, nor are episodes of discrimination in bars, clubs, dances, meetings, and collectives (Bannerji, 1993; Heske, Khayal, and Utsa, 1993). Bannerji (1993) writes:

> Much of the experience of racism is constructed through gender. As a child and adolescent, I not only yearned to be a White girl, . . . I also saw White femaleness through White men's eyes. . . . The first women to whom I was attracted reflected the White male gaze I had obediently eroticized. I found nothing sensual about my own body nor the bodies of black and Indian girls around me [p. 61].

She continues and comments on the parallels between her invisibility as a woman in a patriarchal society and as an Indian lesbian in the broader U.S. lesbian community: "Just as men had silenced me in the solidarity committees and meetings of the left, so too I found White lesbians talking for me and about me as though I was not present" (Bannerji, 1993, p. 60).

Shah (1993) posits that South Asian lesbians have to define themselves because of the extreme lack of awareness of them in both South Asian patriarchal societies and in Western lesbian communities. In the absence of the word *lesbian* in their native languages, they have developed their own names for themselves. The Sanskrit word *anamika* (p. 114), which means "nameless," was taken by a lesbian collective in 1985 and was used to address the lack of names in South Asian languages for lesbian relationships (Shah, 1993). Other names have been developed out of various South Asian languages by lesbians of those cultures who wish to name themselves in affirmative ways.

Like their ethnic counterparts, the relationships between Indian and South Asian lesbians and their families is intense and complex. While there is a strong commitment to family and family bonds may override the family's homophobia, Parmar (cited in Khush, 1993) notes that "coming out" carries the realistic risk of being rejected, to the extreme of being completely shunned.

Latina Lesbians

Espín (1984) and others (Amaro, 1978; Hidalgo and Hidalgo-Christensen, 1976; Morales, 1989; Vasquez, 1979) report that gender roles are well established within Latino families and culture. Women are generally expected to be overtly submissive, virtuous (virginal), respectful of elders, and willing to defer to men, who are considered superior to women (Espín, 1984; Morales, 1989). While women are encouraged to maintain emotional and physical closeness to other women, such behavior is not presumed to be lesbian (Amaro, 1978; Espín, 1984; Hidalgo and Hidalgo-Christensen, 1976). Closeness with female friends is encouraged, particularly during adolescence, and may serve as a way of protecting the virginity of young women by diminishing their contact with males. The open discussion of sex and sexuality between women is not culturally sanctioned, and women are expected to be sexually naive (Espín, 1984). Comas-Diaz (personal communication, Jan. 1993) suggests that there is a known tolerance for same-gender sexual behavior among males, as long as it is not overtly labeled as the person's preferred behavior. This avoidance of adopting a stigmatized identity is explained as a function of the cultural importance of saving face, a key component of maintaining dignity and commanding respect. Being indirect is the culturally prescribed way of managing conflict, since in that way, participants do not lose face. Espín (1987) contends that in labeling themselves lesbian, Latina women force a culture that denies the sexuality of women to confront it. Furthermore, it implies not only a woman's conscious participation in sexual behavior—behavior that is taboo and that is not performed out of duty to her husband but out of her own desire—but also a confrontation of others with the fact that she engages in forbidden behavior. This stance not only violates the taboo against engaging in such behavior but also challenges the cultural directive to be indirect or avoidant in the face of conflict.

According to Trujillo (1991), the majority of Chicano heterosexuals view Chicana lesbians as a threat to the established order of male dominance in Chicano communities. Their existence is viewed as having the potential of raising the consciousness of Chicana women, causing them to question the premises of male dominance and female subordination.

Espín (1984), Hidalgo and Hidalgo-Christensen (1976), and Morales (1992) suggest that disapproval in Latino communities is more intense than the homophobia in the dominant Anglo community. They further suggest that a powerful form of heterosexist oppression takes place within Latin cultures, leaving many lesbian members feeling a pressure to remain closeted. Declaring a lesbian sexual orientation may be experienced as an act of treason against the culture and family. Espín (1984, 1987) and Hidalgo (1984) note that a lesbian family member may maintain a place in the family and be quietly tolerated, but this does not constitute acceptance of her lesbian sexual orientation. It is more likely that such tolerance reflects the family's denial. Generally, only masculine-looking females ("butch") would be perceived as lesbian and challenged.

The extent to which Latina lesbians will present themselves as gender-role stereotyped in their own relationships, or the degree to which they will observe stereotypes learned in a culture where gender roles are somewhat rigid, will be a function of their level of acculturation, as well as of the extent to which their own families engage in traditional gender roles (Morales, 1989). Despite the antilesbian sentiment of their ethnic communities and families, Espín (1987) and Hidalgo (1984) found that there was a deep attachment among Latina lesbians to those communities. Gutierrez (1992) writes:

> It isn't easy to be part of a gay and lesbian culture whose rites and institutions too often consider us to be peripheral or an acquired taste. . . . Our families may reject us but we belong to them nonetheless. . . . The same is true for our friends, neighborhoods, etc. . . . We must not abandon them, . . . they are ours. . . . Even if it is impossible to stay, they remain ours for as long as we claim them [p. 242].

MENTAL HEALTH ISSUES

Lesbian women of color exist within a tangle of multiply devalued identities, surrounded by the oppression and discrimination that accompany institutionalized racism, sexism, and heterosexism. Unlike their White counterparts, lesbians of color bear the additional task involved in integrating major features of their identity when they are conspicuously devalued. Unlike their ethnic identities, their sexual orientation and sometimes their gender may be devalued by those closest to them in their families.

Women of color usually receive positive cultural mirroring during development, generally but not exclusively through their families. This helps to buffer the demeaning messages and distorted, stereotyped images of themselves created and maintained by the dominant culture. Those who do not receive positive cultural mirroring are at risk for internalizing society's racism.

Lesbians of color also learn a range of negative stereotypes about lesbian sexual orientation long before they know that they are lesbian themselves. With the exception of Native Americans, other ethnic groups have either no words in their language for lesbian or only words and names that are degrading. The unquestioned internalization of pernicious attitudes about lesbians, gleaned from loved and trusted figures, complicates the process of lesbian identity development and self-acceptance for women of color in ways that are not as complex for their White counterparts (Gock, 1992).

Regardless of the specific ethnic group to which they belong, lesbian women of color must manage the dominant culture's racism, sexism, and heterosexism, as well as that of their own ethnic group. Although most lesbians of color experience their ethnic communities as being of great practical and emotional significance, the homophobia in these communities makes lesbian members more vulnerable, perhaps more inclined to remain closeted, and therefore invisible to them (Chan, 1992; Espín, 1984; Greene, 1993b, 1996; Mays and Cochran, 1988; Morales, 1989; Moses and Hawkins, 1982). This increases their psychological vulnerability. How important these ties may be to an individual client may vary depending on the degree of her attachment to her cultural background and the degree of acculturation (Falco, 1991). Appropriate, intense ties to ethnic community and family may complicate the coming-out process for lesbians of color in ways that it may not for their White counterparts. Decisions about coming out to family members are already fraught with anxiety for most women who are lesbians, but for lesbians of color, there is often more to lose. Lesbians of color cannot presume acceptance by the broader lesbian community if their families reject them, and they risk giving up an important source of support if this feared rejection occurs.

Just as the oppression created by heterosexism produces greater stressors for lesbians than for heterosexual women, the combined effects of racism, sexism, and heterosexism for lesbians of color intensify and complicate the stressors for them (Morgan and Eliason, 1992). While we may assume that the stress of coming out is intense for lesbians of color, because they must manage multiple oppressions, we must also assume that they may bring unique resources and resiliences to this task. Lesbians of color, unlike their White counterparts, have often been forced to learn useful coping mechanisms against racism and discrimination, long before they ever realized that they were lesbians. When confronted with managing other devalued aspects of their identities, they may call on the mechanisms used against racism to assist them. Psychotherapy can be useful in developing an awareness of these resources in the client and assisting her in their effective use. Problems occur when previously learned coping mechanisms are maladaptive or self-destructive; hence, clients in this category are perhaps more vulnerable to the development of serious pathology. Other variables include not simply the mere presence of other stressors, but their intensity and the amount of attention they require on an ongoing basis. There are no empirical data with significant numbers of lesbians of color to justify more than clinical speculations in this area, but it might be safe to say that it is somewhat more difficult for lesbians of color to be out than for their White counterparts. Further research is needed.

The quiet toleration observed in many ethnic minority families for a lesbian member is generally marked by denial and the need to view lesbian sexual orientations as something whose origins exist outside the culture. Tremble, Schneider, and Appathurai (1989) suggest that attributing lesbian sexual orientation to some outside source may in fact enable some families to accept a family member while removing themselves or that family member from any perceived sense of responsibility. Hence the ubiquitous notion that a lesbian sexual orientation is a Western or White man's disease that is "caught" or chosen. Thus a rationale for rejecting lesbian sexual orientation can be developed by presenting it as if it and ethnic identity were mutually exclusive (Chan, 1992; Espín, 1987; Greene, 1994, 1996; Hidalgo, 1984; Mays and Cochran, 1988; Morales, 1989, 1992; Tremble, Schneider, and Appathurai, 1989). The woman who is lesbian is then presented with the notion that if she were true to her ethnic heritage, she would have no part in such a lifestyle.

Many people of color believe that only heterosexual orientation is natural or normal and, by correlation, that a woman of color who is lesbian has "chosen" her sexual orientation. Thus follows the assumption that she could choose to be heterosexual if she wanted to do so. Some family members may assert that the choice a lesbian family member makes to acknowledge this aspect of her identity is done deliberately to hurt them. When treating a family member of a lesbian of color, it is important to be familiar with these stereotypes, to assist them in understanding that a lesbian relative does not consciously choose her sexual orientation any more than a heterosexual woman does, and to advise them that their support is important to her.

Members of ethnic minority communities as well as White lesbians often choose to view identity as if it were a singular entity. Strong identification with one's ethnic group and, alternately, sexual orientation are often perceived as if they were mutually exclusive of each other as well as other aspects of identity. Hence, being lesbian is often viewed by ethnic heterosexual peers as a repudiation of one's ethnicity. Similarly, lesbians from the dominant culture often lack an appreciation for the ongoing work required to cope adaptively with racism and, concomitantly, the strength and importance of ethnic ties. This can leave lesbians of color feeling poorly understood, as well as guilt ridden about which community to devote their resources to.

Lesbians of color find themselves confronted with racial stereotypes and discrimination in the broader lesbian community. With the exception of large cities, most minority communities are not large enough to maintain a distinct or formal lesbian community of their own (Tremble, Schneider, and Appathurai, 1989). Hence, interactions with members of the mainstream lesbian community become important outlets for social support and for meeting others. However, lesbians of color commonly report discriminatory treatment in lesbian bars, clubs, and social and political gatherings and in individuals within the lesbian community (Chan, 1992; Dyne, 1980; Garnets and Kimmel, 1991; Greene, 1994, 1996; Gutierrez and Dworkin, 1992; Mays and Cochran, 1988; Morales, 1989). They describe feeling an intense sense of conflicting loyalties to two communities, in both of which they are marginalized by the requirement to conceal or minimize important aspects of their identities in order to be accepted.

Lesbians of color frequently experience a sense of never being part of any group completely, leaving them at greater risk for isolation, feelings of estrangement, and increased psychological vulnerability. When in the midst of groups like themselves, there may be a tendency to idealize the group. What often follows is the expectation of a level or similarity, acceptance, being liked, and being understood in ways that never quite live up to the fantasy. Hence, a client may experience a disturbing sense of aloneness or disappointment, or a heightened sense of not fitting in any setting when idealized environments fail to meet all of their expectations, or when their expectations are unrealistic. While the variance within these groups may be as wide as the variance between them and other groups, that variance may be concealed by similarities. Similarities in experiences and characteristics between people are important, but they do not warrant the assumption that they will automatically result in a person's being perfectly understood on all levels.

Some clients with more serious preexisting psychopathology may tend to idealize people who are like them and devalue people who are not like them, rather than make judgments on a person-to-person basis. In some clients, this may reflect a particular stage of lesbian–ethnic minority identity development. However, it may also represent the client's own deeply rooted sense of self-hate. In any case, such a stance actually increases her difficulty getting support from the outside world by restricting the range of people from whom it may be obtained. This difficulty then fuels or confirms a self-fulfilling fear of being unable to get support or of being unworthy. More seriously disturbed clients may rapidly alternate between idealization and devaluation of the group, a particular aspect of themselves about which they feel conflicted, and, if known, that same aspect of the therapist. Ethnicity, gender, and sexual orientation are overdetermined characteristics for idealizing and devaluing stances; such behavior thus may be most acute during the early stages of coming out or at other times of crisis.

Relationship Issues for Lesbian Women of Color

Lesbian women of color find themselves in relationships that are largely unsupported outside the lesbian community. Differences within the lesbian community on preferences for some relationship structures over others are pertinent, but beyond the scope of this chapter. What is clear, however, is that these women may encounter unique challenges in relationships with partners who have the same gender socialization, in a culture that has few open, healthy models of such relationships. That same environment conspicuously devalues their person and devalues their relationships on many levels as well. While lesbian women of color may be accustomed to obtaining family support for their struggles with racism and perhaps sexism, they may not presume the appropriate support of family for their romantic relationships or for their appropriate distress if that relationship is troubled. On seeking professional assistance, they may find few if any therapists who have training in addressing the many nuances of nontraditional relationships.

Lesbians of color are found in relationships with women who are not of their own ethnic group to a significantly greater degree than are their White counterparts (Croom, 1993; Mays and Cochran, 1988; Tafoya and Rowell, 1988), a phenomenon that has been attributed in part to the fact that there are larger numbers of White lesbians to choose from (Tafoya and Rowell, 1988). While heterosexual interracial relationships bring unique challenges and often lack support on both sides of families and communities, for lesbians of color, they provide yet another challenge in a process that is already fraught with difficulty.

An interracial lesbian couple may be more publicly visible as a couple than two women of the same ethnic group. This brings realities of racism that the White partner may have never encountered before. Clunis and Green (1988) observe that because women have tried to avoid racism does not mean that it disappears from their relationships. Lesbians of color have usually developed a variety of coping strategies in addressing racism and often wear a protective psychological armor (Sears, 1987). Because it is a ubiquitous reality and stressor for them, they learn to prioritize their responses to it. A White partner may never have had to do this and may be less prepared (Clunis and Green, 1988). The latter may fail to notice slights that are racist in origin and experience her partner's anger as inappropriate, may overreact (experience her partner as underreactive), or may take on a protective role that her partner does not require or desire, and may even find patronizing.

A White partner may also feel guilty about racism and may be unaware of the distinction she must make between her personal behavior in the relationship and the racism in the outside world. In the latter case, she may attempt to compensate her partner personally for the racism she faces in the world, a task that she cannot do successfully and that will ultimately leave her feeling angry and frustrated. In such relationships, neither the lesbian of color nor her White partner can realistically assume that a White partner is free of racism because of her political beliefs or intentions (Clunis and Green, 1988; Garcia, Kennedy, Pearlman, and Perez, 1987). The lesbian of color in such relationships may also need to be aware of her own jealousy or resentment of her lover's privileged status in the dominant culture and in the lesbian community. Both partners may be perceived as lacking loyalty to their own culture and may even feel ashamed of their involvement with a person who is not of the same race (Clunis and Green, 1988; Falco, 1991; Greene, 1996). This complicates the resolution of issues within the relationship and intensifies the complex web of loyalties and estrangements for lesbian women of color.

While racial issues and cultural differences may contribute to realistic challenges to lesbian relationships, they do not account for all of the problems within them. Racial and cultural differences are often scapegoated as the problem, allowing the couple to avoid looking at more threatening issues. Differences that are most visible lend themselves to be seen as the cause of problems, particularly when simple explanations are desired. At times, racial differences may be the cause of significant difficulties, but other problems may be experienced as if they were about racial or ethnic differences when they have more complex origins within the relationship.

Choices of partners and feelings about those choices may reflect conflicts about intimacy and other interpersonal issues. They may also reflect conflicts about racial and ethnic identity. These conflicts may be expressed by lesbian women of color who choose or are attracted to White women exclusively or who devalue lesbians of color as unsuitable partners.

Lesbians of color who experience themselves as racially or culturally deficient or ambiguous may presume that a partner who is a member of their own ethnic group will somehow compensate for their perceived deficiency or that such a choice will demonstrate their cultural loyalty. There may also be a tendency for a lesbian of color in a relationship with a lesbian from a different minority ethnic group to presume a level of similarity of experience or worldview that is not present. While many of their experiences in the dominant culture as oppressed women of color and lesbians may be similar, their respective views on their roles in a relationship, maintaining a household, and the role of other family members in their lives can be very different.

Some lesbians of color may be appropriately sensitive to what Sears (personal communication, May 1992) refers to as "pony stealing" and Clunis and Green (1988, p. 140) as "ethnic chasing," while Lee (1991, p. 117) describes certain White lesbians as "Asianophiles." These terms are used to identify White women who seek out lesbians of color as partners to assuage their own guilt about being White, to compensate for their lack of a strong ethnic identity, or to prove their liberal attitudes. The ethnosexual stereotypes of lesbians of color as less sexually inhibited than their White counterparts may serve as another determinant of this behavior. An ethnic chaser may seek, usually unconsciously, to gain from proximity to a lesbian of color whatever they perceive to be lacking in themselves. As these attempts at self-repair are doomed to fail, the partner who is not a woman of color may respond by feeling angry, resentful, and somehow betrayed by her partner. In treatment settings, it is helpful to assist women in such relationships to clarify their expectations about being in any relationship. Beyond this general assessment, the kinds of assumptions held about ethnic or White women in an intimate relationship should be explored.

Exclusive choices in this realm may also reflect a woman's tendency to idealize people who are like her and devalue those who are not, or the reverse. When this is the case, the reality often does not live up to the fantasy, resulting in disappointment and self-denigration. It is important to remember that many of these decisions are made without conscious awareness of them and, most important, that they may have many different determinants.

A therapist should not presume that participation in an interracial lesbian relationship is an automatic expression of cultural or racial self-hate in the woman of color. Nor should he or she presume that a relationship between two lesbians of color is necessarily anchored in loyalty or respect for that culture, or in any of the aforementioned problematic premises. What is of significance is that the therapist be aware of a wide range of clinical possibilities and explore them accordingly.

TREATMENT IMPLICATIONS: COUNTERTRANSFERENCE ISSUES

Lesbian sexual orientation, racial differences, and the social conflicts that surround these matters are issues about which most people have intense feelings. Psychotherapists are no exception. The sensitive treatment of lesbian women of color in psychotherapy brings those provocative issues together in a profound way and creates a range of challenges for even the most experienced psychotherapist.

Initially, the therapist must be culturally literate, familiar with the broader characteristics of the client's culture as well as the special strengths and vulnerabilities of clients who are lesbians. A majority of graduate training programs do not routinely offer training in these areas; therefore, therapists must be willing to seek that training elsewhere. This may be accomplished by combining attendance in special workshops or classes with individual or group supervision with clinicians who have training in these respective areas. Failure to do so can result in less-than-adequate treatment to clients (Greene, 1994, 1996).

The interaction among culture, gender, and sexual orientation is not static. Rather, it is dynamic, encompassing major dimensions around which people organize their assumptions about who they are in the world. In therapy, unraveling these issues, their interactions, and the mechanisms developed to adapt to them is complex, to say the least. The therapist who has not taken the time to explore the manifestations of these dilemmas fully will find it difficult, if not impossible, to unravel them successfully. This process must also include the therapist's personal examination of her or his own feelings and responses to women of color and to lesbians, as well as her or his own sexual orientation, gender, and ethnicity. Therapists must also be aware of the stereotypes and beliefs about women of color and lesbians that they have internalized without question. These variables may, if unexamined, predispose the therapist to make a range of inaccurate assumptions about clients and their experiences.

Heterosexual female therapists who are insecure in their own feelings about sexual orientation, or who expect lesbian clients of color to be preoccupied with sexual matters, may be predisposed to have greater expectations of eroticized transferences from lesbian clients of color. In this example, if the therapist has a personal need to see such transferences, she may tend to overlook or minimize issues that are of greater importance to the client. For some heterosexual therapists, such transference reactions are frightening and may be perceived as a threat to the therapist's own sexual orientation, particularly if the therapist is insecure about it. If therapists fear that such transference reactions will occur, they may tend to overlook them, avoid appropriate explorations of material that might expose such feelings in the client, or avoid addressing the client's direct expressions of such material. Heterosexual therapists who are insecure about their own sexual orientation may also find themselves "leaking" personal information to the client, particularly in the midst of eroticized transference reactions, presumably to let clients know that they are not lesbian. The therapist may find that this occurs despite the fact that she does not ordinarily disclose such information without judicious consideration of how it would be helpful to the client to do so or despite being generally neutral about such matters.

Most therapists struggle with the delicate balance involved in urging a client who is a lesbian of color to assume greater personal responsibility for her actions, when appropriate, without seeming insensitive to the realistic barriers that are a result of the many levels of discrimination she faces. The therapist errs, however, if feeling sorry for or admiring the client leads him or her to avoid setting appropriate limits in treatment or to fail to direct the client's attention to her own role in her dilemma. Such a therapist may feel uncomfortable when the situation warrants more than support and validation for the client's struggles.

Therapists who are White and heterosexual, regardless of gender, may inadvertently find themselves bending over backward to accommodate the client who is a lesbian of color, failing to maintain appropriate boundaries or behaving in ways that they would not with other clients. Such behavior may be evoked in the therapist if the client makes him or her feel guilty, angry, uncomfortable, or incompetent. There may be a need to compensate the client in some way for the therapist's feeling of inadequacy. Therapists may also feel guilty about their memberships in dominant and oppressive groups and may seek to compensate the client by being indulgent. Of course, this is never helpful to the client, since it is motivated by the therapist's guilt rather than his or her genuine concern for the client's welfare (Greene, 1994).

Judith White (personal communication, Feb. 1993) observes that sexual behavior, like any other behavior, constitutes a vehicle for communicating feelings and as such warrants exploration in therapy. It is not unusual for the lesbian of color to express reluctance or refusal to explore this area in any detail, if at all, with a heterosexual therapist. Lesbians may be even less likely to agree to discuss such matters with a heterosexual therapist who is a member of the client's ethnic group. Such reluctance is understandable, since many lesbian clients have accurately experienced such inquiries as voyeuristic on the part of homophobic therapists. It is also noted that lesbian clients of color may perceive therapists who are members of their ethnic group and whom they presume are heterosexual as potentially more homophobic than a therapist from the dominant culture (Croom, 1993; Gock, 1992; Tafoya, 1992).

It is important to be sensitive to the client's feelings about making such disclosures, but that does not mean that the material should go unexplored. It is the therapist's responsibility to earn the client's trust and assist her in understanding the importance of such inquiries. It may be helpful to assist the client in understanding by whom she feels sexually excited and why. If the therapist, however, feels uncomfortable with this material, he or she may respond to the client's reluctance by avoiding any further exploration of it. The therapist may believe this is respecting the client's feelings, but avoidance may just as likely be contrary to a client's interests as in them. For example, the therapist may be avoiding what he or she thinks the material will elicit from the client or may not want to challenge any of the client's assumptions or perceptions. This may arise out of some irrational fear of what the client will do in response, worrying that, for example, the client will discontinue therapy. The therapist may fear that the client's departure from therapy would reflect badly on the therapist, confirming the therapist's fears of incompetence. Hence, the therapist's insecurity about treating lesbians of color and anxiety that they may terminate treatment can cripple his or her ability to challenge and explore clients' feelings appropriately.

Similarly, a White heterosexual therapist may have difficulty understanding and accepting the realistic barriers imposed by racism and homophobia in the client's life, just as a male therapist may not fully understand the role of sexism in a woman's life. This does not mean that all White heterosexual or male therapists are destined to respond in this way, but rather that this is a potential occurrence. This dilemma may be responded to by attempting to move too quickly past communications about discrimination by avoiding, dismissing, or minimizing their importance. While clients may unconsciously use realistic problems associated with racism, sexism, and heterosexism to avoid an exploration of material that is even more painful, the realistic magnitude of life stressors associated with these dimensions cannot be underestimated. They warrant the same respectful attention in therapy as intrapsychic explorations (Greene, 1994).

The therapist who is also a lesbian of color may be predisposed to certain countertransference dilemmas. The most obvious is observed in the therapist who is overidentified with the client and as a result tends to overlook or minimize psychopathology. The therapist may attribute all of the client's problems to the barriers that result from institutional oppression and may unconsciously avoid an exploration of other significant aspects of the client's personal life. A therapist who harbors a fear of overidentification or loss of her own boundaries tends to avoid any identification with the client, which can impair the therapist's capacity for empathy.

The therapist who is a lesbian or lesbian of color may face other countertransference issues related to the maintenance of therapeutic boundaries. Most therapists are faced with the challenge of maintaining appropriate distance without seeming aloof and disinterested in the client's dilemma. This is complicated by the tendency for some clients with multiple minority status similar or identical to that of the therapist to harbor idealized expectations of the therapist and of therapy. There may be a tendency to presume that the therapist "knows" exactly how she feels because she is the "same." In this fantasized view of the therapist, the client may presume that the therapist will not need to ask detailed questions about sensitive issues or explore intrapsychic parameters of realistic problems related to ethnicity, gender, sexual orientation, or the discrimination that accompanies them. While such assumptions may be flattering to the therapist initially, one must be careful not to reinforce these erroneous beliefs. Doing so often serves the purpose of blocking or cutting off communication and exploration rather than facilitating it. Furthermore, acting on these beliefs predisposes the therapist to substitute intellectual discussions of social phenomena for therapeutic inquiries. The latter practice should not be confused with validating the client's accurate perception of discriminatory barriers.

Lesbian women of color are often vulnerable to isolation and estrangement. Therapists who are members of these groups are no exception. Therapists who are lesbians of color must be sure that they have developed supportive networks of peers and colleagues and adequate social and emotional support in their own lives, lest they inadvertently seek to gratify these needs, turning to clients with whom they share these important human dimensions. Many aspects of the psychotherapy process can facilitate a client's wish for a personal relationship with the therapist. In this scenario, lesbian of color clients and therapists share significant and realistic experiences and are members of groups that are much smaller than the mainstream. In this context, it can be tempting for the therapist to view clients as potential social acquaintances, friends, or even lovers. This is a natural phenomenon when people share important attributes or life experiences, and particularly when they are members of minority groups in hostile environments. If, however, the therapist succumbs to the temptation to develop a dual relationship with the client, she engages in the unethical practice of abdicating her primary role and responsibility to respond to the needs of the client as a therapist, adopting instead the easier social role. Similarly, therapists who discuss their ambivalence about maintaining the boundaries of the relationship or their own desire for a personal relationship with a client risk being seductive. Discussions of this sort should take place in the therapist's own therapy or supervision. While such behavior gratifies the therapist's personal needs, there is no evidence to suggest that it is ever helpful to the client. In fact, most evidence suggests the contrary (Gartrell, 1993). Furthermore, client requests or even demands for such contacts or relationships do not relieve therapists of responsibility for the negative effects of granting such requests. The failure to maintain boundaries in this area appropriately can effectively undermine the client's treatment.

SUMMARY

Many lesbian women of color in the United States come from ethnic groups that were at some point in history colonized or captured by invaders from countries with patriarchal values. For all of these women, the original values and practices of their cultures were altered by this contact; some were almost obliterated. As a result, many people took on the patriarchal values of their colonizers, and others became more intensely patriarchal than they were prior to contact. In these systems, women who are not subordinate to men and who challenge or do not rigidly adhere to traditional gender roles must be discredited, making lesbian sexuality an affront. Men of color are expected to treat women in accordance with these values. Openly acknowledging or tolerating lesbians of color may be perceived as a failure to keep the women in their culture subordinate. Hence, there are complex roots to homophobia in the groups discussed earlier and in lesbians of color themselves.

In this context, there is the potential for negative effects on the health and psychological well-being of lesbian women of color. Mental health practitioners must make themselves aware of the distinct combinations of stressors and psychological demands impinging on lesbians of color, particularly the potential for isolation, anger, and frustration. Aside from being culturally literate, the practitioner must develop a sense of the unique experience of the client with respect to the importance of their ethnic identity, gender, and sexual orientation and their need to establish priorities in an often confusing and painful maze of loyalties and estrangements.

References

Acosta, E. "Affinity for Black Heritage: Seeking Lifestyle Within a Community." *Blade,* 1989, *11,* A-1, A-25.

AIDS Bhedbar Virodhi Andolan. "Homosexuality in India: Culture and Heritage." In R. Ratti (ed.), *A Lotus of Another Color.* Boston: Alyson, 1993.

Allen, P. G. "Beloved Women: The Lesbian in American Indian Culture." In T. Darty and S. Potter (eds.), *Women Identified Women.* Palo Alto, Calif.: Mayfield, 1984.

Allen, P. G. *The Sacred Hoop: Recovering the Feminine in American Indian Traditions.* Boston: Beacon Press, 1986.

Amaro, H. "Coming Out: Hispanic Lesbians, Their Families and Communities." Paper presented at the National Coalition of Hispanic Mental Health and Human Services Organization, Austin, Tex., 1978.

Bannerji, K. "No Apologies." In R. Ratti (ed.), *A Lotus of Another Color.* Boston: Alyson, 1993.

Bass-Hass, R. "The Lesbian Dyad: Basic Issues and Value Systems." *Journal of Sex Research,* 1968, *4,* 126.

Bell, A., and Weinberg, M. *Homosexualities: A Study of Human Diversity Among Men and Women.* New York: Simon & Schuster, 1978.

Boyd-Franklin, N. *Black Families in Therapy: A Multisystems Approach.* New York: Guilford Press, 1990.

Bradshaw, C. "A Japanese View of Dependency: What Can Amae Psychology Contribute to Feminist Theory and Therapy?" *Women and Therapy,* 1990, *9,* 67–86.

Brownworth, V. A. "Linda Villarosa Speaks Out." *Deneuve,* 1993, *3*(3), 16–19, 56.

Chan, C. "Asian Lesbians: Psychological Issues in the 'Coming Out' Process." *Asian American Psychological Association Journal,* 1987, *12,* 16–18.

Chan, C. "Issues of Identity Development Among Asian American Lesbians and Gay Men." *Journal of Counseling and Development,* 1989, *68*(1), 16–20.

Chan, C. "Cultural Considerations in Counseling Asian American Lesbians and Gay Men." In S. Dworkin and F. Gutierrez (eds.), *Counseling Gay Men and Lesbians.* Alexandria, Va.: American Association for Counseling and Development, 1992.

Christian, B. *Black Feminist Criticism: Perspectives on Black Women Writers.* New York: Pergamon, 1985.

Clarke, C. "The Failure to Transform: Homophobia in the Black Community." In B. Smith (ed.), *Home Girls: A Black Feminist Anthology.* New York: Kitchen Table–Women of Color Press, 1983.

Clarke, C. "Saying the Least Said, Telling the Least Told: The Voices of Black Lesbian Writers." In M. Silvera (ed.), *Piece of My Heart: A Lesbian of Color Anthology.* Toronto, Ontario: Sister Vision Press, 1991.

Claybourne, J. "Blacks and Gay Liberation." In K. Jay and A. Young (eds.), *Lavender Culture.* New York: Jove/Harcourt Brace Jovanovich, 1978.

Clunis, M., and Green, G. D. *Lesbian Couples.* Seattle, Wash.: Seal Press, 1988.

Collins, P. H. *Black Feminist Thought: Knowledge, Consciousness, and the Politics of Empowerment.* Boston: Unwin Hyman, 1990.

Croom, G. "The Effects of a Consolidated Versus Non-Consolidated Identity on Expectations of African American Lesbians Selecting Mates: A Pilot Study." Unpublished doctoral dissertation, Illinois School of Professional Psychology, 1993.

deMonteflores, C. "Notes on the Management of Difference." In T. Stein and C. Cohen (eds.), *Contemporary Perspectives in Psychotherapy with Lesbians and Gay Men.* New York: Plenum, 1986.

Dew, M. A. "The Effects of Attitudes on Inferences of Homosexuality and Perceived Physical Attractiveness in Women." *Sex Roles,* 1985, *12,* 143–155.

Dyne, L. "Is D.C. Becoming the Gay Capital of America?" *Washingtonian,* Sept. 1980, pp. 96–101, 133–141.

Espín, O. "Cultural and Historical Influences on Sexuality in Hispanic/Latina Women: Implications for Psychotherapy." In C. Vance (ed.), *Pleasure and Danger: Exploring Female Sexuality.* London: Routledge and Kegan Paul, 1984.

Espín, O. "Issues of Identity in the Psychology of Latina Lesbians." In Boston Lesbian Psychologies Collective (eds.), *Lesbian Psychologies: Explorations and Challenges.* Urbana: University of Illinois Press, 1987.

Falco, K. L. *Psychotherapy with Lesbian Clients.* New York: Brunner/Mazel, 1991.

Folayan, A. "African American Issues: The Soul of It." In B. Berzon (ed.), *Positively Gay.* Berkeley, Calif.: Celestial Arts, 1992.

Garcia, N., Kennedy, C., Pearlman, S. F., and Perez, J. "The Impact of Race and Culture Differences: Challenges to Intimacy in Lesbian Relationships." In Boston Lesbian Psychologies Collective (eds.), *Lesbian Psychologies: Explorations and Challenges.* Urbana: University of Illinois Press, 1987.

Garnets, L., and Kimmel, D. "Lesbian and Gay Male Dimensions in the Psychological Study of Human Diversity." In J. Goodchilds (ed.), *Psychological Perspectives on Human Diversity in America.* Washington, D.C.: American Psychological Association, 1991.

Gartrell, N. "Boundaries in Lesbian Therapy Relationships." *Women and Therapy,* 1993, *12,* 29–50.

Glassgold, J. "New Directions in Dynamic Theories of Lesbianism: From Psychoanalysis to Social Constructionism." In J. Chrisler and D. Howard (eds.), *New Directions in Feminist Psychology: Practice, Theory and Research.* New York: Springer, 1992.

Gock, T. S. "Psychotherapy with Asian Pacific Gay Men: Psychological Issues, Treatment Approach and Therapeutic Guidelines." Paper presented at the meeting of the Asian American Psychological Association, Los Angeles, Aug. 1985.

Gock, T. S. "Asian-Pacific Islander Issues: Identity Integration and Pride." In B. Berzon (ed.), *Positively Gay.* Berkeley, Calif.: Celestial Arts, 1992.

Gomez, J. "A Cultural Legacy Denied and Discovered: Black Lesbians in Fiction by Women." In B. Smith (ed.), *Home Girls: A Black Feminist Anthology.* New York: Kitchen Table–Women of Color Press, 1983.

Gomez, J., and Smith, B. "Taking the Home out of Homophobia: Black Lesbian Health." In E. C. White (ed.), *The Black Women's Health Book: Speaking for Ourselves.* Seattle, Wash.: Seal Press, 1990.

Grahn, J. *Another Mother Tongue: Gay Words, Gay Worlds.* Boston: Beacon Press, 1984.

Greene, B. "When the Therapist Is White and the Patient Is Black: Considerations for Psychotherapy in the Feminist Heterosexual and Lesbian Communities." *Women and Therapy,* 1986, *5,* 41–66.

Greene, B. "Sturdy Bridges: The Role of African American Mothers in the Socialization of African American Children." *Women and Therapy,* 1990a, *10*(1/2), 205–225.

Greene, B. "African American Lesbians: The Role of Family, Culture and Racism." *BG Magazine,* 1990b, pp. 6, 26.

Greene, B. "Ethnic Minority Lesbians and Gay Men: Mental Health and Treatment Issues." *Journal of Consulting and Clinical Psychology,* Apr. 1992, *62*(2).

Greene, B. "Psychotherapy with African-American Women: Integrating Feminist and Psychodynamic Models." *Journal of Training and Practice in Professional Psychology,* 1993a, *7*(1), 49–66.

Greene, B. "Stereotypes of African American Sexuality: A Commentary." In S. Rathus, J. Nevid, and L. Rathus-Fichner (eds.), *Human Sexuality in a World of Diversity.* Needham Heights, Mass.: Allyn and Bacon, 1993b.

Greene, B. "Lesbian Women of Color: Triple Jeopardy." In L. Comas-Diaz and B. Greene (eds.), *Women of Color: Integrating Ethnic and Gender Identities in Psychotherapy.* New York: Guilford Press, 1994.

Greene, B. "African American Lesbians: Triple Jeopardy." In A. Brown-Collins (ed.), *The Psychology of African American Women.* New York: Guilford Press, 1996.

Gutierrez, E. "Latino Issues: Gay and Lesbian Latinos Claiming La Raza." In B. Berzon (ed.), *Positively Gay.* Berkeley, Calif.: Celestial Arts, 1992.

Gutierrez, F., and Dworkin, S. "Gay, Lesbian, and African American: Managing the Integration of Identities." In S. Dworkin and F. Gutierrez (eds.), *Counseling Gay Men and Lesbians.* Alexandria, Va.: American Association of Counseling and Development, 1992.

H., Pamela. "Asian American Lesbians: An Emerging Voice in the Asian American Community." In Asian Women United of California (eds.), *Making Waves: An Anthology of Writings by and About Asian American Women.* Boston: Beacon Press, 1989.

Heske, S., Khayal, and Utsa. "There Are, Always Have Been, Always Will Be Lesbians in India." *Conditions: 13. International Focus,* 1986, *1,* 135–146.

Hidalgo, H. "The Puerto Rican Lesbian in the United States." In T. Darty and S. Potter (eds.), *Woman Identified Women.* Palo Alto, Calif.: Mayfield, 1984.

Hidalgo, H., and Hidalgo-Christensen, E. "The Puerto-Rican Lesbian and the Puerto-Rican Community." *Journal of Homosexuality,* 1976, *2,* 109–121.

hooks, b. *Ain't I a Woman: Black Women and Feminism.* Boston: South End Press, 1981.

Icard, L. "Black Gay Men and Conflicting Social Identities: Sexual Orientation Versus Racial Identity." *Journal of Social Work and Human Sexuality,* 1986, *4*(1/2), 83–93.

Jayakar, P. *The Children of Barren Women: Essays, Investigations, Stories.* New Delhi: Penguin, 1994.

Jeffries, I. "Strange Fruits at the Purple Manor: Looking Back on 'the Life' in Harlem." *NYQ,* Feb. 23, 1992, pp. 40–45.

Kanuha, V. "Compounding the Triple Jeopardy: Battering in Lesbian of Color Relationships." *Women and Therapy,* 1990, *9*(1/2), 169–183.

Khush. "Fighting Back: An Interview with Pratibha Parmar." In R. Ratti (ed.), *A Lotus of Another Color.* Boston: Alyson, 1993.

Kim. "They Aren't That Primitive Back Home." In R. Ratti (ed.), *A Lotus of Another Color*. Boston: Alyson, 1993.

Kite, M. "When Perceptions Meet Reality: Individual Differences in Reactions to Lesbians and Gay Men." In B. Greene and G. Herek (eds.), *Lesbian and Gay Psychology: Theory, Research, and Clinical Applications*. Thousand Oaks, Calif.: Sage, 1994.

Kite, M., and Deaux, K. "Gender Belief Systems: Homosexuality and the Implicit Inversion Theory." *Psychology of Women Quarterly*, 1987, *11*, 83–96.

LaFromboise, T. D., Heyle, A. M., and Ozer, E. J. "Changing and Diverse Roles of Women in American Indian Cultures." *Sex Roles*, 1990, *22*(7/8), 455–476.

Lee, C. A. "An Asian Lesbian's Struggle." In M. Silvera (ed.), *Piece of My Heart: A Lesbian of Color Anthology*. Toronto, Ontario: Sister Vision Press, 1991.

Mays, V., and Cochran, S. "The Black Women's Relationship Project: A National Survey of Black Lesbians." In M. Shernoff and W. Scott (eds.), *The Sourcebook on Lesbian/Gay Health Care*. (2nd ed.) Washington, D.C.: National Lesbian and Gay Health Foundation, 1988.

Mays, V., Cochran, S., and Rhue, S. "The Impact of Perceived Discrimination on the Intimate Relationships of Black Lesbians." *Journal of Homosexuality*, forthcoming.

Meera. "Working Together: An Interview with Urvashi Vaid." In R. Ratti (ed.), *A Lotus of Another Color*. Boston: Alyson, 1993.

Morales, E. "Ethnic Minority Families and Minority Gays and Lesbians." *Marriage and Family Review*, 1989, *14*(3/4), 217–239.

Morales, E. "Latino Gays and Latina Lesbians." In S. Dworkin and F. Gutierrez (eds.), *Counseling Gay Men and Lesbians: Journey to the End of the Rainbow*. Alexandria, Va.: American Association for Counseling and Development, 1992.

Morgan, K., and Eliason, M. "The Role of Psychotherapy in Caucasian Lesbians' Lives." *Women and Therapy*, 1992, *13*, 27–52.

Moses, A. E., and Hawkins, R. *Counseling Lesbian Women and Gay Men: A Life Issues Approach*. St. Louis, Mo.: Mosby, 1982.

Namjoshi, S. "Flesh and Paper: An Interview." New York: WNET, June 14, 1992. Television program.

Newman, B. S. "The Relative Importance of Gender Role Attitudes to Male and Female Attitudes Toward Lesbians." *Sex Roles*, 1989, *21*, 451–465.

Noda, B., Tsui, K., and Wong, Z. "Coming Out: We Are Here in the Asian Community: A Dialogue with Three Asian Women." *Bridge: An Asian American Perspective*, Spring 1979.

Omosupe, K. "Black/Lesbian/Bulldagger." *Differences: A Journal of Feminist and Cultural Studies*, 1991, *2*(2), 101–111.

Poussaint, A. "An Honest Look at Black Gays and Lesbians." *Ebony*, Sept. 1990, pp. 124, 126, 130–131.

Ratti, R. "Introduction." In R. Ratti (ed.), *A Lotus of Another Color: An Unfolding of the South Asian Gay and Lesbian Experience*. Boston: Alyson, 1993.

Sears, V. L. "Cross-Cultural Ethnic Relationships." Unpublished manuscript, 1987.

Shah, N. "Sexuality, Identity, and the Uses of History." In R. Ratti (ed.), *A Lotus of Another Color*. Boston: Alyson, 1993.

Shockley, A. "The Black Lesbian in American Literature: An Overview." In L. Bethel and B. Smith (eds.), *Conditions: 5. The Black Women's Issue*, 1979, *2*(2), 133–144.

Silvera, M. "Man Royals and Sodomites: Some Thoughts on the Invisibility of Afro-Caribbean Lesbians." In M. Silvera (ed.), *Piece of My Heart: A Lesbian of Color Anthology*. Toronto, Ontario: Sister Vision Press, 1991.

Smith, B. "Toward a Black Feminist Criticism." In G. Hull, P. Scott, and B. Smith (eds.), *All the Women Are White, All the Blacks Are Men, But Some of Us Are Brave*. Old Westbury, N.Y.: Feminist Press, 1982.

Smith, B., and Smith, B. "Across the Kitchen Table: A Sister to Sister Dialogue." In C. Moraga and G. Anzaldúa (eds.), *This Bridge Called My Back: Writings by Radical Women of Color*. Watertown, Mass.: Persephone Press, 1981.

Tafoya, T. "Native Gay and Lesbian Issues: The Two Spirited." In B. Berzon (ed.), *Positively Gay*. Berkeley, Calif.: Celestial Arts, 1992.

Tafoya, T., and Rowell, R. "Counseling Native American Lesbians and Gays." In M. Shernoff and W. A. Scott (eds.), *The Sourcebook on Lesbian/Gay Health Care*. Washington, D.C.: National Lesbian and Gay Health Foundation, 1988.

Taylor, A. T. "Conceptions of Masculinity and Femininity as a Basis for Stereotypes of Male and Female Homosexuals." *Journal of Homosexuality*, 1983, *9*, 37–53.

Tremble, B., Schneider, M., and Appathurai, C. "Growing Up Gay or Lesbian in a Multicultural Context." *Journal of Homosexuality*, 1989, *17*, 253–267.

Trujillo, C. (ed.). *Chicana Lesbians: The Girls Our Mothers Warned Us About*. Berkeley, Calif.: Third Woman Press, 1991.

Vasquez, E. "Homosexuality in the Context of the Mexican American Culture." In D. Kukel (ed.), *Sexual Issues in Social Work: Emerging Concerns in Education and Practice*. Honolulu: University of Hawaii School of Social Work, 1979.

Weinrich, J., and Williams, W. L. "Strange Customs, Familiar Lives: Homosexuality in Other Cultures." In J. Gonsiorek and J. Weinrich (eds.), *Homosexuality: Research Findings for Public Policy*. Thousand Oaks, Calif.: Sage, 1991.

Weston, K. *Families We Choose: Lesbians, Gays and Kinship*. New York: Columbia University Press, 1991.

Whitley, B. E., Jr. "The Relation of Sex Role Orientation to Heterosexual Attitudes Toward Homosexuality." *Sex Roles*, 1987, *17*, 103–113.

Williams, W. L. *The Spirit and the Flesh: Sexual Diversity in American Indian Culture*. Boston: Beacon Press, 1986.

Wooden, W. S., Kawasaki, H., and Mayeda, R. "Lifestyles and Identity Maintenance Among Gay Japanese-American Males." *Alternative Lifestyles*, 1983, *5*, 236–243.

Wyatt, G., Strayer, R., and Lobitz, W. C. "Issues in the Treatment of Sexually Dysfunctioning Couples of African American Descent." *Psychotherapy*, 1976, *13*, 44–50.

CHAPTER TWENTY-SEVEN

Prevalence and Predictors
of Physical Partner Abuse Among
Mexican American Women

E. Anne Lown
William A. Vega

*This chapter, which focuses on a single group of Mexican women
in Fresno, California, is the first large study of intimate partner
violence in a subgroup of Latinas between the ages of 18 and
59. In addition to the insights provided, the findings have
importation implications for prevention and treatment.*

Intimate partner violence (IPV) is recognized as a prevalent problem (Ratner, 1993; Sorenson, Upchurch, and Shen, 1996; Stark and Flitcraft, 1988; Straus and Gelles, 1990) with serious medical and social consequences (Sorenson, Upchurch, and Shen, 1996; Burnam and others, 1987; Drossman and others, 1990; Golding, 1994, 1996; Grisso, Wishner, and Schwarz, 1991; Kellermann and Mercy, 1992; Koss, 1992; Leserman and others, 1996; Walker and others, 1992; Warshaw and others, 1993). Although research on IPV among Hispanics has been published (Ratner, 1993; Sorenson, Upchurch, and Shen, 1996; Caetano and others, 2000; Kantor, Jasinski, and Aldarondo, 1994; Straus and Smith, 1990), little is known about the prevalence of IPV and associated factors among ethnic subgroups such as Mexican Americans.

The study was supported by NIH grants MH5119 and DA12167. Work on the chapter was supported by NIAAA fellowship T32AA07420 and the Alcohol Research Group. We wish to thank Meredith Minkler, Jacqueline Golding, Lorraine Midanik, and Ralph Catalano for many helpful comments, as well as Ezra Susser, whose vision and clarity were invaluable. The research was conducted after appropriate review of the research protocol and interview instrument by the institutional review boards of the University of California, Berkeley, and the California State University, Fresno. All interviews were voluntary and were conducted after the survey was fully explained to potential respondents and subjects gave written consent to be interviewed. Respondents had the right to refuse the interview without any penalty or to terminate the interview at any time. No human subject confidentiality issues arose during the course of the research.

Among Hispanics, reports of IPV during the past year range from 10.5 percent to 17.3 percent (Kantor, Jasinski, and Aldarondo, 1994; Straus and Smith, 1990; Neff, Holamon, and Schluter, 1995), compared with rates among Whites of 3.4 percent to 11.6 percent (Ratner, 1993; Sorenson, Upchurch, and Shen, 1996; Stark and Flitcraft, 1988; Straus and Gelles, 1990). However, debate exists about whether Hispanic families are more violent than Anglo families. Acculturation status may account for differing prevalence rates.

In the National Family Violence Survey (NFVERSUS), past-year IPV was higher among Hispanics than among Whites (17.3 percent versus 10.8 percent) (Straus and Smith, 1990). However, the interview was available only in English, and the survey results may disproportionately describe highly acculturated Hispanics. Other studies report lower rates of physical or sexual violence among Hispanics than among Whites (Sorenson, Upchurch, and Shen, 1996; McFarlane, Parker, Koeken, and Bullock, 1992; Sorenson and others, 1987). These studies provided Spanish interviews and thus may have included a wider range of acculturation levels. Finally, no differences were found between Hispanics and Whites in two population-based studies representing a national sample ($n = 800$) (Kantor, Jasinski, and Aldarondo, 1994) and an urban sample ($n = 379$) (Neff, Holamon, and Schluter, 1995).

Increased acculturation to the United States by Hispanics (for which birthplace is often used as a proxy) has been associated with numerous health and mental health problems (Burnam and others, 1987; English, Kharrazi, and Guendelman, 1997; Guendelman and English, 1995; Guendelman and Abrams, 1995; Vega and others, 1998; Vega, Alderete, Kolody, and Aguilar-Gaxiola, 1998) as well as the perpetration of IPV (Kantor, Jasinski, and Aldarondo, 1994; Sorenson and Telles, 1991). Among Mexicans, acculturation has been described as disruptive to families, resulting in the deterioration of Mexicans' traditionally strong extended family orientation and social support networks (Keefe, 1984; Vega, 1990). New immigrants also face stresses as they adapt to a new language and culture while often lacking key instrumental skills (Rogler, Cortes, and Malgady, 1991). It could be argued that both immigrants and U.S.-born Mexican Americans face family hardships that could result in increased violence.

Disparate findings on the prevalence of abuse among women of Mexican origin may be due to differences in study design and lack of measurement of acculturation. This analysis is unique in that it involves the first large study of IPV to employ a sample of exclusively Mexican American women. In addition, the survey represented urban, town, and rural areas and employed both English and Spanish interviews. Findings from this analysis address two main questions. First, what is the prevalence of IPV by a current partner in a population-based sample of urban, town, and rural Mexican American women? Second, what is the role of birthplace in a woman's risk of physical abuse by her male partner? Since IPV among U.S.-born women may be explained by the higher frequency of characteristics that are common risk factors for abuse, such as young age, greater number of children, poverty, urban residence, social isolation, and lack of church attendance, these characteristics were controlled for in logistic regression analyses.

METHODS

Sample

The analysis includes data for women who were involved in an intimate relationship with a male partner at the time of the interview and who answered questions about violence ($n = 1,155$). These women are a subsample from a larger stratified randomized household survey of 3,012 men and women of Mexican origin. All respondents were aged 18 to 59 years and lived in Fresno County, California, a primarily agricultural county whose population is 38 percent Hispanic. Overall response rates were 90 percent. Subjects were selected in a three-stage stratified cluster sampling design with census blocks as primary sampling units and households as secondary sampling units. The original sample was stratified by sex and place of residence (urban, town, and rural). (For more information about the sampling procedure, see Vega and others, 1998.) To collect data for this study, we used a Computer Assisted Personal Interview (CAPI) system administered by a trained interviewer in the participant's home. Interviews were administered in English or Spanish and took approximately one hour. Weights were applied at the analysis stage to ensure comparability of the final sample to the actual distribution of county residents by urban, town, and rural residence, census block, and household size.

Measures

The outcome variable is physical abuse by a current male partner, measured by asking, "Has your current (spouse/partner) ever pushed you, hit you with a fist, used a knife or gun, tried to choke or burn you?" The question was adapted from the Abuse Assessment Screen (McFarlane, Parker, Koeken, and Bullock, 1992). The primary predictor variable is birthplace (United States versus Mexico). Control variables include age (18–30 years versus 31–59 years), place of residence (urban, town, rural), family income (0–$999 per month versus $1,000 or more per month), church attendance (one or more times per month versus less than one time per month), number of children (zero to three versus four or more), and social support. Social support was measured by asking, "Do you have anyone with whom you can share your innermost thoughts and feelings or problems?" Other variables examined include partner's unemployment (yes/no), a woman's heavy alcohol use (drinking five or more drinks per day at least once a week during any period of her life), and income ratio (a woman's earning more than or as much as her male partner versus less than her partner).

Analysis

All bivariate and logistic regression procedures were first calculated with the statistical software SPSS, version 7.5 (SPSS). SUDAAN30 was used for all analyses to adjust standard errors to reflect stratified and cluster sampling strategies. Prevalence estimates and 95 percent confidence intervals for physical abuse (ever by current partner) were calculated. Univariate and bivariate frequencies were used to describe characteristics of those with and without a history of physical abuse by a current partner. Group differences and crude odds ratios were calculated with a chi-square test or the Fisher exact test, with significance levels set at .05. Logistic regression models were constructed to describe differences between women reporting or not reporting IPV, with factors thought to be associated with abuse controlled for. The final model was built by introducing one predictor at a time and making log-likelihood comparisons to retain variables when the new model was different from the previous model at the .05 level.

RESULTS

Sample Characteristics

The distribution of the sample by demographic characteristics and by abuse status is shown in Table 27.1. A total of 127 women (10.7 percent; 95 percent confidence interval [CI] = 8.03 percent, 13.40 percent) reported physical abuse by a current partner. Approximately two-fifths of the women were born in the United States. The median age was 32 years, with a range of 18 to 59 years. Once the data were weighted, over 60 percent of the sample lived in an urban area, 15 percent lived in small towns, and 25 percent lived in rural areas of Fresno County. Income was low, with 45 percent having family incomes of less than $1,000 per month. Women had a median of two children. Church attendance was common, with 62 percent attending church one or more times a month. Social support was reported by 78 percent of women.

Table 27.2 presents crude and adjusted odds ratios for IPV. In bivariate analyses, the odds of reporting IPV were 2.45 times higher (95 percent CI = 1.38, 4.35) among U.S.-born women than among Mexican-born women. For women living in an urban environment, the odds of reporting IPV were more than two and a half times higher than for women living in rural areas. Living in a town was not associated with significantly elevated risk for IPV compared with rural residence. No church attendance or infrequent church attendance significantly increased the odds of IPV.

Table 27.1. Demographic Characteristics (Weighted) of Mexican American Women with Current Partners, by Physical Abuse Status: Fresno County, California, 1996

	Percentage of Sample (n = 1,188)[a]	Percentage Physically Abused
All respondents	100.00	10.7
Birthplace		
United States	41.7	15.8
Mexico[b]	58.3	7.1
Age, years (median = 32)		
18–30	44.1	12.6
31–59	55.9	9.3
Residence		
Urban	60.5	13.2
Town	14.7	8.6
Rural	24.9	5.8
Income[c]		
$0–999 per month	44.6	10.5
$1,000 or more per month	55.4	10.7
Social support		
No	21.7	14.2
Yes	78.3	9.7
Number of children (median = 2)		
4 or more	39.5	13.4
0–3	60.5	9.0
Church attendance		
Less than once a month	37.9	16.2
Once or more a month	62.1	7.4
Partner unemployed		
Yes	8.1	17.3
No	91.9	10.1
Woman's heavy alcohol use		
Five or more drinks per day once weekly	10.5	15.1
Fewer than five drinks per day once weekly	89.5	10.2
Couple's income ratio		
Woman's earnings equal to or greater than partner's	28.0	12.8
Woman's earnings less than partner's	72.0	9.8

[a]The effective *n* is weighted to updated Fresno County adult population data by residence (urban/town/rural), household size, and census block aggregate. Unweighted *n* = 1,155.
[b]A total of 691 women were born in Mexico, and 1 was born in Honduras.
[c]There were thirty-eight missing values for income.

Table 27.2. Logistic Regression: Crude and Adjusted Odds Ratios for Mexican American Women Reporting Physical Abuse by Their Current Partner

	Crude OR	95% CI	Adjusted OR	95% CI
Birthplace				
United States	2.45**	1.38, 4.35	2.10**	1.24, 3.56
Mexico	1.00	. . . .	1.00	. . .
Age, years				
18–30	1.41	0.83, 2.38	1.81*	1.10, 3.00
31 or more	1.00	. . . .	1.00	. . .
Residence				
Urban	2.57**	1.41, 4.69	2.13*	1.15, 3.93
Town	1.76	0.92, 3.39	1.79	0.90, 3.54
Rural	1.00	. . . .	1.00	. . .
Income, monthly				
$0–$999	0.98	0.56, 1.73	0.91	0.54, 1.55
$1,000 or more	1.00	. . . .	1.00	. . .
Social support				
No	1.53	0.86, 2.75	1.84*	1.05, 3.20
Yes	1.00	. . . .	1.00	. . .
Number of children				
4 or more	1.57	0.93, 2.64	2.6***	. . .
0–3	1.00	. . . .	1.00	
Church attendance				
Less than once a month	2.42**	1.44, 4.07	1.72*	1.05, 2.82
Once or more a month	1.00	. . . .	1.00	. . .
Possible mediating variables[a]				
Partner looking for work	1.85	0.80, 4.26	1.52	0.73, 3.20
Woman's heavy alcohol use (ever)	1.56	0.81, 3.03	1.15	0.59, 2.25
Woman's earnings equal to or more than her partner's	1.35	0.75, 2.45	1.00	0.57, 1.73

Note: OR = odds ratio; CI = confidence interval.
[a]Adjusted odds ratios are reported for each of these three characteristics, after control for the seven characteristics in the above model.
*$p \leq .05$; **$p \leq .01$; ***$p \leq .001$.

The independent effects of birthplace, age, residence, income, social support, number of children, and church attendance on IPV were examined with logistic regression models controlling for all other variables. U.S. birthplace remained associated with IPV (odds ratio [OR] = 2.10; 95 percent CI = 1.24, 3.56) even after the other variables in the model were adjusted for. Young age, living in an urban area, lack of social support, having four or more children, and no or infrequent church attendance all were associated with IPV in a logistic regression model.

To examine possible explanations for the association between birthplace and IPV, a number of characteristics were individually introduced into the model. None of the following characteristics explained the IPV–birthplace association: male partner's unemployment, victim's history of heavy alcohol use, or victim's having a higher income than her partner.

DISCUSSION

Abuse of women by their intimate partners remains a major social and public health problem that has serious physical, psychological, and social consequences. Accurate population-based prevalence estimates combined with information about the predictors of abuse provide important information for treatment and prevention (Davidson, 1996).

The overall prevalence of IPV reported in this study suggests that partner violence is not a rare event. The prevalence of IPV among U.S.-born Mexican American women in this study is similar to the reported prevalence among English-speaking Hispanics in the National Family Violence Survey.

Sociodemographic characteristics associated with IPV in this population are consistent with those reported in previous studies of both Anglo and Hispanic populations, which have identified young age (Ratner, 1993; Stark and Flitcraft, 1988; Kantor, Jasinski, and Aldarondo, 1994; Dearwater and others, 1998; Straus, Gelles, and Steinmetz, 1980; Nielsen, Endo, and Ellington, 1992), living in an urban area (Sorenson, Upchurch, and Shen, 1996; Straus and Smith, 1990), social isolation (Sorenson, Upchurch, and Shen, 1996; Nielsen, Endo, and Ellington, 1992), and having many children as common risk factors (Sorenson, Upchurch, and Shen, 1996; Straus, Gelles, and Steinmetz, 1980). Low income is sometimes reported as a risk factor (Sorenson, Upchurch, and Shen, 1996; Stark and Flitcraft, 1991), but more often no association is found for low-income and partner abuse (Kantor, Jasinski, and Aldarondo, 1994; Straus and Smith, 1990; Fagan and Browne, 1994). Lack of variability in income in our sample (reflecting low income among Hispanics in general) made this relation difficult to assess. Religious involvement has been shown to be protective in previous studies (Sorenson, Upchurch, and Shen, 1996; Straus, Gelles, and Steinmetz, 1980), as it was in our sample.

Results from this analysis of women victims of IPV are consistent with findings from three population-based studies that examined birthplace (or acculturation) among perpetrators of IPV. In a national sample of 609 Hispanics (Kantor, Jasinski, and Aldarondo, 1994), U.S. birthplace was a predictor of husbands' violence against their wives (OR = 2.1; p = .05). Similarly, Sorenson and Telles (1991) described higher rates of self-reported perpetration of IPV among U.S.-born Mexican Americans than among those born in Mexico (31 percent versus

12.8 percent; $p < .05$). Caetano and others (2000) described the highest rates of IPV perpetration among moderately acculturated Hispanic men and women and the second highest among those who are highly acculturated. These studies primarily examined birthplace/acculturation status as a factor associated with the perpetration of violence. The current work examines the association between birthplace and IPV victimization.

Results in this study show a consistent association between IPV and higher acculturation and are not limited to immigration status. Other measures intended to capture aspects of acculturation include years in the United States (ten or more years versus less than ten years), country of schooling (all or some schooling in the United States versus all foreign schooling), and a language-based acculturation scale (English dominant, bilingual, and Spanish dominant). Results are consistent with birthplace analyses, with more than two times the odds of reporting IPV among women in each of the highest acculturation groups.

Other possible explanatory factors for the birthplace–abuse association include a woman's alcohol use (Kantor and Straus, 1989), a woman's higher status (Yllo, 1983), measured by the ratio of her income to her partner's), and her male partner's unemployment (Ratner, 1993; Kantor, Jasinski, and Aldarondo, 1994; Catalano, Novaco, and McConnell, 1997). None of these factors was associated with IPV in our data, and the introduction of these variables into our model did not explain the association between IPV and U.S. birthplace.

This study was limited by the fact that questions about IPV were asked only of women, while it was the men who were carrying out the abuse. The strength of this analysis is that it allows us to characterize women who are at risk for abuse. Information on correlates of IPV among women is important in medical and social service settings, where attempts should be made to identify and address IPV. Failure to identify IPV places a woman at continued risk for abuse and may result in treatment failures and increased health care use (Golding and others, 1988; Koss, Koss, and Woodruff, 1991; Leserman, Li, Drossman, and Hu, 1998; McCauley and others, 1995). An examination of IPV and birthplace in a general population of Mexican American men would make an important contribution toward prevention of violent behavior in this group.

Two factors may have contributed to an underestimation of the true prevalence of IPV. First, recently divorced or separated women without current partners were not asked questions about IPV. This group was shown in earlier studies (Ratner, 1993; Sorenson and Telles, 1991; Bergman and Brismar, 1991; Berrios and Grady, 1991) to be at highest risk. Second, women receiving welfare may have denied having partners (since this would violate welfare requirements) and thus were not asked about IPV.

Although this study did not find an association between welfare and IPV, it is worth noting that welfare eligibility requirements that the father be identified and be involved in child support could place abused Mexican American women and their children at significant risk. This problem is particularly serious for immigrant women, who have been shown to have difficulty gaining access to legal and social services and who may not believe that the protections of the U.S. legal system apply to immigrants (Orloff, Jang, and Klein, 1995). Since data for this study were collected in 1996, before welfare reform was instituted, an examination of the impact of welfare reform on IPV is not possible, although it remains an important area for future research.

This study contains all the usual biases of self-report. Underreporting is more likely to be a concern than overreporting, given the sanctions against discussing private behavior. Abused women, particularly if their immigrant status is undocumented, may fear the consequences of reporting and thus fail to disclose abuse. Questions were phrased so as to ask about specific behaviors (hitting, choking) rather than about abuse generally. This technique is shown to yield more positive answers than questions that ask about abuse or violence in general (Russell, 1982). Despite its limitations, this study contributes to literature on IPV among women of Mexican origin in a population-based sample. The sample was unique in that it included urban, town, and rural residents and did not merge several Hispanic groups. The sample represented a significantly larger number of Mexican Americans (with high response rates) than did previous studies of IPV (Kantor, Jasinski, and Aldarondo, 1994; Neff, Holamon, and Schluter, 1995; Sorenson and Telles, 1991).

In sum, IPV among Mexican-origin women is not a rare event, and U.S.-born women are at highest risk. It seems paradoxical that women who are United States born are the target of more violence, given that known risk factors for violence are lower in this group. For example, U.S.-born women report more social supports, fewer children, higher incomes, and higher education. There may be aspects of traditional Mexican culture that serve a protective function for families. With exposure to the United States, traditional culture may erode and families may experience increased stresses, resulting in violence. Conclusions drawn from this analysis have applications in the identification of women at high risk of IPV for the purposes of prevention and treatment.

Mexican Americans are commonly thought to underuse health care services (Andersen, Lewis, and Giachello, 1981), so we cannot rely solely on screening and identification of abused women in the health care setting. These findings point to the importance of developing effective bilingual messages about warning signs of impending abuse as well as disseminating information on where to seek assistance for women at risk. Programs may need to be developed and implemented at the community level, including in schools, religious institutions, community centers, and the workplace (Davidson, 1996). Results from this study may help to target broader public health prevention programs among U.S.-born Mexican American women and their partners. These programs should be aimed at reinforcing family strengths and social networks while addressing the many social conditions, especially in urban areas, that make life among U.S.-born women more stressful (Rueschenberg and Buriel, 1995). Further research should be done to increase understanding of the impact of immigration on a woman's risk for IPV.

References

Andersen, R., Lewis, S. Z., and Giachello, A. L. "Access to Medical Care Among the Hispanic Population of the Southwestern United States." *Journal of Health and Social Behavior,* 1981, *22,* 78–79.

Bergman, B., and Brismar, B. "A Five-Year Follow-Up Study of 117 Battered Women." *American Journal Public Health,* 1991, *81,* 1486–1489.

Berrios, D., and Grady, D. "Domestic Violence, Risk Factors and Outcomes." *Western Journal of Medicine,* 1991, *155,* 133–135.

Burnam, A. R., and others. "Acculturation and Lifetime Prevalence of Psychiatric Disorders Among Mexican Americans in Los Angeles." *Journal of Health and Social Behavior,* 1987, *28,* 89–102.

Caetano, R., and others. "Intimate Partner Violence, Acculturation, and Alcohol Consumption Among Hispanic Couples in the United States." *Journal of Interpersonal Violence,* 2000, *15,* 30–45.

Catalano, R., Novaco, R., and McConnell, W. "A Model of the Net Effect of Job Loss on Violence." *Journal of Personality and Social Psychology,* 1997, *72,* 1440–1447.

Davidson, L. "Editorial: Preventing Injuries from Violence Towards Women." *American Journal Public Health,* 1996, *86,* 12–14.

Dearwater, S. R., and others. "Prevalence of Intimate Partner Abuse in Women Treated at Community Hospital Emergency Departments." *JAMA,* 1998, *280,* 433–438.

Drossman, D. A., and others. "Sexual and Physical Abuse in Women with Functional or Organic Gastrointestinal Disorders." *Annals of Internal Medicine,* 1990, *113,* 828–833.

English, P., Kharrazi, M., and Guendelman, S. "Pregnancy Outcomes and Risk Factors in Mexican Americans: The Effect of Language Use and Mother's Birthplace." *Ethnicity and Disease,* 1997, *7,* 229–240.

Fagan, J., and Browne, A. "Violence Between Spouses and Intimates: Physical Aggression Between Women and Men in Intimate Relationships." In A. J. Reiss and J. A. Roth (eds.), *Understanding and Preventing Violence.* Washington, D.C.: National Academy Press, 1994.

Golding, J. M. "Sexual Assault History and Physical Health in Randomly Selected Los Angeles Women." *Health Psychology,* 1994, *13,* 130–138.

Golding, J. M. "Sexual Assault History and Limitations in Physical Functioning in Two General Population Samples." *Research in Nursing Health,* 1996, *19,* 33–44.

Golding, J. M., and others. "Sexual Assault History and Use of Health and Mental Health Services." *American Journal of Community Psychology,* 1988, *16,* 625–643.

Grisso, J. A., Wishner, A., and Schwarz, D. "A Population-Based Study of Injuries in Inner-City Women." *American Journal of Epidemiology,* 1991, *134,* 59–68.

Guendelman, S., and Abrams, B. "Nutrient Intake of Mexican-American and Non-Hispanic White Women by Reproductive Status: Results of Two National Studies." *Journal of the American Diet Association,* 1995, *95,* 916–918.

Guendelman, S., and English, P. "Effect of United States Residence on Birth Outcome Among Mexican Immigrants: An Exploratory Study." *American Journal of Epidemiology,* 1995, *142*(Suppl.), S30–S38.

Kantor, G. K., Jasinski, J. L., and Aldarondo, E. "Sociocultural Status and Incidence of Marital Violence in Hispanic Families." *Violence and Victims,* 1994, *9,* 207–222.

Kantor, K. G., and Straus, M. A. "Substance Abuse as a Precipitant of Wife Abuse Victimizations." *American Journal of Drug and Alcohol Abuse,* 1989, *15,* 173–189.

Keefe, S. "Real and Ideal Extended Familism Among Mexican Americans and Anglo Americans: On the Meaning of 'Close' Family Ties." *Human Organization,* 1984, *43,* 65–70.

Kellermann, A. L., and Mercy, J. A. "Men, Women, and Murder: Gender-Specific Differences in Rates of Fatal Violence and Victimization." *Journal of Trauma,* 1992, *33,* 1–5.

Koss, M. P. "Somatic Consequences of Violence Against Women." *Archives of Family Medicine,* 1992, *1,* 53–59.

Koss, M. P., Koss, P. G., and Woodruff, J. "Deleterious Effects of Criminal Victimization on Women's Health and Medical Utilization." *Archives of Internal Medicine,* 1991, *151,* 342–347.

Leserman, J., Li, Z., Drossman, D. A., and Hu, Y.J.B. "Selected Symptoms Associated with Sexual and Physical Abuse History Among Female Patients with Gastrointestinal Disorders: The Impact on Subsequent Health Care Visits." *Psychological Medicine,* 1998, *28,* 417–425.

Leserman, J., and others. "Sexual and Physical Abuse History in Gastroenterology Practice: How Types of Abuse Impact Health Status." *Psychosomatic Medicine,* 1996, *58,* 4–15.

McCauley, J., and others. "The 'Battering Syndrome': Prevalence and Clinical Characteristics of Domestic Violence in Primary Care Internal Medicine Practices." *Annals of Internal Medicine,* 1995, *123,* 737–746.

McFarlane, J., Parker, B., Koeken, K., and Bullock, L. "Assessing for Abuse During Pregnancy." *JAMA,* 1992, *267,* 3176–3178.

Neff, J. A., Holamon, B., and Schluter, T. D. "Spousal Violence Among Anglos, Blacks, and Mexican Americans: The Role of Demographic Variables, Psychosocial Predictors, and Alcohol Consumption." *Journal of Family Violence,* 1995, *19,* 1–21.

Nielsen, J. M., Endo, R. K., and Ellington, B. L. "Social Isolation and Wife Abuse: A Research Report." In E. C. Viano (ed.), *Intimate Violence: Interdisciplinary Perspectives.* Washington, D.C.: Hemisphere, 1992.

Orloff, L., Jang, D., and Klein, C. "With No Place to Turn: Improving Advocacy for Battered Immigrant Women." *Family Law Quarterly,* 1995, *29,* 313.

Ratner, P. A. "The Incidence of Wife Abuse and Mental Health Status in Abused Wives in Edmonton, Alberta." *Canadian Journal of Public Health,* 1993, *84,* 246–249.

Rogler, L. H., Cortes, D. E., and Malgady, R. G. "Acculturation and Mental Health Status Among Hispanics." *American Psychologist,* 1991, *46,* 585–597.

Rueschenberg, E. J., and Buriel, R. "Mexican American Family Functioning and Acculturation: A Family Systems Perspective." In A. Padilla (ed.), *Hispanic Psychology: Critical Issues in Theory and Research.* Thousand Oaks, Calif.: Sage, 1995.

Russell, D.E.H. *Rape in Marriage.* New York: Macmillan, 1982.

Shah, B., Barnwell, B., and Bieler, G. *SUDAAN User's Manual, Version 6.4.* (2nd ed.) Research Triangle Park, N.C.: Research Triangle Institute, 1996.

Sorenson, S. B., and Telles, C. A. "Self-Reports of Spousal Violence in a Mexican-American and Non-Hispanic White Population." *Violence and Victims,* 1991, *6,* 3–15.

Sorenson, S. B., Upchurch, D., and Shen, H. "Violence and Injury in Marital Arguments: Risk Patterns and Gender Differences." *American Journal of Public Health,* 1996, *86,* 35–40.

Sorenson, S. B., and others. "The Prevalence of Adult Sexual Assault: The Los Angeles Epidemiologic Catchment Area Project." *American Journal of Epidemiology,* 1987, *126,* 1154–1164.

Stark, E., and Flitcraft, A. "Violence Among Intimates: An Epidemiologic Review." In V. B. Van Hasselt, R. L. Morrison, A. S. Bellack, and M. Hersen (eds.), *Handbook of Family Violence.* New York: Plenum Press, 1988.

Stark, E., and Flitcraft, A. "Spouse Abuse." In M. Rosenberg and M. A. Fenley (eds.), *Violence in America: A Public Health Approach.* New York: Oxford University Press, 1991.

Straus, M. A., and Gelles, R. J. "How Violent Are American Families? Estimates from the National Family Violence Resurvey and Other Studies." In M. Straus and R. Gelles (eds.), *Physical Violence in American Families: Risk Factors and Adaptations to Violence in 8,145 Families.* New Brunswick, N.J.: Transaction Publishers, 1990.

Straus, M. A., Gelles, R. J., and Steinmetz, S. K. *Behind Closed Doors.* New York: Anchor Books, 1980.

Straus, M., and Smith, C. "Violence in Hispanic Families in the United States: Incidence Rates and Structural Interpretations." In M. A. Straus and R. J. Gelles (eds.), *Physical Violence in American Families: Risk Factors and Adaptations to Violence in 8,145 Families.* New Brunswick, N.J.: Transaction Publishers, 1990.

Suitor, J. J., Pillemer, K., and Straus, M. A. "Marital Violence in a Life-Course Perspective." In M. A. Straus and R. J. Gelles (eds.), *Physical Violence in American Families: Risk Factors and Adaptations to Violence in 8,145 Families.* New Brunswick, N.J.: Transaction Books, 1990.

Vega, W. A. "Hispanic Families in the 1980s: A Decade of Research." *Journal of Marriage and the Family,* 1990, *52,* 1015–1024.

Vega, W. A., Alderete, E., Kolody, B., and Aguilar-Gaxiola, S. "Illicit Drug Use Among Mexicans and Mexican Americans in California: The Effects of Gender and Acculturation." *Addiction,* 1998, *93,* 1839–1850.

Vega, W. A., and others. "Lifetime Prevalence of DSM-III-R Psychiatric Disorders Among Urban and Rural Mexican Americans in California." *Archives of General Psychiatry,* 1998, *55,* 771–778.

Walker, E., and others. "Medical and Psychiatric Symptoms in Women with Childhood Sexual Abuse." *Psychosomatic Medicine,* 1992, *54,* 658–664.

Warshaw, M., and others. "Quality of Life and Dissociation in Anxiety Disorder Patients with Histories of Trauma or PTSD." *American Journal of Psychiatry,* 1993, *150,* 1512–1516.

Yllo, K. "Sexual Equality and Violence Against Wives in American States." *Journal of Comparative Family Studies,* 1983, *1,* 67–86.

CHAPTER TWENTY-EIGHT

Acculturation and Disordered Eating Patterns Among Mexican American Women

Rebeca Chamorro[1]
Yvette Flores-Ortiz

The focus and findings of the study described in this chapter are unique for their attention to the emerging problem of disordered eating patterns among young Latinas. The editors of this book consider this problem to be a "disease of acculturation" that results from conflicting cultural notions of beauty. Although the study is based on a small sample of Mexican American women in the San Francisco Bay Area, it is the best presentation available on the subject to date. It opens the door for developing additional studies that address an emerging problem among Latinas.

A significant problem exists regarding the paucity of cross-cultural research among Hispanics (Cuellar and Roberts, 1984; Rogler, Cortes, and Malgady, 1991). This contrasts with census reviews showing that Hispanics will be the largest minority group in the twenty-first century, with individuals of Mexican descent comprising the majority of this ethnic population (Sue, 1981, as cited in Vega and Amaro, 1994). As an ethnic minority group, Mexican Americans undergo the process of acculturation as they adopt certain traits, attitudes, and behaviors of the dominant culture (Berry, 1980).

For Mexican American women, part of the cultural exchange includes the United States' patriarchal definition of beauty as a means of acknowledging women. These physical requisites involve a lean, svelte, almost prepubescent

---

[1]This chapter is based on a doctoral dissertation by R. Chamorro submitted in partial fulfillment for the doctoral degree at the California School of Professional Psychology–Berkeley/Alameda. Parts of it were presented at the Harvard Medical School, Department of Psychiatry's Sixth Annual Research Day. We acknowledge and thank Debra Franko for her support and help in editing this manuscript.

body image. This is in contrast to the Hispanic Health and Nutrition Examination Survey (HHANES), which found Mexican American women to be heavier than their white and nonwhite counterparts (Delgado, Johnson, Roy, and Trevino, 1990). Thus, the aim of the study presented here was to address the dilemma such women may face: In her attempt toward recognition, is the Mexican American woman at risk of "dissolving" the differences between her body shape and that of the larger societal ideal through restrictive eating?

Studies addressing the relevance of culture to eating attitudes have found that Mexican American junior and high school students have high levels of disordered eating (Pumariega, 1986; Joiner and Kashubeck, 1996). Additionally, Hispanic women appear to stand out in comparison to other ethnic minority females. Hispanic Americans and Caucasians share more weight-related body image disturbances as compared to African Americans and Asian Americans (Altabe, 1998). Researchers have also found more severe binge eating symptoms among Hispanic versus black or white women (Fitzgibbon and others, 1998).

The purpose of this study was to correlate levels of acculturation in Mexican American females and eating attitudes. It incorporated five generation levels of Mexican American women as defined by Cuellar, Harris, and Jasso (1980). This range included first-generation women (subjects born in Mexico) to fifth-generation women (subjects, parents, and grandparents born in the United States).

METHOD

Participants

Participants included 139 Mexican American women drawn through flyers from local undergraduate Chicano studies courses, community agencies, and Latina organizations in the San Francisco Bay Area. The mean age was 29.1 years (SD = 10.0). Most of the women were single (58.7 percent), in the process of completing college (46.8 percent), with income levels of $15,000 or less (49.3 percent), and had been in the United States since birth (57.6 percent). Most women were either first-generation (36.0 percent) or second-generation (37.4 percent) Mexican American.

Measures

A demographic questionnaire was developed to quantify age, height, weight, education level, average income, marital status, occupation, and number of years in the United States. The Acculturation Rating Scale for Mexican Americans

(ARSMA; Cuellar, Harris, and Jasso, 1980) is suitable for Mexican Americans of varying socioeconomic, educational, and linguistic levels. The twenty-item questionnaire distinguishes five types of Mexican Americans ranging from: Type 1, Very Mexican to Type 5, Very Anglicized. The twenty-six-item Eating Attitudes Test (EAT-26; Garner, Olmsted, Bohr, and Garfinkel, 1982) is used to assess eating patterns. It comprises three factors: Factor I: dieting; Factor II: bulimia and food preoccupation; Factor III: oral control and perceived pressure from others to gain weight. These factors significantly distinguish among sub-samples of restricters versus bulimics.

RESULTS

Table 28.1 shows that the relationship between eating attitudes and levels of acculturation was positive ($r = .129$, $p > .05$). A positive, statistically significant relationship was found between total acculturation scores and Factor III of the EAT, $r = .235$, $p < .01$ (significant at the .01 level).

In addition a negative, statistically significant correlation between acculturation level, as measured by the ARSMA, and generation level, $r = -238$, $p < .01$ (significant at the .01 level), was found. Table 28.2 breaks down the relationship among generation level, mean ARSMA acculturation level, and eating attitudes score. This table clearly shows that second-generation Mexican American women, as compared to first-, third-, fourth-, and fifth-generation levels, produced the highest eating attitude scores and the greatest acculturation level scores.

Table 28.1. Mean Total EAT Scores and EAT Factor Scores by Levels of ARSMA Categories as Compared to Standardized Control Group

ARSMA Category	EAT Total M	EAT Total (SD)	EAT FAC01 M	EAT FAC01 (SD)	EAT FAC02 M	EAT FAC02 (SD)	EAT FAC03 M	EAT FAC03 (SD)
1	—	—	—	—	—	—	—	—
2	6.8	(5.9)	5.5	(4.5)	1.3	(1.5)	—	—
3	7.9	(6.2)	6.1	(5.2)	0.4	(1.1)	1.2	(2.0)
4	9.4	(8.7)	5.7	(6.4)	1.1	(2.3)	2.4	(2.8)
5	12.3	(13.0)	8.1	(8.9)	1.5	(3.0)	3.0	(3.5)
ARSMA total	9.6	(9.2)	6.2	(6.7)	1.1	(2.3)	2.2	(2.8)
EAT female control	9.9	(9.2)	7.1	(7.2)	1.0	(2.1)	1.9	(2.1)

Note: EAT = Eating Attitudes Test; ARSMA = Acculturation Rating Scale for Mexican Americans.

Table 28.2. Mean ARSMA scores and Mean EAT Scores by Generation Level

Generation Level	ARSMA		EAT	
	M	(SD)	M	(SD)
All levels	3.6	(0.4)	9.4	(9.1)
1	3.6	(0.5)	9.0	(8.7)
2	3.8	(0.3)	10.0	(10.7)
3	3.5	(0.3)	9.3	(7.7)
4	3.3	(0.2)	8.4	(6.6)
5	3.4	(0.3)	9.6	(5.7)

Note: ARSMA = Acculturation Rating Scale for Mexican Americans; EAT = Eating Attitudes Test.

Thirteen women endorsed EAT-26 profiles beyond the standardized cut-off score and produced greater mean elevations on Factor II. This classified them with profiles specifically of the bulimic type.

DISCUSSION

This research showed that elevated EAT-26 means, reflecting disordered eating, corresponded to ascending acculturation types. In particular, there was a significant, positive correlation between acculturation and Factor III of the EAT-26, which highlights perceived pressure from others to gain weight. Of the three factors, only Factor III incorporates an interpersonal element.

More specifically, the findings show that second-generation Mexican American women—women born in the United States to parents either born in Mexico or other foreign country—were the most acculturated and had the highest disordered eating patterns. Thus, this group may be at greatest risk for disordered eating. It is not surprising that they would represent a worrisome profile when one ponders the strains inherent in being the "first born" to an immigrant family. This position may create special demands as the individual attempts to bridge two worlds.

These women's preferences, beliefs, and behaviors may be different compared to those around them. If such women have adopted U.S. societal values about a thin body ideal, this is likely to clash and create perceived pressure from others, for example, older family members who are less acculturated and still espouse a measure of health that upholds heavier weight and a less restrictive appetite.

Women endorsing the most disordered eating patterns underscored bulimic symptomatology. Such a dynamic manifests the interplay between ideations of receiving/accepting versus rejecting/separating that are inherent in the binge-purge cycle as well as in the acculturating ethnic minority.

FUTURE DIRECTIONS

Given the sample, generalizability of these findings is primarily limited to university students and professional women. A more varied sample may help enhance within-group differences. Future research would benefit from the incorporation of interviews in assessing the complexity of these women's relationship with food, including the familial and systemic components among intergenerational eating patterns and weight ideals. The use of native idioms regarding food may prove revealing with this population, as was recently done with Chinese patients (Lee, Lee, and Leung, 1998).

Interventions and treatment with a minority population, such as with Mexican American women, must assess differing societal and cultural values as they are experienced within the individual's family as well as the manner in which they are internally negotiated by the woman in question.

References

Altabe, M. "Ethnicity and Body Image: Quantitative and Qualitative Analysis." *International Journal of Eating Disorders,* 1998, *23,* 153–160.

Berry, J. W. "Acculturation as Varieties of Adaptation." In A. M. Padilla (ed.), *Acculturation: Theory, Models, and Some New Findings.* Boulder, Colo.: Westview Press, 1980.

Cuellar, I., Harris, L. C., and Jasso, R. "An Acculturation Scale for Mexican-American Normal and Clinical Populations." *Hispanic Journal of Behavioral Sciences,* 1980, *2,* 199–217.

Cuellar, I., and Roberts, R. E. "Psychological Disorders Among Chicanos." In J. L. Martinez and R. H. Mendoza (eds.), *Chicano Psychology.* (2nd ed.) Orlando, Fla.: Academic Press, 1984.

Delgado, J. L., Johnson, C. L., Roy, I., and Trevino, F. M. "Hispanic Health and Nutrition Examination Survey: Methodological Considerations." *American Journal of Public Health,* 1990, *80,* 6–10.

Fitzgibbon, M. L., and others. "Correlates of Binge Eating in Hispanic, Black and White Women." *International Journal of Eating Disorders,* 1998, *24,* 43–52.

Garner, D. M., Olmsted, M. P., Bohr, Y., and Garfinkel, P. E. "The Eating Attitudes Test: Psychometric Features and Clinical Correlates." *Psychological Medicine,* 1982, *12,* 871–878.

Joiner, G. W., and Kashubeck, S. "Acculturation, Body Image, Self-Esteem, and Eating-Disorder Symptomatology in Adolescent Mexican American Women." *Psychology of Women Quarterly,* 1996, *20,* 419–435.

Lee, S., Lee, A. M., and Leung, T. "Cross-Cultural Validity of the Eating Disorder Inventory: A Study of Chinese Patients with Eating Disorders in Hong Kong." *International Journal of Eating Disorders,* 1998, *23,* 177–188.

Pumariega, A. J. "Acculturation and Eating Attitudes in Adolescent Girls: A Comparative and Correlational Study." *Journal of the American Academy of Child Psychiatry,* 1986, *25,* 276–279.

Rogler, L. H., Cortes, D. E., and Malgady, R. G. "Acculturation and Mental Health Status Among Hispanics: Convergence and New Directions for Research." *American Psychologist,* 1991, *46,* 585–597.

Vega, W. A., and Amaro, H. "Latino Outlook: Good Health, Uncertain Prognosis." *Annual Review of Public Health,* 1994, *15,* 39–67.

CHAPTER TWENTY-NINE

Welfare Reform and Its Impact on Latino Families

Diana Romero

The absence of literature on the impact of the 1996 welfare reform legislation on Latinas and their families made it necessary to commission this chapter for this book. The author reviews the existing literature, identifies barriers that Latinas and Latino families face as a result of the welfare system, and explores the consequences of the welfare reform environment on the health of Latina women and children.

Two major policy shifts transpired in 1996: the passage of the Personal Responsibility and Work Opportunity Reconciliation Act (PRWORA) of 1996, also known as welfare reform, and the Illegal Immigrant Reform and Immigrant Responsibility Act (IIRIRA), or immigration reform. Welfare reform marked a dramatic change in social policy toward the poor in the United States. This included increased work and behavioral requirements, a maximum five-year lifetime limit on cash assistance, which emphasized its shift from an entitlement program to temporary cash assistance, and retrenchment of the role of the federal government resulting from devolution of oversight to the states. The legislation also dramatically limited the access of documented and undocumented immigrants to various social programs (for example, cash assistance, Medicaid, and food stamps). Although the federal government and certain states restored some of these benefits over time, this applied to specific groups of immigrants, such as those with specific disabilities (for example, blindness) or those who were either minors or 65 years or older on August 22, 1996 (Haider,

The research reported above was made possible by a seed grant from the Institute for Social and Economic Research and Policy (ISERP) at Columbia University, New York. The author would also like to acknowledge the valuable guidance provided by Wendy Chavkin, M.D., M.P.H., and the assistance with literature research, review, and data entry provided by Lauren Oshman, M.P.H., Barbara Pastrana Pahud, M.D., M.P.H., and Michelle Mulbauer, B.A.

Schoeni, Bao, and Danielson, 2001). Immigration reform also contained many provisions, including a change in the standards for public charge inadmissibility of potential immigrants, as well as more stringent financial requirements for those sponsoring family- and job-related immigrants.

While it is likely that both acts have had an impact on poor and immigrant populations, the focus of this chapter is on the welfare reform act, which has clearly had dramatic results on the overall population of those living in poverty and on Latinos in particular. Welfare caseloads have declined by over 50 percent since 1996 (U.S. Department of Health and Human Services, 2000). Prior to passage of welfare reform, those receiving Aid to Families with Dependent Children were also eligible for food stamps and Medicaid. However, welfare reform administratively separated the new cash assistance program, Temporary Assistance to Needy Families (TANF), from the food assistance and health insurance programs for the poor, purportedly to ensure that poor children and families maintained access to these latter services. This delinking was considered important because receipt of cash assistance was associated with compliance with various work and behavioral requirements. In most cases, noncompliance would result in financial sanctions or entire loss of TANF eligibility. As such, the ability to maintain receipt of food stamps and Medicaid was viewed positively. Actual experience at the state level, however, revealed that many administrative systems had not been changed, and loss of TANF resulted in a concurrent loss of other benefits. In addition, the PRWORA denied benefits to certain categories of documented immigrants. Concurrent changes in immigration law tightened restrictions on new immigration and increased penalties against undocumented immigrants living in the United States. Specific components of these major policy changes had the potential to affect the health of poor Latino populations. Thus, the research reported here addresses whether welfare reform policies implemented over the past five years may have had such an impact.

Various reports indicate that Latinos and African Americans have not left the TANF rolls at the same rate as the White population and instead are remaining on TANF for longer periods of time (Starr, 1999; Swarns, 1998; Rodriguez and Kirk, 2000; DeParle, 1998). Although the experience of poor African Americans with welfare reform policies is very important, this chapter specifically focuses on the experience of poor native- and foreign-born Latinos, two groups that are likely to face barriers to employment as a result of lower educational attainment and, for the latter group, English as a second language. Since implementation of welfare reform, there have also been substantial declines in enrollment in food stamps and Medicaid (Swarns, 1997). The U.S. Census Bureau (2002) recently reported that the proportion of the population without health insurance increased to 41.2 million people—from 14.2 percent in 2000 to 14.6 percent in 2001—an increase of 1.4 million people. Moreover, Latinos (66.8 percent) were less likely than Whites (90.0 percent), African Americans (81.0 percent), and

Asians and Pacific Islanders (81.0 percent) to have health insurance. It may be that some of these changes are associated with welfare reform policies and may have disproportionately burdened certain groups, particularly Latinos.

Although TANF caseloads have dropped in the past several years, the proportion of Latino adults receiving welfare increased from 21 percent of the caseload in 1995/96 to 25 percent in 1998/99 (from 22 percent to 26 percent among children) (Rodriguez and Kirk, 2000). Because the major trend has been in the direction of people leaving the welfare rolls, the higher proportion of Latinos receiving TANF likely reflects those who *remain* on the rolls rather than *new* cases. While Latinos have been historically overrepresented among the poor, the dramatic three-year change in their relative proportion among those receiving cash assistance coincides with the implementation of welfare reform policies. Lack of education appears to be a major obstacle to successfully leaving welfare. Census data for 1999 indicate that only 56 percent of Latinos in the general population had a high school diploma, compared with 85 percent of Whites and 77 percent of African Americans (U.S. Census Bureau, 1999). Within the welfare population, Latinos fare even worse, with two-thirds (64 percent) of Latino recipients not having completed high school (Starr, 1999). In short, Latino women face a host of obstacles to leaving welfare, including lower educational attainment and literacy in English, lack of job skills and training, and unavailability and mistrust of child care. Furthermore, fear of deportation related to new federal public charge rules (U.S. Immigration and Naturalization Service, 1999; U.S. Department of Justice Immigration and Naturalization Service, 1999) may act as a barrier to pursuing other forms of assistance for which they may be eligible, such as Medicaid, food stamps, the Supplemental Program for Women, Infants, and Children, and Supplemental Security Income (SSI).

While the PRWORA intended to reduce welfare dependency and poverty, it may have had the opposite effect on ethnic minorities and immigrant groups. Of particular concern is the extent to which changes in welfare policy have been assessed with regard to poor Latino women and children and what the consequences of such policy changes may have meant for their health. The experience of this group will become increasingly salient as White welfare recipients continue to leave the welfare rolls and the relative proportion of Latino and African American welfare recipients grows. Thus, this chapter reviews the extant literature to identify barriers that Latino women may face in this new welfare system and to explore the consequences of this experience on women and children.

Although the caseload data suggest that the experience of Latino women and other ethnic minorities receiving TANF differs from White recipients, the specific details are not well understood. Furthermore, increased health problems among welfare recipients have been reported (Polit, London, and Martinez, 2001; Philadelphia Citizens for Children and Youth United Way of Southeastern

Pennsylvania, 1998). Thus, the health burden that Latino families suffer should be explored to determine the role that poor health may play in a "reformed" welfare environment, which requires increased work participation and has instituted a limit on the length of time that individuals can receive cash assistance. Many of the sparse data that are available on welfare policies and ethnic minorities derive from specific cities (particularly those with large immigrant and minority populations, such as New York and Los Angeles), vary by research methodology, and in many instances contain no data on health. It is important, however, that the information that has been collected be reviewed, incorporated into ongoing research, and used to inform future research activities.

METHODOLOGY

A comprehensive literature search was conducted to determine both the amount of relevant information on welfare policy changes and Latino groups, as well as the extent to which it addressed health issues. First, fifteen social science, health, and governmental databases were selected from a universe of 297 in the Columbia University Libraries Online electronic database system (Exhibit 29.1). Keyword searches were conducted using select terms (*Latino/Latina, welfare, poverty, health,* and *immigrant*) in different combinations to produce a comprehensive list of potential articles. All database searches were limited to English language articles published between 1994 and 2001.

Exhibit 29.1. Social Science, Health, and Governmental Databases Searched

Sociological Abstracts
Women's Resources International
Anthropological Index Online
Anthropological Literature
Ethnic NewsWatch
Latino American Periodical Index
POPLINE
Social Sciences Abstracts
Social Sciences Citation Index Expanded
Social Work Abstracts
MOCAT/GPO
Access/GPO Gate
ArticleFirst
ClariNews
CINAHL

Exhibit 29.2. Abstract Form Data Fields

Citation information: title, author(s), source, publisher, year, pages	Regular doctor visits
	Trust in health care
Type of article (for example, primary or secondary analysis, editorial)	Confusion (regarding policy changes)
	Immunization
Description of research/article	Family planning
Relevant years	Prenatal care
Keywords	Disease prevention
Relevant variables	Reproductive health care
Population studied	Sexually transmitted disease treatment
Unit of analysis	Dental health
Education	Mental health
Public benefits	Health status (well-being)
Adult Medicaid enrollment	Health care costs
Child Medicaid enrollment	Child abuse
Emergency care	Child neglect
Public insurance eligibility	Welfare reform
Private insurance obtained	Policy recommendations
Percentage uninsured (overall)	Research recommendations
Percentage mothers uninsured	Latino-specific population
Percentage children uninsured	Other/miscellaneous
Preventive services	
Have regular doctor	
Delay in seeking treatment	

(Select publications from 2002 have been included in the discussion so that the information provided in this chapter is as up-to-date and useful as possible.) From a universe of over seven hundred articles identified through the literature search, sixty-seven articles were potentially relevant and therefore selected for further review.

Abstracted data were entered into a database that consisted of forty-five fields, including citation information, source description, research methodology, findings relevant to maternal and child health, health status, receipt of public assistance, and other welfare- and policy-related variables (Exhibit 29.2). The differences across these publications (for example, objectives, time periods, sample characteristics, and welfare versus health focus) make it impossible to aggregate the information so that it could be compared quantitatively. The goal was to identify similar (or disparate) trends, as well as particularly salient findings. In this way, areas that warrant more focused research and attention could be identified and important next steps taken.

FINDINGS

Overall

The sixty-seven articles reviewed fell into four broad categories: general socio-demographic and program information concerning Latino and immigrant populations in the United States (ten articles); effects of welfare and immigration reform (non–health-specific; twenty articles); welfare reform, Latinos and other immigrants, and health issues (eight articles); and Latinos and immigrants and health (not specific to welfare or immigration reform; twenty-nine articles) (Table 29.1). The majority of the articles identified that were related to Latinos and Latinas and welfare reform did not address health issues. Because only a small proportion of the articles (eight of sixty-seven, or 12 percent) directly addressed health issues of Latino populations within the context of welfare reform, it is often unclear whether the factors related to poor health are specific to welfare reform or part of larger, long-standing problems.

Low educational attainment continues to surface as an important factor for overall well-being, yet in the context of new welfare policies, it may have specific implications for one's ability to comply with workfare requirements and ultimately end dependence on TANF. Thus, the lower level of high school completion among Latino citizens and immigrants compared to non-Latinos (Starr, 1999; U.S. Census Bureau, 1999; Newburger and Curry, 1999; Ng, 1999) has serious implications for the successful transition by Latinos from reliance on cash assistance to paid employment that will provide a livable income. This is particularly noteworthy given that among all workers in 1998, Latinos had the lowest average annual income at $22,117, compared to Whites at $33,336 and just slightly less than African American workers at $22,887 (Newburger and Curry, 1999).

A recent analysis of the impact of welfare reform policies on immigrants' use of public assistance programs—TANF, Medicaid, Food Stamps, and SSI programs—showed that use of these programs by documented immigrants, that is, legal permanent residents (LPRs), declined across the board from 1994 to 1999 (Fix and Passel, 1999, 2002). The percentage decline in program participation was as follows: TANF, 60 percent (from 4.9 percent to 2.0 percent); Medicaid, 15 percent (from 19.9 percent to 17 percent); Food Stamps, 48 percent (from 14.8 percent to 7.7 percent); and SSI, 32 percent (from 5.7 percent to 3.9 percent). Except for Medicaid, these rates exceeded declines in program participation experienced by citizens. Furthermore, during this period, neither the rate of naturalizations nor the incomes among immigrants increased, which some might suggest as factors related to decreased program participation among immigrants (Fix and Passel, 2002). This analysis did not stratify the immigrant groups by ethnicity or country of origin; however, it is likely that these findings are at least broadly applicable to Latino immigrants given that half of foreign-born residents in the United States are from Latin America (U.S. Census Bureau, 2000).

Table 29.1. Publications Included in Literature Review by Category

Year	Author	Title
	Demographic and Program Information	
2001	Lollock	"The Foreign-Born Population of the United States: Population Characteristics"
2000	Duncan and Brooks-Gunn	"Family Poverty, Welfare Reform, and Child Development"
2000	U.S. Census Bureau	"Coming from the Americas: A Profile of the Nation's Latin American Foreign Born"
1999	Mills	"Health Insurance Coverage: Consumer Income"
1999	Newburger and Curry	"Educational Attainment in the United States: Population Characteristics"
1999	Zambrana and Capello	"Promoting Latino Child and Family Welfare: Strategies for Strengthening the Child Welfare System"
1998	Zambrana and Dorrington	"Economic and Social Vulnerability of Latino Children and Families by Subgroup: Implications for Child Welfare"
1996	Wilcox, Robbennolt, O'Keeffe, and Pynchon	"Teen Nonmarital Childbearing and Welfare: The Gap Between Research and Political Discourse"
1995	National Research Council Institute of Medicine	"Immigrant Children and Their Families: Issues for Research and Policy"
1995	U.S. Census Bureau	"Mothers Who Receive AFDC Payments: Fertility and Socioeconomic Characteristics"
	Effects of Welfare Reform and/or Immigration Reform (non-health-specific)	
2002	Fix and Passel	"The Scope and Impact of Welfare Reform's Immigrant Provisions"
2002	Fremstad	"Immigrants and Welfare Reauthorization"
2001	Haider, Schoeni, Bao, and Danielson	"Immigrants, Welfare Reform, and the Economy in the 1990s"
2001	Leachman	"Restoring Food Stamp Benefits to Immigrants and Refugees in Oregon"
2000	Cordero-Guzman and Navarro	"Managing Cuts in the "Safety Net": What Do Immigrant Groups, Organizations, and Service Providers Say About the Impacts of Recent Changes in Immigration and Welfare Laws?"

(Continued)

Table 29.1. Publications Included in Literature Review by Category (Continued)

Year	Author	Title
2000	Rodriguez and Kirk	"Welfare Reform, TANF Caseload Changes, and Latinos: A Preliminary Assessment"
1999	Fix and Zimmerman	"All Under One Roof: Mixed Status Families in an Era of Reform"
1999	Fix and Passel	"Trends in Noncitizens' and Citizens' Use of Public Benefits Following Welfare Reform: 1994–1997"
1999	Gaytan and Hernandez	"Beyond a Culture of Fear: "How Welfare Reform Has Failed Immigrants and Public Health in California"
1999	Jessop and others	"The Impact of Recent Immigration Policy Changes on the Receipt of WIC Services: An Aggregate Analysis"
1999	Ng	"From War on Poverty to War on Welfare: The Impact of Welfare Reform on the Lives of Immigrant Women"
1999	Starr	"Left Behind"
1999	U.S. General Accounting Office	"Welfare Reform: Information on Former Recipients' Status"
1999	Zimmerman and Tumlin	"Patchwork Policies: State Assistance for Immigrants Under Welfare Reform"
1998	Ivey	"The Impact of Recent Legislation on the Delivery of Health Care to Immigrants"
1998	Philadelphia Citizens for Children and Youth United Way of Southeastern Pennsylvania	"Watching Out for Children in Changing Times: What 50 Families Have to Say—A Report on Welfare Reform"
1998	Thadani and others	"Impact of Welfare Reform and Illegal Immigration Acts on Immigrants: Access to Health Care, Health-Seeking Behaviors, and Health Outcomes in New York City"
1997	Bane	"Welfare as We Might Know It"
1997	Espenshade, Baraka, and Huber	"Implications of the 1996 Welfare and Immigration Reform Acts for US Immigration"
1997	Keigher	"America's Most Cruel Xenophobia"

Welfare Reform, Latinos/Immigrants, and Health Issues

2000	Currie and Grogger	"Medicaid Expansions and Welfare Contractions: Offsetting Effects on Prenatal Care and Infant Health"

Table 29.1. (Continued)

Year	Author	Title
2000	Ku and Matani	"Immigrants' Access to Health Care and Insurance on the Cusp of Welfare Reform"
2000	New York Immigrant Coalition	"Welfare Reform and Health Care: The Wrong Prescription for Immigrants"
1998	Ellwood and Ku	"Welfare and Immigration Reforms: Unintended Side Effects for Medicaid"
1998	Ivey and Kramer	"Immigrant Women and the Emergency Department: The Juncture with Welfare and Immigration Reform"
1998	Zimmerman and Fix	"Declining Immigrant Applications for Medi-Cal and Welfare Benefits in Los Angeles County"
1997	Carmichael	"Welfare Reform: Strategies to Monitor the Health Impact on Immigrant Women and Their Children in New York City"
1997	Minkoff, Bauer, and Joyce	"Welfare Reform and the Obstetrical Care of Immigrants and Their Newborns"

Latinos/Immigrants and Health (General)

Year	Author	Title
2001	Holahan, Ku, and Pohl	"Is Immigration Responsible for the Growth in the Number of Uninsured?"
2001	Jackson and others	"Women's Health Centers and Minority Women: Addressing Barriers to Care"
2000	Berk, Schur, Chavez, and Frankel	"Health Care Use Among Undocumented Latino Immigrants"
2000	Carrasquillo, Carrasquillo, and Shea	"Health Insurance Coverage of Immigrants Living in the United States: Differences by Citizenship Status and Country of Origin"
2000	Center for Immigration Studies	"Without Coverage: Immigration's Impact on the Size and Growth of the Population Lacking Health Insurance"
2000	Derose and Baker	"Limited English Proficiency and Latinos' Use of Physician Services"
2000	Gilliland and others	"Patterns of Mammography Use Among Latino, American Indian, and Non-Latino White Women in New Mexico 1994–1997"
2000	Henry J. Kaiser Foundation	"Health Insurance Coverage and Access to Care Among Latinos"

(Continued)

Table 29.1. Publications Included in Literature Review by Category (Continued)

Year	Author	Title
2000	Ku and Blaney	"Health Coverage for Legal Immigrant Children: New Census Data Highlight Importance of Restoring Medicaid and SCHIP Coverage"
2000	Ramirez and others	"Latino Women's Breast and Cervical Cancer Knowledge, Attitudes and Screening Behaviors"
2000	Ronsaville and Hakim	"Well Child Care in the United States: Racial Differences in Compliance with Guidelines"
1999	Brown, Wyn, and Ojeda	"Access to Health Insurance and Health Care for Children in Immigrant Families"
1999	Brown, Wyn, and Ojeda	"Noncitizen Children's Rising Uninsured Rates Threaten Access to Health Care"
1999	Center on Budget and Policy Priorities	"Overcoming Barriers Immigrants Face in Accessing Benefits and Services"
1999	Lara, Allen, and Lange	"Physician Perceptions of Barriers to Care for Inner-City Latino Children with Asthma"
1999	Zambrana, Dunkel-Schetter, Collins, and Scrimshaw	"Mediators of Ethnic-Associated Differences in Infant Birth Weight"
1999	Zambrana, Breen, Fox, and Gutierrez-Mohamed	"Use of Cancer Screening Practices by Latino Women: Analyses by Subgroup"
1998	Bechtel, Davidhizar, and Tiller	"Patterns of Mental Health Care Among Mexican Americans"
1998	Ferran	"Model Programs and Cultural Proficiency in Service Delivery: Principles and Pitfalls"
1998	Koshar and others	"The Hispanic Teen Mother's Origin of Birth, Use of Prenatal Care, and Maternal and Neonatal Complication"
1998	Pastore and Diaz	"Cultural and Medical Issues of Latino Adolescents"
1997	American Academy of Pediatrics	"Health Care for Children of Immigrant Families"
1997	Fujiura and Yamaki	"Analysis of Ethnic Variations in Developmental Disability Prevalence and Household Economic Status"
1997	Halfon and others	"Medicaid Enrollment and Health Services Access by Latino Children in Inner-City Los Angeles"

Table 29.1. (Continued)

Year	Author	Title
1996	Chavkin	"Race/Ethnicity and Women's Health"
1996	Gany and De Bocanegra	"Overcoming Barriers to Improving the Health of Immigrant Women"
1996	Moss, Baumeister, and Biewener	"Perspectives of Latina Immigrant Women on Proposition 187"
1996	Norton, Kenney, and Ellwood	"Medicaid Coverage of Maternity Care for Aliens in California"
1994	Zambrana and others	"The Relationship Between Psychosocial Status of Immigrant Latino Mothers and Use of Emergency Pediatric Services"

Latino TANF Recipients and Leavers: Factors Related to Departure from or Continued Receipt of TANF

Relatively few "leaver" studies—that is, assessments of all former TANF recipients—have been conducted, in large part because the PRWORA did not require states to evaluate their welfare programs. The lack of uniformity across the few leaver studies conducted by states and localities limits the utility of the findings for broad-based application (U.S. General Accounting Office, 1999).

A 1999 General Accounting Office report on former welfare recipients' status highlighted the difficulty in assessing and comparing the experiences of former recipients given the divergent approaches that states use to follow up with former clients. None of the seventeen leaver studies reviewed in this report provided specific information by ethnic subgroup or immigration status. As such, it is impossible to determine the impact that the new welfare reform policies have had on former native and immigrant Latino TANF recipients.

An analysis of current and former welfare recipients between 1995 and 1997, however, found that Latinos represented 13 percent of leavers, while 52 percent were White (Loprest, 1999). Thus, compared to Whites, a substantially smaller proportion of individuals leaving TANF are Latino, at a rate that is half their representation in the TANF caseload (Rodriguez and Kirk, 2000). Many reports have identified less education, limited skills, lack of English proficiency, and discrimination toward Latinos—thus, less job readiness and opportunities—as key factors related to their remaining on TANF (Starr, 1999; Swarns, 1998; Rodriguez and Kirk, 2000; Cordero-Guzman and Navarro, 2000; Ng, 1999). This is particularly problematic given the federal five-year time limit on receipt of cash assistance.

Health-Related Data for Latino Women and Children

As was expected (Keigher, 1997; Espenshade, Baraka, and Huber, 1997; Carmichael, 1997), the first and most salient health-related consequence of welfare reform for immigrants has been a decline in health insurance, a development that could result in decreased access to health care services. Since passage of the law in 1996, a series of analyses have consistently documented significant reductions in health insurance (Medicaid) among immigrants (Ku and Matani, 2000; Ellwood and Ku, 1998; New York Immigrant Coalition, 2000; Minkoff, Bauer, and Joyce, 1997; Brown, Wyn, and Ojeda, 1999a, 1999b; Carrasquillo, Carrasquillo, and Shea, 2000; Ku and Blaney, 2000); however, subgroup analyses by ethnic background or country of origin are limited.

In a nationally representative study ($n = 44,461$), Ku and Matani (2000) found that the proportion of low-income immigrants who lack health insurance increased from 54 percent in 1995 to 59 percent in 1998. Noncitizen adults reported both low levels of Medicaid and employer-provided insurance, even after controlling for factors such as income and employment. Compared to native citizens with similar socioeconomic characteristics, this group was also less likely to have a usual source of care, to have visited a medical provider, gone to an emergency room, or received dental care in the past year. It is noteworthy that contrary to findings from other investigations, noncitizen immigrant families in this study received both less primary and less emergency care. A related analysis by Ku and Blaney (2000) of census data covering the period from 1995 to 1999 found a concurrent decline in Medicaid enrollment among low-income noncitizen children (36 percent to 28 percent) and citizen children of noncitizen parents (47 percent to 43 percent).

Brown, Wyn, and Ojeda (1999a) reported findings from a study that used national data sets to examine uninsurance among noncitizen children in the United States (between 1995 and 1998), and conducted a subgroup analysis by ethnic background. It found that more than half (55.9 percent) of noncitizen Latino children did not have health insurance, more than double the rate for noncitizen White children (24.7 percent), and five times the rate of White children whose parents are citizens (10.2 percent). Latino noncitizen children were clearly less likely to be covered by Medicaid: only three in ten had Medicaid, compared with five in ten noncitizen Asian-Pacific Islanders and six in ten noncitizen Whites. Findings from this study also revealed the linear relationship of health insurance across the citizenship gradient, such that lack of child health insurance was lowest among citizen children with citizen parents (17.1 percent) and increased for citizen children with naturalized parents (22.9 percent), citizen children with noncitizen parents (33.4 percent), and noncitizen children with noncitizen parents (53.6 percent).

An analysis by Zimmerman and Fix (1998) of various welfare benefits programs in California between 1996 and 1998 found dramatic declines in new applications and overall caseload pertaining to immigrants. Specifically, approved TANF applications for noncitizens dropped by 52 percent, which accounted for almost one-quarter (23 percent) of the decline in total monthly approvals during this two-year time period. Medi-Cal (California's Medicaid program) applications mirrored the TANF trend: the number of noncitizens applying for "Medi-Cal only" benefits dropped by 24 percent (compared with a 7 percent decline among citizens). Moreover, the number of citizen children (of noncitizen parents) applying for both TANF and Medi-Cal declined by 48 percent (compared with an increase of 6 percent for citizen children of citizen parents). Finally, the number of cases in which the applicant's primary language is Spanish decreased by 46 percent (compared with a 9 percent decline for English speakers). These findings are particularly noteworthy given that despite federal restrictions in the PRWORA barring immigrants who entered the United States after August 22, 1996, from TANF and Medicaid for their first five years in this country, the state of California elected to provide these programs to newly entering immigrants using state funds. It is likely that this was the result of a lack of outreach and dissemination of accurate information for this population; thus, the fears of deportation or other sanctions were not allayed.

The New York Immigrant Coalition (2000) assessed the health-related impact of welfare reform policies on immigrants in New York City, where over one-third of the city's population is foreign born and the Latino population totals over 2 million. Between 1994 and 1998, the proportion of uninsured noncitizens increased from 34.4 percent to 45 percent, while uninsurance among citizens remained virtually unchanged (16.6 percent to 17.7 percent). This analysis projected future health-related costs for immigrants resulting from elimination of access to primary care and limiting Medicaid coverage to emergency care. Specifically, if Medicaid eligibility had been reinstated for documented immigrants in 2000, 52,000 immigrants would have received full Medicaid coverage at an average annual cost per beneficiary of $2,800 (totaling $145 million). By comparison, 12,200 immigrants without coverage received emergency care at an average annual cost per beneficiary of approximately $17,000 (totaling $207 million). By 2005, the cost for full Medicaid benefits would total $1.547 billion compared to $1.679 billion for emergency Medicaid spending for a much smaller number of people. The researchers highlighted both the fiscal argument for reinstating Medicaid eligibility to immigrants as well as the health benefits associated with access to primary care (over emergency care), which have been extensively documented in the public health literature.

Other than health insurance status, the available data most closely related to health status for Latino populations refer to usual source of care and minimum standards for physician visits. During the period between 1995 and 1996, more Latino children and adults did not have a usual source of care when compared with Whites, regardless of insurance status: uninsured, Medicaid, or private

(Henry J. Kaiser Family Foundation, 2000). (Some of the reasons put forth have included systemic and structural barriers such as easy access, availability, and hours of services, as well as receiving appointments in a timely manner.) Similarly, across age and health status groups (0–5 years; 6–17 years; women, 18–64 years, in fair or poor health; all adults, 18–64, in fair or poor health), greater proportions of Latinos had not had the minimum number of annual physician visits (8 percent, 16 percent, 13 percent, and 25 percent, respectively) compared with Whites (5 percent, 7 percent, 6 percent, and 14 percent, respectively) (Henry J. Kaiser Family Foundation, 2000). Again, these disparities persisted across insurance categories. Thus, although these data (and the lack of other health-outcome–specific data for Latinos) do not permit conclusions concerning differences in health status between Latino and other ethnic groups in the United States, they provide some indication of the possible factors related to documented health disparities.

DISCUSSION

In order to address the research questions posed concerning differences between Latino and non-Latino TANF recipients and leavers, as well as factors related to Latinos' departure from TANF for employment, two kinds of data are required. First, we need scientifically rigorous leaver studies. Second, we need subgroup analyses by racial/ethnic groups. This would allow for a more detailed understanding of the experience of Latino recipients with the TANF system and the factors related to their departure from and return to TANF. The majority of leaver studies conducted to date have not reported findings by race/ethnicity. In addition, they are seriously flawed with regard to their inconsistent methodologies (which preclude comparison) and the proportion of respondents lost to follow-up (U.S. General Accounting Office, 1999). The limited information available indicates that Latinos have left the TANF rolls at a slower rate than both Whites and African Americans and suggests that the main reasons are lower educational attainment, language and work skills barriers, immigration status, and possibly cultural differences concerning views of the role of mothers and outside employment. Prolonged TANF membership may reduce the opportunity to enter the workforce and achieve economic self-sufficiency.

As for the potential association between the health status of poor Latino women and children and their experience with departure from TANF, the overwhelming share of health-related data focuses on health insurance status. While this is an important health-related indicator given its correlation with access to health care, it is not a measure of health status or specific health outcomes. Lack of health insurance among citizen and noncitizen Latinos may suggest various scenarios, such as reduced utilization of health services and participation in low-level employment that does not provide benefits. Uninsurance alone, however, does not inform us as to the specific health consequences that vulnerable families might experience.

We have recently published research regarding health barriers related to employment and departure from TANF in a predominantly Latino (62 percent) population. (This was not included in the summary of the literature review provided above because the publication dates were outside the established search criterion for reports published between 1994 and 2000.) Seventy percent of low-income mothers of children with chronic health conditions in San Antonio, Texas, reported suffering from a chronic health condition as well (Romero and others, 2002). Subgroup analyses by TANF status revealed that current or former TANF recipients and applicants were significantly more likely to report physical and mental health problems, visits to the emergency department, and experience with domestic violence than those never involved with TANF. Furthermore, these health factors were also significantly related to employment status—that is, women who were not currently working were more likely to report these problems, including that their health problem made activities of daily living difficult for them.

Additional analyses of these data found that health-related limitations in daily activities were significantly greater among children of current TANF recipients (71 percent) and denied TANF applicants (75 percent) compared with children of nonrecipients (54 percent) (Smith and others, 2002). When the subgroup of children with asthma was examined, children whose mothers had been denied TANF had significantly more asthma symptoms than did children whose mothers had no contact with the welfare system (Wood and others, 2002). In addition, children of mothers with poorer mental health had significantly more asthma symptoms and higher rates of health care utilization. As for departure from TANF, there is some evidence of a language barrier, given that among those who reported Spanish as their primary language (11 percent), significantly fewer (3 percent) had left TANF compared with current recipients (16 percent) (Romero and others, 2002).

From a public health perspective, the presence of health disparities such as those described above (that is, physical and mental health problems among poor Latino mothers) is cause for concern and action. From a welfare perspective, these disparities reflect the differential impact of policies and serve as a harbinger of the next set of issues to be addressed. For example, the five-year lifetime time limit for receipt of federal TANF benefits means that many families may find themselves with no cash assistance and that many states must now cover the cost of assisting these families solely from state funds (which are already stretched in this period of economic recession). The implications of this scenario for citizen and noncitizen Latinos are profound. As Latinos are remaining on TANF longer, they will increasingly confront the five-year time limit with less favorable employment possibilities than experienced by their White and African American counterparts. This is particularly worrisome if their ability to succeed is hindered by poor health and an inability to seek health care given their lower levels of health insurance.

Passage of the PRWORA marked a new era in American history in that, among other things, for the first time, it made a distinction between the two groups of tax-paying residents of this country (U.S. citizens and legal permanent residents)—a country largely defined by its immigrant foundation and history. It allowed citizens access to social benefits programs while barring new documented immigrants from applying for cash assistance and health insurance for five years and further restricting immigrants' eligibility for food stamps and SSI. "By rationing access to benefits in this way, the law elevate[d] the importance of citizenship for societal membership in a manner that is unusual by international standards" (Fix and Passel, 2002, p. 6). One need only look at the documented uninsurance trend across immigrant/citizen categories (concordance or discordance between child and parental status) to see evidence of this country's "citizenship hierarchy" in social policy.

There is not enough information about the specific experiences of citizen and noncitizen Latinos with TANF or of the role that health problems may play in their ability to become self-sufficient. We do know, however, that the largest proportion (51 percent) of immigrants to the United States are from Latin America (Lollock, 2001); that the PRWORA has led to a dramatic decline in immigrants' receipt of benefits; that Latinos have left the TANF rolls at the slowest rate and have the lowest levels of health insurance; and that child and maternal health problems may have caused barriers to maternal employment in one predominantly Latino sample (Romero and others, 2002; Smith and others, 2002; Wood and others, 2002). While the longitudinal nature of the research that produced the latter finding may permit for causal conclusions, the majority of the associations that can be drawn from these other findings are ecological. As such, it is imperative that states conduct and, ideally, the federal government require evaluation of TANF programs with regard to the health status and racial/ethnic makeup of their clients. If the true goal of this policy is to enable poor families to improve economically and become self-sufficient, then barriers to achieving these goals must be addressed. There is ample evidence that both health problems and Latino ethnicity are associated with increased TANF dependency. It is time that the specific barriers at work (such as lack of health care, lack of medically skilled child care, less education, and poor English) be identified and efforts made to remove them. A policy that does not address significant barriers to its achievement is not only flawed but will fail. The recently reported increase in individuals returning to TANF as well as in overall poverty in this country would suggest that the PRWORA is failing not only citizen and noncitizen Latinos specifically, but the population overall (Greenberg, Richer, and Sankarapaudian, 2002; Proctor and Dalaker, 2002).

References

American Academy of Pediatrics. Committee on Community Health Services. "Health Care for Children of Immigrant Families." *American Academy of Pediatrics,* 1997, *100*(1), 153–156.

Bane, M. "Welfare as We Might Know It." *American Prospect,* 1997, *8*(30), 1–9.

Bechtel, G., Davidhizar, R., and Tiller, C. M. "Patterns of Mental Health Care Among Mexican Americans." *Journal of Psychosocial Nursing,* 1998, *36*(11), 20–27.

Berk, M., Schur, C. L., Chavez, L. R., and Frankel, M. "Health Care Use Among Undocumented Latino Immigrants." *Health Affairs,* 2000, *19*(4), 51–64.

Brown, E. R., Wyn, R., and Ojeda, V. D. "Access to Health Insurance and Health Care for Children in Immigrant Families." Los Angeles: UCLA Center for Health Policy Research Policy Report, June 1999a.

Brown, E. R., Wyn, R., and Ojeda, V. D. "Noncitizen Children's Rising Uninsured Rates Threaten Access to Health Care." Los Angeles: UCLA Center for Health Policy Research, June 1999b.

Carmichael, S. "Welfare Reform: Strategies to Monitor the Health Impact on Immigrant Women and Their Children in New York City." New York: Center for Disease Control and Prevention, 1997.

Carrasquillo, O., Carrasquillo, A. I., and Shea, S. "Health Insurance Coverage of Immigrants Living in the United States: Differences by Citizenship Status and Country of Origin." *American Journal of Public Health,* 2000, *90*(6), 917–923.

Center on Budget and Policy Priorities. "Overcoming Barriers Immigrants Face in Accessing Benefits and Services." Washington, D.C.: Center on Budget and Policy Priorities, 1999. Materials packet.

Center for Immigration Studies. "Without Coverage: Immigration's Impact on the Size and Growth of the Population Lacking Health Insurance." Washington, D.C.: Center for Immigration Studies, 2000.

Chavkin, W. "Race/Ethnicity and Women's Health." *Journal of American Medical Women's Association,* 1996, *51*(4), 131–132.

Cordero-Guzman, H., and Navarro, J. "Managing Cuts in the 'Safety Net': What Do Immigrant Groups, Organizations, and Service Providers Say About the Impacts of Recent Changes in Immigration and Welfare Laws?" New York: New School University, 2000.

Currie, J., and Grogger, J. "Medicaid Expansions and Welfare Contractions: Offsetting Effects on Prenatal Care and Infant Health?" Washington, D.C.: National Bureau of Economic Research, 2000.

DeParle, J. "Shrinking Welfare Rolls Leave Record High Share of Minorities." *New York Times,* July 27, 1998, pp. 1, 12.

Derose, K., and Baker, D. "Limited English Proficiency and Latinos' Use of Physician Services." *Medical Care Research and Review,* 2000, *57*(1), 76–91.

Duncan, G., and Brooks-Gunn, J. "Family Poverty, Welfare Reform, and Child Development." *Child Development,* 2000, *71*(1), 188–196.

Ellwood, M., and Ku, L. "Welfare and Immigration Reforms: Unintended Side Effects for Medicaid." *Health Affairs,* 1998, *17*(3), 137–151.

Espenshade, T., Baraka, J. L., and Huber, G. A. "Implications of the 1996 Welfare and Immigration Reform Acts for US Immigration." *Population and Development Review,* 1997, *23*(4), 769–801.

Ferran, E. "Model Programs and Cultural Proficiency in Service Delivery: Principles and Pitfalls." *Journal of Child and Family Studies,* 1998, *70*(3), 263–268.

Fix, M., and Passel, J. "Trends in Noncitizens' and Citizens' Use of Public Benefits Following Welfare Reform: 1994–1997." Washington, D.C.: Urban Institute, 1999.

Fix, M., and Passel, J. "The Scope and Impact of Welfare Reform's Immigrant Provisions." Washington, D.C.: Urban Institute, 2002.

Fix, M., and Zimmerman, W. "All Under One Roof: Mixed Status Families in an Era of Reform." Washington, D.C.: Urban Institute, 1999.

Fremstad, S. "Immigrants and Welfare Reauthorization." Washington, D.C.: Center on Budget and Policy Priorities, 2002.

Fujiura, G., and Yamaki, K. "Analysis of Ethnic Variations in Developmental Disability Prevalence and Household Economic Status." *Mental Retardation,* 1997, *35*(4), 286–294.

Gany, F., and De Bocanegra, H. T. "Overcoming Barriers to Improving the Health of Immigrant Women." *Journal of American Medical Women's Association,* 1996, *51*(4), 155–159.

Gaytan, C., and Hernandez, J. "Beyond a Culture of Fear: How Welfare Reform Has Failed Immigrants and Public Health in California." *Latin Issues Forum,* 1999, 1–24.

Gilliland, F., and others. "Patterns of Mammography Use Among Hispanic, American Indian, and Non-Hispanic White Women in New Mexico, 1994–1997." *American Journal of Epidemiology,* 2000, *152*(5), 432–437.

Greenberg, M., Richer, E., and Sankarapaudian, V. "Welfare Caseloads Are Up in Most States." [http://www.clasp.org/pubs/TANF/Fyo1&20Caseload&20Data.htm]. 2002.

Haider, S., Schoeni, R. F., Bao, Y., and Danielson, C. "Immigrants, Welfare Reform, and the Economy in the 1990s." Santa Monica, Calif.: RAND, 2001.

Halfon, N., and others. "Medicaid Enrollment and Health Services Access by Latino Children in Inner-City Los Angeles." *JAMA,* 1997, *277*(8), 636–641.

Henry J. Kaiser Family Foundation. "Health Insurance Coverage and Access to Care Among Latinos." Washington, D.C.: Kaiser Commission on Medicaid and the Uninsured, June 2000.

Holahan, J., Ku, L., and Pohl, M. "Is Immigration Responsible for the Growth in the Number of Uninsured?" Washington, D.C.: Henry J. Kaiser Family Foundation, 2001.

Ivey, S. "The Impact of Recent Legislation on the Delivery of Health Care to Immigrants: Welfare and Immigration Reforms in 1996 and 1997." In E. Kramer, S. Ivey, and Y.-W. Ying (eds.), *Immigrant Women's Health: Problems and Solutions.* San Francisco: Jossey-Bass, 1998.

Ivey, S., and Kramer, E. "Immigrant Women and the Emergency Department: The Juncture with Welfare and Immigration Reform." *Journal of American Medical Women's Association,* 1998, *53*(2), 94–95.

Jackson, S., and others. "Women's Health Centers and Minority Women: Addressing Barriers to Care—The National Centers of Excellence in Women's Health." *Journal of Women's Health and Gender-Based Medicine,* 2001, *10*(6), 551–559.

Jessop, D., and others. "The Impact of Recent Immigration Policy Changes on the Receipt of WIC Services: An Aggregate Analysis." New York: Medical and Health Research Association of New York City, 1999.

Keigher, S. "America's Most Cruel Xenophobia." *Health and Social Work,* 1997, *22*(3), 232–237.

Koshar, J., and others. "The Hispanic Teen Mother's Origin of Birth, Use of Prenatal Care, and Maternal and Neonatal Complication." *Journal of Pediatric Nursing,* 1998, *13*(3), 151–157.

Ku, L., and Blaney, S. "Health Coverage for Legal Immigrant Children: New Census Data Highlight Importance of Restoring Medicaid and SCHIP Coverage." Washington, D.C.: Center on Budget and Policy Priorities, Oct. 2000.

Ku, L., and Matani, S. "Immigrants' Access to Health Care and Insurance on the Cusp of Welfare Reform." Washington, D.C.: Urban Institute, 2000.

Lara, M., Allen, F., and Lange, L. "Physician Perceptions of Barriers to Care for Inner-City Latino Children with Asthma." *Journal of Health Care for the Poor and Underserved,* 1999, *10*(1), 27–44.

Leachman, M. "Restoring Food Stamp Benefits to Immigrants and Refugees in Oregon." Silverton: Oregon Center for Public Policy, 2001.

Lollock, L. "The Foreign-Born Population of the United States: Population Characteristics." Washington, D.C.: U.S. Census Bureau, 2001.

Loprest, P. "Families Who Left Welfare: Who Are They and How Are They Doing?" Washington, D.C.: Urban Institute, 1999.

Mills, R. "Health Insurance Coverage: Consumer Income." Washington, D.C.: U.S. Census Bureau, 1999.

Minkoff, H., Bauer, T., and Joyce, T. "Welfare Reform and the Obstetrical Care of Immigrants and Their Newborns." *New England Journal of Medicine,* 1997, *337*(10), 705–707.

Moss, N., Baumeister, L., and Biewener, J. "Perspectives of Latina Immigrant Women on Proposition 187." *Journal of American Medical Women's Association,* 1996, *51*(4), 161–165.

National Research Council Institute of Medicine. "Immigrant Children and Their Families: Issues for Research and Policy." *Critical Issues for Children and Youths,* 1995, *5*(2), 72–83.

New York Immigrant Coalition. "Welfare Reform and Health Care: The Wrong Prescription for Immigrants." New York: New York Immigrant Coalition, 2000.

Newburger, E., and Curry, A. "Educational Attainment in the United States: Population Characteristics." Washington, D.C.: U.S. Census Bureau, 1999.

Ng, D. "From War on Poverty to War on Welfare: The Impact of Welfare Reform on the Lives of Immigrant Women." San Francisco: Equal Rights Advocates, 1999.

Norton, S., Kenney, G. M., and Ellwood, M. R. "Medicaid Coverage of Maternity Care for Aliens in California." *Family Planning Perspectives*, 1996, *28*(3), 108–112.

Pastore, D., and Diaz, A. "Cultural and Medical Issues of Latino Adolescents." *Adolescent Medicine*, 1998, *9*(2), 315–322.

Philadelphia Citizens for Children and Youth United Way of Southeastern Pennsylvania. "Watching Out for Children in Changing Times: What 50 Families Have to Say—A Report on Welfare Reform." Philadelphia: Philadelphia Citizens for Children and Youth United Way of Southeastern Pennsylvania, 1998.

Polit, D. F., London, A. S., and Martinez, J. M. "The Health of Poor Urban Women: Findings from the Project on Devolution and Urban Change." New York: Manpower Demonstration Research Corp., 2001.

Population Estimates Bureau. "Resident Population Estimates for the United States by Sex, Race, and Hispanic Origin: April 1, 1990, to July 1, 1999, with Short-Term Projection to August 1, 2000." Washington, D. C.: U.S. Census Bureau, 2000.

Proctor, B. P., and Dalaker, J. "Poverty in the United States: 2001." Washington, D.C.: U.S. Census Bureau, 2002.

Ramirez, A., and others. "Hispanic Women's Breast and Cervical Cancer Knowledge, Attitudes, and Screening Behaviors." *American Journal of Health Promotion*, 2000, *14*(5), 292–300.

Rodriguez, E., and Kirk, K. "Welfare Reform, TANF Caseload Changes, and Latinos: A Preliminary Assessment." Washington, D.C.: *National Council of La Raza*, 2000, *3*, 1–13.

Romero, D., and others. "Welfare to Work? Impact of Maternal Health on Employment." *American Journal of Public Health*, 2002, *92*(9), 1462–1468.

Ronsaville, D., and Hakim, R. "Well Child Care in the United States: Racial Differences in Compliance with Guidelines." *American Journal of Public Health*, 2000, *90*(9), 1436–1443.

Smith, L. A., and others. "Employment Barriers Among Welfare Recipients and Applicants with Chronically Ill Children." *American Journal of Public Health*, 2002, *92*(9), 1453–1457.

Starr, A. "Left Behind." *Washington Monthly*, 1999, *31*(4), 18–22.

Swarns, R. "Denied Food Stamps, Many Immigrants Scrape for Meals." *New York Times*, Dec. 8, 1997, pp. 1, 4.

Swarns, R. "Latino Mothers Lagging as Others Leave Welfare." *New York Times*, Sept. 15, 1998, pp. A1, B8.

Thadani, R., and others. "Impact of Welfare Reform and Illegal Immigration Acts on Immigrants: Access to Health Care, Health-Seeking Behaviors, and Health Outcomes in New York City." Paper presented at MICHEP Workshop, Centers for Disease Control and Prevention, Atlanta, Ga., Dec. 1998.

U.S. Census Bureau. "Mothers Who Receive AFDC Payments: Fertility and Socioeconomic Characteristics." Washington, D.C.: U.S. Department of Commerce, Bureau of the Census, 1995.

U.S. Census Bureau. *Educational Attainment in the United States.* Washington, D.C.: U.S. Census Bureau, 1999.

U.S. Census Bureau. "Coming from the Americas: A Profile of the Nation's Latin American Foreign Born." Washington, D.C.: U.S. Census Bureau, 2000.

U.S. Census Bureau. "Health Insurance Coverage: 2001." [http://www.census.gov/hhes/hlthins/hlthin01/hlth01asc.html]. 2002.

U.S. Department of Health and Human Services. Temporary *Assistance for Needy Families (TANF) Program: Annual Report to Congress.* Washington, D.C.: Department of Health and Human Services, Administration for Children and Families, Office of Planning, Research and Evaluation, 2000.

U.S. Department of Justice, Immigration and Naturalization Service. *Inadmissibility and Deportability on Public Charge Grounds.* Washington, D.C.: U.S. Department of Justice, Immigration and Naturalization Services, 1999.

U.S. General Accounting Office. "Welfare Reform: Information on Former Recipients' Status." Washington, D.C.: General Accounting Office, 1999.

U.S. Immigration and Naturalization Service. "Fact Sheet: Public Charge." Washington, D.C.: U.S. Immigration and Naturalization Service, 1999.

Wilcox, B., Robbennott, J. K., O'Keefe, J. E., and Pynchon, M. E. "Teen Nonmarital Childbearing and Welfare: The Gap Between Research and Political Discourse." *Journal of Social Issues,* 1996, *52*(3), 71–90.

Wood, P., and others. "Relationships Between Welfare Status, Health Insurance Status, and Medical Care Among Children with Asthma." *American Journal of Public Health,* 2002, *92*(9), 1446–1452.

Zambrana, R., Breen, N., Fox, S. A., and Gutierrez-Mohamed, M. L. "Use of Cancer Screening Practices by Latino Women: Analyses by Subgroup." *Preventive Medicine,* 1999, *29,* 466–477.

Zambrana, R., and Capello, D. "Promoting Latino Child and Family Welfare: Strategies for Strengthening the Child Welfare System." Paper presented at the Conference on Los Ninos de Los Barrios, Oct. 1999.

Zambrana, R., and Dorrington, C. "Economic and Social Vulnerability of Latino Children and Families by Subgroup: Implications for Child Welfare." *Child Welfare League of America,* 1998, *75*(1), 5–27.

Zambrana, R., Dunkel-Schetter, C., Collins, N. L., and Scrimshaw, S. "Mediators of Ethnic-Associated Differences in Infant Birth Weight." *Journal of Urban Health: Bulletin of the New York Academy of Medicine,* 1999, *76*(1), 102–116.

Zambrana, R., and others. "The Relationship Between Psychosocial Status of Immigrant Latino Mothers and Use of Emergency Pediatric Services." *Health and Social Work,* 1994, *19*(2), 93–102.

Zimmerman, W., and Fix, M. "Declining Immigrant Applications for Medi-Cal and Welfare Benefits in Los Angeles County." Washington, D.C.: Urban Institute, 1998.

Zimmerman, W., and Tumlin, K. "Patchwork Policies: State Assistance for Immigrants Under Welfare Reform." Washington, D.C.: Urban Institute, 1999.

NAME INDEX

SUBJECT INDEX